Neurosteroids

CONTEMPORARY ENDOCRINOLOGY

P. Michael Conn, SERIES EDITOR

22. *Gene Engineering in Endocrinology,*
     edited by MARGARET A. SHUPNIK, 2000
21. *Neurosteroids: A New Regulatory Function in the Nervous System,*
     edited by ETIENNE-EMILE BAULIEU, PAUL ROBEL, AND MICHAEL SCHUMACHER, 1999
20. *Hormones and the Heart in Health and Disease,* edited by LEONARD SHARE, 1999
19. *Human Growth Hormone: Research and Clinical Practice,* edited by
     ROY G. SMITH AND MICHAEL O. THORNER, 1999
18. *Menopause: Endocrinology and Management,* edited by DAVID B. SEIFER AND
     ELIZABETH A. KENNARD, 1999
17. *The IGF System: Molecular Biology, Physiology, and Clinical Applications,*
     edited by RON G. ROSENFELD AND CHARLES ROBERTS, 1999
16. *Neurosteroids: A New Regulatory Function in the Nervous System,* edited by
     ETIENNE-EMILE BAULIEU, PAUL ROBEL, AND MICHAEL SCHUMACHER, 1999
15. *Autoimmune Endocrinopathies,* edited by ROBERT VOLPÉ, 1999
14. *Hormone Resistance Syndromes,* edited by J. LARRY JAMESON, 1999
13. *Hormone Replacement Therapy,* edited by A. WAYNE MEIKLE, 1999
12. *Insulin Resistance: The Metabolic Syndrome X,* edited by GERALD M. REAVEN
     AND AMI LAWS, 1999
11. *Endocrinology of Breast Cancer,* edited by ANDREA MANNI, 1999
10. *Molecular and Cellular Pediatric Endocrinology,* edited by
     STUART HANDWERGER, 1999
 9. *The Endocrinology of Pregnancy,* edited by FULLER W. BAZER, 1998
 8. *Gastrointestinal Endocrinology,* edited by GEORGE H. GREELEY, 1999
 7. *Clinical Management of Diabetic Neuropathy,* edited by ARISTIDIS VEVES, 1998
 6. *G Protein-Coupled Receptors and Disease,* edited by ALLEN M. SPIEGEL, 1997
 5. *Natriuretic Peptides in Health and Disease,* edited by WILLIS K. SAMSON
     AND ELLIS R. LEVIN, 1997
 4. *Endocrinology of Critical Diseases,* edited by K. PATRICK OBER, 1997
 3. *Diseases of the Pituitary: Diagnosis and Treatment,* edited by
     MARGARET E. WIERMAN, 1997
 2. *Diseases of the Thyroid,* edited by LEWIS E. BRAVERMAN, 1997
 1. *Endocrinology of the Vasculature,* edited by JAMES R. SOWERS, 1996

NEUROSTEROIDS

A NEW REGULATORY FUNCTION IN THE NERVOUS SYSTEM

Edited by

ETIENNE-EMILE BAULIEU, MD, PhD

PAUL ROBEL, MD, PhD

MICHAEL SCHUMACHER, PhD

Collége de France, Le Kremlin-Bicêtre, France

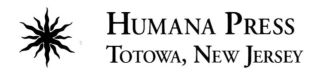 HUMANA PRESS
TOTOWA, NEW JERSEY

For additional copies, pricing for bulk purchases, and/or information about other Humana titles, contact Humana at the above address or at any of the following numbers: Tel: 973-256-1699; Fax: 973-256-8341; E-mail: humana@humanapr.com or visit our Website at http://humanapress.com

This publication is printed on acid-free paper. ∞
ANSI Z39.48-1984 (American National Standards Institute)
Permanence of Paper for Printed Library Materials.

Cover design by Patricia F. Cleary.

Printed in the United States of America. 10 9 8 7 6 5 4 3 2 1

Neurosteroids: a new regulatory function in the nervous system/edited by Etienne-Emile Baulieu, Paul Robel, and Michael Schumacher
    p.   cm.—(Contemporary endocrinology; 21)
    Includes index.
    ISBN 0-89603-545-X (alk. paper)
    1. Neuroendocrinology.   2. Steroid hormones.   3. Neurohormones. I. Baulieu, Etienne-Emile. II.
Robel, Paul. III. Schumacher, Michael. IV. Series: Contemporary endocrinology (Totowa, NJ); 21.
    [DNLM: 1. Steroids—physiology.   2. Receptors, Steroid—physiology.   3.
Central Nervous System—physiology.   QU 85 N4943 1999]
QP356.4.N497 1999
612.8'042—dc21
DNLM/DLC
for Library of Congress   99-10461
                                             CIP

PREFACE

Steroids are remarkable molecules: basically they look almost alike, being derivatives of cholesterol, but the few slight chemical differences suffice to give them the extraordinarily diverse biological specificities that are important in animal physiology and medical therapeutics. The complex array of enzymes involved in their synthesis and metabolism—from many cytochrome P450s to a large number of different oxidoreductases—distributed through the different cell compartments in steroidogenic glands, did not portend that the fine biochemical synthesis of steroids could also be performed by nonendocrine cells. The fact that neurosteroids (1) are synthesized in the neuronal and glial components of the nervous system (2) suggests that Nature, once more, has shown imagination (and economy) by the optimum use of the same chemical mechanisms in different physiological contexts. Indeed, at least in some glial cells, cholesterol may be the source for pregnenolone production, the first key molecule at the gate to the world of other steroids.

On the pathway from cholesterol to the steroid hormones, compounds such as pregnenolone itself and its sulfate, and dehydroepiandrosterone (DHEA) and its sulfate, are formed in endocrine cells. Until recently they have been known only as products/substrates of the successive chemical reactions shaping up the structure of active hormones. Interestingly, they now appear to play a physiological role in the nervous system and have pharmacological activities of their own. The same concept applies to many steroidal molecules derived from hormones by enzymatic reactions, metabolites that were generally considered as detoxification products ready for excretion (3) . In all cases, the steroids thus far designated as neurosteroids have been known chemically for many years, but often remained unrecognized as bioactive molecules. Indeed, in the nervous system, they appear to have some paracrine (possibly also autocrine) function within the networks that they help regulate. This is also true for a classical "steroid hormone," progesterone, which, produced in Schwann cells, loses its status as a sex hormone in its role with respect to the myelination of the sciatic nerve (4).

Receptors that have already been described as mediators of neurosteroid activities are often those of neurotransmitters, for which the neurosteroids appear to be allosteric (positive or negative) modulators. Are there proper (neuro)steroid receptors at the membrane level? Since the first evidence, obtained 20 years ago, for the membrane effect of progesterone in the resumption of meiosis of amphibian oocytes (5), none has been properly described in molecular terms, even if the links between these functionally described ligand receptors and voltage-gated channels and/or transduction systems are often well recognized. Finally, the detailed description of nuclear receptors for neurosteroids, such as that for progesterone in myelinating glial cells (4), still awaits: are there neuro/glial-specific isoforms?

The overall physicochemical properties of steroids—lipidic, neutral, or acidic—and the narrow structure–activity relationships that are clearly demonstrated for neurosteroid activities, open the way towards novel pharmaceutical agents that may be of important therapeutic value. We have already found effects of physiological significance in the fields of neurotrophicity (4) and behavior (6). Pathologically, the steroids involved and the age-related decrease in their levels, may be important factors contributing to the too many cerebral dysfunctions that each of us would like to avoid or repair. To understand first, in order to treat in consequence, is our goal.

Acknowledgments

I thank Dr. Michael Conn and The Humana Press for asking my coeditors and me to produce this book. Paul Robel, my colleague since the beginning of the neurosteroid story; Michael Schumacher, who will conduct our research group toward new discoveries: and I have selected scientists who have, in our judgment, contributed much to this nascent field. I thank them very gratefully for their contributions, as well as Corinne Legris, who diligently took care of the manuscripts.

Emile-Etienne Baulieu,MD, PhD
Paul Robel, MD, PhD
Michael Schumacher, PhD

REFERENCES

1. Baulieu EE. Steroid hormones in the several mechanisms? In: Fuxe K., Gustafsson, J. A., Wetterberg, L., eds. Steroid Hormone Regulation of the Brain. Pergamon, Oxford, UK, 1981, pp. 3–14.

2. Baulieu EE. Neurosteroids: of the nervous system, by the nervous system, for the nervous system. Rec Prog Horm Res 1997;52;1–32.

3. Baulieu EE. The action of hormone metabolites: a new concept in endocrinology. Fertility Sterility 1971; 58–59.

4. Koenig HL, Schumacher M, Ferzaz B, Do Thi AN, Ressouches A, Guennoun R, Jung-Testas I, Robel P, Akwa Y, Baulieu EE. Progesterone synthesis and myelin formation by Schwann cells. Science 1995; 268:1500–1503.

5. Finidori-Lepicard J, Schorderet-Slatkine S, Hanoune J, Baulieu EE. Steroid hormone as regularory agent of adenylate cyclase. Inhibition by progesterone of the membrane bound enzyme in Xenopus laevis oocytes. Nature 1981; 292:255–256.

6. Vallée M. Mayo W, Darnaudéry M, Corpéchot C, Young J, Koehl M, Le Moal M, Baulieu EE, Robel P, Simon H. Neurosteroids: deficient cognitive performance in aged rats depends on low pregnenolone sulfate levels in hippocampus. Proc Natl Acad Sci USA 1997;94:14,865–14,870.

CONTENTS

Preface v

Contributors ix

List of Main Steroids and Enzymes Involved in Steroid Metabolism xiii

1   Neurosteroids: *From Definition and Biochemistry to Physiopathologic Function* 1
    Paul Robel, Michael Schumacher, and Etienne-Emile Baulieu

2   Molecular Biology and Developmental Regulation of the Enzymes Involved in the Biosynthesis and Metabolism of Neurosteroids 27
    Synthia H. Mellon and Nathalie A. Compagnone

3   Cytochrome P450 in the Central Nervous System 51
    Margaret Warner and Jan-Åke Gustafsson

4   Steroidogenic Factor 1 Plays Key Roles in Adrenal and Gonadal Development and in Endocrine Function 67
    Kathleen M. Caron, Yayoi Ikeda, Xunrong Luo, and Keith L. Parker

5   Peripheral-Type Benzodiazepine Receptor: *Role in the Regulation of Steroid and Neurosteroid Biosynthesis* 75
    Caterina Cascio, Patrizia Guarneri, Hua Li, Rachel C. Brown, Hakima Amri, Noureddine Boujrad, Maria Kotoula, Branislav Vidic, Katy Drieu, and Vassilios Papadopoulos

6   Aspects of Hormonal Steroid Metabolism in the Nervous System 97
    Angelo Poletti, Fabio Celotti, Roberto Maggi, Roberto C. Melcangi, Luciano Martini, and Paola Negri-Cesi

7   The Selective Interaction of Neurosteroids with the GABA$_A$ Receptor 125
    Jeremy J. Lambert, Delia Belelli, Susan E. Shepherd, Marco Pistis, and John A. Peters

8   Potentiation of GABAergic Neurotransmission by Steroids 143
    Robert H. Purdy and Steven M. Paul

9   Neurosteroid Antagonists of the GABA$_A$ Receptors 155
    Maria Dorota Majewska

10 Modulation of Ionotropic Glutamate Receptors by Neuroactive Steroids 167
    Terrell T. Gibbs, Nader Yaghoubi, Charles E. Weaver, Jr., Mijeong Park-Chung, Shelley J. Russek, and David H. Farb

11   Steroidal Modulation of Sigma Receptor Function *191*
     Stéphane Bastianetto, François Monnet,
        Jean-Louis Junien, and Rémi Quirion

12   Steroid Modulation of the Nicotinic Acetylcholine Receptor *207*
     Bruno Buisson and Daniel Bertrand

13   Neuroactive Steroid Modulation of Neuronal Voltage-Gated
        Calcium Channels *225*
     Jarlath M. H. ffrench-Mullen

14   Gonadal Hormone Regulation of Synaptic Plasticity in
        the Brain: *What Is the Mechanism?* *233*
     Bruce S. McEwen

15   Steroid Effects on Brain Plasticity: *Role of Glial Cells and
        Trophic Factors* *255*
     *Luis Miguel Garcia-Segura, Julie Ann Chowen,
        Frederick Naftolin, and Ignacio Torres-Aleman*

16   Steroid Receptors in Brain Cell Membranes *269*
     Victor D. Ramírez and Jianbiao Zheng

17   Novel Mechanisms of Estrogen Action in the Developing
        Brain: *Role of Steroid/Neurotrophin Interactions* *293*
     C. Dominique Toran-Allerand

18   Neurosteroids: *Behavioral Studies* *317*
     *Willy Mayo, Monique Vallée, Muriel Darnaudéry, and
        Michel Le Moal*

19   Remarkable Memory-Enhancing Effects of Pregnenolone
        Sulfate with Pheromone-Like Sensitivity: *An Amplificatory
        Hypothesis* *337*
     Eugene Roberts

20   The Neuropsychopharmacological Potential of Neurosteroids ... *349*
     Rainer Rupprecht, Elisabeth Friess, and Florian Holsboer

     Index *365*

CONTRIBUTORS

HAKIMA AMRI, PHD • *Department of Cell Biology, Georgetown Medical Center, Washington, DC*

STÉPHANE BASTIANETTO, MD • *Douglas Hospital Research Center, Neuroscience Division, Verdun, Québec, Canada*

ETIENNE-EMILE BAULIEU, MD, PHD • *Institut National de la Santé et de la Recherche Médicale, Collége de France, Le Kremlin-Bicêtre, France*

DELIA BELELLI, MD • *Department of Pharmacology and Neuroscience, Ninewells Hospital and Medical School, The University of Dundee, Dundee, Scotland*

DANIEL BERTRAND, MD • *Department of Physiology, CMU, Geneva, Switzerland*

NOUREDDINE BOUJRAD, PHD • *Department of Cell Biology, Georgetown Medical Center, Washington, DC*

RACHEL C. BROWN, BSC • *Department of Cell Biology, Georgetown Medical Center, Washington, DC*

BRUNO BUISSON, MD • *Department of Physiology, CMU, Geneva, Switzerland*

KATHLEEN M. CARON, PHD • *Department of Medicine, Duke University Medical Center, Durham, NC*

CATERINA CASCIO, MD • *Department of Cell Biology, Georgetown Medical Center, Washington, DC*

FABIO CELOTTI, MD • *Istituto di Endocrinologia, Milan, Italy*

JULIE ANN CHOWEN, MD • *Istituto Cajal, CSIC, Madrid, Spain*

NATHALIE A. COMPAGNONE, PHD • *Department of Obstetrics, Gynecology & Reproductive Sciences, University of California, San Francisco, CA*

MURIEL DARNAUDÉRY, MD • *University of Bordeaux, Bordeaux Cedex, France*

KATY DRIEU, DPHARM • *Department of Cell Biology, Georgetown Medical Center, Washington, DC*

DAVID H. FARB, MD • *Department of Pharmacology, Boston University School of Medicine, Boston, MA*

JARLATH M. H. FFRENCH-MULLEN, MD • *AstraZeneca Pharmaceuticals, London, UK*

ELISABETH FRIESS, MD • *Max Planck Institute of Psychiatry, Munich, Germany*

LUIS MIGUEL GARCIA-SEGURA, MD • *Istituto Cajal, CSIC, Madrid, Spain*

TERRELL T. GIBBS, MD • *Department of Pharmacology, Boston University School of Medicine, Boston, MA*

PATRIZIA GUARNERI, PHD • *Department of Cell Biology, Georgetown Medical Center, Washington, DC*

JAN-ÅKE GUSTAFSSON, MD, PHD • *Department of Medical Nutrition and Center for Nutrition and Toxicology, Huddinge University Hospital, Huddinge, Sweden*

FLORIAN HOLSBOER, MD • *Max Planck Institute of Psychiatry, Munich, Germany*

YAYOI IKEDA, PHD • *Department of Medicine, Duke University Medical Center, Durham, NC*

JEAN-LOUIS JUNIEN, MD • *Douglas Hospital Research Center, Neuroscience Division, Verdun, Québec, Canada*

MARIA KOTOULA, PHD • *Department of Cell Biology, Georgetown Medical Center, Washington, DC*

JEREMY J. LAMBERT, MD • *Department of Pharmacology and Neuroscience, Ninewells Hospital and Medical School, The University of Dundee, Dundee, Scotland*

MICHEL LE MOAL, MD • *University of Bordeaux, Bordeaux Cedex, France*

HUA LI, MSC • *Department of Cell Biology, Georgetown Medical Center, Washington, DC*

XUNRONG LUO, MD, PHD • *Department of Medicine, Duke University Medical Center, Durham, NC*

ROBERTO MAGGI, MD • *Istituto di Endocrinologia, Milan, Italy*

MARIA DOROTA MAJEWSKA, MD • *Medications Development Division, National Institute on Drug Abuse, National Institutes of Health, Bethesda, MD*

LUCIANO MARTINI, MD • *Istituto di Endocrinologia, Milan, Italy*

WILLY MAYO, MD • *University of Bordeaux, Bordeaux Cedex, France*

BRUCE S. MCEWEN, MD • *Laboratory of Neuroendocrinology, The Rockefeller University, New York, NY*

ROBERTO C. MELCANGI, MD • *Istituto di Endocrinologia, Milan, Italy*

SYNTHIA H. MELLON, MD • *Department of Obstetrics, Gynecology & Reproductive Sciences, University of California, San Francisco, CA*

FRANÇOIS MONNET, MD • *Douglas Hospital Research Center, Neuroscience Division, Verdun, Québec, Canada*

FREDERICK NAFTOLIN, MD • *Istituto Cajal, CSIC, Madrid, Spain*

PAOLA NEGRI-CESI, MD • *Istituto di Endocrinologia, Milan, Italy*

VASSILIOS PAPADOPOULOS, PHD • *Department of Cell Biology, Georgetown Medical Center, Washington, DC*

MIJEONG PARK-CHUNG, MD • *Department of Pharmacology, Boston University School of Medicine, Boston, MA*

KEITH L. PARKER, MD, PHD • *Division of Endocrinology, Department of Internal Medicine, University of Texas Southwestern Medical Center, Dallas, TX*

STEVEN M. PAUL, MD • *Lilly Research Laboratories, Indianapolis, IN*

JOHN A. PETERS, MD • *Department of Pharmacology and Neuroscience, Ninewells Hospital and Medical School, The University of Dundee, Dundee, Scotland*

MARCO PISTIS, MD • *Department of Pharmacology and Neuroscience, Ninewells Hospital and Medical School, The University of Dundee, Dundee, Scotland*

ANGELO POLETTI, MD • *Istituto di Endocrinologia, Milan, Italy*

ROBERT H. PURDY, PHD • *Lilly Research Laboratories, Indianapolis, IN*

RÉMI QUIRION, MD • *Douglas Hospital Research Center, Neuroscience Division, Verdun, Québec, Canada*

VICTOR D. RAMÍREZ, MD • *Department of Molecular and Integrative Physiology, University of Illinois at Urbana-Champaign, Urbana, IL*

PAUL ROBEL, MD, PHD • *Institut National de la Santé et de la Recherche Médicale, Collége de France, Le Kremlin-Bicêtre Cedex, France*

EUGENE ROBERTS, MD • *Department of Neurobiochemistry, Beckman Research Institute of the City of Hope, Duarte, CA*

RAINER RUPPRECHT, MD • *Max Planck Institute of Psychiatry, Munich, Germany*

SHELLEY J. RUSSEK, MD • *Department of Pharmacology, Boston University School of Medicine, Boston, MA*

MICHAEL SCHUMACHER, PHD • *Collége de France, Institut National de la Santé et de la Recherche Médicale, Le Kremlin-Bicêtre, France*

SUSAN E. SHEPHERD, MD • *Department of Pharmacology and Neuroscience, Ninewells Hospital and Medical School, The University of Dundee, Dundee, Scotland*

C. DOMINIQUE TORAN-ALLERAND, MD • *Department of Anatomy and Cell Biology, Columbia University, New York, NY*

IGNACIO TORRES-ALEMAN, MD • *Istituto Cajal, Madrid, Spain*

MONIQUE VALLÉE, MD • *University of Bordeaux, Bordeaux Cedex, France*

BRANISLAV VIDIC, SD • *Department of Cell Biology, Georgetown Medical Center, Washington, DC*

MARGARET WARNER, PHD • *Department of Medical Nutrition and Center for Nutrition and Toxicology, Huddinge University Hospital, Huddinge, Sweden*

CHARLES E. WEAVER, JR., MD • *Department of Pharmacology, Boston University School of Medicine, Boston, MA*

NADER YAGHOUBI, MD • *Department of Pharmacology, Boston University School of Medicine, Boston, MA*

JIANBIAO ZHENG, PHD • *Department of Molecular and Integrative Physiology, University of Illinois at Urbana-Champaign, Urbana, IL*

LIST OF MAIN STEROIDS AND ENZYMES
INVOLVED IN STEROID METABOLISM

Enzymes

Current name	Abbreviation to be used	Abbreviations not to be used
cholesterol side-chain cleavage enzyme	P450scc	P450 11A
17α hydroxylase/17,20 lyase	P450c17	
21 hydroxylase	P450c21	
11β hydroxylase	P450c11β	P45011B1
aldosterone synthase	P450AS	P45011B2
aromatase	P450 aro	P45019
7α hydroxylase	P450c7B	
3β-hydroxy steroid dehydrogenase	3βHSD	
3α-hydroxy steroid oxidoreductase	3αHOR	3αHSD
17β-hydroxy steroid oxidoreductase	17βHOR	17βHSD
11β-hydroxy steroid oxidoreductase	11βHOR	11 oxidoreductase 11βHSD
sulfotransferase	ST	
sulfatase		

Steroids

Chemical name	Current name	Abbreviation to be used	Abbreviations not to be used
3α-hydroxy-5α-pregnan-20-one	allopregnanolone	3α,5α-TH PROG	3α-OH-DHP;5α-pregnane-3α-ol-20-one; THP
3β-hydroxy-5α-pregnan-20-one	epiallopregnanolone	3β,5α-TH PROG	3β-OH-DHP;5α-pregnane-3β-ol-20-one
3α-hydroxy-5β-pregnan-20-one	pregnanolone	3α,5β-TH PROG	5β-pregnane-3α-ol-20-one
3α,20-dihydroxy-5α-pregnan-20-one	tetrahydrodeoxycorticosterone	3α,5α-TH DOC	5α-pregnan-3α,21-diol-20-one;TH DOC; 5α-TH DOC
3β-hydroxy-androst-5-en-17-one	dehydroepiandrosterone	DHEA	D; DHA
3β-hydroxy-androst-5-en-17-one sulfate	dehydroepiandrosterone sulfate	DHEAS	DS
sulfate ester	sulfate	S	
3β-hydroxy-pregna-5-en-20-one	pregnenolone	PREG	P
3β-hydroxy-pregna-5-en-20-one sulfate	pregnenolone sulfate	PREGS	PS
4-pregnene-3,20-dione	progesterone	PROG	P
1,3,5(10)-estratriene-3,17β-diol	estradiol	E	17β-E; E$_2$;17β-E$_2$;17β-estradiol
1,3,5(10)-estratriene-3,17α-diol	17α-estradiol	17α-E	
17β-hydroxy-androst-4-en-3-one	testosterone	T	
11β,21-dihydroxy-pregna-4-ene-20-one	corticosterone	B	

11β,21-dihydroxy-pregna-4-ene-3,18,20-trione	aldosterone	
5α-androstane-3β, 17β-diol	3β-androstanediol	3β, 5α-diol
5α-androstane-3α, 17β-diol	3α-androstanediol	
5α-pregnane-3,20-dione	5α-dihydroprogesterone	5α-DH PROG
3α-hydroxy-5α-androstan-17-one	androsterone	
3α-hydroxy-pregna-4-en-20-one		
3α-hydroxy-5α-preg-9(11)-en-20-one		
3α-hydroxy-3β-trifluoromethyl-5α-pregnan-20-one		
5α-pregnane-3α,20α-diol		
5β-pregnane-3α,20α-diol		
5α-pregnane-3α,20β-diol		
5β-pregnane-3α,20β-diol		
11β,17,21-trihydroxy-pregna-4-ene-3,20-dione	cortisol	F
17,20α,21-trihydroxy-pregna-4-ene-3,11-dione	20α-dihydrocortisone	

Steroids (continued)

5β-pregnane-3α,11β,17,20α,21-pentol	cortol	
3α-hydroxy-5α-pregnane-11,20-dione	alphaxalone	
3β-hydroxy-5α-pregnane-11,20-dione	betaxolone	
3α-hydroxy-3β-methyl-5α-pregnan-20-one	ganaxolone	
2β-ethoxy-3α-hydroxy-11α-dimethylamino-5α-pregnan-20-one	minaxolone	
estrogen	no abbreviation	
1,3,5(10)-estratrienne-3,17β-diol-6-CMO-BSA	estradiol-6-carboxymethyl oxime-BSA	E-6-BSA / 17β-E-6-BSA
1,3,5(10)-estratriene-3,17α-diol-6-CMO-BSA	17α-estradiol-6-carboxymethyl oxime-BSA	17α-E-6-BSA
pregna-4-ene-3,17-dione-3-CMO-BSA	progesterone-3-carboxymethyl oxime-BSA	P-3-BSA / PROG-3-BSA
21-hydroxy-pregna-4-ene-3,20-dione	deoxycorticosterone	DOC

1

Neurosteroids:
From Definition and Biochemistry
to Physiopathologic Function

Paul Robel, MD, PhD, Michael Schumacher, PhD, and Etienne-Emile Baulieu, MD, PhD

CONTENTS

INTRODUCTION
DEFINITION
MEASUREMENT
ENZYMES OF NEUROSTEROIDS BIOSYNTHESIS IN THE RODENT BRAIN
PHYSIOLOGICAL CORRELATES OF NEUROSTEROIDS
REFERENCES

INTRODUCTION

The relationships between steroid hormones and brain function have mostly been envisioned within the framework of endocrine mechanisms as responses elicited by secretory products of steroidogenic endocrine glands, borne by the blood stream, and exerting actions on the brain.

The brain is a target organ for steroid hormones. Intracellular receptors involved in the regulation of specific gene transcription have been identified in neuroendocrine structures, with each class of receptor having a unique distribution pattern in the complex anatomy of the brain *(1,2)*. Mechanisms involving steroid receptors account for most steroid-induced feedback and many behavioral effects; for the regulation of the synthesis of several neurotransmitters, hormone and neuromediator receptors, and hormone-metabolizing enzymes; and also for the organizational effects on neural circuitry that occur during development and persist to adulthood.

However, it is now well established that local target tissue metabolism is an important factor in the action of sex steroid hormones. Not only may such metabolism be involved in the regulation of intracellular hormones levels, but it may also provide an essential contribution to the cellular response. The brain is a site of extensive steroid metabolism, and in the case of androgens aromatization and 5α-reduction give rise to active metabo-

From: *Contemporary Endocrinology: Neurosteroids: A New Regulatory Function in the Nervous System* Edited by: E.-E. Baulieu, P. Robel, and M. Schumacher
© Humana Press Inc., Totowa, NJ

lites, respectively, estradiol and 5α-dihydrotestosterone, which influence neuroendocrine function and behavior (3–5).

Progesterone (PROG) is also a substrate of 5α-reductase, and is converted to several metabolites, particularly 5α-dihydroprogesterone (5α-DH PROG) and 3α-hydroxy -5α pregnan-20-one (allopregnanolone, 3α,5α-TH PROG), which exert progesterone-like effects on neuroendocrine functions such as gonadotropin regulation and sexual behavior (6).

The characterization of pregnenolone (PREG) and dehydroepiandrosterone (DHEA) in the rat brain, as nonconjugated steroids and their sulfate (S) and fatty acid (L) esters, at higher concentrations in brain than in blood, has led to reconsideration of steroid-brain interrelationships (reviewed in ref. 7). The accumulation of DHEA, PREG, and their conjugates in the brain appeared to be at least in part independent of adrenal and gonadal sources, as shown by the persistence of these steroids in the brain for up to 1 mo after gland ablation or pharmacological suppression. This contrasted with testosterone and corticosterone, the concentrations of which readily decline to undetectable levels after removal of corresponding endocrine glands. This observation led to the discovery of a steroid biosynthetic pathway in the nervous system (CNS). Then, research was conducted in order to define some of the physiological function and pharmacological activities of this new class of regulatory molecules, the neurosteroids (8).

DEFINITION

The term "neurosteroid" was proposed in 1981. It applies to the steroids, the accumulation of which in the central and peripheral nervous systems occurs independently, at least in part, of supply by the steroidogenic endocrine glands, and which can be synthesized de novo in the nervous system from sterol precursors (9). All intermediary compounds can be assayed and/or demonstrated to be formed in situ. However in several instances, the precursor of a given neurosteroid, for example, progesterone in the case of 3α, 5α-TH PROG, can be synthesized in the nervous system but is also provided by endocrine sources (ovarian, adrenal, and/or placental). The physiological significance of neurosteroidal PROG is clearly different from that of endocrine PROG; it may act paracrinally (see Subheading "Trophic Effects of Neurosteroids on Neurons and Glial Cells") and in particular the site of formation of 3α, 5α-TH PROG might be different from either source. On the contrary, steroids that are formed exclusively from blood-borne precursors, as, for example, estrogens (estrone and estradiol), which derive by aromatization from blood-borne androstenedione and testosterone, will not be qualified as neurosteroids.

There is a tendency in the scientific literature to regard as neurosteroids all neuroactive steroids, including synthetic, nonnatural molecules. This is unfortunate. We shall restrict our study to steroids that are still present in the nervous system long after the removal of steroidogenic glands, and the biosynthesis of which can be demonstrated, by pathways that have been previously documented in endocrine glands, eventually by mechanisms proper to the nervous system. Alone, none of these two conditions suffices to qualify a steroid present in the nervous system as a neurosteroid.

MEASUREMENT

The Rodent Brain

Brain samples from adult male rats of the Sprague Dawley strain (11–12 wk old) were generally used. Plasma and tissue homogenates were processed as previously described

Table 1
Neurosteroids in the Adult Male Rat Brain and Plasma

Location	Concentration (ng/g or ng/mL)(mean ± SD)					
	DHEA	DHEA S	DHEAL	PREG	PREG S	PREG L
Brain	0.24 ± 0.33	1.70 ± 0.32	0.41 ± 0.13	9.5 ± 2.7	15.1 ± 1.8	10.5 ± 0.4
Plasma	0.06 ± 0.06	0.20 ± 0.08	0.18 ± 0.05	0.9 ± 0.5	2.5 ± 0.7	2.9 ± 1.5

Rats of the Sprague Dawley Ofa strain (Iffa-Credo, L'Arbresles, France) were killed by decapitation when they were approx 11 wk old (200–220 g body weight), 2–3 h after lights were on. The entire brain was quickly removed, weighed, and immediately processed. Trunk blood was collected in heparinized tubes and centrifuged at 4°C. Results are expressed in terms of ng steroid either unconjugated or released from the sulfate or lipoidal esters. [Data from Young et al. *(18)*]

(9–11). The extracts containing unconjugated steroids were prepared by a differential extraction procedure. The water phase containing steroid sulfates was solvolyzed. The organic phase was taken to dryness and defatted by solvent partition. The 90% methanol phases containing unconjugated steroids were further purified by reverse-phase chromatography on C18 microcolumns. The isooctane phases containing lipoidal derivatives were taken to dryness, saponified, and the steroids released were further purified as were those in the unconjugated fractions.

The steroids recovered from the unconjugated, solvolyzed, and saponified fractions were separated by partition chromatography on a celite microcolumn, thus allowing the separation and radioimmunoassay of PROG, 5α DH-PROG, 3α,5α-TH PROG, dehydroepiandrosterone (DHEA), pregnenolone (PREG), and corticosterone (B) *(12)*. Definitive identification of the steroid moiety was made by gas chromatography/ mass spectrometry.

The quantitation of brain neurosteroids appeared to depend on several environmental and methodological factors. Some factors have been partly documented in rodents, as being lighting schedules, hour of killing, housing conditions (number of animals per cage, rats of the other sex in the same room), and stress. The workup conditions for the removal and initial processing of brain tissue was also critical. Therefore, all physiological and pharmacological experiments were conducted under strictly defined conditions.

The concentration of DHEA (mainly in the form of the sulfate ester) is about 2.5 ng (10/pmol)/g tissue, whereas the concentration of PREG (both unconjugated and esterified) is about 35 ng (100 pmol)/g tissue (*see* Table 1). Although we found differences in neurosteroid concentrations between selected brains areas, the lack of sensitivity of radioimmunoassays precluded any definitive statement.

Concentrations of both neurosteroids were definitely larger in the rat brain than in plasma, and even, in the case of DHEA S, larger in the posterior brain than in the adrenal glands. This led us to assume that there are independent mechanisms for the formation and/or accumulation of brain 3β-hydroxy-Δ5-steroids *(11)*. Neither DHEA nor PREG disappeared in the brain 15–45 d after combined adrenalectomy (ADX) and orchiectomy (ORX) (*see* Fig.1). Brain DHEA S was also unchanged after administration of corticotropin (ACTH) for 3 d.

Further work has described additional neurosteroids. PROG concentrations were measured in several brain areas of immature female rats before and after induction of ovulation with pregnant mare serum gonadotropin *(14)*. The highest preovulatory PROG

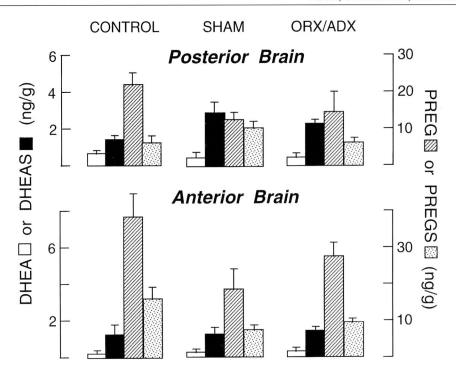

Fig. 1. Persistent DHEA and PREG after removal of steroidogenic glands. Male Sprague-Dawley rats were killed at the age of 77 ± 3 d. Groups of five males either intact (CONTROL), or castrated and adrenalectomized (ORX/ADX) 15 d before killing or sham-operated controls (SHAM) were used. Decapitation was performed 2–3 h after lights were on. Individual brains were divided in the posterior part (cerebellum, pons, medulla oblongata) and anterior part (cortex cerebri and mesencephalon). Brain samples were processed for RIA of DHEA, DHEAS, PREG, and PREGS. Results are expressed in ng/g (mean $\pm$ SD, $n = 5$). Fifteen days after the removal of steroidogenic glands, the concentrations of neurosteroids in brain were quite similar in ADX and in SHAM groups (adapted from ref. *11*).

concentrations were found in the hypothalamus and the striatum (3.5 ± 0.7 and 4.6 ± 0.9 ng/g, respectively). After ovulation, PROG concentrations in the hypothalamus were increased almost tenfold (27 ± 5.2 ng/g), and there was a significant positive correlation between PROG plasma levels and the concentration in the cerebral cortex in the postovulatory, but not in the preovulatory, rat, although the adrenal gland is a documented source of PROG in the female rat *(15)*. Therefore, PROG was measured in the brain of male and female rats before and after combined ADX + gonadectomy *(13,16)*. Residual brain PROG levels in the 1–2 ng/g range were measured in operated rats of both sexes, whereas plasma levels were undetectable, thus strongly suggesting that PREG is converted to significant amounts of PROG in the brain. Similar observations were made in the peripheral nervous system *(17)*. This conclusion was also supported by the administration of trilostane, a 3β-hydroxy steroid dehydrogenase inhibitor, to operated males, which resulted in a large decrease of PROG and increase of PREG in the brain in accordance with a precursor-to-product relationship *(18)*.

The biosynthesis and metabolism of PROG are reviewed in Chapter 2 in this book by Mellon and Compagnone *(19)* and Chapter 6 by Poletti et al. *(20)*. PROG is mainly converted to its 5α-reduced metabolite 5α-DH PROG, which is in turn converted to

3α- and 3β-hydroxy-5α-pregnan-20-ones. The 3α, 5α-reduced metabolites of PROG (3α,5α-TH PROG) and of deoxycorticosterone (3α,5α-THDOC) have raised considerable interest because they are potent allosteric modulators of gamma-aminobutyric acid A (GABA$_A$) receptors, with sedative, anxiolytic and anesthetic properties (review in refs. 21–24).

Radioimmunoassay and gas chromatographic-mass fragmentographic methods (26) have been developed for the measurement of allopregnolone and its precursors in the brain.

There is no consensus about the basal levels of 3α, 5α-TH PROG in the young adult male rat brain, whereas Corpéchot et al. (13) report barely detectable levels, other reports using sham-operated and/or restrained males, indicate concentrations of 1–3 ng/g (16,27). In these 2 reports, adrenalectomy induced only a partial decrease of 3α, 5α-TH PROG in the brain. Allopregnanolone levels have also been measured in the brain of female rats and found to parallel PROG levels, i.e, to be strongly dependent on estrus cycle or pregnancy, when they reach approx 12 ng/g (13,22). Allopregnanolone was still detectable after combined adrenalectomy and ovariectomy. The intermediate compound between PROG and 3α, 5α-THPROG (5α-DH PROG) has also been measured in the rat brain, and found at concentrations approaching those of PROG (13) or of -3α-, 5α-TH PROG (16).

The concentrations of neurosteroids have also been measured in castrated adult male Swiss mice (28). The concentrations of DHEA, PREG, PREG S, PROG, 5α-DH PROG, and 3α, 5α-TH PROG were similar to those of intact male rats. However, injection of DHEA (80 μg daily for 2 wk) to castrated mice markedly increased the concentrations of 5α-DH PROG (approx 5 ng/g) and 3α, 5α-TH PROG (approx 2 ng/g). This was attributed to an androgenic effect, as it was also observed after injection of testosterone (40 ng daily for 5d) and counteracted by coadministration of an antiandrogen (J. Young and P. Robel, unpublished results).

Neurosteroids Variations in the Rodent Brain

Changes in neurosteroid levels have been observed in several situations, such as ontogenesis, biological rhythms, heterosexual exposure, or stress. In most instances, the relative contributions of locally synthesized neurosteroids and blood-borne steroids has not been established.

ONTOGENESIS

In newborn rats of both sexes, PREG(S) (as the sum PREG + PREG S) and corticosterone (B) are high at the time of delivery in both rat brain and plasma. Brain PREG decreases steadily during the first day of life (postnatal day 1, PN 1), then remains within the range of adult levels, whereas B decreases to insignificant levels between days PN 1 and PN 10 (29). Contrary to B, brain PREG was unchanged when 4-d-old rats were treated with ACTH or dexamethasone for 2 d. The concentrations of DHEA(S) (as the sum DHEA + DHEA S) were very stable between birth and PN 22, in the 1.8–3.4 ng/g range not different from the values found in adults (30).

CIRCADIAN AND INFRADIAN RHYTHMS

In adult male Sprague-Dawley rats, timing of the removal of the brain, as related to the light-dark cycle, demonstrated prominent circadian rhythms of 3β-hydroxy-Δ5-steroids in plasma and brain. When the data were represented by the cosinor method, the acrophases of PREG(S) in brain and of DHEA(S) in plasma significantly preceded the acrophase of B, suggesting partly separate coordinatory mechanisms (31). Fifteen days after ADX + ORX, a significant rhythm of brain DHEA(S) persisted with an acrophase at the beginning of the dark period and a similar trend was observed for PREG (32).

In female Holtzman rats, data were collected over 11 d. The variations of brain DHEA(S), DHEA L, and PREG L followed a complex pattern that could best be approximated by the concomitant fit of cosine functions with about 5- and 1-d periods (33).

Concentrations of PROG, of 5α-DH PROG, and of $3\alpha,5\alpha$-TH PROG have been measured in the mouse brain throughout the estrous cycle. Plasma PROG concentrations were also measured for comparison. At each stage, circadian fluctuations were found in the concentrations of brain PROG and its metabolites (34). Such fluctuations were greater than those attributable to any particular stage of the estrous cycle. Over the entire cycle, a significant correlation was found between brain 5α-DH PROG or $3\alpha,5\alpha$-TH PROG and PROG concentrations. Brain PREG S also underwent circadian variations during the estrous cycle that unexpectedly were in phase with plasma PROG but not brain PROG concentrations. Results suggested that circadian and ovarian influences on the concentrations of PROG and its 5α-reduced metabolites in female whole mouse brain were caused predominantly by changes in the supply of PROG from within the tissue, whatever the contribution of peripheral sources.

HETEROSEXUAL EXPOSURE

When intact male rats were exposed to the scent of estrous females for 7 d, a significant decrease of PREG(S) concentrations occurred in the olfactory bulbs but not in any other brain structure. Moreover, DHEA(S) concentrations tended to increase in the hypothalamus (30) (Fig. 2). When male rats were exposed to the scent and view of female rats, PREG(S) decreased significantly in the olfactory bulb, whereas DHEA(S) increased significantly in the olfactory bulb and the retina, and PROG decreased in the hypothalamus, amygdala, and parietal cortex (35).

STRESS

The transient increase of brain DHEA S that occurs in the brain of male rats 2 d after adrenalectomy or the corresponding sham operation has been related to the heavy stress following anesthesia and surgery (10). Several later reports have provided interesting informations about the effect of stress on the levels of neurosteroids in the rat brain. In rats habituated to the manipulation that precedes killing, the cerebral cortical concentration of PREG and PROG were about 2-fold lower than in naive animals (36). Rapid (25 min) and robust (4- to 20-fold) increases of $3\alpha,5\alpha$-TH PROG, and $3\alpha,5\alpha$-TH DOC were detected in the brain and plasma of naive male rats after exposure to ambient temperature swim stress (27). Adrenalectomy essentially obliterated the response to stress, with the notable exception of brain $3\alpha,5\alpha$-TH PROG. Another type of acute stress, CO_2 inhalation, elicited a marked increase in the concentrations of PREG, PROG, and DOC in the brain cortex and hippocampus of handling habituated rats, whereas DHEA levels were unchanged (36). Foot shock also increased the concentrations of PREG, PROG, and $3\alpha,5\alpha$-TH PROG in both brain and plasma of intact rats (37).

ACUTE ETHANOL INTOXICATION

Sprague-Dawley male rats (175 g) were given ethanol (16% in saline) by intraperitoneal injection to obtain a blood alcohol level of approx 50 mg/100 mL. Control rats were given an equal volume of saline. Ethanol injection resulted in a dramatic decrease

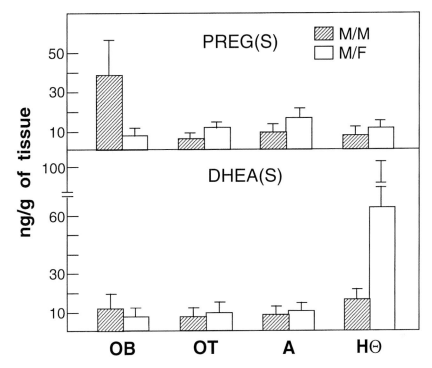

Fig. 2. PREG(S) decreases in the olfactory bulb of male rats exposed to the scent of females. PREG(S) (as the sum PREG + PREGS) and DHEA(S) were measured in the limbic system of male rats exposed to the scent of either males (M/M) or estrous females (M/F). OB, olfactory bulb; OT, olfactory tubercle; A, amydala; HYP, hypothalamus. The only significant differences were the decrease of PREG(S) in the OB and the increase of DHEA(S) in the HYP of M/F groups vs M/M ones (adapted from ref. *30*).

of DHEA(S) concentrations in the brain. This decrease occurred rapidly, DHEA(S) had completely disappeared after 30 min and reappeared progressively to reach control values after 4 h. All brain areas investigated were similarly affected. PREG and PREG S did not change *(23)*.

To gain some insight into the mechanisms involved in the depletion of brain DHEA, 2.5 mg of the steroid were injected intramuscularly in sesame oil, 4 h before killing, to control or ethanol-treated rats. DHEA was cleared much more rapidly from the brain under the influence of ethanol, thus suggesting that ethanol induces a rapid metabolic conversion of DHEA and DHEA S. It was previously reported that ethanol markedly increases the metabolic conversion of DHEA to Androst-5ene-3β, 17β-diol in humans *(38)*.

Other Mammalian Species

MONKEYS

In primates, contrary to rodents, the adrenal secretes large amounts of DHEA S, which is the most abundant steroid in plasma. DHEA(S), PREG(S), and PREG L concentrations have been measured in the brain of *Macaca fascicularis* without or with suppression of adrenocortical steroid secretion by dexamethasone (DEX) *(39)*. Two control adult spayed females and two DEX-treated females (4 mg DEX daily for 3 d) were studied. The effectiveness of adrenal suppression was indicated by the decrease of plasma cortisol to undetectable levels 20 h after the last injection of DEX. Concentrations of DHEA(S) in plasma were also much smaller after DEX treatment (91.5–93.5 ng/mL before DEX and 4.5–19.3 ng/mL after DEX, respectively). DHEA(S) concentrations in the brain were about threefold smaller than in plasma. Adrenal suppression resulted in about twofold smaller brain concentration, but the fraction of DHEA(S) remaining in the brain after adrenal suppression was much larger than the corresponding fraction in plasma, suggesting that the accumulation of DHEA(S) in monkey brain is, at least in part, independent of peripheral endocrine glands, as previously shown in the rat.

PREG(S) concentrations were severalfold larger in brain than in plasma but about twofold smaller than those of DHEA(S); and did not seem to be influenced by adrenal suppression.

The impermeability of the blood-brain barrier to DHEA S had been previously investigated in the Rhesus monkey (39). Two brains were perfused in vivo either with [^{14}C]DHEA and [^{3}H]DHEA S, or with [^{3}H]DHEA. Plasma from the jugular vein and the brain were analyzed for free and conjugated metabolites. Much more free than sulfoconjugated DHEA was withdrawn from the blood. Slight conversion of [^{14}C]DHEA to [^{14}C]DHEA S and of [^{3}H]DHEA S to [^{3}H]DHEA occurred in the brain.

HUMANS

The concentrations of Δ5-3β-hydroxysteroids have been measured in specific regions of the human brain (41,42). The tissue samples were obtained by routine craniotomy from cadavers that had been stored at 4°C until autopsy within 24 h.

The overall mean of PREG was 120.7 nmol/kg or 38.2 ng/g, the overall mean of PROG was 10.1 nmol/kg or 3.2 ng/g, and the overall mean of DHEA was 19.6 nmol/kg or 5.6 ng/g (41). The concentrations of the free steroids generally exceeded those of the sulfate esters (41), and were much higher than those of the sex steroid hormones and in the same range as those reported in the rat.

The ratios of PREG and DHEA concentrations in the brain to the corresponding plasma concentration typically found in aged subjects were 74 and 6.5, respectively. Hence it is tempting to speculate that the human brain is capable of de novo biosynthesis of steroids. With the immunoperoxidase technique, P450$_{scc}$, adrenodoxin and adrenodoxin reductase have been detected in the human brain (43). The human brain possesses DHEA sulfotransferase and sulfatase activities (40).

Postmortem concentrations of PROG, 5α-DH PROG, and 3α,5α-TH PROG were measured in the brain and serum of fertile women in the luteal phase and postmenopausal women (44). There were regional differences in brain concentrations of all three steroids and in their relative amounts. Theses concentrations were significantly higher in the womens' luteal phase compared to their postmenopausal control subjects, thus showing that the levels of those neurosteroids were at least in part related to ovarian steroid (PROG) production.

CONCLUSION

Despite the prominent diversity of adrenal DHEA(S) secretion among mammalian species, from almost nil in rodents to more abundant than cortisol in primates, it remains that the pattern of Δ5-3β-hydroxysteroids in the brain is quite constant, in particular with PREG(S) predominating over DHEA(S). The biosynthesis of PREG in mammalian brain seems firmly established, whereas that of DHEA, although likely, may not follow the classical $\xrightarrow{\text{P450c17}}$ DHEA pathway (*see* Subheading "Biosynthesis of DHEA"). Because DHEAS hardly crosses the blood-brain barrier, and because DHEA sulfotransferase activity has been measured, although at a low level, it appears that, whatever the origin of DHEA, the formation of DHEA S is likely to occur directly in the brain, thus corresponding to the definition of "neurosteroids."

Regulatory Mechanisms

Little is known about the mechanisms regulating neurosteroid formation. Both cAMP and glucocorticosteroids have been shown to enhance PREG formation from [^{3}H]mevalonate, precursor of cholesterol, in mixed glial cell cultures, but these effects might be related to an acceleration of cell differentiation in vitro *(45)*. Cholesterol side-chain cleavage activity is regulated in the C6 glioma cell line by the mitochondrial benzodiazepine receptor, which is involved in intramitochondrial cholesterol transport, thereby increasing the substrate availability to P-450 as previously described for adrenals and gonads *(46)*.

The concentrations of PREG, PROG, and DOC were significantly increased by db-cAMP and forskolin. The forskolin effect was prevented by preexposing the rat brain cortex minces to PK 11195, a high-affinity ligand for the mitochondrial benzodiazepine receptor endowed with antagonistic properties, suggesting that the rapid effect of cAMP on neurosteroid synthesis was related to the diazepam-binding inhibitor-receptor system *(47)*. In addition, cAMP has a delayed action on neurosteroid synthesis, owing probably to the stimulation of P450$_{scc}$ synthesis *(48,49)*.

Rat retina also has the ability to synthesize pregnenolone and other neurosteroids, and the cytochrome P450$_{scc}$ was located in retinal ganglion cells *(50)*. Ganglion cells possess GABA$_A$ receptors. Agonists of the GABA$_A$ receptors, or benzodiazepines that preferentially bind to central-type receptors, possess effective steroidogenic activities correlated with their affinities for those receptors *(51)*. This effect was reversed by the GABAergic antagonists bicuculline and picrotoxinin. Unexpectedly, isoniazid, a drug that decreases GABA synthesis, and hence GABA$_A$ receptor-mediated transmission, has been shown to elicit a time-dependent increase of PREG, PROG, and 3α,5α-TH DOC concentrations in rat brain and plasma *(52)*. Because this effect of isoniazid was accompanied by an increase of plasma corticosterone, it was likely linked to a stimulation of adrenal secretion, since it was indeed by abecarnil, an anxiolytic β-carboline, and was abolished by adrenalectomy and castration *(37)*.

ENZYMES OF NEUROSTEROID BIOSYNTHESIS IN THE RODENT BRAIN

Current View of Neurosteroid Biosynthesis

The definition *stricto sensu* of neurosteroids applies to PREG, DHEA, and their sulfate and fatty acid esters and to PROG and its 5α-reduced metabolites (5α-DH PROG, 3α,5α-TH PROG, and 3β,5α-TH PROG). It is not our purpose to provide a detailed description of the biosynthetic and metabolic enzymes, as they are accounted for extensively in other chapters of this book (refs. *19, 20*, and *53*) We mainly wish to provide a critical appraisal of present knowledge. Our current view of neurosteroid biosynthesis and metabolism in the rat brain is summarized on Fig. 3.

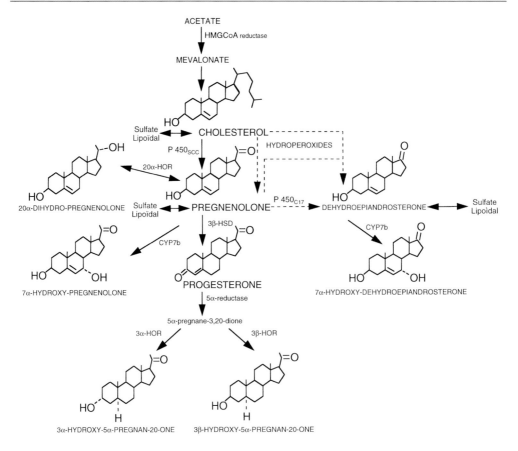

Fig. 3. Neurosteroid biosynthesis and metabolism in the rat brain. Dotted arrows indicate metabolic conversions not yet formally demonstrated. Other metabolic reactions are not indicated such as the possible formation of 17β-hydroxylated steroids (e.g., Δ5-androstene-3β,17β-diol and testosterone), C19-steroids of the 5α series (e.g., androsterone and epiandrosterone), and phenolsteroids (e.g., estrogens).

Biosynthesis of Pregnenolone

Solid evidence has been provided for the biosynthesis of PREG in the nervous system. Incubation of primary cultures of newborn rat forebrain glial cells (a mixture of mature oligodendrocytes and astrocytes after 20 d of culture) with [³H]mevalonolactone, a precursor of cholesterol, led to the formation of cholesterol, PREG, PROG, and 2α-DH-PREG *(45)*, and incubation of rat oligodendrocyte mitochondria with [³H] cholesterol yielded pregnenolone *(54)*.

There is only one cholesterol side-chain cleavage enzyme, cytochrome P450$_{scc}$ with strong structural homology between rodent, bovine, and human species. The presence of immunoreactive P450scc protein in the rat brain has been established in the white matter and in primary cultures of newborn rat forebrain glial cells *(45,55)*. However, the abundance of P45Oscc mRNA is exceedingly low and could be demonstrated only by reverse transcription polymerase chain reaction (RT-PCR) *(56–58)*.

Biosynthesis of DHEA

DHEA BIOSYNTHESIS IN THE ADULT RAT BRAIN

Incubations of [^{3}H]-PREG (and sulfate or acetyl esters) with brain slices, homogenates, or microsomes; with primary cultures of mixed glial cells, or with astrocytes and neurons of rat and mouse embryos never produced a radioactive metabolite with the chromatographic behavior of [^{3}H]-DHEA *(7)*. Moreover, all attempts to demonstrate the P450c17 antigen immunohistochemically in the rat brain with antibodies to the enzyme purified from pig testis and in the guinea pig brain with specific antibodies to the enzyme from guinea pig adrenal were unsuccessful *(59)*. Accordingly, Mellon and Deschepper failed to detect the mRNA for P450c17 by RNAase protection assays and RT-PCR *(56)*. Only a transient expression of the mRNA for this enzyme during embryonic life was reported *(60)*, however a conflicting report indicated its presence was also in the adult rat brain *(57)*. Thus, the pathway(s) by which DHEA biosynthesis occurs in the brain remain(s) controversial.

THE RAT RETINA

The biosynthesis of PREG also occurs in the rat retina where it is the most abundant steroid. Although suggested by Guarneri et al., the presence and activity of P450c17 in retina has not been conclusively demonstrated *(50)*.

THE HYDROPEROXIDE PATHWAY

We also failed to demonstrate the direct conversion of radioactive cholesterol or sesterpene to DHEA *(61)*. However, Prasad et al. have been able to generate PREG and DHEA from organic solvent extracts of rat brain by reactions with various reagents *(62)*. They have suggested the intermediate formation of cholesterol 17,20-cycloperoxide or 17-hydroperoxide in an hypothetical biochemical pathway from cholesterol to DHEA. Their results are supported by a recent report of Cascio et al. *(63)*. Previous reports had indicated that C6 rat glioma cells in culture biosynthesize both PREG and DHEA, despite the complete lack of expression of P450c17. Adding FeS04 to the culture medium increased the synthesis of both neurosteroids, even in the presence of specific inhibitors of P450$_{scc}$ and/or P450c17. These results were interpreted as caused by the fragmentation of *in situ*-formed tertiary hydroperoxides ("hydroperoxide pathway") (Fig. 3). Namely, the precursor of brain DHEA might be a steroid where both C-17 and C-20 are oxygenated. The enzyme(s) responsible for these conversions is (are) unknown.

Sulfotransferases and Sulfatases

In the rat brain, the concentrations of PREG S and DHEA S (in mol/g) are significantly higher than those in plasma (in mol/mL) and are maintained for several weeks after adrenalectomy and castration.

These observations, together with the blood-brain barrier's low permeability to steroid sulfates *(64)* argue for the changes in brain PREG S and DHEA S levels being independent of direct uptake from the circulation. This would mean that they are either synthesized *in situ* or stored in some other form, possibly analogous to the labile sulfolipid derivative(s), for which indirect evidence has been obtained *(65)*.

SULFOTRANSFERASES

Where estrogen sulfotransferase activity in mammalian brain is ascertained, the search for Δ5-3β-hydrosteroid sulfotransferase activity has been disappointing *(66)*. Low hydroxysteroid sulfotransferase activity was detected in all regions of the rat brain, with the highest one in the hypothalamus *(67)*. The cytosolic enzyme has different properties from those of hepatic isozymes, with a pH optimum of 6.5 and a high K_m of 2.8 mM for DHEA. The enzyme was equally active with PREG as the substrate. The specific activity (per mg cytosolic protein) in the brain was approximately 300-fold lower than in the liver and was higher in females than in males. Relatively high activities were found in the fetal brain and these declined at birth. There was a major peak in activity in pubertal female brain and a less important one in males. The low brain hydroxysteroid sulfotransferase activity explains the lack of information in the literature, and it is not known whether the enzyme cloned from rat liver is the one expressed in brain *(68)*. There is still the question as to whether such low activity is adequate to explain the origin of DHEA S and PREG S in the brain. With a number of assumptions, it was calculated that it would take the rat brain over 5 d to synthesize 6 ng DHEA S/g *(67)*. These data are compatible with the lack of increase of DHEA S in the brain after subcutaneous injection of DHEA in oil solution *(12)*.

SULFATASE

Steroid sulfatase (STS) activity in the rat brain is associated with the nuclear and cytosolic fractions *(69)*. Purification of the murine enzyme allowed to measure the protein by enzyme-linked immunosorbent assay (ELISA) in the brain *(70)*. Rat and mouse STS have been cloned *(70,71)*. Expression of STS was investigated in mouse brain during embryogenesis (E) *(72)*. On days E16.5–E18.5, an *in situ* hybridization signal was found in the thalamus, hippoccampus, cerebellum, and spinal chord, and expression in these regions persisted 9 d after birth. Expression was also observed in the peripheral nervous system.

STS activity may be involved in the regulation of steroid sulfate concentrations in the brain, although no direct measurement has been reported. Inhibition of sulfatase activity by selective sulfatase inhibitors might increase DHEA S (and PREG S) concentrations in brain and might be involved in the slow effect of selective STS inhibitors on memory performance, as they were shown to increase plasma DHEA S and counteract scopolamine-induced amnesia as measured by a passive avoidance test *(73)*.

Acyltransferase

Because DHEA and PREG were also characterized in the rat brain as unpolar complexes converted to the respective unconjugated steroids by saponification, which is known to split fatty acid esters *(39)*, the characterization of a Δ5-3β-hydroxysteroid acyltransferase activity in rat brain microsomes was undertaken *(74)*.

Endogenous fatty acids in the microsomal fraction served for the esterification of steroids. The enzyme system had a pH optimum of 4.5 with [^{3}H]DHEA as the substrate. The apparent K_m was 92 ± 31 μM and the V_{max} was 18.6 ± 3.4 nmol/h per mg protein (mean ± standard error of the mean). The highest activity in 1-to 3-wk-old rats may be related to the development of the brain, particularly to myelin formation which occurs at that stage.

The inhibition constants of PREG and testosterone for the sulfonation of [^{3}H]DHEA were 123 and 64 μM, respectively, and results were compatible with a competitive type of inhibition. The main endogenous fatty acids coupled to DHEA and PREG were palmitate, oleate, linoleate, stearate, and myristate.

It may be envisioned that the persistent accumulation of PREG and DHEA observed in the rat brain after combined orchiectomy and adrenalectomy occurs at the expenses of PREG L and DHEA L stores. In fact, the concentrations of lipoidal derivatives did not decrease significantly in the brain of operated rats, thus excluding the possibility that they serve as storage molecules *(62)*.

3β-*Hydroxysteroid Dehydrogenase* Δ5 → 4 *Isomerase (3β-HSD)*

The rat brain can convert [^{3}H]PREG into [^{3}H]progesterone *(75)* and [^{3}H]DHEA into [^{3}H]androstenedione *(38)*. Converting PREG to PROG was demonstrated in cultured rodent glia *(45)*, neurons *(76)*, and astrocytes *(77)*. Four different isoforms (I–IV) of rat 3β-HSD have been thus far characterized *(78)*. An *in situ* hybridization study, using an oligonucleotide probe common to the four known isoforms, demonstrated 3β-HSD mRNA in neurons of several brain regions *(79)* and in rat sensory neurons and Schwann cells *(80)*. Using selective RNA probes, *in situ* hybridization indicated that 3β-HSD isoforms I, II, and IV are expressed throughout the brain at a low level and mainly in white matter *(58)*.

Cell culture experiments showed that 3β-HSD activity may be regulated by cell density. Purified type 1 astrocytes were obtained from fetal rat forebrain, plated at low, intermediate or high density and maintained for 21 d. They were then incubated with [^{14}C]DHEA or [^{3}H] PREG for 24 h and the radioactive metabolites formed (androstenedione or PROG, respectively) were analyzed *(81)*. It appeared that the 3β-HSD activity observed at low cell density was almost completely inhibited at high density. Another example of regulation 3β-HSD activity by cellular interaction has been observed in the peripheral nervous system. Schwann cells can synthesize PROG from [^{3}H]PREG, but only in response to a diffusible factor produced by dorsal root ganglia sensory neurons *(80)*. In accordance with this finding, neurons induced a 20-fold increase of 3β-HSD mRNA levels in Schwann cells. The dependence of 3β-HSD expression on a neuronal signal could also be demonstrated in vivo: its RNA was easily detected by RT-PCR in the intact rat sciatic nerve but was down-regulated to undetectable levels 3 d after cryolesion when axons have degenerated. By 6 d when Schwann cells made new contact with the regenerating axons, 3β-HSD mRNA was again present. After cutting and ligating the nerve fibers, thus preventing their regeneration, 3β-HSD mRNA was not reexpressed (F. Robert, R. Guennoun, F. Désarnaud, A. D. Thi, U. Sueter, E.-E. Baulieu, and M. Schumacher, unpublished results).

DHEA and DHEA S did not increase in the brain of male rats treated for 7 d with trilostane, an inhibitor of 3β-HSD, thus suggesting that the DHEA → androstenedione conversion is very low in the CNS in vivo *(82)*. Conversely, PREG and PREG S were increased, mostly as a result of increased ardrenocortical secretion.

7α-*Hydroxylase (CYP 7b)*

DHEA and PREG are converted by rat brain microsomes into polar metabolites, identified as the respective 7α-hydroxylated (7α-OH) derivatives by gas chromatography mass spectrometry (GC-MS) of deuterated substrates *(83)*. Under optimal conditions, the K_m values for DHEA and PREG are 13.8 and 4.41 μM and the V_{max} values are 322 and 38.8 pmol/min/mg of microsomal protein, respectively. Formation of 7α-hydroxylated metabolites is low in prepubertal rats and increases fivefold in adults. Activity might decrease with aging *(84)*. The biochemical properties of the brain microsomal enzyme were reminiscent of those of 5α-androstane-3β, 17β-diol hydroxy-lase *(85)*, and of 27-hydroxy cholesterol 7α-hydroxylase *(86)* measured in the rat brain. Indeed, a novel cytochrome P450 was cloned from rat hippocampus *(87)*, and later identified as the neurosteroid 7α-hydroxylase and designated as CYP 7b, distinct from the previously cloned liver cholesterol 7α-hydroxylase *(88)*. Extracts from Hela cells infected with a recombinant virus were very active on DHEA and PREG and less active on 25-hydroxycholesterol, 17β-estradiol, and 5α-androstane-3β,17β-diol, with low to undectable activity toward steroids devoid of a 3β-hydroxyl. 7α-Hydroxylation might serve as a control mechanism of neuroactive neurosteroids in brain *(83,89)*. Moreover 7α-OH DHEA and 7α-OH PREG might have activities of their own. Stimulation of immune responses has been reported *(90,91)*.

Pregnenolone-7β-hydroxylating activity has been assigned to another enzyme, cyto-chrome P450-1A1 *(92)*.

20α-Hydroxysteroid Oxidoreductase

Pregnenolone and progesterone can be converted to the respective 20α-dihydro-derivatives by cultures of rat brain glial cells and neurons *(20)*. The yields vary according to experimental conditions. For example, after the release of aminoglutethimide block-ade, which inhibits $P450_{scc}$ activity and thus produces the accumulation of [^{3}H]choles-terol in cultured glial cells, [^{3}H]Pregn-5-ene-3β, 20α-diol (20α-dihydro-PREG) was the major steroid released in culture medium *(93)*.

20α-Hydroxysteroid oxidoreductase has been mainly investigated in rat corpus luteum, where it serves to regulate the concentration of PROG. The ovarian enzyme was cloned, sequenced, and shown to belong to the NADP aldo-keto reductase family *(94)*. Its expression and distribution in brain have not yet been reported.

5α-Reductase and 3α-Hydroxysteroid Oxido Reductase (3α-HOR)

These enzymes are responsible for the conversion of PROG and deoxycorticosterone into their neuroactive metabolites 3α,5α-TH PROG and 3α,5α-TH DOC, respectively. They have been the subject of extensive reviews *(5,95,96)* and are described in two other chapters of this book *(19,20)*. Although 5α-reductase is found both in neurons and glial cells, the reductive form of 3α-HOR is expressed mainly in glial cells *(23)*. Therefore, the neuroactive 3α,5α-TH PROG seems provided to neurons by surrounding astrocytes in a paracrine mode of action.

PHYSIOLOGICAL CORRELATES OF NEUROSTEROIDS

Pregnenolone Sulfate and Progesterone

Although it was already known that there are steroids active on the nervous system (neuroactive), the discovery of neurosteroids gave a big boost to pharmacological stud-ies of neuroactive steroids since the early 1980s, and a new physiological role for steroids in the nervous system was envisioned.

The pharmacology of neurosteroids is the subject of several chapters in this book, dealing with their effects on $GABA_A$ receptors *(24,97)*, glutamate receptors *(98)*, Sigma receptors *(99)*, or calcium channels *(100)*.

However, there are still little functional correlates of neurosteroids suggesting their physiological implication in the functioning of the nervous system. Here we review three such examples. Two of them deal with the implication of PREG S in a particular type of aggressive behavior and in memory performance, the third one relates to the role of progesterone in peripheral nerve regeneration.

Pregnenolone Sulfate and the Aggressive Behavior of Mice Against Lactating Female Intruders

This peculiar model of aggressiveness has been discovered and characterized by Marc Haug *(101)*. This behavior is triggered by a pheromonal signal emitted in the urine of lactating mice *(102)*. It is influenced by the genotype of the mice *(103)* and by their sex: females are more aggressive than males *(103)*. Moreover, castration of males triggers a marked increase of aggressiveness, suggesting an inhibitory role of male gonadal hormones *(104)*. Indeed, treatment of castrated males with testosterone or estradiol counteracts the effect of castration.

DHEA INHIBITS THE AGGRESSIVENESS OF CASTRATED MALE MICE

DHEA also inhibits the aggressiveness of castrated male mice *(105)*. This effect was mimicked neither by DHEAS nor by its estrogenic metabolite androst-5-ene-3β, 17β-diol. It is well known that DHEA can be converted in vivo into active androgens and/or estrogens *(106)*. However, the conversion of the injected amounts of DHEA (280 nmol daily in oil vehicle for 2 wk) to testosterone in the brain was extremely small *(105)*: the concentration of testosterone in intact mice was 2.8 ± 1.2 ng/g (mean $\pm$ standard deviation), in castrated mice it was 0.04 ± 0.02 ng/g, and in DHEA treated castrated mice it was 0.16 ± 0.06 ng/g. To completely eliminate the possibility of an androgenic action of DHEA, the effect of its analog 3β-methyl-androst-5-en-17-one (CH$_3$-DHEA) was investigated. This molecule cannot be metabolized into sex steroids and is not demonstrably estrogenic or androgenic *(12)*. Nevertheless, it inhibited the aggressive behavior of castrated mice dose relatedly, at least as efficiently as DHEA itself *(107)*.

DHEA AND CH$_3$-DHEA DECREASE THE CONCENTRATION OF PREG S IN THE BRAIN OF CASTRATED MALE MICE

Both DHEA and CH$_3$-DHEA (280 nmol/day for 2 wk) produced a marked and significant decrease of PREG S concentrations (more than twofold) in the brain of treated castrated mice *(12)*. Neither testosterone nor estradiol mimicked this effect of DHEA and CH$_3$-DHEA. We have speculated that the decrease of PREG S levels might increase the calming GABAergic tone, which has repeadly been implicated in the control of aggressiveness, and possibly may decrease also the activity of excitatory NMDA receptors *(98)*.

The time-course of PREG S decrease in brain following DHEA administration supports this conclusion. Indeed, the castrated mice had to be treated for 2 wk with DHEA before getting a clear-cut, significant inhibitory effect on aggressiveness. Accordingly, the decrease of PREG S in the brain was gradual and became significant only 15 d after the onset of treatment *(108)*.

DHEA INHIBITS THE AGGRESSIVENESS OF FEMALE MICE

Adult female mice display an aggressive behavior toward lactating intruders, which does not depend on ovarian hormones, as it persists after ovariectomy and is not corrected by estradiol in spayed females *(109)*. Because differences in sensitivity of aggressive behavior of males and females to sex steroid hormones may be related to the neonatal imprinting, spontaneously provoked by testosterone in males, the influence of DHEA treatment was investigated in females together with its eventual modulation by testosterone injected to the newborn *(110)*. Indeed, the females that had been androgenized at birth, then treated as adults with DHEA, were much less aggressive towards lactating intruders than mice from any other experimental subgroup.

In accordance with this observation, the decrease in the concentration of PREGS produced by DHEA, already significant in the group of spayed mice treated with DHEA, was significantly larger in the subgroup of neonatally androgenized females treated with DHEA *(110)*.

The mechanisms by which DHEA or CH_3-DHEA decrease PREG S concentrations in brain are unknown. An inhibition of sulfotransferase activity might be involved.

Pregnenolone Sulfate and Memory Performance of Aged Rats

The effects of neurosteroids on memory performance are reviewed elsewhere in this book and are very briefly reviewed in this section *(111)*. The suggestion of neurosteroid induced improvement in aged mice *(112)* led to investigations of the physiological role of PREG S in relationship with age-related cognitive impairments. Cognitive abilities exhibit a natural decline with age, although with considerable interindividual differences, which have been exploited in the search for relationships between the performance of each approx 2-yr-old rat and PREG S content in several areas of its brain, particularly in the hippocampus *(113)*. The spatial memory performances of aged rats were investigated in two different spatial memory tasks, the Morris water maze and the Y maze. Performances in both tests were correlated and, accompanied by appropriate controls, were considered to evaluate genuine memory function.

The fundamental observation was that individual hippocampal PREG S levels and distance to reach the platform in the water maze were linked by a significant negative correlation, i.e., these rats with no or minimal memory deficits had the highest PREG S levels, whereas no relationship was found with PREG S content in other brain areas (amygdala, prefrontal cortex, parietal cortex, striatum).

As a confirmation for the role of PREG S, the memory deficit of cognitively impaired aged rats was transiently corrected after either intraperitoneal or bilateral intrahippocampal injection of PREG S.

In conclusion, it was proposed that the hippocampal content of PREG S plays a physiological role in preserving and/or enhancing cognitive abilities in old animals, possibly via an interaction with central cholinergic systems. Thus, neurosteroids should be further studied in the context of prevention and/or treatment of age-related memory disorders. For that purpose, methods should be developed to produce a sustained correction of PREG S deficits in the hippocampus of aged rodents.

Trophic Effects of Neurosteroids on Neurons and Glial Cells

EFFECTS OF NEUROSTEROIDS ON NEURONS AND ASTROCYTES

In addition to their neuromodulatory and behavioral actions, neurosteroids also exert trophic effects on neurons and glial cells. Thus, when added to the culture medium, both DHEA and DHEA S greatly enhance the survival and differentiation of neurons prepared from embryonic mouse brain *(114)*. In hippocampal slice cultures from adult male rats, DHEA as well as PREG and PREG S influence the morphology of astrocytes *(115)*. Whereas DHEA induces the formation of hypertrophic cells, which are highly immunoreactive for glial fibrillary acid protein (GFA), and which have the appearance of reactive astroglia, PREG and PREG S increase the number of GFAP-immunoreactive processes. Administering PROG to gonadectomized rats significantly decreases the proliferation of astrocytes in response to lesions made in the cerebral cortex or hippocampus *(116)*. As astrocytes can synthesize PROG from PREG *(81)*, this neurosteroid may be an autocrine regulator of astroglial proliferation.

Pregnenolone and Progesterone Neuronal Regeneration

Neurotrophic or neuroprotective effects of PREG and PROG have been documented by in vivo studies. An important role has been attributed to PREG during the recovery from spinal cord injury. After compressive injury of the rat spinal cord, immediate treatment with subcutaneous pellets of PREG was found to reduce histopathological changes of the nervous tissue, to spare the tissue from secondary injury, and to increase the recovery of motor functions *(117)*. Whether these are direct effects of PREG or whether they are mediated by its metabolites, such as PROG, remains to be determined. These observations suggest that neurosteroids may be therapeutically useful for attenuating the consequences of traumatic brain and spinal cord injuries.

Following axotomy, the treatment of adult rats with PROG increases the survival of motoneurons *(118)*. This neurosteroid also reduces cerebral edema, secondary neuronal degeneration, and behavioral impairment that accompany contusion lesions of the frontal cortex *(119)*. This beneficial effect of PROG was first suggested by observations that males have significantly more edema than females after cortical contusion and that edema is almost absent in pseudopregnant female rats.

Effects of Steroid Hormones and Neurosteroids on Myelinating Glial Cells

Several studies have shown that the myelinating glial cells, oligodendrocytes in the CNS, and Schwann cells in the peripheral nervous system (PNS) are a target for gonadal and adrenal steroid hormones, such as estrogens and glucocorticosteroids and express receptors for these steroids *(120,121)*. Estradiol, at nanomolar concentrations, increases the proliferation of rat Schwann cells in synergy with cAMP *(122)*, a finding that may explain the pathogenesis of neurofibromas, which are tumors of the peripheral nerves *(123)*. The potency of Schwann cell mitogens is enhanced by the synthetic glucocorticosteroid dexamethasone *(124)*, which also activates promoters of the genes coding for the myelin proteins protein zero (P0) and peripheral myelin protein-22 (PMP-22) *(125)*. In cultured rat oligodendrocytes, glucocorticosteroids also activate the genes encoding glycerol phosphate dehydrogenase, myelin basic protein, and proteolipid protein as well as the synthesis of lipids *(126,127)*. In vivo, acceleration of spontaneous remyelination after lysolecithin-induced demyelination has been observed in the mouse spinal cord in response to treatment with the glucocorticosteroid methylprednisolone. These results were interpreted in terms of modulation of the inflammatory response and stimulation of myelin sheath formation by the steroid *(128)*.

PROG also promotes myelin formation, as shown in explant cultures of embryonic rat dorsal root ganglia, in which Schwann cells myelinate the axons of sensory neurons. Adding low concentration of PROG (20 n*M*) to the culture medium dramatically increases the number of myelinated fibers *(17)*. By studying the incorporation of a fluorescent ceramide analog into myelin lipids, it has recently been shown that PROG or its synthetic analogue R5020 accelerate the time of initiation and enhance the rate of myelin synthesis in cocultures of Schwann cells and sensory neurons *(129)*. Levels of mRNAs for the cytochrome P450$_{scc}$, the 3β-HSD and the PROG receptor were found to be markedly increased during peak myelin formation in these cocultures, strongly suggesting that *de novo* synthesis of PROG by the cells may play an important role in myelin formation *(129)*. Schwann cells and sensory neurons can indeed synthesize PROG from its tritiated precursor (*see* Subheading 3β-Hydroxysteroid Dehydrogenase Δ5 → 4 Isomerase [3β-HSD]).

Locally Synthesized Progesterone Promotes Myelination in Peripheral Nerves

That locally synthesized endogenous PROG indeed plays an important role in myelin repair has recently been demonstrated in the male mouse sciatic nerve after lesion by local freezing *(17)*. Peripheral nerves are particularly well suited to explore the trophic functions of neurosteroids because of their relatively simple structure, their great plasticity and their remarkable regenerative capacity *(130)* In response to a cryolesion, axons and their myelin sheaths distal to the lesioned site rapidly degenerate by a process known as Wallerian degeneration, but Schwann cells survive and proliferate. Such lesion leaves basal lamina tubes of the nerve fibers intact and provides an appropriate environment for a rapid regeneration of the damaged axons, which are then remyelinated by Schwann cells and eventually make new functional neuromuscular connections.

In the intact regenerating nerve, concentrations of PROG are about sixfold larger than in plasma (plasma: 1.3 ± 0.1 ng/mL nerve: 8.5 ± 0.9 ng/g). Blocking either its local synthesis or action by repeated applications of either trilostane (an inhibitor of the 3β-HSD) or RU486 to the regenerating nerve inhibits the formation of new myelin sheaths after cryolesion. Conversely, repeated local administration of a high dose of PROG or its direct precursor PREG (100 µg), accelerates the process of remyelination (Fig. 4). In these experiments, the width of myelin sheaths was analyzed by electron microscopy on cross sections 2 wk after lesioning *(17)*.

Mechanisms by Which Progesterone Promotes Myelination

PROG acts as an autocrine/paracrine signaling molecule in the PNS. In fact, Schwann cells not only have the capacity to synthesize PROG from PREG, they also express an intracellular receptor for the neurosteroid *(131)*. In addition, PROG activates the expression of genes in Schwann cells encoding the peripheral myelin proteins P0 and PMP-22 *(125)*. This was shown by transiently transfecting rat Schwann cells with gene constructs where the promoter region of either myelin gene was linked to the luciferase reporter gene (P0 promoter: 1 kb upstream of the start site, PMP-22 promoter 1: 2.5 kb, promoter 2: 3.4 kb). Progesterone stimulates the P0 promoter and the promoter 1, but not promoter 2, of PMP-22 in a dose-dependent manner and its effect is hormone- and Schwann cell-specific. As dosage of P0 and PMP-22 gene expression plays an important role in peripheral neuropathies, their reduced or increased expression leading to demyelination and eventually axonal degeneration *(132)*, PROG may play a significant role in the pathophysiology of these diseases and may provide opportunities for their treatment.

Several observations support a role of the 5α-reduced metabolites of PROG in myelination: high 5α-reductase activity is present in the white matter of brain and peripheral nerves *(133)* and a low concentration of 3α,5α-TH PROG very efficiently increased the expression of P0 when added to cultures of newborn rat Schwann cells *(134)*. However, studies using selective inhibitors are required to clarify the role of the 5α-reduced metabolites of PROG in myelination because 3α,5α-TH PROG can be converted back to 5α-DH

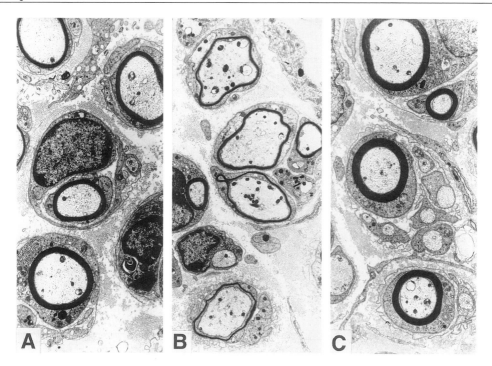

Fig. 4. Role of locally synthesized progesterone in the formation of myelin sheaths. The thickness of myelin sheaths was quantified by electron microscopy on cross sections of sciatic nerves from male mice 15 days after cryolesion. **(A)** Spontaneous regeneration, **(B)** effect of trilostane (3β-HSD inhibitor), **(C)** the inhibitory effect of trilostane was prevented by the simultaneous administration of progesterone. Trilostane without or with progesterone was directly applied to the regenerating nerves every 5 d (100 μg of the compound). (Adapted from ref. *17.*)

PROG, which binds to the intracellular PROG receptor and activates the transcription of PROG-sensitive genes *(135)*. Interestingly, repeated treatment with 5α-DH PROG partially restores the decreased PO gene expression in the sciatic nerve of aged rats *(134)*.

PROGESTERONE MAY PROMOTE MYELINATION IN THE CENTRAL NERVOUS SYSTEM

An important question is whether PROG also potentiates the formation of myelin in the brain and spinal cord, which are affected by demyelinating diseases such as multiple sclerosis and Pelizaeus-Merzbacher disease. One has indeed to be cautious when extrapolating results obtained in peripheral nerves to the CNS, because the process of myelination is different: axons are myelinated in the PNS by Schwann cells and in the CNS by oligodendrocytes, the protein composition of peripheral and central myelin is different, and distinct transcription factors activate and coordinate the expression of myelin genes in Schwann cells and oligodendrocytes *(136)*. Nevertheless, preliminary findings strongly suggest that PROG may also promote myelination in the CNS. Like Schwann cells, oligodendrocytes express 3β-HSD and intracellular PROG receptors and, in cultures of glial cells prepared from newborn rat brain, the number of oligodendrocytes expressing the myelin basic protein is increased by PROG *(137,138)*. PROG synthesized by oligodendrocyte progenitors may promote their maturation by autocrine actions: the mRNAs for cytochrome P450scc and 3β-HSD are induced during the differentiation of oligodendrocyte progenitors *(129)*.

REFERENCES

1. Fuxe K, Gustafsson JA, eds. Wetterberg L. Steroid Hormone Regulation of the Brain, Pergamon, Oxford, UK, 1981.
2. McEwen BS. Steroid hormones are multifunctional messengers to the brain. Trends Endocrinol Metab 1991;2:62–67.
3. Naftolin F, Ryan KJ, Davies IJ, Reddy VV, Flores F, Petro Z, Kuhn M, White RJ, Takaoka Y, Wolin L. The transformation of estrogens by central neuroendocrine tissues. Recent Progr Horm Res 1975;31:295–319.
4. Celotti F, Melcangi RC, Martini LJ. The 5α-reductase in the brain: molecular aspects and relation to brain function. Frontiers Neuroendocrinol 1992;13:163–215.
5. Mac Lusky NJ, Philip A, Hurlburt C, Naftolin F. Estrogen metabolism in neuroendocrine structures. In: Celotti F, Naftolin F, Martini L, eds. Metabolism of Hormonal Steroids in the Neuroendocrine Structures. Raven, New York, 1984, pp. 103–116.
6. Cheng YJ, Karavolas HJ. Conversion of progesterone to 5α-pregnane-3,20-dione and 3α-hydroxy-5α-pregnan-20-one by rat medial basal hypothalami and the effects of estradiol and stage of estrous cycle on the conversion. Endocrinology 1973;93:1157–1162.
7. Robel P, Akwa Y, Corpechot C, Hu ZY, Jung-Testas I, Kabbadj K, Le Goascogne C, Morfin R, Vourc'h C, Young J, Baulieu EE. Neurosteroids: Biosynthesis and function of pregnenolone and dehydroepiandrosterone in the brain. In: Motta M, ed. Brain Endocrinology. Raven, New York, 1991, pp. 105–131.
8. Baulieu EE. Steroid hormones in the brain: several mechanisms? In: Fuxe K, Gustafsson JA, Wetterberg L, eds. Steroid Hormones Regulation of the Brain. Pergamon Press, Oxford, UK, 1981, pp. 3–14.
9. Baulieu EE. Neurosteroids: of the nervous system, by the nervous system, for the nervous system. Rec Prog Horm Res 1997;52:1–32.
10. Corpechot C, Robel P, Axelson M, Sjövall J, Baulieu EE. Characterization and measurement of dehydroepiandrosterone sulfate in the rat brain. Proc Natl Acad Sci USA 1981;78:4704–4707.
11. Corpechot C, Synguelakis M, Tahla S, Axelson M, Sjövall J, Vihko R, Baulieu EE, Robel P. Pregnenolone and its sulfate ester in the rat brain. Brain Res 1983;270:119–125.
12. Young J, Corpechot C, Haug M, Gobaille S, Baulieu EE, Robel P. Suppressive effects of dehydroepiandrosterone and 3β-methyl-androst-5-en-17-one on attack towards lactating female intruders by castrated male mice. II Brain neurosteroids. Biochem Biophys Res Commun 1991;174:892–897.
13. Corpechot C, Young J, Calvel M, Wehrey C, Veltz JN, Touyer G, Mouren M, Prasad VVK, Banner C, Sjövall J, Baulieu EE, Robel P. Neurosteroids: 3α-hydroxy-5α-pregnan-20-one and its precursors in the brain, plasma and steroidogenic glands of male and female rats. Endocrinology 1993;133:1003–1009.
14. Bixo M, Backström T, Winblad B, Selstam G, Andersson A. Comparison between pre- and postovulatory distributions of oestradiol and progesterone in the brain of the PMSG treated rat. Acta Physiol Scand 1986;128:241–246.
15. Fajar AB, Holzbauer M, Newport HM. The contribution of the adrenal gland to the total amount of progesterone produced in the female rat. J Physiol 1971;214:115–126.
16. Cheney DL, Uzunov D, Costa B, Guidotti A. Gas chromatographic mass fragmentographic quantitation of 3α-hydroxy-5α-pregnan 20-one (allopregnanolone) and its precursors in blood and brain of adrenalectomized castrated rats. J Neurosci 1995;15:4641–4650.
17. Koenig HL, Schumacher M, Ferzaz B, Do Thi A, Ressouches A, Guennoun R, Jung-Testas I, Robel P, Akwa Y, Baulieu EE. Progesterone synthesis and myelin formation by Schwann cells. Science 1995;268:1500–1503.
18. Young J, Corpechot C, Perché F, Haug M, Baulieu EE, Robel P. Neurosteroids: pharmacological effects of a 3β-hydroxy-steroid dehydrogenase inhibitor. Endocrine 1994;2:505–509.
19. Mellon SH, Compagnone NA. Molecular biology and developmental regulation of the enzymes involved in the biosynthesis, and metabolism of neurosteroids. In: Baulieu EE, Robel P, Schumacher M, eds. Contemporary Endocrinology Series. Neurosteroids: A New Regulatory Function in the Nervous System. Humana Press, Totowa, NJ, 1999, pp. 27–50.
20. Poletti A, Celotti F, Maggi R, Melcangi RC, Martini L, Negri-Cesi P. Aspects of hormonal steroid metabolism in the nervous sytem. In: Baulieu EE, Robel P, Schumacher M, eds. Contemporary Endocrinology Series. Neurosteroids: A New Regulatory Function in the Nervous System. Humana Press, Totowa, NJ, 1999, pp. 97–124.

21. Majewska MD. Neurosteroids: endogenous bimodal modulators of the $GABA_A$ receptor: Mechanism of action and physiological significance. Prog Neurobiol 1992;38:379–395.

22. Paul SM, Purdy RH. Neuroactive steroids. FASEB J 1992;6:2311–2322.

23. Robel P, Baulieu EE. Neurosteroids: Biosynthesis and function. Trends Endocrinol Metab 1994;5:1–8.

24. Lambert J, Belelli D, Shepherd SE, Pistis M, Peters JA. The selective interaction of neurosteroids with the $GABA_A$ receptor. In: Baulieu EE, Robel P, Schumacher M, eds. Contemporary Endocrinology series. Neurosteroids: A New Regulatory Function in the Nervous System. Humana Press, Totowa, NJ, 1999, pp. 125–142.

25. Purdy RH, Moore PH Jr, Rao PN, Hagino N, Yamaguchi T, Schmidt P, Rubinow DR, Morrow AL, Paul SM. Radioimmunoassay of 3α-hydroxy-5α-pregnan-20-one in rat and human plasma. Steroids 1990;55:290–296.

26. Uzunov DP, Cooper TB, Costa E, Guidotti A. Fluoxetine elicited changes in brain neurosteroid content measured by negative ion mass fragmentography. Proc Natl Acad Sci USA 1996;93: 12,599–12,604.

27. Purdy RH, Morrow AL, Moore PH Jr, Paul S. Stress-induced elevations of gamma aminobutyric type A receptor-active steroids in the rat brain. Proc Natl Acad Sci USA 1991;88:4553–4557.

28. Young J, Corpechot C, Perch F, Eychenne B, Haug M, Baulieu EE, Robel P. Neurosteroids in the mouse brain: Behavioral and pharmacological effects of a 3β-hydroxy steroid dehydrogenase inhibitor. Steroids 1996;61:144–149.

29. Robel P, Corpechot C, Clarke C, Groyer A, Synguelakis M, Vourc'h C, Baulieu EE. Neurosteroids: 3β-Hydroxy-$\Delta5$-derivatives in the rat brain. In: Fink G, Harmar AJ, McKerns KW, eds. Neuroendocrine Molecular Biology. Plenum Press, New York, 1986, pp. 367–377.

30. Baulieu EE, Robel P, Vatier O, Haug M, Le Goascogne C, Bourreau E. Neurosteroids: Pregnenolone and déhydroépiandrosterone in the brain. In: Fuxe K, Agnati F, eds. Receptor-Receptor Interactions. Macmillan, Basingstoke, UK 1987, pp. 89–104.

31. Synguelakis M, Halberg F, Baulieu EE, Robel P. Evolution circadienne de D5-3b-hydroxystéroïdes et de glucocorticostéroïdes dans le plasma et le cerveau de rat. CR Acad Sci Paris 1985;301:823–826.

32. Robel P, Synguelakis M, Halberg F, Baulieu EE. Persistance d'un rythme circadien de la dehydroepiandrosterone dans le cerveau, mais non dans le plasma, de rats castrés et adrénalectomisés. CR Acad Sci Paris 1986;303:235–238.

33. Jo DH, Sanchez de la Pena S, Halberg F, Ungar F, Baulieu EE, Robel P, Circadian infradian rhythmic variation of brain neurosteroids in the female rat. Prog Clin Biol Res 1990;341B:125–134.

34. Corpéchot C, Collins BE, Carey MP, Tzouros T, Robel P, Fry JP. Brain neurosteroids during the mouse estrous cycle. Brain Res 1997;766:276–280.

35. Lanthier A, Patwardhan VV. Effect of heterosexual olfactory and visual stimulation on 5α-en-3β-hydroxysteroids and progesterone in the male rat brain. J Steroid Biochem 1987;28:697–701.

36. Barbaccia ML, Roscetti G, Trabucchi M, Cuccheddu T, Concas A, Biggio G. Neurosteroids in the brain of handling habituated and naive rats: effect of CO_2 inhalation. Eur J Pharmacol 1994;261:317–320.

37. Barbaccia ML, Roscetti G, Trabucchi M, Purdy RH, Mostallino MC, Concas A, Biggio G. The effects of inhibitors of GABAergic transmission and stress on brain and plasma allopregnanolone concentrations. Br J Pharmacol 1997;120:1582–1588.

38. Andersson S, Crönholm F, Sjövall J. Redox effects of ethanol on steroid metabolism. Alcohol Clin Exper Res 1986;10:555–615.

39. Robel P, Bourreau E, Corpéchot C, Dang DC, Halberg F, Clarke C, Haug M, Schlegel ML, Synguelakis M, Vourc'h C, Baulieu EE. Neurosteroids: 3β-hydroxy-$\Delta5$-derivatives in rat and monkey brain. J Steroid Biochem 1987;27:649–655.

40. Knapstein P, David A, Wu CH, Archer DF, Flickinger GL, Touchstone JC. Metabolism of free and sulfoconjugated DHEA in brain tissue *in vivo* and *in vitro*. Steroids 1968;11 :885-896.

41. Lanthier A, Patwardhan VV. Sex steroids and 5-en-3β- hydroxysteroids in specific regions of the human brain and cranial nerves. J Steroid Biochem 1986;25:445–449.

42. Lacroix C, Fiet J, Benais JP, Gueux B, Bonete R, Villette JM, Gourmel B, Dreux C. Simultaneous radioimmunoassay of progesterone, androst-4-enedione, pregnenolone, dehydroepiandrosterone and 17-hydroxy progesterone in specific regions of human brain. J Steroid Biochem 1987;28:317–325.

43. Le Goascogne C, Gouézou M, Robel P, Defaye G, Chambaz E, Waterman MR, Baulieu EE. The cholesterol side-chain cleavage complex in human brain white matter. J Neuroendocrinol 1989;1:153–156.

44. Bixo M, Andersson A, Winblad B, Purdy RH, Backström T. Progesterone, 5α-pregnane-3, 20-dione and 3α-hydroxy-5α-pregnan-20-one in specific regions of the human female brain in different endocrine states. Brain Res 1997;764:173–178.

45. Jung-Testas I, Hu ZY, Robel P, Baulieu EE. Biosynthesis of pregnenolone and progesterone in primary cultures of rat glial cells. Endocrinology 1989;125:2003–2091.

46. Guarneri P, Papadopoulos V, Pan B, Costa E. Regulation of pregnenolone synthesis in C6-2B glioma cells by 4'-chlorodiazepam. Proc Natl Acad Sci USA 1992;89:5118–5122.

47. Roscetti G, Ambrosio C, Trabucchi M, Massotti M, Barbaccia ML. Modulatory mechanisms of cyclic AMP-stimulated steroid content in rat brain cortex. Eur J Pharmacol 1994;269:17–24.

48. Papadopoulos V, Guarneri P. Regulation of C6 glioma cell steroidogenesis by adenosine –3',5' cyclic monophosphate. Glia 1994;10:75–78.

49. Zhang O, Rodriguez H, Mellon SH. Transcriptional regulation of $P450_{scc}$ gene expression in neural and steroidogenic cells: implications for regulation of neurosteroidogenesis. Mol Endocrinol 1995;9:1571–1582.

50. Guarneri P, Guarneri R, Cascio C, Pavasant P, Piccoli F, Papadopoulos V. Neurosteroidogenesis in rat retinas. J Neurochem 1994;63:83–96.

51. Guarneri P, Guarneri R, Cascio C, Piccoli F, Papadopoulos V. Gamma-aminobutyric acid type A/benzodiazepine receptors regulate rat retina neurosteroidogenesis. Brain Res 1995;683:65–72.

52. Barbaccia ML, Roscetti G, Trabucchi M, Purdy RH, Mostallino MC, Puva C, Concas A, Biggio G. Isoniazid-induced inhibition of GABAergic transmission enhances neurosteroid content in the rat brain. Neuropharmacology 1996;35:1299–1305.

53. Warner M, Gustafsson JA. Cytochrome P450 in the central nervous system. In: Baulieu EE, Robel P, Schumacher M, eds. Contemporary Endocrinology Series. Neurosteroids: A New Regulatory Function in the Nervous System. Humana Press, Totowa, NJ, 1999, pp. xxx–xxx.

54. Hu ZY, Bourreau E, Jung-Testas I, Robel P, Baulieu EE. Neurosteroids: oligodendrocyte mitochondria convert cholesterol to pregnenolone. Proc Natl Acad Sci USA 1987;84:8215–8219.

55. Le Goascogne C, Robel P, Gouézou M, Sananès N, Baulieu EE, Waterman M. Neurosteroids: Cytochrome $P450_{scc}$ in rat brain. Science 1987;237:1212–1215.

56. Mellon SH, Deschepper CF. Neurosteroid biosynthesis: genes for adrenal steroidogenic enzymes are expressed in the brain. Brain Res 1993;629:283–292.

57. Strömstedt M, Waterman MR. Messenger RNA encoding steroidogenic enzymes are expressed in rodent brain. Mol Brain Res 1995;4:75–84.

58. Sanne JL, Krueger KE. Expression of cytochrome P450 side-chain cleavage enzyme and 3β-hydroxy-steroid dehydrogenase in the rat central nervous system: A study by polymerase chain reaction and in situ hybridization. J Neurochem 1995;65:528–536.

59. Le Goascogne C, Sananès N, Gouézou M, Takemori S, Kominami S, Baulieu EE, Robel P. Immunoreactive cytochrome $P450_{17α}$ in rat and guinea-pig gonads, adrenal glands and brain. J Reprod Fertil 1991;93:609–622.

60. Compagnone NA, Bulfone A, Rubenstein JLR, Mellon SH. Steroidogenic enzyme P450c17 is expressed in the embryonic central nervous system. Endocrinology 1995;136:5212–5223.

61. Baulieu EE, Robel P. Dehydroepiandrosterone and dehydroepiandrosterone sulfate as neuroactive steroids. J Endocrinol 1996;150:5221–5239.

62. Prasad VVK, Vegesna SR, Welch M, Lieberman S. Precursors of the neurosteroids. Proc Natl Acad Sci USA 1994;91:3220–3223.

63. Cascio C, Prasad VVK, Lin YY, Lieberman S, Papadopoulos V. Detection of P450c17-independent pathways for dehydroepiandrosterone (DHEA) biosynthesis in brain glial tumor cells. Proc Natl Acad Sci USA 1998;95:2862–2867.

64. Kishimoto Y, Hoshi M. Dehydroepiandrosterone sulphate in rat brain: Incorporation from blood and metabolism in vivo. J Neurochem 1972;19:2207–2215.

65. Mathur C, Prasad VVK, Raju VS, Welch M, Lieberman S. Steroids and their conjugates in the mammalian brain. Proc Natl Acad Sci USA 1993;90:85–88.

66. Hobkirk R. Steroid sulfation. Current concepts. Trends Endocrinol Metab 1993;4:69–74.

67. Rajkowski K, Robel P, Baulieu EE. Hydroxysteroid sulfotransferase activity in the rat brain and liver as a function of age and sex. Steroids 1997;62:427–436.

68. Strott CA. Steroid sulfotransferases. Endocrine Rev 1996;17:670–696.

69. Hobkirk R. Steroid sulfotransferases and steroid sulfate sulfatases: Characteristics and biological roles. Can J Biochem Cell Biol 1985;63:1127–1144.

70. Li XM, Salido EC, Goug Y, Kitada K, Serikawa T, Yen PH, Shapiro LJ. Cloning of the rat steroid sulfatase gene (Sts), a non-pseudoautosomal X-linked gene that undergoes X inactivation. Mamm Genome 1996;7:420–424.

71. Salido EC, Li XM, Yen PH, Martin N, Mohandas TK, Shapiro J. Cloning and expression of the mouse pseudoautosomal steroid sulphatase gene (Sts). Nat Genet 1996;13:83–86.

72. Compagnone NA, Salido E, Shapiro I, Mellon SA. Expression of steroid sulfatase during embryogenesis. Endocrinology 1997;138:4768–4773.

73. Rhodes ME, Li PK, Burke AM, Johnson DA. Enhanced plasma DHEAS, brain acetylcholine and memory mediated by steroid sulfatase inhibition. Brain Res 1997;773:28–32.

74. Vourc'h C, Eychenne B, Jo DH, Raulin J, Lapous D, Baulieu EE, Robel P. Δ5-3β-hydroxysteroids acyl transferase activity in the rat brain. Steroids 1992;57:210–215.

75. Weindenfeld J, Siegel RA, Chowers I. *In vitro* conversion of pregnenolone to progesterone by discrete areas of the male rat. J Steroid Biochem 1980;13:961–963.

76. Bauer HC, Bauer H. Micromethod for the determination of 3-beta-HSD activity in cultured cells. J Steroid Biochem 1989;33:643–646.

77. Kabbadj K, El Etr M, Baulieu EE, Robel P. Pregnenolone metabolism in rodent embryonic neurons and astrocytes. Glia 1993;7:170–175.

78. Pelletier G, Dupont E, Simard J, Luu-The V, Bélanger A, Labrie F. Ontogeny and subcellular localization of 3β-hydroxysteroid dehydrogenase (3β-HSD) in the human and rat adrenal, ovary and testis. J Steroid Biochem Mol Biol 1992;43:451–467.

79. Guennoun R, Fiddes RJ, Gouézou M, Lombès M, Baulieu EE. A key enzyme in the biosynthesis of neurosteroids, 3β-hydroxysteroid dehydrogenase/Δ5-Δ4-isomerase (3β -HSD), is expressed in rat brain. Mol Brain Res 1995;30:287–300.

80. Guennoun R, Schumacher M, Robert F, Delespierre B, Gouézou M, Eychenne B, Akwa Y, Robel P, Baulieu EE. Neurosteroids: Expression of functional 3β-hydroxysteroid dehydrogenase by rat sensory neurons and Schwann cells. Eur J Neurosci 1997;9:2236–2247.

81. Akwa Y, Sananès N, Gouézou M, Robel P, Baulieu EE, Le Goascogne C. Astrocytes and neurosteroids: metabolism of pregnenolone and dehydroepiandrosterone. Regulation by cell density. J Cell Biol 1993;121:135–143.

82. Young J, Corpechot C, Perché F, Haug M, Baulieu EE, Robel P. Neurosteroids: Pharmacological effects of a 3β-hydroxysteroid dehydrogenase inhibitor. Endocrine 1994;2:505–509.

83. Akwa Y, Morfin RF, Robel P, Baulieu EE. Neurosteroid metabolism. 7α-Hydroxylation of dehydroepiandrosterone and pregnenolone by rat brain microsomes. Biochem J 1992;288:954–964.

84. Doostzadeh J, Morfin R. Studies of the enzyme complex responsible for pregnenolone and dehydroepiandrosterone 7α-hydroxylation in mouse tissues. Steroids 1996;61:613–620.

85. Warner M, Strömstedt M, Möller L, Gustafsson JA. Distribution and regulation of 5α-androstane-3β,17β-diol hydroxylase in the rat central nervous system. Endocrinology 1989;124:2699–2706.

86. Zhang J, Akwa Y, Baulieu EE, Sjövall J. 7α-hydroxylation of 27-hydroxycholesterol in rat brain microsomes. CR Acad Sci Paris 1995;318:345–349.

87. Stapleton G, Steel M, Richardson M, Mason JO, Rose KA, Morris RGM, Lathe R. A novel cytochrome P450 expressed primarily in brain. J Biol Chem 1995;270:29,739–29,745.

88. Rose KA, Stapleton G, Dott K, Kieny MP, Best R, Schwarz M, Russell DW, Björkhem I, Seckl J, Lathe R.Cyp 7b, a novel brain cytochrome P450, catalyzes the synthesis of neurosteroids 7a-hydroxy dehydroepiandrosterone and 7a-hydroxy pregnenolone. Proc Natl Acad Sci USA 1997;94:4925–4930.

89. Strömstedt M, Warner M, Banner CD, Macdonald PC, Gustafsson JA. Role of brain cytochrome P450 in regulation of the level of anesthetic steroids in the brain. Mol Pharmacol 1993;44:1077–1083.

90. Morfin R, Courchay G. Pregnenolone and dehydroepiandrosterone as precursors of native 7-hydroxylated metabolites which increase the immune response in mice. J Steroid Biochem Mol Biol 1994;50:91–100.

91. Padgett DA, Loria RM. In vitro potentiation of lymphocyte activation by dehydroepiandrosterone, androstenediol, and androstenetriol. J Immunol 1994;153:1544–1552.

92. Doostzadeh J, Flinois JP, Beaune P, Morfin R. Pregnenolone 7β-hydroxylating activity of human cytochrome P450-1A1. J Ster Biochem Mol Biol 1997;60:147–152.

93. Hu ZY, Bourreau E, Jung-Testas I, Robel P, Baulieu EE. Neurosteroids: steroidogenesis in primary cultures of rat glial cells after release of aminoglutethimide blockade. Biochem Biophys Res Commun 1989;161:917–922.

94. Mao J, Duan WR, Albarrain CT, Parrner TG, Gibori G. Isolation and characterization of a rat luteal cDNA encoding 20α-hydroxysteroid dehydrogenase. Biochem Biophys Res Commun 1994;201: 1289–1295.

95. Cheng KC, Lee J, Khanna M, Qin K-N. Distribution and ontogeny of 3α-hydroxysteroid dehydrogenase in the rat brain. J Steroid Biochem Mol Biol 1994;50:85–89.

96. Li X, Bertics PJ, Karavolas HJ. Regional distribution of cytosolic and particulate 5α-dihydroprogesterone 3α-hydroxysteroid oxidoreductases in female rat brain. J Steroid Biochem Mol Biol 1997;60:311–318.

97. Majewska MD. Neurosteroid antagonists of the $GABA_A$ receptors. In: Baulieu EE, Robel P, Schumacher M, eds. Contemporary Endocrinology series. Neurosteroids: A New Regulatory Function in the Nervous System. Humana Press, Totowa, NJ, 1999, pp. 155–166.

98. Gibbs TT, Yaghoubi N, Weaver CE Jr., Park-Chung M, Russek S, Farb DH. Modulation of ionotropic glutamate receptors by neuroactive steroids. In: Baulieu EE, Robel P, Schumacher M, eds. Contemporary Endocrinology series. Neurosteroids: A New Regulatory Function in the Nervous System. Humana Press, Totowa, NJ, 1999, pp. 167–190.

99. Bastianetto S, Monnet F, Junien JL, Quirion R. Steroidal modulation of sigma receptor function. In: Baulieu EE, Robel P, Schumacher M, eds. Contemporary Endocrinology series. Neurosteroids: A New Regulatory Function in the Nervous System. Humana Press, Totowa, NJ, 1999, pp. 191–205.

100. French-Mullen JMH. Neuroactive steroid modulation of neuronal voltage-gated calcium channels. In: Baulieu EE, Robel P, Schumacher M, eds. Contemporary Endocrinology series. Neurosteroids: A New Regulatory Function in the Nervous System. Humana Press, Totowa, NJ, 1999, pp. 225–232.

101. Haug M. Phénomène d'agression lié à l'introduction d'une femelle étrangère vierge ou allaitante au sein d'un groupe de souris femelles. CR Acad Sci Paris 1972;275:2729–2732.

102. Haug M, Brain PF. Attack directed by groups of castrated male mice towards lactating or no lactating intruders: a urine dependent phenomenon. Physiol Behav 1978;21:549–552.

103. Haug M, Brain PF. Attack directed by groups of gonadectomized male and female mice towards lactating intruders. Physiol Behav 1979;23:397–400.

104. Haug M, Brain PF. The effects of differential housing, castration, and steroidal hormone replacement on attacks directed by resident mice towards lactating intruders. Physiol Behav 1983;30:557–560.

105. Schlegel ML, Spetz JF, Robel P, Haug M. Studies on the effects of dehydrepiandrosterone and its metabolites on attack by castrated mice on lactating intruders. Physiol Behav 1985;34:867–870.

106. Parker CR, Mahesh VB. Dehydroepiandrosterone induced precocious ovulation: Correlative changes in blood steroids, gonadotropins, and cytosol estradiol receptors of anterior pituitary gland and hypothalamus. J Steroid Biochem 1977;8:173–177.

107. Haug M, Schlegel ML, Spetz JF, Brain PF, Simon V, Baulieu EE, Robel P. Suppressive effect of dehydroepiandrosterone and 3β-methyl androst-5-en-17-one on attack towards lactating female intruders by castrated male mice. Physiol Behav 1988;46:955–959.

108. Robel P, Young J, Corpéchot C, Mayo W, Perché F, Haug M, Simon H, Baulieu EE. Biosynthesis and assay of neurosteroids in rats and mice: functional correlates. J Steroid Biochem Mol Biol 1995,53:355–360.

109. Haug M, Brain PF, Kamis AB. A brief review comparing the effects of sex steroids on two forms of agression in laboratory mice. Neurosci Biobehav Rev 1986;10:463–468.

110. Haug M, Young J, Robel P, Baulieu EE. L'inhibition par la déhydroépiandrostérone des réponses agressives de souris femelles castrées vis-à-vis d'intruses allaitantes est potentialisée par l'androgénisation néonatale. CR Acad Sci Paris 1991;312:511–516.

111. Mayo W, Vallée M, Darnaudéry M, Le Moal M. Neurosteroids: behavioral studies. In: Baulieu EE, Robel P, Schumacher M, eds. Contemporary Endocrinology series. Neurosteroids: A New Regulatory Function in the Nervous System. Humana Press, Totowa, NJ, 1999, pp. 317–335.

112. Flood JF, Roberts E. Dehydroepiandrosterone sulfate improves memory in aging mice. Brain Res 1998;448:178–181.

113. Vallée M, Mayo W, Darnaudéry M, Corpéchot C, Young J, Koehl M, Le Moal M, Baulieu EE, Robel P, Simon H. Neurosteroids: deficient cognitive performance in aged rats depends on low pregnenolone sulfate levels in the hippocampus. Proc Natl Acad Sci USA 1997;94:14,865–14,870.

114. Bologa L, Sharma J, Roberts E. Dehydroepiandrosterone and its sulfated derivative reduce neuronal death and enhance astrocytic differentiation in brain cell cultures. J Neurosci Res 1987;17:225–234.

115. Del Cerro S, Garcia-Estrada J, Garcia-Segura LM. Neuroactive steroids regulate astroglia morphology in hippocampal cultures from adult rats. Glia 1995;14:65-71.

116. Garcia-Estrada J, Del Rio JA, Luquin S, Soriano E, Garcia-Segura LM. Gonadal hormones down-regulate reactive gliosis and astrocyte proliferation after penetrating brain injury. Brain Res 1993;628:271–278.

117. Guth L, Zhang Z, Roberts E. Key role for pregnenolone in combination therapy promotes recovery after spinal cord injury. Proc Natl Acad Sci USA 1994;91:12,308–12,312.

118. Yu WH. Survival of motoneurons following axotomy is enhanced by lactation or by progesterone treatment. Brain Res 1989;491:379–382.

119. Roof RL, Duvdevani R, Stein DG. Gender influences outcome of brain injury—Progesterone plays a protective role. Brain Res 1993;607:333–336.

120. Warembourg M, Otten U, Schwab ME. Labelling of Schwann and satellite cells by [^{3}H] dexamethasone in a rat sympathetic ganglion and sciatic nerve. Neuroscience 1981;6:1139–1143.

121. Jung-Testas I, Schumacher M, Robel P, Baulieu EE. Demonstration of progesterone receptors in rat Schwann cells. J Steroid Biochem Mol Biol 1996;58:77–82.

122. Jung-Testas I, Schumacher M, Bugnard H, Baulieu EE. Stimulation of rat Schwann cell proliferation by estradiol: synergism between the estrogen and cAMP. Dev Brain Res 1993;72:282–290.

123. Jay JR, MacLaughlin DT, Badger TM, Miller DC, Martuza RL. Hormonal modulation of Schwann cell tumors. Ann NY Acad Sci 1986;486:371–382.

124. Neuberger TJ, Kalimi O, Regelson W, Kalimi M, De Vries GH. Glucocorticoids enhance the potency of Schwann cell mitogens. J Neurosci Res 1994;38:300–313.

125. Désarnaud F, Do Thi AN, Brown A, Lemke G, Suter U, Baulieu EE, Schumacher M. Progesterone stimulates the activity of the promoters of peripheral myelin protein-22 and P0 genes in Schwann cells. J Neurochem 1998;71:1765–1768.

126. Kumar S, Cole R, Chiappelli F, de Vellis J. Differential regulation of oligodendrocyte markers by glucocorticoids: post-transcriptional regulation of both proteolipid protein and myelin basic protein and transcriptional regulation of glycerol phosphate dehydrogenase. Proc Natl Acad Sci USA 1989;86:6807–6811.

127. Warringa RAJ, Hoeben RC, Koper JW, Sykes JEC, Van Golde LMG, Lopes-Cardozo M. Hydrocortisone stimulates the development of oligodendrocytes in primary glial cultures and affects glucose metabolism and lipid synthesis in these cultures. Dev Brain Res 1987;34:79–86.

128. Pavelko KD, van Engelen BGM., Rodriguez M. Acceleration in the rate of CNS remyelination in Iysolecithin-induced demyelination. J Neurosci 1998;18:2498–2505.

129. Chan JR, Phillips LJ, Glaser M. Glucocorticoids and progestins signal the initiation and enhance the rate of myelin formation. Proc Natl Acad Sci USA 1998;95:10,459–10,464.

130. Fawcett JW, Keynes RJ. Peripheral nerve regeneration. Annu Rev Neurosci 1990;13:43–60.

131. Jung-Testas I, Schumacher M, Robel P, Baulieu EE. Actions of steroid hormones and growth factors on glial cells of the central and peripheral nervous system. J Steroid Biochem Mol Biol 1994;48:145–154.

132. Suter U, Snipes GJ. Biology and genetics of hereditary motor and sensory neuropathies. Ann Rev Neurosci 1998;18:45–75.

133. Celotti F, Melcangi RC, Martini L. The 5α-reductase in the brain: molecular aspects and relation to brain function. Front Neuroendocrinol 1992;13:163–215.

134. Melcangi RC, Magnagi V, Cavarretta L, Martini L, Piva F. Age-induced decrease of glycoprotein P0 and myelin basic protein gene expression in the rat sciatic nerve. Repair by steroid derivatives. Neuroscience 1998;85:569–578.

135. Rupprecht R, Reul JMHM, Trapp T, Van Steensel B, Wetzel C, Damm K, Ziegelgänsberger W, Holsboer F. Progesterone receptor-mediated effects of neuroactive steroids. Neuron 1993;11:523–530.

136. Lemke G. The molecular genetics of myelination: An update. Glia 1993;7:263–271.

137. Jung-Testas I, Renoir JM, Gasc JM, Baulieu EE. Estrogen-inducible progesterone receptor in primary cultures of rat glial cells. Exp Cell Res 1991;193:12–19.

138. Jung-Testas I, Schumacher M, Robel P, Baulieu EE. The neurosteroid progesterone increases the expression of myelin proteins (MBP and CNPase) in rat oligodendrocytes in primary culture. Cell Mol Neurobiol 1996;16:439–443.

2

Molecular Biology and Developmental Regulation of the Enzymes Involved in the Biosynthesis and Metabolism of Neurosteroids

Synthia H. Mellon, PhD
and Nathalie A. Compagnone, PhD

CONTENTS

INTRODUCTION
STEROIDOGENIC CYTOCHROMES P450
NON-P450 STEROIDOGENIC ENZYMES
CONCLUSION
REFERENCES

INTRODUCTION

The synthesis of steroid hormones in the adrenal, gonad, and placenta, considered "classic" endocrine tissues, results from a series of enzymatic steps that involves both P450 and non-P450 enzymes. The tissue-specific expression of the different enzymes dictates which steroids will be synthesized. However, the initial steps in the synthesis of all steroids are common to all steroidogenic tissues. Recent demonstration of steroid synthesis in the brain suggests that these steroids may be synthesized using the same steroidogenic enzymes found in classic steroidogenic tissue. The cloning of cDNAs and genes for all the steroidogenic enzymes over the past decade has enabled investigators to establish unequivocally that the brain expresses the same steroidogenic genes as classic steroidogenic tissues. Furthermore, through the work of many investigators, it has been established that the genes encoding the steroidogenic enzymes are expressed in multiple species, from frogs to human beings, in a developmental, regional, and tissue-specific fashion in the central and peripheral nervous systems. Although the genes expressed in neural and in classic steroidogenic tissues may be the same, recent work indicates that the nuclear factors regulating the transcription of the genes for one steroidogenic enzyme are different in neural vs classic steroidogenic tissue.

From: *Contemporary Endocrinology: Neurosteroids: A New Regulatory Function in the Nervous System* Edited by: E.-E. Baulieu, P. Robel, and M. Schumacher
© Humana Press Inc., Totowa, NJ

STEROIDOGENIC CYTOCHROMES P450

Most steroidogenic enzymes are members of the cytochrome P450 group of oxidases *(1,2)*. All of these enzymes have molecular weights about 50 kDa and contain a single heme group. They are called "P450" ("pigment" 450) because they all exhibit a characteristic absorbance at 450 nm upon reduction with carbon monoxide *(3)*. The mechanism by which all the steroidogenic P450s function is identical. They all reduce atmospheric oxygen with electrons from nicotinamide-adenine-dinucleotide phosphate (NADPH). These electrons reach the P450 by one or more protein intermediates. For the mitochondrial P450s, two protein intermediates, adrenodoxin reductase and adrenodoxin, are involved. For the microsomal P450s, one protein intermediate, P450 reductase, is involved.

The adrenal, gonadal, and placental synthesis of all steroid hormones from cholesterol involves six distinct cytochromes P450 (Fig. 1), while the synthesis of neurosteroids involves three cytochromes P450 (Fig. 2). P450scc is the cholesterol side chain cleavage enzyme; P450c17 is 17α hydroxylase/17,20 lyase; P450c21 is 21 hydroxylase; P450c11β is 11β hydroxylase, P450c11AS is aldosterone synthase and P450aro is aromatase. P450scc, P450c11β, and P450c11AS are mitochondrial enzymes; P450c21, P450c17, and P450aro are microsomal enzymes. The synthesis of specific steroid hormones in the adrenal, gonads, and placenta is dependent on the tissue-specific expression of these various enzymes. Thus, P450c11β and P450c11AS are expressed in the adrenal and not the gonads or placenta, resulting in glucocorticoid and mineralocorticoid production, whereas expression of P450c17 in the testes results in androgen production, and P450aro expression in the gonads results in estrogen production.

As is evident from the reactions shown in Fig. 1, many of the steroid hydroxylases have multiple enzymatic activities. Purification of the proteins and cloning of the cDNAs encoding these proteins has rigorously demonstrated that these activities indeed reside within single proteins.

The synthesis of neurosteroids probably proceeds through pathways both similar to and different from those used in the adrenals, gonads, and placenta. The brain contains additional steroid metabolizing enzymes that convert classic steroid hormones to a variety of neuroactive compounds, shown in Fig. 2. Pregnenolone (PREG), dehydroeplandrosterone (DHEA), and metabolites of progesterone (PROG) and 20α hydroxyprogesterone have been identified in the brains of many species. These metabolites include 5α dihydroprogesterone and 3α,5α-tetrahydroprogesterone (allopregnanolone), suggesting that the brain metabolizes PROG in a fashion different from adrenals and gonads. Just as in the adrenals, gonads, and placenta, the expression of the steroidogenic enzymes in the central and peripheral nervous systems is developmentally, regionally, and cell-specifically regulated, ensuring the regulated synthesis of specific neurosteroids.

P450scc

The first, rate-limiting, and hormonally regulated step in the synthesis of all steroid hormones is the conversion of cholesterol to PREG. This reaction is catalyzed the mitochondrial enzyme cholesterol side-chain cleavage, P450scc. The conversion of cholesterol to PREG involves three chemical reactions: 20α hydroxylation, 22 hydroxylation, and scission of the C20 C22 carbon bond. The products of this reaction are pregnenolone

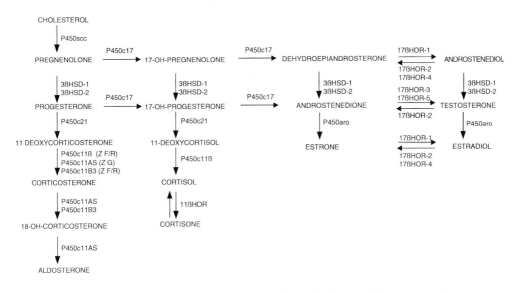

Fig. 1. Steroid hormone synthesis in "classic" steroidogenic tissues. The names of the enzymes are shown for each reaction. P450scc, cholesterol side-chain cleavage; 3βHSD, 3β hydroxysteroid dehydrogenase/isomerase; P450c17, 17α hydroxylase/c17,20 lyase; P450c21, 21 hydroxylase; P450c11β, 11β hydroxylase; P450c11AS, aldosterone synthase; P450c11B3, developmentally-regulated 11β hydroxylase/18 hydroxylase; 17βHSD, 17β hydroxysteroid dehydrogenase/17 ketosteroid reductase; P450aro, aromatase. "ZF/R" refers to the adrenal zona fasciculata/reticularis and "ZG" refers to the adrenal zona glomerulosa. The numbers next to 3βHSD and 17βHSD refer to the enzyme type that mediates the particular conversion in human beings. P450scc, P450c11β and P450c11AS are mitochondrial enzymes; P450c21, P450c17, and P450aro are microsomal enzymes. The synthesis of specific steroid hormones in the adrenal, gonads and placenta is dependent on the tissue-specific expression of these various enzymes. P450c11β and P450c11AS are expressed in the human and rat adrenal and not in the gonads or placenta, resulting in glucocorticoid and mineralocorticoid production; P450c11B3 is developmentally expressed only in the rat adrenal. P450c17 is expressed in the human adrenal (which synthesizes abundant quantities of DHEA and the glucocorticoid cortisol) but not in the rodent adrenal (which synthesizes the glucocorticoid corticosterone, and does not synthesize DHEA). P450c17 is expressed in the rat placenta, but not in the human placenta, and hence the human adrenal provides androgen substrates for estrogen synthesis. P450c17 expression in the testes and ovarian theca cells results in androgen production, and P450aro expression in the ovaries converts androgens into estrogens.

and isocaproic acid. Protein purification and cDNA cloning have demonstrated that a single protein is responsible for these three reactions, and that the same protein is found in all steroidogenic tissue, including the brain *(4,5)*.

P450scc is the rate-limiting step in steroidogenesis, and is one of the slowest enzymes known, with a V_{max} of ~1 mol cholesterol/mol enzyme/s. The slowest part of this reaction may be the entry of cholesterol into the mitochondria and binding to the active site of P450scc.

The human and rat genomes contain a single gene encoding P450scc *(9)* which is about 20 kb long, contains nine exons, and in humans is located on chromosome 15. This gene encodes an mRNA about 2.0 kb, which encodes a 521-amino-acid protein. This protein is proteolytically cleaved, removing a 39-amino-acid leader peptide that directs the protein to the mitochondria.

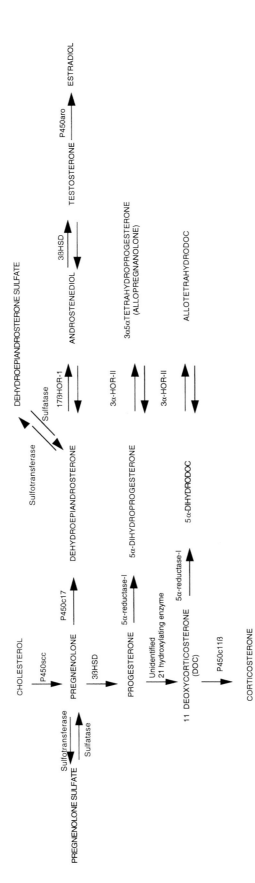

Fig. 2. Pathways of neurosteroid hormone synthesis in the central and peripheral nervous systems. The presence of most the enzymes listed have been identified at the enzymatic, protein, and mRNA levels.

Transcription of the P450scc gene is regulated by tropic hormones: adrenocorticotropic hormone (ACTH) in the adrenal, gonadotropins in the testes and ovaries, and by an unknown factor in the placenta, all working through cAMP as second messenger. In the brain, the P450scc gene is also transcriptionally regulated by mechanisms involving cAMP *(10)*. In the adrenal glomerulosa, P450scc is regulated by angiotensin II, which works through the calcium and protein kinase C system. While the effects of ACTH on increasing steroidogenesis are rapid, its effect on transcription, while fast at the molecular level, results in the chronic, persistent effect of ACTH. The transcriptional regulation of the P450scc gene in the various steroidogenic tissues involves both similar and different, tissue-specific nuclear proteins. For example, the nuclear protein Steroidogenic Factor-1 (SF-1) is involved in the transcriptional activation of P450scc in the adrenal and gonads, but not in the placenta or brain. The brain contains an additional factor not found in the adrenal or testis that appears to bind to the rat P450scc promoter, and may increase its basal and cAMP-mediated transcription *(10)*.

Expression of P450scc in the Adult Rat Brain

The demonstration of P450scc activity in the adult rat brain and in cultured oligodendrocytes suggested that these tissues may use the same enzyme, P450scc, as do classical endocrine tissues, to mediate synthesis of PREG from PROG. Rat brains can mimic adrenal steroidogenesis, because primary cultures of neonatal rat forebrain glial cells, like mouse adrenocortical Y-1 cells, convert ^{3}H mevalonolactone, a precursor of cholesterol, to ^{3}H cholesterol, ^{3}H PREG, and ^{3}H 20-OH PREG *(11)*.

Immunocytochemical analysis also suggested that P450scc protein was expressed in the white matter of the adult rat brain *(12)*. To determine whether P450scc mediated this conversion, we analyzed RNA from rat brains, primary cultures of glial cells, and C6 glioma cells for P450scc mRNA *(4)*. Using RNase protection assays, we did not detect P450scc mRNA in any of the tissues analyzed. However P450c11β mRNA (11β hydroxylase), but not the mRNAs for P450c11AS (aldosterone synthase) or P450c17 (17α hydroxylase), was detected by RNase protection assays. We could only detect P450scc mRNA, but not P450c17 nor P450c11AS mRNA, in our primary glial cultures or rat brains after amplification of RNA by polymerase chain reaction (PCR) and Southern blotting, thus indicating that the abundance of this mRNA was extremely low. In the adult rat, P450scc and P450c11β mRNAs were most abundant in the cortex, but were also found in the amygdala, hippocampus, and midbrain of both male and female rats. P450c11β was found in greater quantities in the hippocampus in females than in males. Purification of our mixed primary glial cultures showed that type-1 astrocytes synthesized P450scc mRNA. Western blotting and immunocytochemistry showed that P450scc protein was almost as abundant in our cultures as in Y-1 cells, whereas P450scc mRNA was orders of magnitude less abundant, suggesting that the protein was very stable in the brain.

Transcriptional Regulation of P450scc in Glia

Regulation of steroidogenesis is also mediated by transcriptional regulation of the P450scc gene *(13–18)*. Although only a few hundred bases of DNA flanking the start of transcription were necessary for the tissue-specific and cAMP-mediated regulation of this gene, different regions of the P450scc 5' flanking region were functional in different steroidogenic tissues. The extremely low abundance of P450scc mRNA in the brain suggested that its transcriptional regulation was likely to be different in the brain. We determined if the P450scc gene was transcriptionally regulated in neural cells, and whether the brain used the same DNA sequences and nuclear proteins as traditional steroidogenic tissues. In MA-10 and in Y-1 cells, but not in C6 cells, basal and cAMP-responsive elements were within 94 bp of the transcriptional start site. This site is bound the orphan nuclear receptor SF-1. In both MA-10 and C6 cells, another element that increased both basal and cAMP-mediated transcription was between –130/–94 bp. A third *cis*-acting region was between –230/–130 in all three cell types. DNA sequences beyond 450 bp did not increase transcriptional activity further. The 2.5 kb P450scc promoter/regulatory region was transcriptionally inactive in rat GC somatotrope and mouse GT1-7 neuro-secretory cells, indicating that neural expression of P450scc is most likely cell-type- and region-specific.

Gel shift analysis of the –130/–94 region showed two protein/DNA complexes with nuclear extracts from C6 glioma cells, one protein/DNA complex with extract from MA-10 cells, and no complexes with extracts from four different adrenal cell lines. Therefore, this region of the rat P450scc gene may be regulated in a tissue-specific fashion. Methylation interference assays indicated that proteins from C6 cells bind to a sequence GGGCGGG, resembling an Sp1 site. However, these C6 proteins did not bind to a consensus Sp1 sequence *(19)*. Nevertheless, mutations of either group of triplet Gs resulted in loss of C6 nuclear protein binding. Functional assays indicated that the –130/–94 P450scc DNA-mediated basal and cAMP-induced transcription in C6 cells, but only basal transcription in MA-10 cells. Thus, the P450scc gene is transcriptionally active in C6 glioma cells, and its transcription is regulable by cAMP. Furthermore, this transcriptional regulation may involve nuclear factors distinct from those involved in its transcriptional regulation in adrenals and gonads. The factors that cause increased cAMP production in the glia are currently unknown.

Developmental Regulation of P450scc Expression in the Central and Peripheral Nervous Systems

In the adult rat brain, P450scc mRNA was expressed in specific regions at very low levels, even though immunoassayable P450scc protein appeared to be relatively abundant *(4)*. We analyzed rat embryos throughout gestation (from embryonic d 7.5 to birth) to determine when P450scc was expressed *(20)*. By RNase protection assays, we found that P450scc mRNA was present as early as embryonic d 7.5 (E7.5) and increased until E9.5. Much of this expression was due to increased expression in the placenta, which increased until d 12 *(21)*. After this time, most of the expression of P450scc mRNA was in the trunk of the mouse or rat, consistent with its increasing expression in the adrenals and gonads *(22,23)*. Due to the low level of P450scc mRNA expression, *in situ* hybridization on whole embryos was difficult. Therefore, we analyzed P450scc protein in mice and rat embryos by immunocytochemistry.

We first observed immunocytochemical staining in the mouse embryo on E9.5 in cells in the neural crest. On E11.5, we could detect immunopositive cells in the entrance to Rathke's pouch and in cells derived from the neural crest, including the dorsal root ganglia. On E13.5, we detected immunopositive cells in the peripheral nervous system (mainly in the dorsal root ganglia) and in the trigeminal and facio-acoustic preganglia, in tissues derived from the cranial neural crest, in the midbrain, and in the ventral part of the spinal cord. Thus P450scc is expressed both in the central and in the peripheral nervous systems.

From E16.5 to E18.5 (mouse) or E17.5 to E19.5 (rat), we observed increased immuno-cytochemical staining in the peripheral nervous system, including the dorsal root ganglia, trigeminal ganglia, superior cervical ganglia, and retina (ganglion layer). We detected increased expression of P450scc in motor neurons in the spinal tract, and in sensory structures such as the retina, nasal epithelium, and subcutaneous tissue. In the brain, we detected only faint labeling in the forebrain, the thalamic region of the diencephalon, the pituitary, and the hippocampus. In the brain, the immunostaining was greatest 1 d before birth, and decreased thereafter. However, the immunostaining persisted after birth.

P450scc is expressed in several cell types. In the sympathetic and cranial ganglia, some P450scc-containing cells also contained the neuronal marker neuron-specific enolase (NSE). In the central nervous system (CNS), cells that expressed the oligodendrocyte marker galactocerebroside C (GC) were not immunopositive for P450scc, although others had detected P450scc activity in oligodendrocytes *(11)*. We previously demonstrated that in cells cultured from neonatal forebrains, P450scc was found in type I astrocytes *(4)*. In the subcutaneous tissue, we co-localized P450scc and substance P, which is found in sensory neurons. However, P450scc and substance P were not co-localized in the sensory ganglia. Thus, P450scc can be found in multiple different cell types, depending upon the particular location in the nervous system.

Adrenodoxin Reductase/Adrenodoxin

P450scc functions as the terminal oxidase in a mitochondrial electron transport system. As described above, electrons from NADPH are first accepted by a flavoprotein, adrenodoxin reductase, which is loosely associated with the inner mitochondrial membrane *(24–26)*. Adrenodoxin reductase transfers the electrons to an iron/sulfur protein, adrenodoxin. This protein is not associated with the mitochondrial membrane, and is found in solution in the inner mitochondrial matrix. Adrenodoxin first forms a complex with adrenodoxin reductase, dissociates, and then forms another complex with P450scc (or with P450c11). Both adrenodoxin reductase and adrenodoxin serve the same role for all mitochondrial P450s, not just steroidogenic P450s. Thus, these proteins are often called "ferredoxin oxidoreductase" and "ferredoxin." There is one gene encoding adrenodoxin reductase, found in humans on chromosome 17, and multiple functional human adrenodoxin genes on chromosome 11, encoding identical mRNAs and proteins and two nonfunctional human adrenodoxin pseudogenes on chromosome 20. Adrenodoxin, but not adrenodoxin reductase, is transcriptionally regulated by tropic hormones, acting though cAMP.

Adrenodoxin mRNA was found in virtually all rodent tissues examined *(27)*, including the brain. This was not surprising, as this protein functions with all mitochondrial P450s, not just the steroidogenic P450s. Similarly, as expected, adrenodoxin protein was also found in brain homogenates *(28)*.

P450c17

PREG and PROG may undergo 17α hydroxylation to 17α hydroxypregnenolone and 17α hydroxyprogesterone. These steroids may then undergo scission of the C17,20 bond to form dehydroepiandrosterone and androstenedione. All four of these reactions are mediated by a single P450c17 enzyme. P450c17 is bound to the smooth endoplasmic reticulum, and accepts electrons from P450 reductase. Because P450c17 has both 17α hydroxylase and 17,20 lyase activities, it is a key branch point in steroidogenesis. In the absence of both activities (human adrenal zona glomerulosa), PREG is directed to mineralocorticoids; in the presence of 17α hydroxylase activity alone (human adrenal fasciculata), PREG is directed to glucocorticoids; and in the presence of both 17α hydroxylase and 17,20 lyase activities (human adrenal reticularis/gonads of most species), PREG is directed to sex steroids. Several factors are important in determining whether a steroid will undergo 17,20 bond scission after 17 hydroxylation. The 17α hydroxylase reaction occurs more readily than the 17,20 lyase reaction. P450c17 prefers Δ5 substrates, especially for 17,20 bond scission, accounting for the large concentrations of DHEA in the adrenal. Phosphorylation of P450c17 may be important for lyase activity *(29)*. Finally, hydroxylase and lyase activities are regulated by the factors that regulate electron transport to P450c17, P450 reductase, and cytochrome b5.

The single human gene encoding P450c17 is located on chromosome 10, and contains eight exons. Transcriptional regulation of P450c17 is mediated by cAMP, and involves some of the same nuclear proteins that regulate P450scc gene transcription *(10,20–32)*.

Developmental Regulation of P450c17 Expression in the Nervous System

Initial studies using adult rat brains failed to detect expression of P450c17 mRNA in any region of the adult rat brain, using highly sensitive reverse transcriptase-polymerase chain reaction (RT/PCR) analyses *(4)*. Those studies also indicated that the steroidogenic enzyme proteins may be more easily detected than their mRNAs. We therefore determined where P450c17 was expressed in the mouse and rat embryo using immunocytochemistry on embryonic (E) 7.5–19.5 embryos, and in adult rat brains as well *(33)*. Unlike P450scc, no P450c17 immunoreactivity was detected in embryos from E7.5–E9.5. We first observed P450c17 in the E10.5 mouse in cells migrating from the neural crest. At this time, P450c17 was found in neurons, in both cell bodies and in fibers. By E13.5 (rat), P450c17 immunoreactivity could be seen in condensed dorsal and spinal root ganglia. From E15.5–E19.5 (rat) or E14–E18.5 (mouse), P450c17 was found in neurons in the peripheral nervous system in structures derived from the spinal neural crest, including the dorsal root sympathetic, and parasympathetic ganglia, but not in the adrenal medulla, which also derives from the spinal neural crest.

P450c17 was also found in neurons in structures derived from the cranial neural crest, including the trigeminal, most cranial sensory, and enteric ganglias, but was not found in non-neural tissues derived from the cranial neural crest (e.g., bone, teeth, cartilage, meninges, and blood vessels). In all these neurons, P450c17 was found both in cell bodies and in fibers.

P450c17 was also found in structures not derived from the cranial neural crest including the tongue, nerve fiber layer and amacrine cells in the retina, around the whiskers, diaphragm, intestine, bladder, sensory endings in the skin, and innervating the vestibular sensory epithelium.

In the CNS, P450c17 was expressed in the medulla, the pontine nucleus, in the region of the locus coeruleus, and in the ventral part of the spinal cord. In these regions, P450c17 was found in cell bodies. In other regions of the CNS, P450c17 was found in fibers. Beginning at E16, there was very strong staining in the fibers of the internal capsule, which extended to the cortical area at E18.5. In the region of the subplate (the junction of the intermediate zone and the cortical plate), P450c17 immunostaining could be seen in a rostro-caudal gradient of thickness, consistent with the "age" of the neurons in this region. Immunopositive fibers were also found in the subiculum/entorhinal cortex and hippocampus, as well as in the cerebellum.

P450c17-immunopositive cell bodies and fibers continued to decrease after birth. In the neonatal mouse and rat (d 0–7), P450c17 was mainly detected only in fibers in the brainstem and in the cerebellum, internal capsule, olfactory tract, hippocampus, stria terminalis, and thalamus. No immunopositive cell bodies were detected in any region of the adult rat brain, but were still detected in the dorsal root ganglia. Thus, unlike P450scc, P450c17 is expressed in the CNS only during development, but persists in the peripheral nervous system throughout life.

P450c21 (and Extra-Adrenal 21-Hydroxylase Activity)

Both PROG and 17 hydroxyprogesterone can be hydroxylated at C21 to yield 11-deoxy-corticosterone (DOC) and 11-deoxycortisol. This enzyme has been of great clinical interest because mutations in this enzyme result in complex and devastating symptoms, called congenital adrenal hyperplasia (CAH). 21-hydroxylation is mediated by P450c21 found in the smooth endoplasmic reticulum. Like P450c17, P450c21 uses P450 reductase to transport electrons from NADPH. There are two P450c21 genes that lie in the middle of the HLA locus on human chromosome 6. Only one gene is functional in both human beings and mice, but both genes are expressed in cows.

21-hydroxylase activity has been shown in a large number of extra-adrenal tissues, especially in the fetus and in pregnant women, resulting in the conversion of PROG to 11-DOC (34,35). Analysis of RNA from various human fetal tissues using RNase protection assays demonstrated that P450c21 mRNA was not found in these tissues (36). Thus this activity is not mediated by P450c21. The presence of an additional enzyme with 21-hydroxylase activity was demonstrated by persistence of this activity even in humans who lack a functional P450c21 gene. The enzyme responsible for this activity has not been identified.

P450 Reductase

Both P450c17 and P450c21 receive electrons from a membrane-bound flavoprotein, P450 reductase. This protein is distinct from the mitochondrial flavoprotein adrenodoxin reductase. P450 reductase receives both electrons from NADPH and transfers them one at a time to the microsomal P450. The second electron can also be provided by cytochrome b5. The amount of microsomal P450 reductase is less than that of both P450c21 and P450c17, resulting in competition for this protein. Therefore, factors that influence the association of a specific P450 with the reductase will likely influence the pathway that will be followed , e.g., c17 vs c21-hydroxylation of progesterone or c17,20 lyase vs c21-hydroxylation. Electron abundance also influences the activity of P450c17; increasing electron abundance favors both 17α hydroxylase and 17,20 lyase activities, whereas limiting electron abundance favors only 17α hydroxylase activity. Therefore, the ratio of P450 reductase to P450c17 seems to be critical in determining the pathway of steroidogenesis.

Expression of P450 Reductase in the Brain

P450 reductase activity, protein *(37)* and mRNA *(37,38)* have been reported in the brain. Cytochrome P450 reductase immunoreactivity was detected mainly in neurons, but was also found in some glial populations, and it appears to be expressed widely in the rat CNS *(37)*. Immunocytochemistry and in situ hybridization detected P450 reductase protein and mRNA in many forebrain areas including the olfactory bulb, the cerebral cortex, caudate putamen, globus pallidus, hypothalamus, thalamus, and hippocampus. Cytochrome P450 reductase was also detected in the nucleus of the posterior commissure, superior colliculus, intermediate gray layer, periaqueductal gray, and in the molecular, Purkinje, and granular layers of the cerebellum. In the brain stem, cytochrome P450 reductase was detected in the substantia nigra, nucleus locus coeruleus and raphe nucleus. These are many of the same regions that express P450c17 in the developing rodent CNS *(33)*. As P450c17 activity requires NAPDH reductase as an electron donor, co-expression of these two proteins suggests that P450c17 is functionally active.

P450c11

The final steps in the synthesis of glucocorticoids and mineralocorticoids are mediated by two distinct adrenocortical enzymes, P450c11β and P450c11AS, encoded by two different genes on human chromosome 8. The conversion of 11-DOC and 11-deoxy-cortisol to corticosterone and cortisol is mediated by the mitochondrial P450c11β, 11β hydroxylase. This enzyme is found specifically in the zona fasciculata/reticularis, is not found in the zona glomerulosa, and is regulated by ACTH. P450c11AS, aldosterone synthase, is found exclusively in the zona glomerulosa, and has three distinct activities: 11β hydroxylase, 18 hydroxylase, and 18 oxidase. It therefore converts 11-DOC to aldosterone. This enzyme is mainly regulated by the renin/angiotensin system. Like P450scc, both P450c11β and P450c11AS are found in the inner mitochondrial membrane and use adrenodoxin reductase and adrenodoxin to receive electrons from NADPH. Recently, mRNA derived from a third P450c11 gene, called P450c11B3, was isolated from rat adrenals. P450c11B3 mRNA was only expressed during the early neonatal period, and was not expressed in the fetal or adult adrenal *(39)*. Like P450c11β, P450c11B3 was expressed in the zona fasciculata/reticularis and was regulated by ACTH. However, P450c11B3 enzymatic activity was intermediate between P450c11β and P450c11AS. It had both 11β and 18 hydroxylase activities, but had no 18 oxidase activity, and therefore could synthesize both corticosterone and 18-OH DOC (from DOC) and 18-OH corticosterone (from corticosterone). A third P450c11 gene was not found in human beings *(40)*.

Expression of the P450c11 Genes in the Brain

Analysis of RNA from different regions of the adult rat brain indicated that P450c11β, but not P450c11AS, was region-specifically expressed in the brain *(4)*. The abundance of P450c11β mRNA was greater than that of P450scc mRNA, because it could be detected readily by RNase protection assays. We showed that P450c11β mRNA was found in virtually all regions analyzed (amygdala, cerebellum, cortex, hippocampus, hypothalamus, and midbrain) with the greatest amount in the cortex. We also found that there may be differences between male and female rats in the expression of P450c11β mRNA in the hippocampus, because it appeared to be found in greater amounts in the female than in the male hippocampus.

Unlike P450c11β, P450c11AS mRNA was not detected in any region of the adult rat brain, analyzing RNA by both RNase protection assays, or by RT-PCR (4). A recent preliminary report by others showed expression of P450c11AS mRNA in adult rat brains, and showed aldosterone synthase activity in those regions (41). Thus, expression of P450c11AS in the adult rat brain is not completely resolved.

P450aro

The aromatization of C18 estrogenic steroids from C19 androgenic steroids is mediated by the enzyme aromatase, P450aro, found in the endoplasmic reticulum. P450aro converts androgens to estrogens by two hydroxylations at the C19 methyl and a third hydroxylation at C2. These three hydroxylations result in the loss of C19 and aromatization of the A ring of the steroid. These reactions, all occurring on a single active site of P450aro, utilize three pairs of electrons, donated by three molecules of NADPH and P450 reductase (42,43).

The gene for P450aro has been cloned, is over 75 kb, and is located on human chromosome 15 (44–46). This gene encodes two mRNAs that differ in the length of their 3' untranslated regions (44). Transcription initiates from several different alternative untranslated first exons, and occurs in a tissue-specific fashion in the placenta, ovary, and adipose tissue (reviewed in 47). Thus, the same protein is produced in different tissues, using different regulatory regions of the P450aro gene.

Expression of P450aro in the Brain

There are several lines of evidence that demonstrate that testosterone is aromatized to estradiol in the brain of many species, from frogs and songbirds to human beings (reviewed in 48,49). Aromatase activity in the rat brain was shown to be limited to discrete regions, including the preoptic, hypothalamic, and limbic structures (50). Activity in the rat was greatest in the medial and periventricular preoptic nuclei, the suprachiasmatic nucleus, anterior and ventromedial hypothalamic nuclei, the bed nucleus of the stria terminalis, and the medial and cortical amygdaloid nuclei. Aromatase activity in the rat was first detected on embryonic d 15, increased up to embryonic d 19, and then declined to adult levels (51–53).

Although three distinct P450aro mRNA species of 2.7, 2.2, and 1.7 kb exist in many tissues, only the 2.7 kb P450aro mRNA was found in the rat brain (53). The regulation of P450aro mRNA expression during rodent development was studied by in situ hybridization (54). P450aro mRNA appeared to parallel aromatase activity, but was also found in regions not previously associated with activity. Both aromatase activity and P450aro mRNA were found only in neurons. During development, P450aro mRNA was found in the preoptic/hypothalamic area on embryonic d 16. By embryonic d 18–20, P450aro mRNA was expressed more abundantly and was more widely distributed. P450aro mRNA was detected in the medial preoptic nucleus, the sexually dimorphic nucleus of the preoptic area, the bed nucleus of the stria terminalis, and the medial amygdala. P450aro mRNA was found in lower abundance in the periventricular preoptic nucleus and the ventromedial hypothalamic nucleus. By postnatal d 2 to adulthood, P450aro mRNA abundance decreased in the preoptic area, but remained constant in other areas. In the adult rat, P450aro mRNA was still present in the bed nucleus of the stria terminalis, medial preoptic nucleus, ventromedial nucleus, medial amygdala, and cortical amygdala. Female rats had the same distribution of P450aro mRNA, but the number of cells expressing P450aro mRNA in each region was less than in males rats *(55)*.

The regions of the brain that contained P450aro mRNA, but did not contain activity or were not examined include the mediodorsal thalamus, subfornical organ, cingulate cortex, and hippocampus. P450aro immunoreactivity was demonstrated in the same areas in which P450aro mRNA was detected *(56)*, indicating that the lack of aromatase activity may be owing to the sensitivity of the assay.

NON-P450 STEROIDOGENIC ENZYMES

3β Hydroxysteroid Dehydrogenase

PREG produced from cholesterol can undergo one of two conversions: it may undergo 17α hydroxylation to 17α hydroxypregnenolone, or it may be converted to PROG. The conversion of PREG to PROG is catalyzed by the enzyme 3β hydroxysteroid dehydrogenase. This enzyme has two distinct enzymatic activities: 3β dehydrogenation and isomerization of the double bond from C5,6 in the B ring (Δ5 steroids) to C4,5 in the A ring (Δ4 steroids) *(57–59)*. This enzyme is encoded by multiple distinct genes that are expressed in a tissue-specific manner. The enzymes can be classified in two groups: those that function as dehydrogenase/isomerases and those that function as 3-ketosteroid reductases (reviewed in *60*). Human beings have two 3βHSD isoforms, types I and II, and these two enzymes share greater than 90% amino-acid sequence identity. Expression of these two isoforms in transient transfection assays demonstrated that the catalytic efficiency (V_{max}/K_m) of type I is 5.9-, 4.5-, and 2.8-fold higher than that of type II, using PREG, dehydroepiandrosterone, and dihydrotestosterone as substrates *(61)*. The genes for 3β HSD are each 7.8 kb in length, contain four exons that encode mRNAs of 1.7 kb, are found on human chromosome 1.

Four different rat 3βHSDs have been cloned, and have been given the names type I–IV. Unfortunately, the numbers of these isoforms were assigned in order of discovery, and hence the rat isoforms do not correspond to the human isoforms by number. Rat types I and II share 94% sequence identity, but the rat type I isoform has a specific activity that is 64- and 46-fold higher than the type II enzyme for PREG and DHEA, respectively. These isoforms are related to human type II (adrenal form of 3βHSD). Rat type III is found exclusively in the liver where it functions mainly as a 3-ketoreductase to inactivate steroids *(62)*. Rat type IV is found in the skin and is the predominant form in the placenta, and is equivalent to human type I (placental form of 3βHSD).

3βHSD Expression in the Adult Nervous System

Demonstration of the conversion of PREG to PROG in cultured rat oligodendrocytes *(11)*, astrocytes *(63)*, cultured rodent glia and neurons *(64)*, and discrete regions of the rat and monkey brain *(65,66)* suggested that 3βHSD was expressed in those regions. Expression of 3βHSD protein and mRNA was studied in brains from rats *(68)* and in considerable detail in frogs *(69)*, demonstrating that this enzyme is expressed in the brains from both mammalian and non mammalian vertebrates.

There are conflicting reports as to whether 3βHSD type I alone *(68)* or whether types I, II, and IV *(70)* are the isoforms that are expressed in the adult rat brain. Although 3βHSD activity was reported in both neurons and glia, 3βHSD mRNA and protein were only expressed in neurons *(68,71)*. 3βHSD mRNA was found in the brain in much lower amounts than in the ovary, adrenal, and liver. By short-term exposure of *in situ* hybridization reactions (2 wk), 3βHSD mRNA was detected only in an area near the fourth ventricle, which contains four nuclei: the nucleus prepositus hypoglossi, medial and lateral vestibularis nuclei, and the nucleus ventribularis spinalis *(71)*. By long-term exposure of *in situ* hybridization reactions (10 wk), 3βHSD mRNA was detected in neurons in the olfactory bulb, caudate-putamen, accumbens nucleus, olfactory tubercle, cortex, thalamus, hypothalamus, hippocampus, medial habenular nucleus, and cerebellum *(68)*. In the olfactory bulb, 3βHSD mRNA was detected in granular, mitral, and glomerular layers. In the cerebral cortex, there was no apparent regionalization in its expression. In the hippocampus, 3βHSD mRNA was detected in granule cells in the dentate gyrus and pyramidal cells of CA3 and CA4. The cerebellum showed a greater signal than in the rest of the brain. In the cerebellum, 3βHSD mRNA was detected in the granular and molecular layers.

In another study, expression of 3βHSD protein was extensively analyzed in different regions of the frog CNS by immunocytochemistry *(69)*. As in the rodent brain, 3βHSD was detected only in neurons. However, it was detected both in cell bodies and in fibers in different regions of the brain. In the telencephalon, 3βHSD was only expressed in fibers. These immunopositive fibers were restricted to the lateral ventricles in the nucleus accumbens septi (as in the rat), pars ventralis of the striatum, the medial forebrain bundle, the nucleus of the diagonal band of Broca, the pars lateralis of the amygdala, and the nucleus entopenducularis. In the diencephalon, cell bodies were all found in the three discreet hypothalamic nuclei: the rostral part of the preoptic nucleus (homologous to the supraoptic and paraventricular nuclei of mammals), and the dorsal and ventral infundibular nuclei. (The ventral infundibular nucleus is anatomically and functionally homologous to the arcuate nucleus in mammals.) 3βHSD fibers were mostly found in the ventral hypothalamic nuclei and in the dorsal region of the diencephalon (corpus geniculatus lateralis and the nucleus posterolateralis thalami). The metencephalon, rhombencephalon, spinal cord, and pituitary contained virtually no 3βHSD immunopositive staining.

Reports of 3βHSD activity did not always correlate with expression of 3βHSD. The lack of significant activity in the rat cerebellum and cortex *(65,66)* correlated with the lack of 3βHSD protein found in these regions in the frog *(69)*, but not with the presence of 3βHSD mRNA found in the rat *(68)*. High levels of 3βHSD activity were reported in the rat amygdala and hippocampus *(65)* and 3βHSD mRNA was detected in the rat hippocampus, but 3βHSD protein was not detected in this region in the frog. These differences may be due to the sensitivity of the assays and to species differences.

17β *Hydroxysteriod Oxidoreductase (17βHOR)*

In the adrenal, DHEA is converted to Δ5 androstenediol and Δ4 androsterone is converted to testosterone by 17-ketosteroid reductase (17KSR). In the ovary, estrone is converted to estradiol by similar mechanisms. These reactions are reversible, but although the reverse reactions are mediated by the same enzyme, they are given the name

17β hydroxysteroid dehydrogenase (17β HSD). Like the multiple 3βHSD enzymes, the three 17-KSR/17β HSD reactions are catalyzed by more than one enzyme (reviewed in *60,72*). 17β HSD is an NADPH-dependent, non-P450 enzyme that is bound to the endoplasmic reticulum. It is widely found in both steroidogenic and non-steroidogenic tissues (reviewed in *72*).

Thus far, five types of human 17β HSD have been cloned, and have been given the name types I, II, III, IV, and V, according to the order in which their cDNAs were cloned. Human type I is found on chromosome 17, type II on chromosome 16, type III on chromosome 9, and type V on chromosome 10. Types I, III, and V function as reductases and convert "inactive" to "active" steroids, whereas types II and IV function as oxidases and convert "active" to "inactive" steroids. Type I mainly catalyzes the reductive conversion of estrone to estradiol but also catalyzes the conversion of DHEA to androstenediol, whereas type IV mainly catalyzes the oxidative conversion of estradiol to estrone. Type II catalyzes the conversion of testosterone to androstenedione, androstenediol to DHEA, and estradiol to estrone. Types III and V are "androgenic" because they mainly catalyze the conversion of androstenedione to testosterone.

Type I 17β HSD was originally cloned from human placental cDNA libraries *(73–75)*, but was also found in ovaries and in mammary gland. Type II 17β HSD was first isolated from prostatic and placental cDNA libraries *(76)*, and was also found in the liver, small intestine, endometrium, kidney, pancreas, and colon *(77)*. Type III 17β HSD was found only in testis *(78)*, and mutations in this gene cause pseudohermaphroditism. Type IV 17β HSD has been cloned from humans and pigs *(79,80)*, and was found to be expressed in virtually all human tissues studied, suggesting it may play a role in inactivating estrogens in peripheral tissues.

Expression of 17βHSD in the Brain

Demonstration of 17βHSD activity in the brain of rats and monkeys *(81,82)* indicated that 17βHSD protein and mRNA would also be present. Recent analysis of both rat and frog brains has demonstrated that 17βHSD type I was expressed in the brain *(83,84)*. In adult rat brains, 17βHSD protein was detected in non-neuronal cells (GFAP-positive cells) in the hypothalamus, hippocampus, thalamus, cortex, cerebellum, caudate putamen, and pineal gland *(83)*. In the hypothalamus, 17βHSD immunoreactivity was detected in astrocytes in the paraventricular, arcuate, and supraoptic nuclei. Immunoreactivity was detected in all pyramidal layers of the hippocampus, paraventricular nucleus in the thalamus, all layers of the cortex, and all layers of the cerebellum.

In the frog brain, 17βHSD was also found in glia *(84)*. Immunopositive cell bodies were found exclusively in the telencephalon (pallium mediale) and in the rostral part of the diencephalon. Immunoreactive processes were found in the amygdala, dorsal part of the striatum, nucleus accumbens septi, and the lateral nucleus of the septum. Sparse processes were found in the medial forebrain bundle, the nucleus of the diagonal band of Broca, and the nucleus entopeduncularis. In the diencephalon, 17βHSD immunoreactive processes were found in the corpus geniculatus lateralis, and in the lateral forebrain bundle. All other brain regions, including the mesencephalon, the metencephalon, the rhombencephalon, spinal cord, and pituitary contained no 17βHSD immunoreactivity.

11β Hydroxysteroid Oxidoreductase (11βHOR)

The conversion of cortisol to cortisone is mediated by 11β-hydroxysteroid dehydrogenase (11βHSD, 11βHOR), and the reverse reaction is mediated by an 11-oxidoreductase activity. Enzymologic studies suggest that these reactions are mediated by two different proteins, but cloning and expression of 11βHSD cDNA showed that one protein has both 11β dehydrogenase and 11-oxidoreductase activities (reviewed in *85*). Two isoforms of 11βHSD have been described. 11βHSD-1 is a low-affinity NADPH-dependent enzyme *(86,87)*, and is found mainly in human liver, decidua, lung, gonad, pituitary and cerebellum *(88,89)*. In contrast to 11βHSD1, 11βHSD2 is an NAD-dependent enzyme, localized to the placenta and to mineralocorticoid target tissues (kidney, colon, and salivary gland) *(87,89–91)*. Because 11βHSD converts cortisol to cortisone, it is thought to protect mineralocorticoid receptors—which can be bound by both glucocorticoids and mineralocorticoids—from occupation by glucocorticoids. It is also thought to protect glucocorticoid receptors from occupation by glucocorticoids.

Expression of 11βHOR in the Brain

Both 11βHSD1 (93,94)and 11βHSD2 *(95–97)* activities and mRNA have been detected in adult rat brains. 11βHSD1 mRNA was detected in the hippocampus (highest in CA3) and cortex (layer IV, parietal cortex), medial preoptic area of the hypothalamus, arcuate nucleus, and anterior pituitary *(93)*. By contrast, 11βHSD2 mRNA was not detected in the hippocampus, an area that does not distinguish between aldosterone and corticosterone. It was found in the commissural portion of the nucleus tractus solitarius and the subcommissural organ, and the ventrolateral portion of the ventromedial hypothalamus *(95)*.

During rat development, 11βHSD2 mRNA was widely expressed in the CNS throughout the neuroepithelium, thalamus, and spinal cord up to embryonic day 12.5, and declined thereafter *(97)*. By embryonic day 15.5, 11βHSD2 mRNA was restricted to the thalamus, cerebellar primordia, roof of midbrain, and regions of pontine neuroepithelia, a region next to the tip of the posterior horn of the lateral ventricle. Expression in the thalamus and cerebellum persisted postnatally.

5α Reductase

Testosterone is converted to the more potent androgen dihydrotestosterone (DHT) by 5α reductase. In the brain, PROG is converted to 5α dihydroprogesterone, and 11-DOC is likewise reduced at the 5α position. This membrane-bound, non-P450 enzyme is found mainly in peripheral target tissues such as genital skin and hair follicles.

Cloning and expression of two 5 α reductases have been reported *(98,99)*. The gene for type I is found on human chromosome 5, is about 35 kb, and encodes a 29 kDa protein found in the scalp, but does not encode the protein that is required for sexual differentiation *(100)*. The gene for type II is found on human chromosome 2 and has the same intron/exon structure as the gene for the type I enzyme *(100)*. Mutations in the gene for 5α reductase type II cause classic 5α reductase deficiency.

Expression of 5α Reductase in the Brain

The rat CNS is capable of converting PROG into 5α-reduced metabolites (reviewed in *102*), indicating that this enzyme is present in the CNS. 5α reductase activity, protein, and mRNA have been detected in neurons, astrocytes, and glia *(102–106)*, and the predominant isoform is type I *(107)*. In the adult rat, immunocytochemical staining detected 5α reductase protein throughout the brain, with no differences between male and female rats. Immunostaining was observed in the hypothalamus (paraventricular, arcuate, and supraoptic nuclei), hippocampus, thalamus (paraventricular nucleus), cortex (all cell layers), cerebellum (Bergmann cells), and white matter (corpus callosum) *(105)*. In the cortex and hypothalamus, immunostaining was located in astrocytes, without any association with organelles. This is consistent with a microsomal localization of 5α reductase protein.

Expression of 5α reductase mRNA during rat development was assessed by *in situ* hybridization *(106)*. At embryonic d 12 (E12) , 5α reductase mRNA was detected in the spinal cord and neuroepithelial walls of the brain ventricular system. At E14, the distribution of this mRNA was the same, but the abundance increased in the spinal cord and neuroepithelium. At this time, a signal was observed in the pituitary and in the spinal ganglia, and expression in the brain was greatest above the proliferating zones close to the ventricular wall. At E16, 5α reductase mRNA was detected in the cortex (innermost layers), thalamus, cerebellum, medulla and spinal cord, and spinal ganglia, with lesser amounts found in the trigeminal ganglia and inferior ganglia of the nodose-petrosal nerves (IX and X). At E18, 5α reductase mRNA expression in the brain was more diffuse. Labeling could be detected in the spinal cord, brain stem, cerebellum, pituitary, striatum, amygdala, caudate-putamen, nucleus accumbens, and septum. At E20, 5α reductase mRNA expression was similar, but reduced in all areas except the trigeminal ganglion and the ventricular zones of striatum and amygdala, and the thalamus. In the neonatal rat (d 2), 5α reductase mRNA was expressed most abundantly in the trigeminal ganglion and the ventral part of the striatal ventricular zone, with lesser amounts found in the cortical plate, posterior part of the cerebral neuroepithelium, ventricular zone of the amygdala, thalamus, and hippocampus. Labeling in the hippocampus was greatest in the 6-d old rat. By 2 wk of age, 5α reductase mRNA expression changed completely, and was evenly distributed throughout the brain. At this time, white matter structures (e.g., optic chiasm, lateral olfactory tract, internal capsule, and corpus callosum) were highly positive for 5α reductase mRNA, but other regions (hippocampus, striatal neuroepithelium) were also positive. Thus, 5α reductase mRNA was expressed in three distinct patterns in the rat:

1. During embryonic and early postnatal development, 5α reductase mRNA was found in regions of proliferating cells;
2. 5α reductase mRNA was expressed in regions containing more differentiated cells;
3. In the adult, 5α reductase mRNA was found mainly in white matter structures.

3α HOR

cDNA cloning has revealed that most hydroxysteroid dehydrogenases belong to one of two families: the short-chain dehydrogenase/reductase family (also known as short-chain alcohol dehydrogenases) and the aldo-keto reductase family *(108–110)*.

Mammalian 3αHSDs are members of the aldo-keto reductase family. The reactions catalyzed by 3α HSD are stereospecific, and involve the interconversion of a carbonyl with a hydroxyl group. In the prostate, 3αHSD is involved in inactivating dihydrotestosterone, by conversion to a the weak androgen 3α-androstanediol, whereas in the nervous system, 3αHSD is involved in activating 5α reduced steroids such as 5α dihydroprogesterone to the potent neurosteroid tetrahydroprogesterone. Thus, this enzyme is a key regulator of both steroid hormone receptor and ion-gated channel receptor occupancy and action.

Most biochemical studies have used the rat liver enzyme for purification, biochemical analysis, generation of antibodies, cDNA cloning, and enzyme structure (reviewed in *(110)*. cDNAs from rat liver were cloned *(109,111–113)*, had an open reading frame of 966 nucleotides, and predicted a protein of 322 amino acids. Rat liver 3α HSD cDNA has high sequence identity (>70%) with the clone for human liver type I 3α HSD (DD4 or chlordecone reductase), human liver DD1 (which is both a 3α- and 20α-HSD), and human liver DD2 (human bile-acid binding protein) *(114,115)*. A human liver type II 3α HSD *(116)* and human prostatic 3αHSD cDNAs have also been cloned. Human type I and type II 3α HSDs differ in their K_m values for 5α-DHT, with the type I enzyme having a lower K_m. All 3αHSD cDNAs share high sequence identity. The genes encoding the type I and II enzymes spanned approximately 20 and 16 kb, and both contain 9 exons of the same size and intron/exon boundaries *(116)*.

Expression of 3α HOR in the Brain

Expression of 3αHSD was studied in rat tissues, including brain. Human 3αHSD type II mRNA, but not type I mRNA, was found in the brain, kidney, liver, lung, placenta, and testis, and type I mRNA was found only in the liver *(116)*. Extensive biochemical studies by Karavolas and colleagues demonstrated rat 3αHSD activity in various regions of the brain, and its regulation by estrogens and lactation *(117,118)*. Rat 3αHSD activity was detected in the rat anterior pituitary, medial basal hypothalamus, thalamus, tectum, tegmentum, cerebellum, medulla, and pineal gland *(119)*. Using a monoclonal antibody against liver 3αHSD, Western blots of proteins extracted from different rat brain regions demonstrated that the olfactory bulb contained the greatest abundance of 3αHSD protein *(120)* 3αHSD protein and activity were found in the rat amygdala, brain stem, caudate putamen, cingulate cortex, hippocampus, midbrain, and thalamus *(120)*. 3αHSD activity was found mainly in type I astrocytes, but was also detected in oligodendrocytes *(104)*.

CONCLUSION

The distribution of the neurosteroidogenic enzymes in the central and peripheral nervous systems suggests that neurosteroidogenesis will be developmentally and regionally regulated. The presence of the enzymes in similar locations in brains from frogs, birds, rodents, monkeys, and humans further suggests that the function of neurosteroids may be conserved throughout recent evolution. Because all the enzymes are found neither in identical locations nor at the same time in development, the data further indicate that different neurosteroids will be synthesized in different regions of the adult brain and throughout development. Thus it is apparent that neurosteroids will have many different actions *(5)*. Clearly, effects on some behaviors in adult animals have been established, but other effects on neurotransmitter synthesis, and release, and neuronal growth and migration, have only begun to be explored. It is hoped that laying out a "map" of the neurosteroidogenic enzymes in the adult brain and in the developing nervous system, as well as studying the regulation of these enzymes in the nervous system, will give us insight into the roles these compounds may play throughout life.

ACKNOWLEDGMENTS

This work was supported by NIH grants HD27970 (to SHM) and HD11979 (to the Reproductive Endocrinology Center, Dept. of Ob, Gyn, UCSF), and by a grant from the National Niemann-Pick Foundation (to SHM).

REFERENCES

1. Miller WL. Molecular biology of steroid hormone synthesis. Endocr Rev 1988;9:295–318.
2. Nebert DW, Gonzalez FJ. P-450 genes: structure, evolution and regulation. Annu Rev Biochem 1987;56:945.
3. Hall PF. Cytochromes P-450 and the regulation of steroid synthesis. Steroids 1986;48:131–196.
4. Mellon SH, Deschepper CF. Neurosteroid biosynthesis: genes for adrenal steroidogenic enzymes are expressed in the brain. Brain Res 1933;629:283–292.
5. Mellon SH. Neurosteroids: biochemistry, modes of action, and clinical relevance. J Clin Endocrinol Metab 1994;78:1003–1008.
6. Matteson KJ, Chung B, Urdea MS, Miller WL. Study of cholesterol side chain cleavage (20,22 desmolase) deficiency causing congenital lipoid adrenal hyperplasia using bovine-sequence P450scc oligodeoxyribonucleotide probes. Endocrinology 1986;118:1296–1305.
7. Chung B, Matteson KJ, Voutilainen R, Mohandas TK, Miller WL. Human cholesterol side-chain cleavage enzyme, P450scc: cDNA cloning, assignment of the gene to chromosome 15, and expression in the placenta. Proc Natl Acad Sci USA 1986;83:8962.
8. Morohashi K, Sogawa K, Omura T, Fujii-Kuriyama Y. Gene structure of human cytochrome P-450(SCC), cholesterol desmolase. J Biochem 1987;101:879–887.
9. Oonk RB, Parker KL, Gibson JL, Richards JS. Rat cholesterol side-chain cleavage cytochrome P-450 (P-450scc) gene. Structure and regulation by cAMP in vitro. J Biol Chem 1990;265:22392–22401.
10. Zhang P, Rodriguez H, Mellon SH. Transcriptional regulation of P450scc gene expression in neural and in steroidogenic cells: implications for regulation of neurosteroidogenesis. Mol Endocrinol 1995;9:1571–1582.
11. Jung-Testas I, Hu ZY, Baulieu EE, Robel P. Neurosteroids: biosynthesis of pregnenolone and progesterone in primary cultures of rat glial cells. Endocrinology 1989;125:2083–2091.
12. Le Goascogne C, Robel P, Gouezou M, Sananes N, Baulieu EE, Waterman M. Neurosteroids: cytochrome P-450scc in rat brain. Science 1987;237:1212–1215.
13. Oonk RB, Krasnow JS, Beattie WG, Richards JS. Cyclic AMP-dependent and -independent regulation of cholesterol side chain cleavage cytochrome P-450 (P-450scc) in rat ovarian granulosa cells and corpora lutea. cDNA and deduced amino acid sequence of rat P-450scc. J Biol Chem 1989;264:21934–21942.
14. Moore CCD, Brentano ST, Miller WL. Human P450scc gene transcription is induced by cyclic AMP and repressed by 12-O-tetradecanoylphorbol-13-acetate and A23187 through independent cis elements. Mol Cell Biol 1990;10:6013–6023.
15. Rice DA, Kirkman MS, Aitken LD, Mouw AR, Schimmer BP, Parker KL. Analysis of the promoter region of the gene encoding mouse cholesterol side-chain cleavage enzyme. J Biol Chem 1990;265:11713–11720.
16. Ahlgren R, Simpson ER, Waterman MR, Lund J. Characterization of the promoter/regulatory region of the bovine CYP11A (P-450scc) gene. Basal and cAMP-dependent expression. J Biol Chem 1990;265:3313–3319.
17. Lynch JP, Lala DS, Peluso JJ, Luo W, Parker KL, White BA. Steroidogenic factor 1, an orphan nuclear receptor, regulates the expression of the rat aromatase gene in gonadal tissues. Mol E ndocrinol 1993;7:776–786.
18. Hum DW, Staels B, Black SM, Miller WL. Basal transcriptional activity and cyclic adenosine 3',5'-monophosphate responsiveness of the human cytochrome P450scc promoter transfected into MA-10 Leydig cells. Endocrinology 1993;132:546–552.
19. Dynan WS, Tjian R. The promoter-specific transcription factor Sp1 binds to upstream sequences in the SV40 early promoter. Cell 1983;35:79–87.
20. Compagnone NA, Bulfone A, Rubenstein JLR, Mellon SH. Expression of the steroidogenic enzyme P450scc in the central and peripheral nervous systems during rodent embryogenesis. Endocrinology 1995;136:2689–2696.

21. Durkee TJ, McLean MP, Hales DB, Payne AH, Waterman MR, Khan I, Gibori G. P450(17 alpha) and P450SCC gene expression and regulation in the rat placenta. Endocrinology 1992;130: 1309–1317.

22. Rogler LE, Pintar JE. Expression of the P450 side-chain cleavage and adrenodoxin genes begins during early stages of adrenal cortex development. Mol Endocrinol 1993;7:453–461.

23. Greco TL, Payne AH. Ontogeny of expression of the genes for steroidogenic enzymes P450 side-chain cleavage, 3 beta-hydroxysteroid dehydrogenase, P450 17 alpha-hydroxylase/C17-20 lyase, and P450 aromatase in fetal mouse gonads. Endocrinology 1994;135:262–268.

24. Omura T, Sanders S, Estabrook RW, Cooper DY, Rosenthal O. Isolation from adrenal cortex of a non-heme iron protein and a flavoprotein functional as a reduced triphosphopyridine nucleotide-cytochrome P-450 reductase. Arch Biochem Biophys 1996;117:660–673.

25. Nakamura Y, Otsuka H, Tamaoki B. Requirement of a new flavoprotein and a non-heme iron-containing protein in the steroid 11β- and 18-hydroxylase system. Biochim Biophys Acta 1966;122:34–42.

26. Kimura T, Suzuki K. Components of the electron transport system in adrenal steroid hydroxylase. J Biol Chem 1967;242:485–491.

27. Mellon SH, Kushner JA, Vaisse C. Expression and regulation of adrenodoxin and P450scc mRNA in rodent tissues. DNA Cell Biol 1991;10:339–347.

28. Oftebro H, Stormer FC, Pedersen JL. The presence of an adrenodoxin-like ferredoxin and cytochrome P-450 in brain mitochondria. J Biol Chem 1979;254:4331–4334.

29. Zhang LH, Rodriguez H, Ohno S, Miller WL. Serine phosphorylation of human P450c17 increases 17,20-lyase activity: Implications for adrenarche and the polycystic ovary syndrome. Proc Natl Acad Sci USA 1995;92:10619–10623.

30. Givens C, Zhang P, Bair S, Mellon S. Transcriptional regulation of rat cytochrome P450c17 expression in mouse Leydig MA-10 and adrenal Y-1 cells: identification of a single protein that mediates both basal and cAMP-induced activities. DNA Cell Biol 1994;13:1087–1098.

31. Zhang P, Mellon SH. The orphan nuclear receptor steroidogenic factor-1 regulates the cAMP-mediated transcriptional activation of rat cytochrome P450c17. Mol Endocrinol 1996;10:147–158.

32. Zhang P, Mellon SH. The rat P450c17 gene is regulated by multiple orphan nuclear receptors. Mol Endocrinol 1997;11:891–904.

33. Compagnone NA, Bulfone A, Rubenstein JLR, Mellon SH. Steroidogenic enzyme P450c17 is expressed in the embryonic central nervous system. Endocrinology 1995;136:5212–5223.

34. Casey ML, Winkel CA, MacDonald PC. Conversion of progesterone to deoxycorticosterone in the human fetus: steroid 21-hydroxylase activity in fetal tissues. J Steroid Biochem 1983;18:449–452.

35. Casey ML, MacDonald PC. Extraadrenal formation of a mineralocorticosteroid: deoxycorticosterone and deoxycorticosterone sulfate biosynthesis and metabolism. Endocr Rev 1982;3:396–403.

36. Mellon SH, Miller WL. Extraadrenal steroid 21-hydroxylation is not mediated by P450c21. J Clin Invest 1989;84:1497–1502.

37. Norris PJ, Hardwick JP, Emson PC. Localization of NADPH cytochrome P450 oxidoreductase in rat brain by immunohistochemistry and in situ hybridization and a comparison with the distribution of neuronal NADPH-diaphorase staining. Neuroscience 1994;61:331–350.

38. Simmons DL, Kasper CB. Quantitation of mRNAs specific for the mixed-function oxidase system in rat liver and extrahepatic tissues during development. Arch Biochem Biophys 1989;271:10–20.

39. Mellon SH, Bair SR, Monis H. P450c11B3 mRNA, transcribed from a third P450c11 gene, is expressed in a tissue-specific, developmentally, and hormonally regulated fashion in the rodent adrenal, and encodes a protein with both 11 hydroxylase and 18 hydroxylase activities. J Biol Chem 1995;270:1643–1649.

40. Zhang G, Miller WL. The human genome contains only two CYP11B (P450c11) genes. J Clin Endocrinol Metab 1996;81:3254–3256.

41. Gomez-Sanchez CE, Zhou M, Cozza EN, Morita H, Foecking MF, Gomez-Sanchez EP. Aldosterone synthesis in the rat brain. Endocrinology 1997;138:3369–3373.

42. Thompson EA, Siiteri PK. Studies on the aromatization of C-19 androgens. Ann N Y Acad Sci 1973;212:378–391.

43. Thompson EA Jr., Siiteri PK. The involvement of human placental microsomal cytochrome P-450 in aromatization. J Biol Chem 1974;249:5373–5378.

44. Means GD, Mahendroo MS, Corbin CJ, Mathis JM, Powell FE, Mendelson CR, Simpson ER. Structural analysis of the gene encoding human aromatase cytochrome P-450, the enzyme responsible for estrogen biosynthesis. J Biol Chem 1989;264:19385–19391.

45. Chen SA, Besman MJ, Sparkes RS, Zollman S, Klisak I, Mohandas T, Hall PF, Shively JE. Human aromatase: cDNA cloning, Southern blot analysis, and assignment of the gene to chromosome 15. DNA 1988;7:27–38.

46. Mahendroo MS, Means GD, Mendelson CR, Simpson ER. Tissue-specific expression of human P-450AROM. The promoter responsible for expression in adipose tissue is different from that utilized in placenta. J Biol Chem 1991;266:11276–11281.

47. Simpson ER, Mahendroo MS, Means GD, Kilgore MW, Hinshelwood MM, Graham-Lorence S, Amarneh B, Ito Y, Fisher CR, Michael MD, et al. Aromatase cytochrome P450, the enzyme responsible for estrogen biosynthesis. Endocr Rev 1994;15:342–55.

48. Lephart ED. A review of brain aromatase cytochrome P450. Brain Res Rev 1996;22:1–26.

49. Hutchison JB, Wozniak A, Beyer C, Hutchison RE. Regulation of sex-specific formation of oestrogen in brain development: endogenous inhibitors of aromatase. J Steroid Biochem Mol Biol 1996;56:201–207.

50. Roselli CE, Horton LE, Resko JA. Distribution and regulation of aromatase activity in the rat hypothalamus and limbic system. Endocrinology 1985;117:2471–2477.

51. George FW, Ojeda SR. Changes in aromatase activity in the rat brain during embryonic, neonatal, and infantile development. Endocrinology 1982;111:522–529.

52. MacLusky NJ, Philip A, Hurlburt C, Naftolin F. Estrogen formation in the developing rat brain: sex differences in aromatase activity during early post-natal life. Psychoneuroendocrinology 1985;10:355–361.

53. Lephart ED, Simpson ER, McPhaul MJ, Kilgore MW, Wilson JD, Ojeda SR. Brain aromatase cytochrome P-450 messenger RNA levels and enzyme activity during prenatal and perinatal development in the rat. Brain Res Mol Brain Res 1992;16:187–192.

54. Lauber ME, Lichtensteiger W. Pre- and postnatal ontogeny of aromatase cytochrome P450 messenger ribonucleic acid expression in the male rat brain studied by in situ hybridization. Endocrinology 1994;135:1661–1668.

55. Wagner CK, Morrell JI. Distribution and steroid hormone regulation of aromatase mRNA expression in the forebrain of adult male and female rats: a cellular-level analysis using in situ hybridization. J Comp Neurol 1996;370:71–84.

56. Sanghera MK, Simpson ER, McPhaul MJ, Kozlowski G, Conley AJ, Lephart ED. Immunocytochemical distribution of aromatase cytochrome P450 in the rat brain using peptide-generated polyclonal antibodies. Endocrinology 1991;129:2834–2844.

57. Thomas JL, Myers RP, Strickler RC. Human placental 3 beta-hydroxy-5-ene-steroid dehydrogenase and steroid 5-4-ene-isomerase: purification from mitochondria and kinetic profiles, biophysical characterization of the purified mitochondrial and microsomal enzymes. J Steroid Biochem 1989;33:209–217.

58. Luu-The V, Lachance Y, Labrie C, Leblanc G, Thomas JL, Strickler RC, Labrie F. Full length cDNA structure and deduced amino acid sequence of human 3 beta-hydroxy-5-ene steroid dehydrogenase. Mol Endocrinol 1989;3:1310–1312.

59. Lorence MC, Murry BA, Trant JM, Mason JI 1990 Human 3 beta-hydroxysteroid dehydrogenase/delta 4–5-isomerase from placenta: expression in nonsteroidogenic cells of a protein that catalyzes the dehydrogenation/isomerization of C21 and C19 steroids. Endocrinology 1990;126:2493–2498.

60. Penning TM. Molecular endocrinology of hydroxysteroid dehydrogenases. Endocr Rev 1997;18:281–305.

61. Rheaume E, Lachance Y, Zhao HF, Breton N, Dumont M, de Launoit Y, Trudel C, Luu-The V, Simard J, Labrie F. Structure and expression of a new complementary DNA encoding the almost exclusive 3β-hydroxysteroid dehydrogenase/Δ^5-Δ^4-isomerase in human adrenals and gonads. Mol. Endocrinol. 1991;5:1147–1157.

62. de Launoit Y, Zhao H, Belanger A, Labrie F, Simard J. Expression of liver-specific member of the 3β-hydroxysteroid dehydrogenase family, and isoform possessing an almost exclusive 3-ketosteroid reductase activity. J Biol Chem 1992;267:4513–4517.

63. Kabbadj K, el-Etr M, Baulieu EE, Robel P. Pregnenolone metabolism in rodent embryonic neurons and astrocytes. Glia 1993;7:170–175.

64. Bauer HC, Bauer H. Micromethod for the determination of 3-beta-HSD activity in cultured cells. J Steroid Biochem 1989;33:643–646.

65. Weidenfeld J, Siegel RA, Chowers I 1980 In vitro conversion of pregnenolone to progesterone by discrete brain areas of the male rat. J Steroid Biochem 1980;13:961–963.

66. Robel P, Bourreau E, Corpechot C, Dang DC, Halberg F, Clarke C, Haug M, Schlegel ML, Synguelakis M, Vourch C, Baulieu EE. Neuro-steroids: 3 beta-hydroxy-delta 5-derivatives in rat and monkey brain. J Steroid Biochem 19887;27:649–655.

67. Dupont E, Simard J, Luu-The V, Labrie F, Pelletier G. Localization of 3 beta-hydroxysteroid dehydrogenase in rat brain as studied by in situ hybridization. Mol Cell Neurosci 1994;5:119–123.

68. Guennoun R, Fiddes RJ, Gouezou M, Lombes M, Baulieu EE. A key enzyme in the biosynthesis of neurosteroids, 3 beta-hydroxysteroid dehydrogenase/delta 5-delta 4-isomerase (3 beta-HSD), is expressed in rat brain. Brain Res Mol Brain Res 1995;30:287–300.

69. Mensah-Nyagan AG, Feuilloley M, Dupont E, Do-Rego JL, Leboulenger F, Pelletier G, Vaudry H. Immunocytochemical localization and biological activity of 3 beta-hydroxysteroid dehydrogenase in the central nervous system of the frog. J Neurosci 1994;14:7306–7318.

70. Sanne JL, Krueger KE. Expression of cytochrome P450 side-chain cleavage enzyme and 3 beta-hydroxysteroid dehydrogenase in the rat central nervous system: a study by polymerase chain reaction and in situ hybridization. J Neurochem 1995;65:528–536.

71. Dupont E, Rheaume E, Simard J, Luu-The V, Labrie F, Pelletier G. Ontogenesis of 3 beta-hydroxysteroid dehydrogenase/delta 5-delta 4 isomerase in the rat adrenal as revealed by immunocytochemistry and in situ hybridization. Endocrinology 1991;129:2687–2692.

72. Labrie F, Luu-The V, Lin S-H, Labrie C, Simard J, Breton R, BÈlanger A. The key role of 17β-hydroxysteroid dehydrogenases in sex steroid biology. Steroids 1997;62:148–159.

73. Luu-The V, Labrie C, Zhao HF, Couet J, Lachance Y, Simard J, Leblanc G, Cote J, Berube D, Gagne R, et al. Characterization of cDNAs for human estradiol 17 beta-dehydrogenase and assignment of the gene to chromosome 17: evidence of two mRNA species with distinct 5'-termini in human placenta. Mol Endocrinol 1989;3:1301–1309.

74. Peltoketo H, Isomaa V, Maentausta O, Vihko R. Complete amino acid sequence of human placental 17 beta-hydroxysteroid dehydrogenase deduced from cDNA. FEBS Lett 1988;239:73–77.

75. Tremblay Y, Ringler GE, Morel Y, Mohandas TK, Labrie F, Strauss JFd, Miller WL. Regulation of the gene for estrogenic 17-ketosteroid reductase lying on chromosome 17cen-q25. J Biol Chem 1989;264:20458–20462.

76. Wu L, Einstein M, Geissler WM, Chan HK, Elliston KO, Andersson S. Expression cloning and characterization of human 17 beta-hydroxysteroid dehydrogenase type 2, a microsomal enzyme possessing 20 alpha-hydroxysteroid dehydrogenase activity. J Biol Chem 1993;268:12964–12969.

77. Casey ML, MacDonald PC, Andersson S. 17. beta-Hydroxysteroid dehydrogenase type 2: chromosomal assignment and progestin regulation of gene expression in human endometrium. J Clin Invest 1994;94:2135–2141.

78. Geissler WM, Davis DL, Wu L, Bradshaw KD, Patel S, Mendonca BB, Elliston KO, Wilson JD, Russell DW, Andersson S. Male pseudohermaphroditism caused by mutations of testicular 17 beta-hydroxysteroid dehydrogenase 3. Nat Genet 1994;7:34–39.

79. Adamski J, Carstensen J, Husen B, Kaufmann M, de Launoit Y, Leenders F, Markus M, Jungblut PW. New 17 beta-hydroxysteroid dehydrogenases. Molecular and cell biology of the type IV porcine and human enzymes. Ann N Y Acad Sci 1996;784:124–136.

80. Leenders F, Adamski J, Husen B, Thole HH, Jungblut PW. Molecular cloning and amino acid sequence of the porcine 17 beta-estradiol dehydrogenase. Eur J Biochem 1994;222:221–227.

81. Reddy VV. Estrogen metabolism in neural tissues of rabbits: 17 beta - hydroxysteroid oxidoreductase activity. Steroids 1979;34:207–215.

82. Resko JA, Stadelman HL, Norman RL. 17 beta-hydroxysteroid dehydrogenase activity in the pituitary gland and neural tissue of Rhesus monkeys. J Steroid Biochem 1979;11:1429–1434.

83. Pelletier G, Luu-The V, Labrie F. Immunocytochemical localization of type I 17 beta-hydroxysteroid dehydrogenase in the rat brain. Brain Res 1995;704:233–239.

84. Mensah-Nyagan AM, Feuilloley M, Do-Rego JL, Marcual A, Lange C, Tonon MC, Pelletier G, Vaudry H. Localization of 17beta-hydroxysteroid dehydrogenase and characterization of testosterone in the brain of the male frog. Proc Natl Acad Sci USA 1996;93:1423–1428.

85. Bujalska I, Shimojo M, Howie A, Stewart PM. Human 11β-hydroxysteroid dehydrogenase: studies on the stably transfected isoforms and localization of the type 2 isozyme within renal tissue. Steroids 1997;62:77–82.

86. Moore CCD, Mellon SH, Murai J, Siiteri PK, Miller WL. Structure and function of the hepatic form of 11 beta-hydroxysteroid dehydrogenase in the squirrel monkey, an animal model of glucocorticoid resistance. Endocrinology 1993;133:368–375.

87. Stewart PM, Murry BA, Mason JI. Human kidney 11 beta-hydroxysteroid dehydrogenase is a high affinity nicotinamide adenine dinucleotide-dependent enzyme and differs from the cloned type I isoform. J Clin Endocrinol Metab 1994;79:480–484.

88. Tannin GM, Agarwal AK, Monder C, New MI, White PC. The human gene for 11 beta-hydroxysteroid dehydrogenase. Structure, tissue distribution, and chromosomal localization. J Biol Chem 1991;266:16653–16658.

89. Whorwood CB, Mason JI, Ricketts ML, Howie AJ, Stewart PM. Detection of human 11 beta-hydroxysteroid dehydrogenase isoforms using reverse-transcriptase-polymerase chain reaction and localization of the type 2 isoform to renal collecting ducts. Mol Cell Endocrinol 1995;110:R7–R12.

90. Brown RW, Chapman KE, Edwards CR, Seckl JR. Human placental 11 beta-hydroxysteroid dehydrogenase: evidence for and partial purification of a distinct NAD-dependent isoform. Endocrinology 1993;132:2614–2621.

91. Brown RW, Chapman KE, Kotelevtsev Y, Yau JL, Lindsay RS, Brett L, Leckie C, Murad P, Lyons V, Mullins JJ, Edwards CR, Seckl JR. Cloning and production of antisera to human placental 11 beta-hydroxysteroid dehydrogenase type 2. Biochem J 1996;313:1007–1017.

92. Albiston AL, Obeyesekere VR, Smith RE, Krozowski ZS. Cloning and tissue distribution of the human 11 beta-hydroxysteroid dehydrogenase type 2 enzyme. Mol Cell Endocrinol 1994;105:R11–R17.

93. Moisan MP, Seckl JR, Edwards CR. 11 beta-hydroxysteroid dehydrogenase bioactivity and messenger RNA expression in rat forebrain: localization in hypothalamus, hippocampus, and cortex. Endocrinology 1990;127:1450–1455.

94. Lakshmi V, Sakai RR, McEwen BS, Monder C. Regional distribution of 11 beta-hydroxysteroid dehydrogenase in rat brain Endocrinology 1991;128:1741–1748.

95. Roland BL, Li KX, Funder JW. Hybridization histochemical localization of 11 beta-hydroxysteroid dehydrogenase type 2 in rat brain. Endocrinology 1995;136:4697–4700.

96. Zhou MY, Gomez-Sanchez EP, Cox DL, Cosby D, Gomez-Sanchez CE. Cloning, expression, and tissue distribution of the rat nicotinamide adenine dinucleotide-dependent 11 beta-hydroxysteroid dehydrogenase. Endocrinology 1995;136:3729–3734.

97. Brown RW, Diaz R, Robson AC, Kotelevtsev YV, Mullins JJ, Kaufman MH, Seckl JR. The ontogeny of 11 beta-hydroxysteroid dehydrogenase type 2 and mineralocorticoid receptor gene expression reveal intricate control of glucocorticoid action in development. Endocrinology 1996;137:794–797.

98. Andersson S, Russell DW. Structural and biochemical properties of cloned and expressed human and rat steroid 5 alpha-reductases. Proc Natl Acad Sci USA 1990;87:3640–3644.

99. Andersson S, Berman DM, Jenkins EP, Russell DW. Deletion of steroid 5 alpha-reductase 2 gene in male pseudohermaphroditism. Nature 1991;354:159–161.

100. Jenkins EP, Andersson S, Imperato-McGinley J, Wilson JD, Russell DW. Genetic and pharmacological evidence for more than one human steroid 5 alpha-reductase. J Clin Invest 1992;89:293–300.

101. Thigpen AE, Davis DL, Milatovich A, Mendonca BB, Imperato-McGinley J, Griffin JE, Francke U, Wilson JD, Russell DW. Molecular genetics of steroid 5 alpha-reductase 2 deficiency. J Clin Invest 1992;90:799–809.

102. Celotti F, Melcangi RC, Martini L. The 5 alpha-reductase in the brain: molecular aspects and relation to brain function. Front Neuroendocrinol 1992;13:163–215.

103. Melcangi RC, Celotti F, Castano P, Martini L. Differential localization of the 5 alpha-reductase and the 3 alpha-hydroxysteroid dehydrogenase in neuronal and glial cultures. Endocrinology 1993;132:1252–1259.

104. Melcangi RC, Celotti F, Martini L. Progesterone 5-alpha-reduction in neuronal and in different types of glial cell cultures: type 1 and 2 astrocytes and oligodendrocytes. Brain Res 1994;639:202–206.

105. Pelletier G, Luu-The V, Labrie F. Immunocytochemical localization of 5 alpha-reductase in rat brain. Mol Cell Neurosci 1994;5:394–399.

106. Lauber ME, Lichtensteiger W. Ontogeny of 5 alpha-reductase (type 1) messenger ribonucleic acid expression in rat brain: early presence in germinal zones. Endocrinology 1995;137:2718–2730.

107. Normington K, Russell DW. Tissue distribution and kinetic characteristics of rat steroid 5 alpha-reductase isozymes. Evidence for distinct physiological functions. J Biol Chem 1992;267:19548–19554.

108. Krozowski Z. The short-chain alcohol dehydrogenase superfamily: variations on a common theme. J Steroid Biochem Mol Biol 1994;51:125–130.

109. Pawlowski JE, Huizinga M, Penning TM. Cloning and sequencing of the cDNA for rat liver 3 alpha-hydroxysteroid/dihydrodiol dehydrogenase. J Biol Chem 1991;266:8820–8825.

110. Penning TM, Bennett MJ, Smith-Hoog S, Schlegel BP, Jez JM, Lewis M. Structure and function of 3α-hydroxysteroid dehydrogenase. Steroids 1997;62:101–111.

111. Cheng KC, White PC, Qin KN. Molecular cloning and expression of rat liver 3 alpha-hydroxysteroid dehydrogenase. Mol Endocrinol 1991;5:823–828.

112. Stolz A, Rahimi-Kiani M, Ameis D, Chan E, Ronk M, Shively JE. Molecular structure of rat hepatic 3 alpha-hydroxysteroid dehydrogenase. A member of the oxidoreductase gene family. J Biol Chem 1991;266:15253–15257.

113. Usui E, Okuda K, Kato Y, Noshiro M. Rat hepatic 3 alpha-hydroxysteroid dehydrogenase: expression of cDNA and physiological function in bile acid biosynthetic pathway. J Biochem (Tokyo) 1994;115:230–237.

114. Deyashiki Y, Ogasawara A, Nakayama T, Nakanishi M, Miyabe Y, Sato K, Hara A. Molecular cloning of two human liver 3 alpha-hydroxysteroid/dihydrodiol dehydrogenase isoenzymes that are identical with chlordecone reductase and bile-acid binder. Biochem J 1993;299:545–552.

115. Hara A, Matsuura K, Tamada Y, Sato K, Miyabe Y, Deyashiki Y, Ishida N. Relationship of human liver dihydrodiol dehydrogenases to hepatic bile-acid-binding protein and an oxidoreductase of human colon cells. Biochem J 1996;313:373–376.

116. Khanna M, Qin KN, Wang RW, Cheng KC. Substrate specificity, gene structure, and tissue-specific distribution of multiple human 3 alpha-hydroxysteroid dehydrogenases. J Biol Chem 1995;270:20162–20168.

117. Karavolas HJ, Hodges DR. Neuroendocrine metabolism of progesterone and related progestins. Ciba Found Symp 1990;153:22–55.

118. Karavolas HJ, Hodges DR. Metabolism of progesterone and related steroids by neural and neuroendocrine structures. In: Costa, E, Paul SM, eds. Neurosteroids and Brain Function, vol. 8. Thieme, New York, NY, 1991, pp. 135–145.

119. Hanukoglu I, Karavolas HJ, Goy RW. Progesterone metabolism in the pineal, brain stem, thalamus and corpus callosum of the female rat. Brain Res 1977;125:313–324.

120. Khanna M, Qin KN, Cheng KC. Distribution of 3 alpha-hydroxysteroid dehydrogenase in rat brain and molecular cloning of multiple cDNAs encoding structurally related proteins in humans. J Steroid Biochem Mol Biol 1995;53:41–36.

3

Cytochrome P450 in the Central Nervous System

Margaret Warner, PhD
and Jan-Åke Gustafsson, MD, PhD

CONTENTS

INTRODUCTION
P450 NOMENCLATURE
PROBLEMS OF DETECTION OF P450 IN THE BRAIN
INDIVIDUAL FORMS OF P450 IN THE BRAIN
CONCLUSIONS ABOUT BRAIN STEROIDOGENESIS FROM THE P450 DATA
DRUG, STEROID, AND FATTY ACID METABOLIZING P450S
   IN THE BRAIN
CONCLUSIONS
REFERENCES

INTRODUCTION

The brain is a major target for the action of steroids. These molecules regulate many aspects of brain function, including imprinting of sexual behavior *(1)*, learning and memory *(2)*, and mood and sleep/wakefulness *(3)*. They are also thought to modulate neurodegenerative processes *(4,5)*. The brain is, of course, also the target of many pharmaceutical agents, fatty acid metabolites, and organic solvents. Synthesis and degradation of steroid hormones, as well as the activation and inactivation of therapeutic agents and fatty acids involve several members of the cytochrome P450 super gene family *(6,7)*. P450s are abundant in the adrenals, gonads, and liver, however, when measurable, most P450s are expressed at very low levels in the brain *(8)*. The capacity of the brain to metabolize pharmaceuticals is so low that it is most unlikely that P450 in the brain plays any role in the overall clearance of pharmaceuticals from the body. However, those P450s that are selectively localized at high concentrations in limited numbers of brain cells, can play important roles in the physiology, pharmacology, and toxicology of those cells.

Two key observations have inspired an intensive effort to characterize the P450 in the brain. The first of these observations is that there is much more P450 in the brain than can be accounted for by the known steroid and drug metabolizing P450s *(8)*. This suggests

From: *Contemporary Endocrinology: Neurosteroids: A New Regulatory Function
in the Nervous System* Edited by: E.-E. Baulieu, P. Robel, and M. Schumacher
© Humana Press Inc., Totowa, NJ

that there are novel forms of P450 in the brain. The second is that steroid hormone metabolites and precursors play a role in neuromodulation through interaction with neurotransmitter (as opposed to steroid hormone) receptors *(9–11)* and that these molecules could be synthesized in the brain *(12)*. The effort to characterize the forms of P450 in the brain has led to the discovery of the presence of several steroidogenic forms of P450 in the brain *(13–17)* as well as several novel P450s *(18–23)*, some that could be involved in regulation of the levels of neurosteroids (18), and some that can influence neurotransmission in other ways e.g., synthesis and degradation of fatty acid metabolites *(23–26)*. Many forms of P450 in the brain have only been detected by reverse transcriptase-polymerase chain reaction (RT-PCR) and their physiological functions, regulation and localization have not yet been determined.

In this chapter we will analyze the information available on P450s in the brain and discuss the possible role of some of these enzymes in modulation of neurotransmission. We will not focus on data obtained from neuronal or glial cell lines nor will we discuss evidence that is based solely on immunohistochemical staining of the brain. The cell lines, although interesting model systems for regulation studies, do not necessarily reflect the P450 content or profile of the brain and may unnecessarily complicate our attempt to characterize the physiological role of P450s in the brain. Studies where immunohistochemical localization of P450 in the brain is the sole method of identification of brain P450 are considered to be too preliminary to be included in this review. There are many such studies in the literature *(27–33)* and although many of these staining patterns may reflect P450 containing cells, the widespread staining seen, despite the extremely low levels of the corresponding catalytic activities, raises serious questions about whether all of the staining seen can be attributed to P450.

P450 NOMENCLATURE

In 1987, the use of trivial names for P450 enzymes was replaced by a more systematic nomenclature *(34)*. P450s were classified, on the basis of their amino-acid sequence similarities, into families (40% sequence similarity) and subfamilies (55% sequence similarity). In mammals, families 1–4 are xenobiotic, fatty acid, and steroid hydroxylases (Table 1). Families 5, 7, 11, 17, 19, 21, 24, 27, and 51 are biosynthetic enzymes involved in the synthesis of thromboxane, bile acids, steroid hormones, and cholesterol (Table 2). The latest update (35) reveals that there are 14 families and 26 subfamilies in mammals.

PROBLEMS OF DETECTION OF P450 IN THE BRAIN

As is evident from Table 1, several known forms of P450 can be detected in the brain by RT-PCR. Because of the extreme sensitivity of this method, it is not easy to evaluate the biological relevance of the mRNA detected by RT-PCR. This is not to say that transcripts expressed at low levels in the brain are of no physiological relevance. Because of the division of labor in brain cells, it is to be expected that some genes are expressed in a small specific population of cells and measurement of their expression in whole brain will produce a deceptively low value. In order for biological relevance to be considered, RT-PCR data must be accompanied by evidence that the protein is expressed in the brain and that it is localized in a limited number of cells rather than being present at trace levels in all cells.

Table 1

Xenobiotic, Steroid, and Fatty-Acid Metabolizing P450S in the Rat[a]

Family	1		2								3	4		
Subfamily	1A	1B	2A	2B	2C	2D	2E	2F	2G	2J	3A	4A	4B	4F
Number of known members	2	1	3	6	27	5	1	1	1	1	4	4	1	4
RT-PCR detection in the brain	1A1 1A2			2B1 2B2 2C11 2C12 2C13 2C22	2C6 2C7 2D5	2D1 2D4	2E1				3A1 4A8	4A2 4A3		4F4 4
Reference	20			20	36	37	36				20	23		38
Detection in the brain by Western blot and protein sequencing					2C22	2D1 2D4	2E1					4A3		
Reference					39	40,41	42					42		

[a]Summary of data on members of P450 families 1–4 that have been detected in the brain. Literature data was taken from the references cited.

53

Table 2
Thromboxane, Steroid, and Bile Acid Synthesizing P450s in the Rat Brain[a]

Family	5	7		11		17	19	21	24	27	51
Subfamily		7A	7B	11A	11B						
Members	1	1	1	2	3	1	1	1	1	1	1
RNA detection in Brain			+	+		+	+				
Reference		14	19	14		14	13,45				
Protein detection in brain				+			+	+			
Reference				17			43–46	16			

[a]Summary of the literature data on P450s involved in steroid, thromboxane, and bile acid synthesis in the rat brain.

Detection of P450 protein in the brain is not a simple task. The P450 content of the brain is 20–50 pmol/g wet weight or 2–5 pmol/mg brain microsomal protein. This should be compared with the liver level which is 1 nmol/mg microsomal protein. In tissues where it is abundant, P450 can be quantitated in microsomal fractions by its CO difference spectrum *(47)* or by Western blotting. In the brain, the low levels of the enzyme causes several problems. With a good spectrophotometer, 10 pmol P450/mL is about the lower limit of detection. This means 2 mg brain microsomal protein/mL. In most laboratories, problems of turbidity and interference by other chromophores makes quantitation impossible. Similar limitations occur with Western blotting of brain microsomes. With a very good antibody 0.5 pmol P450/lane can be detected. If there were only one or two forms of P450 in the brain there would be no problem. However, there are multiple forms of P450 in the brain, and in order to detect a P450 which represents 10% of the total brain P450, 1 mg of microsomal protein would have to be loaded onto each lane. The result is usually a very poor signal to noise ratio. Another problem with brain P450 is the difficulty of separating microsomal and mitochondrial fractions. A large part of brain microsomes sediments with the mitochondrial fraction and this reduces the yield of P450 in microsomes. The obvious solution to these technical problems is the use of *in situ* hybridization of mRNA to identify cells in which the P450 genes are transcribed and immunohistochemical techniques to localize the proteins. Both of these techniques are also associated with artefacts and must be combined with other methods of detection for definitive evidence for the presence of specific forms of P450. One of the major drawbacks of the *in situ* hybridization technique is that it cannot detect post transcriptional regulation of genes. As will be discussed later this appears to be a major mechanism for the regulation of brain P450. With immunohistochemical staining, the major problem is the amount of cross reaction with irrelevant proteins. Such staining is called specific when it is completely eliminated by pre-adsorption of the antibody with the antigen. This, of course, is not evidence that the correct protein is recognized in the tissue section. We feel that immunohistochemistry must be accompanied with Western blots, N-terminal sequencing of the protein or catalytic activity. In addition, for each P450 there has to be some reasonable correlation between the amount of immunohistochemical staining and the amount of signal quantitated on Western blots or the amount of catalytic activity. We have chosen to get around these problems of P450 quantitation by solubilizing and partially purifying P450 from a total membrane fraction prepared from brain homogenates. The P450 so obtained contains both microsomal and mitochondrial forms of the enzyme which can be spectrally quantitated, characterized by N-terminal sequencing after SDS PAGE, and by reconstitution of catalytic activities (8). This method has led to the identification of several P450 proteins in the brain (23,7,39–41).

INDIVIDUAL FORMS OF P450 IN THE BRAIN
P450s Identified Only by Catalytic Activities

3β, 5α-DIOL HYDROXYLASE

Interestingly, one of the major constitutive forms of P450 in the brain is not listed in either Table 1 or 2 because its cDNA has not yet been cloned. This P450 that is known to metabolize steroids with 3β, 5α configuration, is abundantly expressed in prostate (48), brain (18), and pituitary gland (49), but is absent in liver and kidney (18). It is distributed evenly throughout the brain, is not sexually differentiated, and is not regulated by the adrenal or gonads. It does not metabolize steroids such as testosterone, corticosterone, aldosterone or estradiol. It catalyses the 6α and 7α hydroxylation of 5α-androstane-3β,17β-diol (3β, 5α-diol) and its catalytic activity in the brain (300 nmol triols formed/h/g tissue) is much higher than that of any other microsomal steroid hydroxylase measured in the brain to date. In the prostate, it is the 3β- and not the 3α, 5α-diol that represents the major pathway for the formation of more polar metabolites and thus the elimination of dihydrotestosterone (DHT) (48). We have shown that a similar pathway exists for the elimination of 5α-reduced metabolites of progesterone from the brain (50). No polar metabolites are formed when 3α-hydroxy-5α-pregnan-20-one, (3α, 5α-THPROG) is incubated with microsomal fractions prepared from rat brain, but 3β-hydroxy-5α-pregnan-20-one (3β, 5α-THPROG) is hydroxylated at the 6α- and 7α-positions. These 3β-diols are not formed to any detectable extent in the liver or kidney, but are formed in prostate, pituitary, brain and breast. These hydroxylations were confirmed to be P450 catalyzed reactions by solubilizing the cytochrome P450 from pituitary, brain, and prostate microsomes and reconstituting the catalytic activity with nicotinamide-adenine-denucleotide phosphate (NADPH)-cytochrome P450 reductase and lipid.

Competition experiments, performed to determine whether the same form of P450 in the brain is involved in the elimination of 3β, 5α-diol and 3β, 5α-THPROG confirmed that these two substrates compete with each other for metabolism in microsomal fractions and in reconstitution experiments with P450 extracted from the brain and prostate.

To test our hypothesis that the hydroxylation of 3β, 5α-THPROG represents a pathway for regulation of the level of the potent anesthetic neurosteroid, 3α, 5α-THPROG in the brain, the effect of inhibition of the hydroxylation of 3β, 5α-THPROG on the duration of 3α, 5α-THPROG-induced anaesthesia was examined. The nonanesthetic steroid, 3β, 5α-diol was used as a competitive inhibitor of the metabolism of 3β, 5α-THPROG. The duration of anaesthesia upon intravenous administration of 3α, 5α-THPROG was increased by 33% when 3β, 5α-diol was coadministered. Although this is a very widespread and abundant P450 in the brain, it can account for only 10% of the P450 in the brain.

Epoxygenases

The cyclooxygenase and lipoxygenase activity of the brain has been studied extensively *(51,52)*. More recently it was shown that epoxygenase metabolites of arachidonic acid are synthesized in the brain by cytochromes P450 *(24–26)*. These metabolites, 5,6, 8,9-, and 14,15- epoxyeicosatrienoic acids and their hydrolytic products, the dihydroxyeicosatrienoic acids have been shown to be potent vasodilators of cerebral arterioles, to mobilize intracellular stores of calcium and to influence dopamine receptor-mediated release of somatostatin. Arachidonic acid epoxygenase activity appears to be due to P450s of the 2 family. In the human heart, CYP 2J2 *(53)*, in the rabbit kidney P450 2C2 *(54)* and in the rat kidney, 2C23 *(55)* have been identified as epoxygenases. The P450s involved in formation of arachidonic acid epoxides in the brain remain to be identified.

P450s Listed in Table 2

P4507B

If we start with the P450s in Table 2, i.e., those P450s in families involved in well known physiological pathways, the most unique of these is P4507B. Unlike the other P450s in Table 2, it is predominantly expressed in the brain and neither its substrate nor its function is known. This P450 and was cloned from a rat hippocampal cDNA library in 1995 *(19)*. By sequence comparison, it was found to be most similar to P4507A, the 7α hydroxylase of cholesterol, but it was different enough to be put into a new subfamily. It is not detectable in the adrenals or gonads. It is possible that because of the similarity to P4507α, cholesterol or one of its derivatives might be natural substrates. One question that arose immediately upon the cloning of P4507B was whether this represented the cDNA of 3β-diol hydroxylase. When the distribution of P450 7B mRNA in the rat brain was examined with Northern blot analysis, a high level of expression in the hippocampus and much lower levels in other brain regions was observed. This distribution is very different from that of 3β-diol hydroxylase, whose catalytic activity was evenly distributed throughout the brain. Of course, catalytic activity is not always directly related to mRNA content so the relationship between P4507B and 3β-diol hydroxylase remains to be clarified. Although no catalytic activity and no evidence for the presence of the protein in the brain has been reported, the abundance of this transcript and its selective localization in a specific brain region suggests that this P450 is of physiological relevance in the brain.

P45011A (P450scc)

Of the other P450s in Table 2, all of those involved in steroid biosynthesis have been found in the brain by RT-PCR. However, the quantitative significance of these P450s in the synthesis of neurosteroids from the precursor, cholesterol within the brain, remains unresolved (reviewed in *56*). P450scc, the first and rate limiting step in the conversion of cholesterol to steroids has been detected in the brain by catalytic activity *(57)*, immunohistochemistry *(13)*, and RT-PCR *(14,15)*. Before a physiological role for P450scc in the brain can be definitely established, the differences in the quantitation of this enzyme in the brain in different laboratories and the discrepancies in the reported abundance of the protein, its mRNA and catalytic activity must be resolved.

Two careful studies have been published on the RT-PCR detection of mRNAs of steroidogenic P450s in the brain *(14,15)*. In both studies the conclusion is that the level of these mRNAs is very low in the brain. Strömstedt and Waterman *(14)*, using 35 cycles of amplification, find P450scc in the cerebellum and brain stem, whereas Mellon and Deschepper *(15)*, with 50 cycles, find it mainly in the cortex. Mellon and Deschepper estimate the level of P450scc mRNA in the brain to be 0.1–0.01% of that in the adrenal. They also find P450scc mRNA and protein in both oligodendrocytes and astrocytes in culture. The protein in the primary cultures as estimated on Western blots is approximately 1% of that in adrenal Y-1 cells. This low level of enzyme is compatible with the data of Le Gascogne et al. *(13)* who could not detect P450scc catalytic activity in brain but could detect it in glial cells in culture *(58)*. However, it is difficult to reconcile these data with those of Korneyev et al. *(57)*, who found that P450scc catalytic activities in brain mitochondria of adrenalectomized and castrated rats as high as those in adrenal Y-1 and glioma cells.

It is quite clear that P450scc mRNA is expressed in the brain and in glial cells in culture. An unresolved issue is the role of brain P450scc in brain steroidogenesis. In order to resolve this issue, it is necessary to know:

1. whether the low level of mRNA and its distribution can account for the widespread distribution of the protein in white matter throughout the brain detected by immunohistochemical staining *(13)*, or whether the P450scc antibodies are detecting some other proteins in the brain;
2. whether this mRNA can result in sufficient quantities of enzyme to account for the accumulation of pregnenolone (PREG) in the brain after the adrenals and gonads have been removed:
3. whether P450scc in glial cells in culture and glioma cell lines reflects the situation in the brain.

Compagnone et. al. *(59)* found that though no mRNA could be detected, P450scc protein is expressed in the nervous system of the developing rodent embryo in cell lineages derived from the neural crest. In order to understand some of these data, more information is needed about the stability of the P450scc protein and its mRNA in the brain, the regulation of brain P450scc in the brains of animals that have been adrenalectomized and gonadectomized, and the quantitative relationship between P450scc in freshly isolated glial cells and glial cells in culture and the specificities of the various antibodies used for Western blotting and immunohistochemistry.

P450 11B1 (11β-Hydroxylase) and 11B2 (Aldosterone Synthase)

In 1991 Ozaki et al. *(17)* reported the presence of P450 11B1 in myelinated areas of the rat brain. The enzyme was detected by its catalytic activity, immunohistochemical localization and by Western blotting of brain homogenates. The concentration of the enzyme as judged by Western blots was 16% of the adrenal level (1.4 pmol/mg protein in the cortical white matter) and catalytic activity was 37% of that in the rat adrenal. These studies fulfilled all of the criteria for positive identification of functional P450 in the brain. It was, therefore, very surprising, when PCR studies were done, to find extremely low levels of the mRNA and lack of correlation between distribution of the protein and mRNA.

RT-PCR studies from Strömstedt and Waterman *(14)* and Mellon and Deschepper *(15)* confirmed the presence of P450 11B mRNA in the rat brain cortex. P450 11B2 was detected at low levels all over the brain by Strömstedt and Waterman but could not be detected by Mellon and Deschepper. As was the case with P450scc, the mRNA levels of P450 11B1 were much lower than could be predicted from the protein levels. In addition, the cerebellum and brainstem which were strongly labeled in the immuno-histochemical study of Ozaki et al. *(17)* had very low or undetectable levels of 11B1 mRNA. The reasons for these discrepancies are not clear. It may be one more indi-cation that the brain regulates its P450 at a post-transcriptional level. However, it cannot yet be ruled out that, in the brain, there is an 11β-hydroxylase enzyme similar enough to be recognized by the antibody raised against adrenal 11B1, yet different enough that it is not detected by PCR primers and/or probe specific for 11B1. Interest-ingly, Strömstedt and Waterman *(14)* found no evidence for P45011B1 or 11B2 mRNA in the mouse brain. It could be very informative to determine whether immu-nohistochemical signals and catalytic activity are also absent from the mouse brain. Such information could help to clarify whether the catalytic activity observed in the rat brain is due to 11B1 or is due to some other enzyme. If, on the other hand, there is no synthesis of glucocorticoids in the mouse brain, comparison of the two species might shed some light on the physiological role of brain-synthesized glucocorticoids. It is difficult to predict what such functions might be, since the known roles of gluco-corticoids in the brain, i.e., in memory and learning *(2)* as well as production of GABA receptor active ligands appear to be depend on a supply of steroids from the adrenal gland *(60)*.

Progesterone 21-Hydroxylase (CYP 21)

Iwahashi et al. *(16)* found CYP 21 catalytic activity in the reticular formation of the thalamus. It was 2.0% of that in the adrenal. A specific antibody raised against purified adrenal CYP21, inhibited this catalytic activity and stained cells and ascending fibers of the reticulothalamicus. No information is available about this mRNA in the rat brain but the mRNA for CYP21 was detectable at low levels in the mouse brain stem by RT-PCR *(14)*.

17α Hydroxylase/17, 20-Lyase (P45017)

No 17α hydroxylase activity has been detected in the brain but its activity in this tissue has been inferred from the accumulation of dehydroepiandrosterone (DHEA) and its sulfate ester in brains of adrenalectomized and castrated rats *(12)*. RT-PCR revealed the presence of P45017 mRNA throughout the brain at very low levels *(14)*. According to the criteria previously listed, there is not enough information available to assign a physi-ological meaning of this RT-PCR detection. The relevance of the PCR detection is particularly troubling because there was a signal, larger than that in the brain regions, detected in the liver. The liver has no measurable 17α hydroxylase activity. One possible explanation for the presence of P45017 mRNA and not protein could be that P45017 was functional early in embryogenesis and is no longer necessary in the adult. In agreement with this concept, Compagnone et al. *(61)* have found that P45017 is expressed in the nervous system of the developing rodent embryo. In this case the mRNA could be detected by RT-PCR in the head of E15.5 to E19.5 rat embryos and immunocytochemically detectable P450c17 protein was expressed in the nervous system as early as embryonic d E10.5

Aromatase (P45019)

Of all the steroidogenic P450s, P45019 is the best studied. Its catalytic activity in the brain has been known since 1975 *(1)* and has been measured in several laboratories over the past years *(42–46)*. Today the enzyme, its mRNA, and its catalytic activity have been localized in the rat brain. Immunohistochemical studies revealed that P45019 is localized in neurons in the amygdala and supraoptic nucleus, regions high in aromatase activity *(46)*. In addition, several brain regions not previously known to contain the enzyme were positively stained. These included the reticular thalamic nucleus, the olfactory tract, and the piriform cortex. From studies conducted in several laboratories two very interesting pieces of information about brain P45019 have emerged that may help to clarify some of the puzzling information about other brain P450s. These are:

1. A significant part of the regulation of the enzyme is post-transcriptional. As will be evident at the end of this chapter, many P450s in the brain appear to be regulated post-transcriptionally, although this phenomenon is not as clearly documented with other P450s as it has been for P45019. The mechanisms involved in such regulation need to be examined. It may well be that increase in translatability or stabilization of protein is a mechanism used by the brain to rapidly increase the amounts of enzyme. The use of post transcriptional mechanisms in the brain means that the relationship between mRNA and corresponding protein is not constant. This could be part of the explanation for the lower than expected levels of mRNA in certain brain regions where the protein levels are relatively high.
2. P45019 may be localized at nerve terminals *(46)*. Such a localization strongly indicates a role in neurotransmission or neuromodulation. It also means that there will be differences in the localization of the mRNAs, which should be confined to the cell body, and the protein, which could be in the terminals far away from the cell body.

CONCLUSIONS ABOUT BRAIN STEROIDOGENESIS FROM THE P450 DATA

Reliable quantitative assessments of the level of catalytic activity and mRNAs of the various steroidogenic enzymes, as well as their localization, is not a purely academic exercise. If regulation of these enzymes is mostly post-transcriptional, mRNA levels would not be expected to reflect changes in catalytic activity and the extremely low levels of the mRNAs might not be so surprising. In the matter of synthesis of steroids from cholesterol, regardless of what the mRNA levels are, the accumulation of pregnenolone and DHEA in the brain in animals where the gonads and adrenals are removed needs to be explained. The extremely low levels of P450scc and 17 catalytic activity found in the brain in normal animals, is unlikely to account for either the accumulation in the brain or for the maintenance of the relatively high plasma levels of these steroids in the absence of gonads and adrenals. There can only be two possible explanations. Either there is a large increase in P450scc and 17 catalytic activities in the brains of adrenalectomized and gonadectomized rats or the plasma level, and thus the brain level of these steroids are maintained by some other tissue through synthesis, or release from tissue stores.

DRUG, STEROID, AND FATTY ACID METABOLIZING P450S IN THE BRAIN

Constitutive Forms of Drug Metabolizing P450s in the Brain

Identification of the drug metabolizing P450s in the brain is even more complicated than identification of the steroidogenic forms. Some of the reasons for this are: the large number of members in each subfamily; the overlapping substrate specificities even in members belonging to distinct subfamilies; cross reactivity of antibodies; and the fact that novel members of known families are constantly being discovered. There is, in addition, further complication of the issue by data from one laboratory, which reports very much higher levels of P450 and hepatic microsomal forms of P450 in the brain. These data, which are very different from those found in other laboratories, have been analyzed in a recent review (8) and will not be included in the present discussion. As is evident from Table 1, many members of family 1–4 have been detected by RT-PCR in the brain. Very few fulfill the criteria qualifying them as P450s of physiological or pharmacological relevance in the brain. Although there are many published studies on P450 catalytic activities in the brain, the overall picture of the level of hepatic P450s in the brain can best be illustrated by a very careful study by Jayyosi et al. published in 1992 (62). This lab has a long reputation in analyzing P450-catalyzed steroid metabolites and using testosterone as a model substrate for characterization of hepatic P450s (63). The position of hydroxylation on the testosterone molecule can be used to identify the form of P450 involved. In Table 3, data from the Jayyosi et al. paper has been used to calculate the contribution of individual forms of P450 to the P450 content of brain microsomes.

There are two main messages to be drawn from this table:

1. The brain has a very low capacity to hydroxylate steroids. This conclusion can be made because the same P450s that catalyze hydroxylations of testosterone also utilize estradiol, progesterone, glucocorticoids, and DHEA.
2. The forms of P450 in the table represent a very small fraction of the P450 in the brain. The brain P450 content is 3–5 pmol/mg microsomal protein. This means that the highest testosterone hydroxylase activity, i.e., production of 2β hydroxy testosterone can only account for 10% of the P450 and forms like 2B1 and 2A2 less than 0.5%. Similar calculations can be made for P450s of family 1A (64), 2D (67), 2E (68), and 4A (23). These are all families whose members have been detected by RT-PCR in the brain.

P450 4A3 is one of the few identified constitutive forms of P450 in the brain. It has been identified in the brain by the presence of its mRNA (RT-PCR) and protein (Western blotting and N-terminal sequencing) (23,41). Available antibodies were not suitable for immunohistochemical localization so the cellular distribution is not yet known. Members of the 4A subfamily are of physiological interest because they terminate the activity of many active metabolites of arachidonic acid (69).

Induction of Brain P450

Although constitutive forms have proven to be elusive, the level of cytochrome P450 in the rat brain can be increased 2–7 fold by exposure of rats to ethanol, organic solvents, and certain neuroactive drugs. After such treatment, multiple forms can be identified in the brain.

Table 3
P450 Isoforms Involved in Testosterone Metabolism in the Rat Brain[a]

P450 isoform in liver	2C12	3A2	2A1	3A2 2A2	2A1	2A2	2B1		2C12	2B1
Testosterone metabolite	2α	2β	6α	6β	7α	15α	1β	15β	16α	16β
Activity in brain (pmol/min/mg microsomal protein)[b]	0	0.70	2.2	0.2	0	0.6	0.15	0.31	0	0.21
Liver content of individual P450 form in male rat liver (pmol/mg microsomal protein)[c]	300	50	50	50 3.2	50	20			300	20
Testosterone hydroxylase activity of individual P450 form (pmol min^{-1}/pmol P450)[d]	9.5	2		12	0	19.6				5.3
Calculated amount of enzyme in brain (pmol/mg microsomal protein)	0	0.35		0.016	0	0.03				0.04

[a]Metabolism of testosterone in the rat brain and calculation of the contribution of specific P450 isoforms to this activity.
[b]Adapted with permission from ref. 62.
[c]Adapted with permission from ref. 65.
[d]Adapted with permission from ref. 66.

Ethanol (1 mL/kg intraperitoneally [ip]) or toluene given as a single ip dose of 100 μL or when presented to rats in the atmosphere at a concentration of 100 ppm increases the P450 content of the brain 2–5 fold. Six distinct forms of P450 could be identified in the brain after ethanol administration (41). These were all microsomal forms and were identified by Western blots and N-terminal sequencing of the individual proteins as 2C11, 4A3, 4A8, 2E1, and 2D1/5. Toluene also induced P450 2E1, a 2C member that has not been identified and 2D4.

Upon daily administration of the neuroleptic drugs clozapine and chlorpromazine for 3 wk, the overall P450 content of the brain increased seven- and threefold, respectively, over control levels. With haloperidol treatment the P450 content of the brain remained unchanged (40). Mianserin, a serotonin receptor blocker and sulpiride, a dopamine D2 receptor blocker (40); phenytoin, an anticonvulsant (70); imipramine, a tricyclic antidepressant (71); nicotine, a nicotinic-adrenergic receptor agonist (72); and also induced P450 in the brain.

One of the P450s induced by both clozapine and toluene, P4502D4, has been studied in more detail. The 2D4 mRNA was detected in various brain regions and localized by in situ hybridization. A specific antipeptide antibody was raised and characterized. It was specific for P4502D4 and, in addition, could selectively immunoprecipitate in vitro-synthesized P450 2D4 (37). This antibody was used for quantitation on Western blots and immunohistochemical localization of P450 2D4 in the brains of untreated, toluene-, and clozapine-treated rats (40). We found that P4502D4 is a small fraction (less than 1%) of the P450 in both untreated and induced animals. Most of the P450 induced by toluene and clozapine is not 2D4. The immunohistochemical studies revealed that induction of P4502D4 occurred in a limited population of neurons in the substantia nigra, olfactory bulb, locus coeruleus and cerebellum. The changes in the protein were not accompanied by any change in the quantity or distribution of the mRNA in the brain.

The studies with P4502D4 have shown that specific forms of P450 that are expressed at low levels in the brain are highly localized in a limited number of neurons and that their levels can be rapidly increased without an increase in transcription. The study also raises many questions, e.g., Why does induction occur in specific cells? Is this a protective or defensive response of the brain? Is the induction involved in the toxic or therapeutic effects of the inducers? Are the cerebellum, olfactory lobes, and substantia nigra regions that respond to all xenobiotics? Does this make these regions more sensitive to neurotoxins and/or oxidative stress? Are all P450s induced in the same population of cells? Do the induced P450s affect physiological pathways?

CONCLUSIONS

Much work needs to be done on the characterization of novel P450s in the brain as well as on the regulation and localization of the known forms before the importance of P450 in the brain becomes clear. All evidence indicates that P450 in the brain is most likely playing some important roles in brain physiology and toxicology. We conclude this chapter with the hope that more investigators will be stimulated by the challenges rather than daunted by the difficulties of pursuing some of the issues raised in this summary.

ACKNOWLEDGMENTS

Our studies on Brain P450 are supported by grants from the Swedish Medical Research Council (13X-06807), the Swedish Work Health Fund, and Hoffman-La Roche, Basel, Switzerland.

REFERENCES

1. MacLusky NJ, Naftolin F. Sexual differentiation of the central nervous system. Science 1981; 211:1294–302.
2. McEwen BS, Sapolsky RM. Stress and cognitive function. Curr Opin Neurobiol 1995;5:205–216.
3. Majewska MD, Harrison NL, Schwartz RD, Barker JL, Paul SM. Steroid hormone metabolites are barbiturate-like modulators of the GABA receptor. Science 1986;232:1004–1007.
4. Magarinos AM, McEwen BS. Stress-induced atrophy of apical dendrites of hippocampal CA3c neurons: involvement of glucocorticoid secretion and excitatory amino acid receptors. Neuroscience 1995;69:89–98.
5. McEwen BS., Gould E., Orchinik M., Weil, NG, Woolley CS. Oestrogens and the structural and functional plasticity of neurons: implications for memory, ageing and neurodegenerative processes. Ciba Foundation Symp 1995;191:52–66.
6. Gonzalez, FJ. Human Cytochromes P450 problems and prospects. TIPS 1992;131:346–352.
7. Wolf CR. Cytochrome P450s: polymorphic gene families involved in carcinogen activation. TIG 1986;2:209–214.
8. Warner M, Wyss A, Yoshida S, Gustafsson J-Å. Cytochromes P450 in the brain. Methods Neurosci 1994;22:51–66.
9. Mok WM, Herschkowitz S, Krieger NR. In vivo studies identify 5α-pregnan–3α-ol–20-one as an active anesthetic agent. J Neurochem 1991;57:1296–1301.

10. Bitran D, Purdy RH, Kellogg CK. Anxiolytic effect of progesterone is associated with increases in cortical allopregnanolone and GABAA receptor function. Pharmacol Biochem Behav 1993;45:423–428.

11. Park-Chung M, Wu F-S, Farb DH. 3α-hydroxy–5β-pregnan–20-one sulfate: a negative modulator of the NMDA-induced current in cultured neurons. Mol Pharmacol 1994;46:146–150.

12. Corpechot C, Robel P, Axelson M, Sjövall J, Baulieu E-E. Characterization and measurement of dehydroepiandrosterone sulfate in the rat brain. Proc Natl Acad Sci USA 1981;78:4704–4707.

13. Le Gascogne C, Robel P, Gouezow M, Snanes N, Baulieu E-E, Waterman M. Neurosteroids: Cytochrome P450scc in the rat brain. Science 1987;237:1212–1214.

14. Strömstedt M, Waterman MR. Messenger RNAs encoding steroidogenic enzymes are expressed in rodent brain. Mol Brain Res 1995;34:75–88.

15. Mellon SH, Deschepper CF. Neurosteroid biosynthesis: genes for adrenal steroidogenic enzymes are expressed in the brain. Brain Res 1993;629:283–292.

16. Iwahashi K, Kawai Y, Suwaki H, Hosokawa K, Ichikawa Y. A localization study of the cytochrome P-450(21)-linked monooxygenase system in adult rat brain. J Steroid Biochem Mol Biol 1993;44:163–169.

17. Ozaki HS, Iwahashi K, Tsubaki M, Fukui Y, Ichikawa Y, Takeuchi Y. Cytochrome P-45011 beta in rat brain. J Neurosci Res 1991;28:518–24.

18. Warner M, Strömstedt M, Möller L, Gustafsson J-Å. Distribution and regulation of 5α-androstane–3β,17β-diol hydroxylase in the rat central nervous system. Endocrinology 1989;124:2699–2706.

19. Stapleton G, Steel M, Richardson M, Mason JO, Rose KA, Morris RGM, Lathe R. A Novel cytochrome P450 expressed primarily in brain J Biol Chem 1993;270:29739–29745.

20. Schilter B, Omiecinski CJ. Regional distribution and expression modulation of cytochrome P-450 and epoxide hydrolase mRNAs in the rat brain. Mol Pharmacol 1993;44:990–996.

21. Farin FM, Omiecinski CJ. Regiospecific expression of cytochrome P-450s and microsomal epoxide hydrolase in human brain tissue. J Toxicol Environ Health 1993;40:317–335.

22. Hodgson AV, White TB, White JW, Strobel HW. Expression analysis of the mixed function oxidase system in rat brain by the polymerase chain reaction. Mol Cell Biochem 1993;120:171–179.

23. Strömstedt M, Warner M, Gustafsson, J-Å. Cytochrome P450 of the 4A subfamily in the brain. J Neurochem 1994;63:671–67.

24. Amruthesh SC, FLack JR, Ellis EF. Brain synthesis and cerebrovascular action of epoxygenase metabolites of arachidonic acid. J Neurochem 992;58:503–510.

25. Junier M-P, Dray F, Blair I, Capdevilla J, Dishman E, Flack J.R, Ojeda SR. Epoxygenase products of arachidonic acid are endogenous constituents of the hypothalamus involved in D2 receptor-mediated dopamine-induced release of somatostatin. Endocrinology 1990;126:1534–1540.

26. Capdevilla J, Chacos N, Flack JR, Manna S, Negro-Vilar A, Ojeda SR. Novel hypothalamic arachidonate products stimulate somatostatin release from the median eminence. Endocrinology 1983;113:421–423.

27. Anandatheerthavarada, HK, ShankarSK, Ravindranath V. Rat brain cytochromes P450:catalytic, immunochemical properties and inducibility of multiple forms. Brain Res 1990;536:339–343.

28. Hansson T, Tindberg N, Ingelman-Sundberg M, Köhler C. Regional distribution of ethanol-inducible cytochrome P450 2E1 in the rat central nervous system. Neuroscience 1990;34:451–463.

29. Cammer W, Downing M, Clarke W Schenkman, J B. Immunocytochemical staining of the RLM6 form of cytochrome P450 in oligodendrocytes and myelin of rat brain. J Histochem Cytochem 1991;39:1089–1094.

30. Kapitulnik J, Gelboin HV, Guengerich FP, Jacobowitz, D.M. Immunohistochemical localization of cytochrome P450 in the rat brain. Neuroscience 1987;20:829–833.

31. Köhler C, Eriksson LG. Hansson T, Warner M, Gustafsson J-Å Immunohistochemical localization of cytochrome P450 in the rat brain. Neurosci Lett 1988;20:829–832.

32. Hagihara K, Shiosaka S, Lee Y, Kato J, Hatano O, Takakusu A, Emi Y, Omura T, Toyama M. Presence of sex difference of cytochrome P450 in the rat preoptic area and hypothalamus with reference to coexistence with oxytocin. Brain Res 1990;515:69–78.

33. Lin L-P, Lee Y, Tohyama M, Shiosaka S. A sex-specific cytochrome P450(F-1) colocalized with various neuropeptides in the paraventricular and supraoptic nuclei of female rats. Neuroendocrinology 1991;54:127–135.

34. Nebert DW, Adesnik M, Coon MJ, Estabrook RW, Gonzalez FJ, Guengerich FP, Gunsalus IC, Johnson EF, Kemper B, Levin W, et al. The P450 gene superfamily: recommended nomenclature. DNA 1987;6:1–11.

35. Nelson DR, Tetsuya K, Waxman DJ, Guengerich FP, Estabrook RW, Feyereisen R, Gonzalez FJ, Coon, MJ Gunsalus IC, Gotoh O, Okuda K, Nebert DW. The P450 superfamily: Update on new sequences, gene mapping, accession numbers, early trivial names of enzymes, and nomenclature. DNA Cell Biol 1993;12:1–51.

36. Zaphiropoulos PG, Wood T. Identification of the major cytochromes P450 of the 2C subfamily that are expressed in brain of female and in olfactory lobes of ethanol treated male rats. Biochem Biophys Res Commun 1993;193:1006–1013.

37. Wyss A, Gustafsson J-Å, Warner M. Cytochromes P450 of the 2D subfamily in rat brain. Mol Pharmacol 1995;47:1148–1155.

38. Kawashima H, Strobel HW. cDNA cloning of three new forms of rat brain cytochrome P450 belonging to the CYP4F subfamily. Biochem Biophys Res Commun 1995;217:1137–1144.

39. Hedlund E, Yoshida S, Gustafsson J-Å, Warner, M. Identification of cytochromes P450 2C22, 2E1 and 4A3 as toluene-induced P450s in the rat brain. Unpublished data

40. Hedlund E, Wyss A, Kainu T, Backlund M, Köhler C, Pelto-Huikko M, Gustafsson J-Å, Warner M. Cytochrome P450 2D4 in the brain: specific neuronal regulation by clozapine and toluene. Mol Pharmacol 1996;50:342–350.

41. Warner M, Gustafsson, J-Å. Induction of Cytochrome P450 in the rat brain by ethanol. PNAS 1994;91:1019–102.

42. Foidart A, Harada N, Balthazart J. Aromatase-immunoreactive cells are present in mouse brain areas that are known to express high levels of aromatase activity. Cell Tissue Res 1995;280:561–74.

43. Lauber ME., Lichtensteiger W. Pre- and postnatal ontogeny of aromatase cytochrome P450 messenger ribonucleic acid expression in the male rat brain studied by in situ hybridization. Endocrinology 1994;135:1661–1668.

44. Roselli CE, Horton LE, Resko JA. Distribution and regulation of aromatase activity in the rat hypothalamus and limbic system. Endocrinology 1985;117:2471–2477.

45. Harada N, Yamada K. Ontogeny of aromatase messenger ribonucleic acid in mouse brain: fluorometrical quantitation by polymerase chain reaction. Endocrinology 1992;131:2306–12.

46. Sanghera MK, Simpson ER, McPhaul MJ, Kozlowski G, Conley AJ, Lephart ED. Immunocytochemical distribution of aromatase cytochrome P450 in the rat brain using peptide-generated polyclonal antibodies. Endocrinology 1991;129:2834–2844.

47. Omura T, Sato R. The carbon monoxide-binding pigment of liver microsomes I. Evidence for its hemoprotein nature. J Biol Chem 1964;239:2370–2378.

48. Sundin M, Warner M, Haaparanta T, Gustafsson J-Å. Isolation and catalytic activity of cytochrome P450 from ventral prostate of control rats. J Biol Chem 1987;262:12293–12297.

49. Guiraud, Morfin R, Ducouret B, Samperez S, Jouan P. Pituitary metabolism of 5alpha-androstane-3beta-17beta-diol: intense and rapid conversion into 5alpha-androstane-3beta,6alpha,17beta-triol and 5alpha-androstane-3beta,7alpha, 17beta-triol. Steroids 1979;34:241–248.

50. Strömstedt M, Warner M, Banner C, Gustafsson J-Å. Role of brain P450 in regulation of the level of anaesthetic steroids in the brain. Mol Pharmacol 1993;44:1077–1083.

51. Birkle DL, Bazan NG. Effect of bicuculline-induced status epilepticus on prostaglandins and hydroxyeicosatetraenoic acids in rat brain subcellular fractions. J Neurochem 1987;48:1768–78.

52. Wolfe LS. Eicosanoids: prostaglandins, thromboxanes, leukotrienes, and other derivatives of carbon–20 unsaturated fatty acids. J Neurochem 1982;38:1–14.

53. Wu S, Moomaw CR, Tomer KB, Falck JR, Zeldin DC. Molecular cloning and expression of CYP2J2, a human cytochrome P450 arachidonic acid epoxygenase highly expressed in heart. J Biol Chem 1996;271:3460–3468.

54. Laethem RM, Koop DR. Identification of rabbit cytochromes P450 2C1 and 2C2 as arachidonic acid epoxygenases. Mol Pharmacol 1992;42:958–963.

55. Imaoka S, Wedlund PJ, Ogawa H, Kimura S, Gonzalez FJ, Kim HY. Identification of CYP2C23 expressed in rat kidney as an arachidonic acid epoxygenase. J Pharmacol Exp Therapeut 1993;267:1012–1016.

56. Warner M, Gustafsson J-A. Cytochrome P450 in the brain: neuroendocrine functions. Front Neuroendocrinol 1995;16:224–236.

57. Korneyev A, Pan BS, Polo A, Romer E, Guidotti A, Costa E. Stimulation of brain pregnenolone synthesis by mitochondrial diazepam binding inhibitor receptor ligands in vivo. J Neurochem 1993;61:1515–11524.

58. Hu ZY, Bourreau, Jung-Testas I, Robel P, Baulieu EE. Neurosteroids: oligodendrocyte mitochondria convert cholesterol to pregnenolone. Proc Natl Acad Sci USA 1987;84:8215–19.

59. Compagnone NA, Bulfone A, Rubenstein JL, Mellon SH. Expression of the steroidogenic enzyme P450scc in the central and peripheral nervous systems during rodent embryogenesis. Endocrinology 1995;136:2689–2696.

60. Purdy RH, Morrow AL, Moore PH, Paul SM. Stress-induced elevations of γ-aminobutyric acid type A receptor-active steroids in the rat brain. Proc Natl Acad Sci USA 1991;88:4553–4557.

61. Compagnone NA, Bulfone A, Rubenstein JL, Mellon SH. Steroidogenic enzyme P450c17 is expressed in the embryonic central nervous system. Endocrinology 1995:136:5212–23.

62. Jayyosi Z, Cooper KO, Thomas PE. Brain cytochrome P450 and testosterone metabolism by rat brain subcellular fractions: presence of cytochrome P450 3A immunoreactive protein in rat brain mitochondria. Arch Biochem Biophys 1992;298:265–70.

63. Walther B, Ghersi-Egea J-F, Jayyosi Z, Minn A, Seist G. Ethoxyresorufin O-deethylase activity in rat brain subcellular fractions. Neurosci Lett 1987;76:58–62.

64. Suchar LA, Chang RL, Thomas PE, Rosen RT, Lech J, Conney AH. Effects of phenobarbital, dexamethasone, and 3-methylcholanthrene administration on the metabolism of 17 beta-estradiol by liver microsomes from female rats. Endocrinology 1996;137:663–676.

65. Arlotto MP, Trant JM, Estabrook RW. Measurement of steroid hydroxylation reactions by high-performance liquid chromatography as indicator of P450 identity and function. Methods Enzymol 1991;206:454–462.

66. Funae Y, Imaoka S. Cytochrome P450 in rodents. Handbook Exp Pharmacol 1992;105:221–237.

67. Tyndale RF, Sunahara R, Inaba T, Kalow W, Gonzalez FJ, Niznik HB. Neuronal cytochrome P450IID1 (debrisoquine/sparteine-type): potent inhibition of activity by cocaine and nucleotide sequence identity to human hepatic P450 gene CYP2D6. Mol Pharmacol 1991;40:63–68.

68. Roberts B.J, Shoaf SE, Jeong K-S, Song BL. Induction of CYP 2E1 in liver, kidney, brain and intestine during chronic ethanol administration and withdrawal: evidence that CYP 2E1 possesses a rapid phase half-life of 6 hours or less. Biochem Biophys Res Commun 1994;205:1064–1070.

69. Roman LJ, Palmer CN, Clark JE, Muerhoff AS, Griffin KJ, Johnson EF, Masters BS. Expression of rabbit cytochromes P4504A which catalyze the omega-hydroxylation of arachidonic acid, fatty acids, and prostaglandins. Arch Biochem Biophys 1993;307;57–65.

70. Volk B, Amelizad Z, Anagnostopoulos J, Knoth R, Oesch F. First evidence of cytochrome P-450 induction in the mouse brain by phenytoin. Neurosci Lett 1988;84;219–24.

71. Sequeira DJ, Strobel HW. High-performance liquid chromatographic method for the analysis of imipramine metabolism in vitro by liver and brain microsomes. J Chromatogr B: Biomed Appli 1995;673;251–258.

72. Anandatheerthavarada HK, Williams JF, Wecker L. Differential effect of chronic nicotine administration on brain cytochrome P4501A1/2 and P4502E1 Biochem Biophys Res Comm 1993;194:312–318.

4

Steroidogenic Factor 1 Plays Key Roles in Adrenal and Gonadal Development and in Endocrine Function

Kathleen M. Caron, PhD,

Yayoi Ikeda, PhD, Xunrong Luo, MD, PhD,

and Keith L. Parker, MD, PhD

CONTENTS

INTRODUCTION
STEROIDOGENIC FACTOR 1: A KEY REGULATOR
   OF STEROID HYDROXYLASE EXPRESSION
PROFILES OF SF-1 EXPRESSION
THE ROLES OF SF-1 IN VIVO: KNOCKOUT MOUSE STUDIES
PERSPECTIVES AND FUTURE DIRECTIONS
REFERENCES

INTRODUCTION

The orphan nuclear receptor steroidogenic factor 1 (SF-1) has emerged as a critical regulator of steroidogenic cell function within the adrenal cortex and gonads. SF-1 also contributes to endocrine development and function at all three levels of the hypothalamic-pituitary-gonadal axis. First identified as a regulator of the tissue-specific expression of the cytochrome P450 steroid hydroxylases, SF-1 subsequently was shown to play considerably broader roles in endocrine function. Knockout mice deficient in SF-1 lacked adrenal glands and gonads and exhibited male-to-female sex reversal of their internal and external genitalia; moreover, they had impaired gonadotrope function and agenesis of the ventromedial hypothalamic nucleus (VMH). These studies delineated multiple essential roles of SF-1 in regulating endocrine differentiation and function. However, the molecular basis underlying these profound consequences of the SF-1 knockout remains to be determined. Moreover, with respect to the biosynthesis of steroids in sites other than the adrenal cortex and gonads, including the neurosteroids, an important goal for further studies is to identify the mechanisms that regulate expression of the steroidogenic enzymes in the absence of SF-1.

From: *Contemporary Endocrinology: Neurosteroids: A New Regulatory Function
in the Nervous System* Edited by: E.-E. Baulieu, P. Robel, and M. Schumacher
© Humana Press Inc., Totowa, NJ

STEROIDOGENIC FACTOR 1 (SF-1): A KEY REGULATOR
OF STEROID HYDROXYLASE EXPRESSION

The biosynthesis of steroid hormones by the adrenal cortex and gonads requires the sequential action of the steroid hydroxylases, many of which are members of the cytochrome P450 family of mixed-function oxidases (reviewed in *1*). As discussed in Chapters 3 and 5, many of these same enzymes are implicated in neurosteroid production. A number of laboratories have sought to define the mechanisms that regulate the expression of the steroid hydroxylases within the classical steroidogenic tissues (reviewed in 2). These studies led to the identification of regulatory elements, sharing similar AGGTCA motifs, that regulated promoter activity of several steroid hydroxylases *(3,4)*. These elements all interacted with a protein that was apparently restricted to steroidogenic cells of the adrenal cortex and gonads, raising the possibility that a shared transcriptional activator regulated the coordinate, cell-specific expression of these related genes. Based on this model, two groups independently isolated cDNAs encoding the protein that interacted with these elements *(5,6)*, which was designated either steroidogenic factor 1 (SF-1) or adrenal 4-binding protein (Ad4BP).

Analysis of the sequence of the SF-1 cDNA revealed that SF-1 belongs to the nuclear hormone receptor superfamily—structurally related transcriptional regulators that mediate the actions of small, hydrophobic ligands such as steroid hormones, thyroid hormone, vitamin D, and retinoids *(7,8)*. This superfamily also includes members for which no ligand is yet known, the orphan nuclear receptors *(9)*. Furthermore, the SF-1 cDNA resembled most closely a cDNA isolated from embryonal carcinoma cells, designated embryonal long-terminal, repeat-binding protein, or ELP *(10)*. The basis for this similarity became apparent when the mouse gene encoding SF-1 was isolated and characterized; both SF-1 and ELP transcripts arise from the same structural gene by alternative promoter usage and 3'-splicing *(11)*. The mouse gene encoding SF-1 and ELP also closely resembles the *Drosophila FTZ-F1* gene that encodes two developmentally regulated nuclear receptors *(12,13)*. Subsequent mapping studies localized the mouse gene to the proximal region of chromosome 2 *(14,15)* and the human homolog to the long arm of chromosome 9 (9q33, ref. *14*).

Profiles of SF-1 Expression

As suggested by the initial gel mobility shift experiments, Northern-blotting analyses showed that SF-1 was selectively expressed in steroidogenic cells of the adrenal cortex and gonads *(5)*. Using more sensitive reverse transcription-polymerase chain reaction (RT-PCR) assays, SF-1 transcripts also were detected in the pituitary, placenta, brain, and spleen *(16)*. To identify the specific cell types expressing SF-1, several laboratories used *in situ* hybridization and immunohistochemical analyses to localize SF-1 expression (reviewed in *17,18*). In these studies, SF-1 expression generally correlated with known sites of primary steroidogenesis, including adrenocortical cells, testicular Leydig cells, and ovarian theca and granulosa cells. These findings again were consistent with an important role of SF-1 in tissue-specific expression of the steroid hydroxylases. Surprisingly, SF-1 was not expressed at appreciable levels in the placenta, despite its known role in steroid hormone production. Finally, as predicted by the RT-PCR studies, SF-1 was also expressed in other cells, including pituitary gonadotropes and neurons comprising

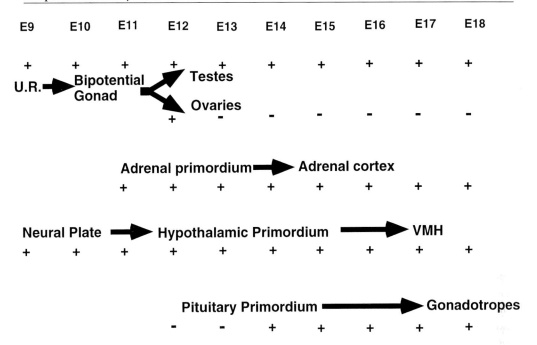

Fig. 1. Ontogeny of SF-1 expression. The ontogeny of expression of SF-1 in developing mouse embryos is summarized schematically. (+), SF-1 transcripts were detected; (–), SF-1 transcripts were not detected. The arrows denote the approximate transition times between the different developmental stages. UR, urogenital ridge. Reprinted with permission from ref. *17*.

the VMH. These findings suggested that SF-1 might also play additional roles beyond regulating the steroid hydroxylases.

To delineate potential roles of SF-1 in mammalian development, similar approaches were used to examine the spatial and temporal profile of SF-1 expression during embryogenesis *(19–22)*. These studies defined intriguing profiles of SF-1 expression (Fig. 1). SF-1 transcripts were detected in the adrenal primordium and gonads from the inception of their development. The initiation of SF-1 expression in these sites before the onset of steroid hydroxylase expression is consistent with the model that SF-1 activates steroid hydroxylase gene expression.

The earliest detectable sign of gonadogenesis begins in mice at ~E9, when the intermediate mesoderm condenses into a urogenital ridge that ultimately contributes to the gonads, adrenal glands, and kidneys. Up until ~E12.5, testes and ovaries cannot be distinguished histologically, and are referred to as indifferent or bipotential gonads. Thereafter, formation of the testicular cords, which contain fetal Sertoli cells that produce Müllerian-inhibiting substance (MIS) and primordial germ cells, allows the testis to be recognized. Interspersed around these cords is the interstitial region, which contains the steroidogenic Leydig cells where androgens are produced. SF-1 initially was expressed in the indifferent gonads of all embryos, and this expression persisted throughout the indifferent stage. Coincident with sexual differentiation and the formation of the testicular cords at E12.5, SF-1 expression increased in the testes but was extinguished in ovaries. Unexpectedly, although SF-1 in the adult testis is expressed primarily by the steroidogenic Leydig cells, SF-1 transcripts were detected in both compartments of the fetal testes: the interstitial region and the testicular cords.

Consistent with the RT-PCR analyses of adult tissues *(16)*, SF-1 transcripts also were detected in the embryonic diencephalon, which ultimately contributes to the endocrine hypothalamus, and the anterior pituitary gland. These findings suggested that SF-1 acts at multiple levels of the hypothalamic-pituitary-steroidogenic organ axis, playing roles that extend beyond regulating the expression of steroidogenic enzymes.

THE ROLES OF SF-1 IN VIVO: KNOCKOUT MOUSE STUDIES

To define the roles of SF-1 in vivo, targeted gene disruption in embryonic stem cells was used to generate SF-1 knockout mice. Three groups independently produced SF-1 knockout mice, with generally congruent results. SF-1 knockout mice had female external genitalia irrespective of genetic sex, and died shortly after birth from adrenocortical insufficiency *(23,24)*, supporting an essential role for SF-1 in androgen and corticosteroid biosynthesis. Surprisingly (Fig. 2), their adrenal glands and gonads were completely absent, revealing obligatory roles for SF-1 in the development of the primary steroidogenic tissues. Developmental studies showed that the earliest stages of adrenal and gonadal development still occurred in the absence of SF-1; subsequently, these structures manifested features characteristic of programmed cell death, and degenerated.

The expression of SF-1 in the anterior pituitary and hypothalamus suggested that the SF-1 knockout mice might also exhibit abnormalities at these sites. Consistent with this model, pituitaries of SF-1 knockout mice were deficient in immunoreactivity for luteinizing hormone (LH) and follicle-stimulating hormone (FSH) *(25,26)*, two separate markers of gonadotropes. Promoter analyses showed that SF-1 interacts with regulatory elements upstream of the genes encoding the α-subunit of glycoprotein hormones *(25,27)*, the β-subunit of luteinizing hormone *(28,29)*, and the GnRH receptor *(30)*, thereby activating their expression. These findings linked SF-1 to gonadotrope function, and thus to a second level of the endocrine axis. Finally, the region corresponding to the VMH was absent from the hypothalamus of the knockout mice (Fig. 3) *(26,31)*, also implicating SF-1 at the hypothalamic level. Similar to the adrenal gland and gonads, developmental studies suggested that early stages of VMH development were initiated in the absence of SF-1, with subsequent degeneration. This link between SF-1 and the VMH is intriguing because this hypothalamic nucleus has been linked to reproductive behavior in experimental model systems *(32)*, again supporting an intimate relationship between SF-1 and reproduction.

PERSPECTIVES AND FUTURE DIRECTIONS

The studies reviewed here have defined essential roles of SF-1 at multiple levels of endocrine differentiation and function, particularly with respect to the reproductive axis. A large number of target genes of SF-1 have already been defined, many of which play key roles in endocrine function (Table 1). There remain, however, gaps in our understanding of the roles of SF-1 in endocrine development and function. Important areas for future studies include: the mechanisms that regulate the expression of SF-1, the potential roles of ligands in mediating SF-1 transcriptional activation, and the identification of additional genes that interact with SF-1 to specify endocrine development. (*See* ref. *17*

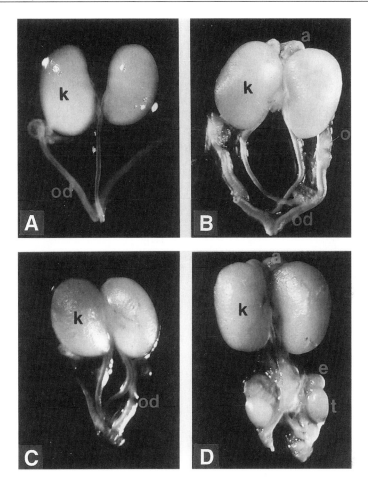

Fig. 2. Adrenal and gonadal agenesis in SF-1 knockout mice. SF-1 knockout mice and wild-type littermates were killed and the genitourinary tracts were dissected. (**A**) SF-1 knockout female; (**B**) Wild-type female; (**C**) SF-1 knockout male; (**D**). Wild-type male. k, kidney; a, adrenal; o, ovary; od, oviduct; e, epididymis; t, testis. Reprinted with permission from ref. *23.*

and *18* for discussions of approaches currently being taken to extend our understanding of SF-1's roles in endocrine development and function.)

With respect to neurosteroids, we understand very little about the processes that regulate their biosynthesis. Unlike adrenocortical and gonadal steroids, whose production is controlled predominantly by pituitary trophic hormones, the factors that modulate neurosteroid production have yet to be defined. Similarly, the factors that determine tissue-selective expression of steroidogenic enzymes within the brain are poorly understood. SF-1 expression in the brain is restricted to neurons of the VMH, whereas steroidogenic enzymes are distributed more widely and are produced by glial cells. Thus, although SF-1 may contribute to neurosteroid biosynthesis—especially to the extent that biologically active neurosteroids are derived from adrenocortical and gonadal precursors—it is unlikely that SF-1 regulates steroidogenic enzyme expression in presumptive sites of *de novo* neurosteroid biosynthesis. This, then, raises the question of what mechanisms regulate steroid hydroxylase expression at nonadrenal and gonadal sites. Conceiv-

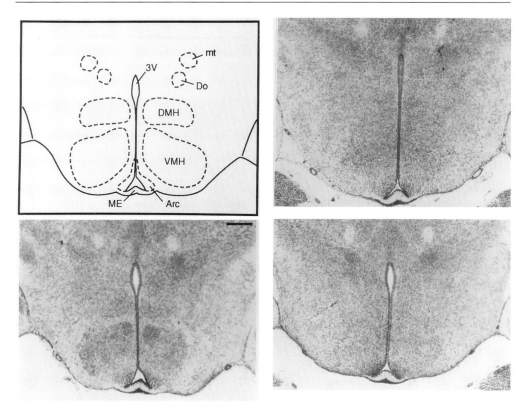

Fig. 3. SF-1 knockout mice have agenesis of the VMH. A drawing of the relevant neuroanatomy of the mouse hypothalamus is shown (upper left). Serial coronal sections from wild-type (lower left) and SF-1 knockout male (lower right) and female (upper right) mice were stained with cresyl violet and analyzed histologically. ME, median eminence; Arc, arcuate nucleus; VMH, ventrome-dial hypothalamic nucleus; DMH, dorsomedial hypothalamic nucleus; Do, dorsal hypothalamic nucleus; mt, mammilothalamic tract; 3V, Third ventricle. Modified with permission from ref.*31.*

ably, different promoters direct their expression at various sites (e.g., the adrenal cortex and gonads vs sites such as the brain and placenta), with only the promoter expressed in the adrenal cortex and gonads utilizing SF-1-responsive elements. This mechanism apparently underlies aromatase expression in different tissues *(33)*. Alternatively, the same promoter may be active in multiple sites, with distinct promoter elements directing transcription in each tissue. In this case, SF-1-responsive elements would regulate expression in the adrenal cortex and gonads, whereas other elements—interacting with yet-to-be-identified transcriptional regulatory proteins—would regulate transcription in sites such as the placenta and brain. Ongoing efforts to explore these questions should provide novel insights into the complex regulation of steroid hormone production, both in classical steroidogenic tissues such as the adrenal cortex and gonads and in the "non-classical" sites such as the brain. One intriguing possibility is that a better definition of the promoter elements that direct steroid hydroxylase expression, coupled with tech-niques for targeted gene modification, may provide a means to abolish *de novo* produc-tion of neurosteroids by blocking selectively steroidogenic enzyme expression in the brain. This would provide a powerful model system to elucidate the roles of neurosteroids in various physiological processes.

Table 1
Sites of Action and Target Genes for SF-1

VMH:	?
Gonadotropes:	α-subunit of glycoprotein hormones β-subunit of luteinizing hormone GnRH receptor
Adrenal cortex:	Cytochrome P450 steroid hydroxylases 3β-hydroxysteroid dehydrogenase Steroidogenic Acute Regulatory Protein ACTH receptor
Gonads: Leydig cells	Cytochrome P450 steroid hydroxylases Steroidogenic acute regulatory protein
Sertoli cells	Müllerian-inhibiting substance
Theca and granulosa cells	Cytochrome P450 steroid hydroxylases Steroidogenic acute regulatory protein, oxytocin

ACKNOWLEDGMENTS

This work was supported by the Howard Hughes Medical Institute and by grant HL48460 from the National Institutes of Health. We thank Dr. Bernard Schimmer for helpful comments about the manuscript.

REFERENCES

1. Miller WL. Molecular biology of steroid hormone biosynthesis. Endocrine Rev 1988;9:295–318.
2. Parker KL, Schimmer BP. Transcriptional regulation of the genes encoding the cytochrome P450 steroid hydroxylases. Vitam Horm 1995;51:339–370.
3. Rice DA, Mouw AR, Bogerd A, Parker KL. A shared promoter element regulates the expression of three steroidogenic enzymes. Mol Endocrinol 1991;5:1552–1561.
4. Morohashi K, Honda S, Inomata Y, Handa H, Omura T. A common trans-acting factor, Ad4-binding protein, to the promoters of steroidogenic P-450s. J Biol Chem 1992;267:17913–17919.
5. Lala DS, Rice DA, Parker KL. Steroidogenic factor I, a key regulator of steroidogenic enzyme expression, is the mouse homolog of fushi tarazu-factor I. Mol Endocrinol 1992;6:1249–1258.
6. Honda S-I, Morohashi K-I, Nomura M, Takeya H, Kitajima M, Omura T. Ad4BP regulating steroidogenic P-450 gene is a member of steroid hormone receptor superfamily. J Biol Chem 1993;268:7494–7502.
7. Evans RM. The steroid and thyroid hormone receptor superfamily. Science 1988;240:889–895.
8. Mangelsdorf DJ, Thummel C, Beato M, Herrlich P, Schutz G, Umesono K, Blumberg B, Kastner P, Mark M, Chambon P, Evans RM. The nuclear receptor superfamily: the second decade. Cell 1995;83:835–839.
9. Enmark E, Gustafsson J-A. Orphan nuclear receptors—the first eight years. Mol Endocrinol 1996;10:1293–1307.
10. Tsukiyama T, Ueda H, Hirose S, Niwa O. Embryonal long terminal repeat-binding protein is a murine homolog of FTZ-F1, a member of the steroid receptor superfamily. Mol Cell Biol 1992;12:1286–1291.
11. Ikeda Y, Lala DS, Luo X, Kim E, Moisan M-P, Parker KL. Characterization of the mouse FTZ-F1 gene, which encodes a key regulator of steroid hydroxylase gene expression. Mol Endocrinol 1993;7:852–860.
12. Ueda H, Sonoda S, Brown JL, Scott MP, Wu C. A sequence specific DNA-binding protein that activates fushi tarazu segmentation gene expression. Genes Dev 1990;4:624–635.

13. Lavorgna G, Ueda H, Clos J, Wu C. FTZ-F1, a steroid hormone receptor-like protein implicated in the activation of fushi tarazu. Science 1991;252:848–851.

14. Taketo M, Parker KL, Howard TA, Tsukiyama T, Wong M, Niwa O, Morton CC, Miron PM, Seldin MF. Homologs of Drosophila fushi tarazu factor 1 map to mouse chromosome 2 and human chromosome 9q33. Genomics 1995;25:565–567.

15. Swift S, Ashworth A. The mouse Ftzf1 gene required for gonadal and adrenal development maps to mouse chromosome 2. Genomics 1995;28:609–610.

16. Morohashi K, Lida H, Nomura M, Hatano O, Honda S, Tsukiyama T, Niwa O, Hara T, Takakusu A, Shibata Y, Omura T. Functional difference between Ad4BP and ELP, and their distributions in steroidogenic tissues. Mol Endocrinol 1994;8:643–653.

17. Parker KL, Schimmer BP. Steroidogenic factor 1: a key determinant of endocrine development and function. Endocrine Rev 1997;18:361–377.

18. Morohashi KI, Omura T. Ad4BP/SF–1, a transcription factor essential for the transcription of steroidogenic cytochrome P450 genes and for the establishment of the reproductive function. FASEB J 1996;10:1569–1577.

19. Ikeda Y, Shen W-H, Ingraham HA, Parker KL. Developmental expression of mouse steroidogenic factor 1, an essential regulator of the steroid hydroxylases. Mol Endocrinol 1994;8:654–662.

20. Hatano O, Takakusu A, Nomura M, Morohashi K-I. Identical origin of adrenal cortex and gonad revealed by expression profiles of Ad4BP/SF-1. Genes Cells 1996;1:663–671.

21. Shen W-H, Moore CCD, Ikeda Y, Parker KL, Ingraham HA. Nuclear receptor steroidogenic factor 1 regulates MIS gene expression: a link to the sex determination cascade. Cell 1994;77:651–661.

22. Hatano O, Takayama K, Imai T, Waterman MR, Takakusu A, Omura T, Morohashi K. Sex-dependent expression of a transcription factor, Ad4BP, regulating steroidogenic P-450 genes in the gonads during prenatal and postnatal rat development. Development 1994;120:2787–2797.

23. Luo X, Ikeda Y, Parker KL. A cell-specific nuclear receptor is essential for adrenal and gonadal development and sexual differentiation. Cell 1994;77:481–490.

24. Sadovsky Y, Crawford PA, Woodson KG, Polish JA, Clements MA, Tourtellotte LM, Simburger K, Milbrandt J. Mice deficient in the orphan receptor steroidogenic factor 1 lack adrenal glands and gonads but express P450 side-chain-cleavage enzyme in the placenta and have normal embryonic serum levels of corticosteroids. Proc Natl Acad Sci USA 1995;92:10939–10943.

25. Ingraham HA, Lala DS, Ikeda Y, Luo X, Shen W-H, Nachtigal MW, Abbud R, Nilson JH, Parker KL. The nuclear receptor steroidogenic factor 1 acts at multiple levels of the reproductive axis. Genes Dev 1994;8:2302–2312.

26. Shinoda K, Lei H, Yoshii H, Nomura M, Nagano M, Shiba H, Sasaki H, Osawa Y, Ninomiya Y, Niwa O, Morohashi K-I. Developmental defects of the ventromedial hypothalamic nucleus and pituitary gonadotroph in the Ftz-F1-disrupted mice. Devel Dynamics 1995;204:22–29.

27. Barnhart KM, Mellon PM. The orphan nuclear receptor, steroidogenic factor 1, regulates the glycoprotein hormone α-subunit gene in pituitary gonadotropes. Mol Endocrinol 1994;9:878–885.

28. Halvorson LM, Kaiser UB, Chin WW. Stimulation of luteinizing hormone beta gene promoter activity by the orphan nuclear receptor, steroidogenic factor-1. J Biol Chem 1996;271:6645–6650.

29. Keri RA, Nilson JH. A steroidogenic factor-1 binding site is required for activity of the luteinizing hormone beta subunit promoter in gonadotropes of transgenic mice. J Biol Chem 1996;271:10782–10785.

30. Duval DL, Nelson SE, Clay CM. A binding site for steroidogenic factor-1 is part of a complex enhancer that mediates expression of the murine gonadotropin-releasing hormone receptor gene. Biol Reprod 1997;56:160–168.

31. Ikeda Y, Luo X, Abbud R, Nilson JH, Parker KL. The nuclear receptor steroidogenic factor 1 is essential for the formation of the ventromedial hypothalamic nucleus. Mol Endocrinol 1995;9:478–486.

32. Pfaff DW, Schwartz-Giblin S, McCarthy MM, Kow L-M. Cellular and molecular mechanisms of female reproductive behaviors. In: Knobil E, Neill JD, eds. The Physiology of Reproduction, 2nd ed. Raven, New York, 1994, pp 107–120.

33. Hinshelwood MM, Liu Z, Conley AJ, Simpson ER. Demonstration of tissue-specific promoters in nonprimate species that express aromatase P450 in placentae. Biol Reprod 1995;53:1151–1159.

5

Peripheral-Type Benzodiazepine Receptor

Role in the Regulation of Steroid and Neurosteroid Biosynthesis

Caterina Cascio, MD, Patrizia Guarneri, PhD, Hua Li, MSc, Rachel C. Brown, BSc, Hakima Amri, PhD, Noureddine Boujrad, PhD, Maria Kotoula, PhD, Branislav Vidic, SD, Katy Drieu, DPHARM, and Vassilios Papadopoulos, PhD

CONTENTS

INTRODUCTION
PERIPHERAL-TYPE BENZODIAZEPINE RECEPTORS (PBRs)
STEROID BIOSYNTHESIS
PBR IN STEROID BIOSYNTHESIS
NEUROSTEROID BIOSYNTHESIS
ENDOGENOUS LIGANDS OF PBR
CONCLUSION
REFERENCES

INTRODUCTION

Eukaryotic steroid hormones, derived from cholesterol, are involved in the maintenance of the organism's homeostasis, adaptability to the environment, and developmental and reproductive functions. In addition to the well-defined actions in peripheral tissues, steroids have pleiotropic actions on the central nervous system (CNS), where they control a number of neuroendocrine and behavioral functions. Thus, comprehension of the molecular systems underlying the control of steroid hormone biosynthesis is essential for the study and treatment of a multitude of physiological disorders.

From: *Contemporary Endocrinology: Neurosteroids: A New Regulatory Function in the Nervous System* Edited by: E.-E. Baulieu, P. Robel, and M. Schumacher
© Humana Press Inc., Totowa, NJ

PERIPHERAL-TYPE BENZODIAZEPINE RECEPTORS (PBRs)

Pharmacological and Biochemical Characteristics

Benzodiazepines are widely used for their anxiolytic, anticonvulsant, and hypnotic actions. It has been well established that the major pharmacological effects of benzodiazepines are mediated by the γ-aminobutyric acid $(GABA)_A$ receptors in the CNS *(1,2)*. However, in search of specific binding sites for benzodiazepines outside the CNS another class of binding sites was first observed in the kidney *(3)* and later determined to be present in apparently all tissues including the CNS *(4–7)*. This class of binding sites is commonly referred to as the peripheral-type benzodiazepine recognition sites or receptors (PBRs) owing to its initial discovery in peripheral tissues.

PBRs were distinguished from $GABA_A$/benzodiazepine receptors by several criteria. Although both receptors bind diazepam with relatively high affinity, they exhibited very different binding specificities. In rodent species, PBRs bind 4'-chlorodiazepam with high affinity, whereas $GABA_A$ receptors show low affinity for this benzodiazepine *(6,7)*. Conversely, clonazepam and flumazenil, which bind with high affinity to $GABA_A$ receptors, exhibit very low affinities for PBR. PBR also bind with high affinity the imidazopyridine alpidem and has a low affinity for the imidazopyridine zolpidem *(8)*. On the contrary, $GABA_A$ receptors bind with high-affinity zolpidem and have low affinity for alpidem. In addition, PBRs have high affinity for three classes of compounds, isoquinoline *(9)*, indoleacetamide *(10)*, and pyrrolobenzoxazepine *(11)* derivatives, which do not bind to the $GABA_A$ receptors *(10,11)*. Isoquinolines were the major tool used for the identification and characterization of PBR *(5–7)*. In addition to these differences in drug specificity, it has been well-established that $GABA_A$/benzodiazepine receptors, composed of 50–55 kDa protein subunits, are coupled to synaptosomal chloride channels whereas PBR, an 18 kDa protein associated with other mitochondrial proteins, are not coupled to GABA recognition sites and their function will be addressed in this review. Subcellular fractionation studies demonstrated that PBRs were primarily localized on mitochondria *(12–14)*, and more specifically on the outer mitochondrial membrane *(15)*, although it is likely that they are not exclusive to this organelle. A plasma membrane location for this receptor was recently identified *(16–18)*.

The first identification of a molecular component associated with PBRs was made possible by the development of a photoaffinity probe, the isoquinoline propanamide PK 14105 *(19)*. This probe specifically labeled an 18 kDa protein, which was subsequently purified *(20,21)*, and the corresponding cDNA cloned from rat *(22)*, human *(23,24)*, bovine *(25)*, and murine *(26)* species. The cDNA sequence of the 18 kDa protein specifies an open reading frame of 169 aminoacids rich in tryptophan residues, with high-sequence homology (>80%) across species. Expression studies with the cDNA probes demonstrated that the 18 kDa protein contains the binding domains for PBR ligands although, owing to the constitutive expression of PBRs in all cells used for transfections, the presence of other (PBR-associated) proteins important for PBR ligand-binding expression cannot be excluded. In support of this hypothesis, we should consider that although high-affinity isoquinoline binding is diagnostic for PBRs, the affinity of benzodiazepines for PBRs is species-specific, varying from high affinity (rodents) to low affinity (bovine) *(6,7)*. These species differences in benzodiazepine binding may be also owing to either structural differences in the 18 kDa protein or to differences in the components comprising the PBR complex in the mitochondrial membranes.

No other mammalian protein sharing homology with the 18 kDa protein was identified. However, a 32% amino-acid identity (66% when accounting for conserved substitutions) was found with the tryptophan-rich-sensory-protein *tspO* (also called *crtK*), involved in carotenoid biosynthesis in *Rhodobacter capsulatus* and *Rhodobacter sphaeroides* photosynthetic bacteria *(27,28)*. The gene encoding the 18 kDa PBR protein has been isolated and characterized for rat *(29)* and human *(24)*. In both species, the gene contains four exons spanning 10–13 kb and the locations of the introns are identical.

One of the interesting features of the 18 kDa PBR protein is the observation that, although this protein is targeted to the mitochondria, it does not contain a typical mitochondria-targeting signal sequence. The amino-terminal sequence of the 18 kDa PBR protein is hydrophobic and resembles a signal peptide, but it is not cleaved when the protein is incorporated in the mitochondrial membrane. In contrast, the carboxy-terminal sequence is hydrophilic, suggesting that it is exposed to the cytoplasmic environment.

We isolated and characterized the 18 kDa PBR cDNA from MA-10 Leydig cells *(26)*. Expression of this cDNA in mammalian cells resulted in an increase in the density of both benzodiazepine and isoquinoline binding sites. In order to examine whether the increased drug binding is owing to the 18 kDa PBR protein alone or to other constitutively expressed components of the receptor, an in vitro system was developed using recombinant PBR protein *(26)*. Isolated maltose-binding protein (MBP)-PBR recombinant fusion protein incorporated into liposomes—formed using lipids found in steroidogenic outer mitochondrial membranes, but not MBP alone—maintained its ability to bind isoquinolines, but not benzodiazepines. Addition of mitochondrial extracts in the liposomes resulted in the restoration of benzodiazepine binding. The protein responsible for this effect was then purified and identified as the 34 kDa voltage-dependent anion channel (VDAC) protein, which by itself does not express any drug binding. Interestingly, a number of laboratories have identified a 30–35 kDa protein, nonspecifically labeled using irreversible isoquinolines and benzodiazepines, to be associated with PBR *(4–7)*. Among the ligands used to identify this 30–35 kDa protein was flunitrazepam *(4–7)*. Based on the observation that the 35 kDa protein photolabeled with flunitrazepam could also bind radiolabeled dicyclohexylcarbodiimide, a reagent that covalently binds to VDAC, and that specific reagents which inhibit VDAC function were able to abolish PBR ligand binding, the hypothesis that VDAC was part of PBR was advanced *(4)*. Moreover, we observed that, among the PBR ligands tested, only flunitrazepam could specifically antagonize the hormone-stimulated cholesterol transport and steroidogenesis, acting via PBR *(30)*. Furthermore, the observation that the 18 kDa PBR was isolated as a complex with the 34 kDa VDAC and the inner mitochondrial membrane adenine nucleotide carrier (ADC) *(31)* suggested that PBR is not a single protein receptor but a multimeric complex.

These studies demonstrated that VDAC is associated functionally to the 18 kDa PBR and is part of the benzodiazepine binding site in the PBR. Benzodiazepine binding, however, will be expressed only in the presence of the 18 kDa PBR protein that confers the other part of the recognition site. This model is also in agreement with the finding that the species difference in benzodiazepine binding may be owing to a five nonconserved amino acids in the C-terminal end of the 18 kDa PBR protein *(32)*. Although the 18 kDa PBR and VDAC are required for drug binding, we cannot exclude the possibility that in vivo other proteins may be transiently or permanently associated with the PBR complex and modulate drug binding in an "allosteric" manner.

VDAC is a large-conductance large-diameter, about 3nm, ion channel with thin walls formed by a β-sheet structure and located in the outer mitochondrial membrane, especially in the junctions between outer and inner membranes (contact sites) where it may complex with the adenine nucleotide carrier, hexokinase, and creatine kinase *(33)*. VDAC forms a slightly anion-selective channel with complex voltage dependence and has been referred to as "mitochondrial porin" by analogy to bacterial porins. VDAC is believed to allow transport of metabolites and small molecules between the cytoplasm and the inner mitochondrial membrane *(33,34)*.

Considering the interaction of 18 kDa PBR with VDAC at the contact site level, we will have to consider a potential role of other proteins shown to participate in contact site formation. The inner mitochondrial membrane ADC was previously shown to be structurally associated with PBR components *(31)*. The inner mitochondrial megachannel (IMC) is also located in the inner membrane of the contact sites and represents activities regulated by voltage and ion (i.e., calcium) changes that result in pore opening and permeability increases *(35,36)*. IMC is inhibited by PBR ligands *(37)* and is sensitive to the immunosuppressant cyclosporin A *(35)*. Interestingly, we observed that cyclosporin A is a noncompetitive inhibitor of PBR, suggesting that IMC may regulate PBR in an "allosteric" manner (Papadopoulos, unpublished data). Taken together, these observations we propose a model of the PBR complex, present at the contact sites of mitochondrial membranes, composed of the 18 kDa PBR protein, VDAC, and two inner membrane proteins, ADC and IMC.

PBR Topography in Mitochondrial Membranes

Native MA-10 Leydig tumor cell mitochondrial preparations were examined by transmission electron and atomic force microscopic (AFM) procedures in order to investigate the topography and organization of PBR. Mitochondria were immunolabeled with an anti-PBR antiserum coupled to gold-labeled secondary antibodies. Results obtained indicated that the 18 kDa PBR protein is organized in clusters of 4–6 molecules *(38)*. Moreover, in many occasions, the interrelationship among the PBR molecules was found to favor the formation of a single pore. Because the 18 kDa PBR protein is associated functionally with the pore-forming 34 kDa VDAC, which is preferentially located in the contact sites of the two mitochondrial membranes, these results suggest that the mitochondrial PBR complex may function as a pore. We then examined whether the hormone-induced biochemical changes—increased PBR binding—correlated with appropriate morphological changes. Fifteen-s treatment with hCG induced the appearance of large clusters of gold labeled PBR varying from 15–25 gold particles or more, in contrast to the 4–6 particle clusters present in mitochondria from control cells. AFM analysis of these areas further demonstrated the reorganization of the membrane at these mitochondrial membrane sites *(39)*. The specificity of the effect of hCG was determined by treating cells with hCG and the selective inhibitor of cAMP-dependent protein kinase H-89, shown to block the hormone-induced PBR binding and steroid formation. H-89 also blocked the effect of hCG on PBR topography. In addition, flunitrazepam also blocked the effect of hCG on PBR distribution on mitochondrial membranes *(39)*. Thus, it seems that hormones induce the rapid reorganization of mitochondrial membranes, favoring the formation of contact sites that may facilitate cholesterol transfer from the outer to the inner mitochondrial membrane. An increase in the formation of contact sites between the mitochondrial membranes has been previously reported *(40)*. Thus, free cholesterol from the outer mitochondrial membrane would transfer freely via the contact sites to the inner membrane where the P-450scc is located. It should be also noted that intra-mitochondrial translocation of phospholipids occurs in a similar manner through mito-chondrial contact sites *(41)*.

Molecular Modeling of PBR

Based on the known amino-acid sequence of the human and mouse 18 kDa PBR protein, a three-dimensional model of this receptor protein was recently developed using molecular dynamics simulations *(42,43)*. According to this model, the five transmem-brane domains of PBR were modeled as five α helices that span one phospholipid bilayer of the outer mitochondrial membrane. This receptor model was then tested as a carrier for a number of molecules and it was shown that it can accommodate a cholesterol molecule and function as a channel. Thus, it was suggested that the receptor's function is to carry cholesterol molecules from the outer lipid monolayer to the inner lipid monolayer of the outer membrane, thus acting as "shield," hiding the cholesterol from the hydrophobic membrane inner medium. Considering the PBR complex formation at the level of the contact sites, this cholesterol movement could end in the inner mitochondrial membrane. Thus, this theoretical model further supports our experimental data, presented in the section "PBR in Steroid Biosynthesis," on the role of PBR in the intramitochondrial cholesterol transport.

STEROID BIOSYNTHESIS

Trophic hormone regulation of steroid synthesis can be thought as being either "acute"—occurring within minutes and results in the rapid synthesis of steroids, or "chronic"—occurring over a long period of time and resulting in continued steroid pro-duction. The primary point of control in the acute stimulation of steroidogenesis by hormones involves the first step in this biosynthetic pathway, where the substrate cho-lesterol is converted to pregnenolone (PREG) by the cholesterol side-chain cleavage cytochrome P-450 enzyme (P-450scc) and auxiliary electron-transferring proteins, localized on inner mitochondrial membranes *(44–47)*. More detailed studies have shown that the reaction catalyzed by P-450scc is not the rate-limiting step in the synthesis of steroid hormones, but rather it is the transport of the precursor—cholesterol—from intracellular sources to the inner mitochondrial membrane and the subsequent loading of cholesterol in the P450scc active site *(44–47)*. This hormone-dependent transport mecha-nism was shown to be mediated by cyclic adenosine monophosphate (cAMP), to be regulated by a cytoplasmic protein, and to be localized in the mitochondrion, where it regulates the intramitochondrial transport of cholesterol *(44–47)*. Although a number of molecules have been proposed as potential candidates mediating this intramitochondrial cholesterol transfer *(46,47)*, no clear evidence has been presented on the identity of this mechanism. During the last decade, however, a new cholesterol-transport mechanism was identified and characterized as mediating the acute stimulation of steroidogenesis by hormones, the PBR protein *(6)*.

PBR IN STEROID BIOSYNTHESIS

Effects of Drug Ligands

Two important observations indicated that PBR are likely to play a role in steroido-genesis: first, PBR are found primarily on outer mitochondrial membranes, and second, we and others showed that PBR are extremely abundant in steroidogenic cells *(5,6)*. We then reported that a spectrum of ligands that bind to PBR with affinities ranging from nM to mM stimulate steroid biosynthesis in various cell systems *(48,49)*. The relationship between the affinities of these compounds for PBR and the concentrations of each compound required to stimulate steroidogenesis was examined and showed an excellent correlation, with a coefficient $r = 0.9$, suggesting that these drugs, via binding to PBR, stimulate steroidogenesis. However, the stimulatory effect of PBR ligands was not additive to the stimulation by hormones and cAMP *(50)*. Considering the mitochondrial localization of PBR, we then examined the direct effect of PBR ligands on mitochondrial steroid formation. PBR ligands were found to stimulate PREG production by isolated mitochondria *(49)*. This effect was greater with "cholesterol-loaded" mitochondria prepared from cells treated with hormone and the protein-synthesis inhibitor cycloheximide *(50)*. This treatment increases the amount of cholesterol present in the outer mitochondrial membrane *(45,47)*. The stimulatory effect of PBR ligands on intact mitochondria was not observed with mitoplasts (mitochondria devoid of the outer membrane) in agreement with the outer mitochondrial membrane localization of the receptor *(49)*. In these studies, we concluded that PBR are implicated in the acute stimulation of adrenocortical and Leydig-cell steroidogenesis, possibly by mediating the entry, distribution, and/or availability of cholesterol within mitochondria.

In order to identify the exact step in mitochondrial PREG formation activated by PBR ligands, we quantified the amount of cholesterol present in the outer and inner mitochondrial membranes before and after treatment with PBR ligands. The results obtained clearly demonstrated that the PBR ligand-induced stimulation of PREG formation was owing to PBR-mediated translocation of cholesterol from the outer to the inner mitochondrial membrane *(50)*. PBR ligands, however, induced a massive translocation of cholesterol: 10 μg/mg of protein. Considering that only approx 10–20% of this cholesterol will be used for steroidogenesis, these data indicate that PBR-mediated lipid translocation may be also involved in a more general mechanism, such as mitochondrial membrane biogenesis. Thus, the abundance of PBR in steroidogenic tissues, together with the tissue-specific cholesterol transport, make PBR a regulator of this rate-determining process. Studies by different laboratories have corroborated these observations *(51,52)* and extended them to placental *(53)* and ovarian granulosa cells *(54)*. Moreover, we showed that a similar mechanism regulates brain glial cell neurosteroid synthesis *(55; see* the section "PBR in Neurosteroid Biosynthesis"). Recently a PBR-mediated cholesterol transport mechanism was also identified in rat liver mitochondria *(56)*. Thus, it seems that the regulation of intramitochondrial cholesterol transport may be a general function of PBR.

PBR in Hormone-Stimulated Steroidogenesis

Despite the data presented on the effect of PBR ligands on basal steroid synthesis, it was still unclear whether PBR participate in the hormone-stimulated steroidogenesis. In search of a PBR drug ligand that may affect hormone-stimulated steroid production we found that flunitrazepam—a benzodiazepine that binds to PBR with high nanomolar affinity—inhibited hormone and cAMP-stimulated steroidogenesis *(30)*. Radioligand-binding studies revealed a single class of binding sites for flunitrazepam which was verified as being PBR by displacement studies using a series of PBR ligands. Furthermore, this drug caused an inhibition in mitochondrial PREG formation, which was determined to result from a reduction of cholesterol transport to the inner mitochondrial membrane P-450scc. These observations demonstrated that the antagonistic action of flunitrazepam on hormone-stimulated steroidogenesis is mediated through the interaction of this compound with PBR. It should be noted, however, that flunitrazepam is also a weak stimulator of basal steroid production, suggesting that it acts as a partial agonist of the receptor-mediated steroid-synthesis process. In conclusion, these studies suggested that hormone-induced steroidogenesis involves, at least in part, the participation of PBR.

Hormonal Regulation of PBR

We examined whether hCG or cAMP regulates PBR expression in Leydig cells measured by ligand binding and RNA (Northern-) blot analysis. Treatment of MA-10 cells from 10 min up to 24 h with hCG was without any effect on PBR binding or message levels *(57)*. However, addition of hCG to MA-10 cells resulted in a very rapid increase of PBR binding capacity (threefold increase within 15 s). This rapid increase gradually returned to basal levels within 60 s. This stimulatory effect of hCG was dose-dependent and the concentrations required were similar to those reported by us and others to stimulate steroidogenesis *(57)*. Scatchard analysis revealed that in addition to the known high affinity (5.0 nM) benzodiazepine binding site, a second higher affinity (0.2 nM), hormone-induced, benzodiazepine binding site appeared. We then examined whether steroid synthesis could be detected in a similar time frame. MA-10 cells were incubated for 15 s with aminoglutethimide, an inhibitor of P-450scc, together with hCG. Mitochondria were isolated from these cells, and after incubation in aminoglutethimide-free buffer, an increase in the rate of PREG formation was observed. Addition of a selective inhibitor of cAMP-dependent protein kinase blocked not only the hormone-induced PBR binding, but also steroid formation. Furthermore, addition of flunitrazepam abolished the hCG-induced rapid stimulation of steroid synthesis. These results demonstrate that, in Leydig cells, the most rapid effect of hCG and cAMP, is the transient induction of a higher-affinity benzodiazepine binding site, which occurs concomitantly with an increase in the rate of steroid formation *(57)*. It should be noted that this biochemical evidence for the hormonal regulation of PBR is in agreement with the data previously presented on the hormone-induced changes in PBR topography seen over the same time frame *(39)*. This, in turn, suggests that hormones alter PBR to activate cholesterol delivery to the inner mitochondrial membrane and subsequent steroid formation.

In search of the mechanism underlying the effect of hCG and cAMP on PBR ligand binding, and considering the well-documented role of protein phosphorylation in the regulation of steroid biosynthesis, we identified putative phosphorylation motifs at the C-terminal domain of the cloned rat, bovine, and murine PBR protein. In mitochondrial preparations, the cAMP-dependent protein kinase, but not other purified protein kinases, was found to phosphorylate the 18 kDa PBR protein *(58)*. In addition, the 18 kDa PBR protein was found to be phosphorylated in digitonin-permeabilized Leydig cells and its phosphorylation was stimulated by cAMP *(58)*, suggesting that PBR is an in vitro and *in situ* substrate of PKA. However, cloning of the human 18 kDa PBR protein predicted an amino-acid sequence missing the phosphorylation motif identified in the rat, mouse, and bovine sequences, thus suggesting that phosphorylation of the 18 kDa PBR protein may not be an ubiquitous mechanism of regulation of PBR function. Thus, we have now turned our efforts in identifying PBR-associated proteins substrates of PKA.

PBR in a Constitutive Steroid-Producing Cell Model

In Leydig cell-derived tumors, steroid synthesis occurs independently of hormonal control, because pituitary LH secretion is suppressed by the excessive amount of steroids produced *(59)*. R2C cells are derived from rat Leydig tumors and maintain their in vitro capacity to synthesize steroids constitutively in a hormone-independent manner *(60)*. Thus, one can expect that constitutive steroidogenesis is driven by the unregulated expression of the hormonal mechanism that controls steroid synthesis or by an unknown separate mechanism. Radioligand binding assays on intact R2C cells revealed the presence of a single class of PBR binding sites with an affinity 10-times higher (Kd = 0.5 nM) than that displayed by the MA-10 PBR (Kd = 5 nM) *(61)*. Photolabeling of R2C and MA-10 cell mitochondria with a photoactivatable PBR ligand showed that the 18 kDa PBR protein was specifically labeled. This indicates that the R2C cells express a PBR protein that has properties similar to the MA-10 PBR. Moreover, a PBR synthetic ligand was able to increase steroid production in isolated mitochondria from R2C cells that express the 5 nM affinity receptor. Interestingly, mitochondrial PBR binding was increased sixfold upon addition of the post-mitochondrial fraction, suggesting that a cytosolic factor modulates the binding properties of PBR in R2C cells and is responsible for the 0.5 nM affinity receptor seen in intact cells *(61)*. In conclusion, these data demonstrate that ligand binding to the mitochondrial higher affinity PBR is involved in maintaining R2C constitutive steroidogenesis.

PBR-Mediated Cholesterol Transport in Bacteria

Bacteria is a model system without endogenous cholesterol. In addition, bacteria do not express PBR protein and ligand binding. *Escherichia coli* were transformed with mouse PBR cDNA in a pET vector. Addition of isopropyl-1-thiol-β-D-galactopyranoside (IPTG) to transfected bacteria resulted in the expression of the 18 kDa PBR protein and ligand binding with similar pharmacological characteristics to that previously described for PBR *(61a)*. IPTG-induced PBR expression resulted in a protein-, time-, and temperature-dependent uptake of radiolabeled cholesterol. No uptake of other radiolabeled steroid could be seen. When IPTG-induced, cholesterol-loaded, bacterial membranes were treated with PK 11195, cholesterol was liberated from the membranes, suggesting that cholesterol is captured by PBR, which releases cholesterol upon ligand binding. Thus, PBR serves a channel function where cholesterol can freely enter and reside stored within the membrane, without being incorporated in the lipid bilayer. PBR ligand binding controls the opening/release state of the channel, thus mediating cholesterol movement across membranes.

Targeted Disruption of the PBR Gene in Steroidogenic Cells

In order to investigate further the role of PBR in steroidogenesis, we developed a molecular approach based on the disruption of PBR gene in the constitutive steroid producing R2C rat Leydig cell line by homologous recombination *(61b)*. On the basis of the known rat PBR gene sequence, we designed two sets of primers that allowed us to amplify two fragments of the PBR gene from R2C cells genomic DNA by PCR. These PBR genomic DNA fragments were cloned and used to design the targeting construct. The targeting vector was constructed by positioning (i) the *neo* gene, conferring the neomycin resistance that allows for a positive selection of cells that have undergone homologous recombination, in between the two PBR genomic DNA fragments; and (ii) the Herpes Simplex Virus-tyrosine kinase gene, for the negative selection against cells that have randomly integrated the targeting construct, at the 3'-end of the second PBR genomic DNA fragment. The targeting vector was then transfected in R2C cells and selection was performed with G418 and ganciclovir *(62)*. Four G418/Ganc-resistant cell lines were generated. PBR expression, examined by ligand binding, was absent in all four cell lines. In addition, the PBR-negative R2C cells produced minimal amounts (10%) of steroids compared with normal R2C cells. However, incubation with the hydrosoluble analog of cholesterol, 22R-hydroxycholesterol, increased the steroid production by the PBR-negative R2C cells, indicating that the cholesterol-transport mechanism was impaired. The genomic DNA characterization of the PBR-negative R2C cells is under investigation.

Role of PBR in In Vivo Steroidogenesis

Glucocorticoid excess has broad pathogenic potential, including neurotoxicity, neuroendangerment, and immunosuppression. Glucocorticoid synthesis is regulated by ACTH, which acts by accelerating the transport of the precursor cholesterol to the mitochondria, where steroidogenesis begins. *Ginkgo biloba* is one of the most ancient trees known, and extracts from its leaves have been used in traditional medicine *(63)*. A standardized extract of Ginkgo biloba leaves, termed EGb 761 (EGb), has been shown to have neuroprotective and "antistress" effects. In vivo treatment of rats with EGb, and its bioactive components ginkgolides A and B, specifically reduces the ligand-binding capacity, protein, and mRNA expression of the adrenocortical mitochondrial PBR *(64)*. As expected, the ginkgolide-induced decrease in glucocorticoid levels resulted in increased ACTH release which in turn induced the expression of the steroidogenic acute regulatory protein (StAR). Because ginkgolides reduced the adrenal PBR expression and corticosterone synthesis despite the presence of high levels of StAR, these data demonstrate that PBR is indispensable for normal adrenal function. Moreover, these results suggest that manipulation of PBR expression could control circulating glucocorticoid levels, and that the antistress and neuroprotective effects of EGb are owing to its effect on glucocorticoid biosynthesis. In addition, these data indicate that EGb and isolated ginkgolides may serve as the prototypes of a new generation of compounds regulating PBR expression.

NEUROSTEROID BIOSYNTHESIS

The specific interactions of steroids with binding sites at neuronal membranes and the ability of various steroids to modulate the brain function has prompted the investigation of the steroidogenic potential of CNS structures. The pioneering work of Baulieu et al. *(65)* demonstrated that glial cells can convert cholesterol to PREG and give origin to steroid metabolites, which are potential modulators of neuronal function. It has been shown that oligodendrocytes, a glioma cell line, and Schwann cells have the ability to metabolize cholesterol to PREG, the first step in steroid biosynthesis. However, discrepancies exist among the levels of the enzymatic activity, the amount of immunoreactive protein, and mRNA of the P450scc present in brain. In addition, despite the high levels of DHEA (the first neurosteroid described) found in brain, no one has demonstrated the presence of the 17α-hydroxylase cytochrome P450 activity in brain (P450c17). Thus, it seems that brain steroid synthesis may not fit the well-defined scheme of adrenal, gonadal, and placental steroidogenesis, and that new pathways should be explored. Understanding the mechanisms of PREG and DHEA formation is paramount to all speculation and hypotheses about neurosteroids and their role in brain function. The levels of these steroids and their sulfated and lipoidal forms in brain are distinct from the peripheral steroid levels *(66,67)*, and their function as neuroactive steroids at the $GABA_A$ and NMDA receptor level has been well-established *(68)*.

We examined neurosteroid synthesis using the C6-2B subclone of the rat C6 glioma cell line. Figure 1 shows that these cells express both the glial fibrillary acidic protein (GFAP), a general marker for glial cells in culture, and galactocerebroside C (Gal C), a specific cell-surface marker for oligodendrocytes in culture. In agreement with our previous findings, using isolated mitochondria in immunoblot studies *(55)*, C6-2B cells also express P450scc protein, but not the P450c17 protein. We then demonstrated that these cells were able to synthesize PREG from the substrates mevanolactone and cholesterol *(69)*.

In order to examine the activity of the P-450scc present in C6 cells hydroxylated analogs of cholesterol were used, which will freely cross the mitochondrial membranes thus accessing the P-450scc in the inner membrane. Three different hydroxylated cholesterols (25-, 22-, and 20-OH-cholesterol) stimulated mitochondrial production of PREG by three to fivefold. Glial-cell P-450scc activity was also tested with hydroxylated cholesterol analogs in the presence of aminoglutethimide, an inhibitor of adrenal, testis, and ovarian P-450scc. Aminoglutethimide inhibited the PREG formation in a concentration-dependent manner from 25- and 22-OH-cholesterol, but failed to affect the conversion of 20-OH-cholesterol into PREG *(55)*. These findings suggest a functional analogy between adrenal and glial P-450scc. Thus, in addition to the P450scc protein, C6-2B cells also express P450scc activity. More recently, we demonstrated that human glioma cells in culture are also able to synthesize neurosteroids in a similar manner to C6-2B cells, thus validating the use of the C6-2B cell model system. Although C6-2B glial cell P450scc protein levels closely correlated those found in the adrenal gland, the P450scc mRNA was undetectable by Northern-blot and RNase protection assays. P450scc mRNA could be detected only after 35 cycles of PCR. Furthermore, the P450scc enzymatic activity in glial cells was 10-fold less than the activity of the adrenal enzyme. These discrepancies may be owing to differences in transcriptional regulation, mRNA stability, and antibody specificity and affinity. Alternatively, the possibility exists that neurosteroids, all or in part, may be formed from alternative precursors using alternative pathways *(70,71)*.

It is important to note that P450scc activity is related to the oligodendrocyte differentiation process *(72)*. Cholesterol accumulation in brain is also related to differentiation *(73)* and coincides with the rate of myelinization *(74)*. Interestingly, all three activities reach their maximum in the rat at 20 d of age and cholesterol accumulation in brain declines after maturation of the CNS structures, such as myelin and nerve endings. These findings demonstrate a temporal relationship among cholesterol accumulation, steroid synthesis, myelinization, and nerve-ending formation. The functional consequence(s) of this relationship is under investigation.

Despite the overwhelming evidence that P450scc activity is localized to glial cells of the brain, an earlier study demonstrated the presence of P450scc immunoreactivity in select neuronal populations *(75)* and more recently P450scc mRNA was detected by the

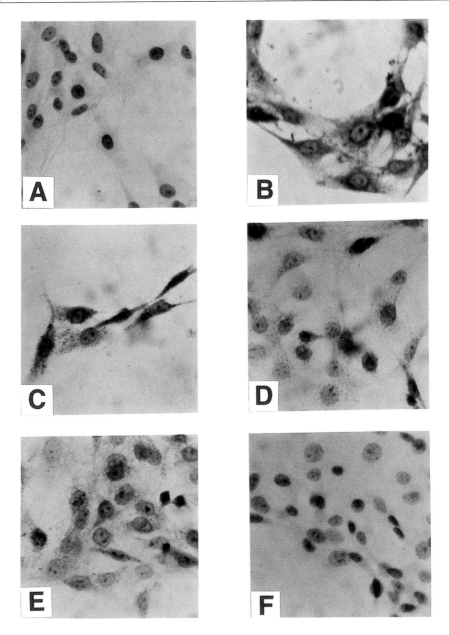

Fig. 1. Characterization of C6-2B rat tumor glioma cells. Cells were immunostained with antibodies: **(B)** anti-GFAP(1:160); **(C)** anti-GALC (1:100); **(D)** anti-PBR (1:200); **(E)** anti-P450scc (1:200); and **(F)** anti-P450c17 (1:200). Normal rabbit serum control is shown in **(A)**. Horseradish-peroxidase conjugated secondary antibody was used for the detection of the anti-serum-antigen complex.

polymerase chain reaction (PCR) technique in primary cerebellar granule neurons *(76)*. In addition, using isolated adult rat retina as a model system, we observed that the neuronal ganglion cells express P450scc protein and activity, and thus are able to synthesize steroids *(77)*.

Regulation of Neurosteroid Biosynthesis by cAMP

In order to understand the mechanisms of neurosteroid synthesis, we looked at well-established mechanisms in peripheral steroidogenic tissues. As previously noted, the regulation of steroid synthesis can be thought of as being either "acute," (occurring within minutes), or "chronic," (occurring over a long period of time). In the chronic regulation, peptide hormones and cAMP act by inducing the expression of steroidogenic enzymes. In acute regulation, the rate of steroid formation depends on the rate of cholesterol transport from intracellular stores to the inner mitochondrial membrane and loading of the P450scc with cholesterol. Using the C6-2B glioma cell line, we demonstrated the presence of both regulatory mechanisms—cAMP and mitochondrial PBR—in the control of neurosteroid synthesis.

Mitochondria isolated from C6-2B cells incubated with the P450scc inhibitor aminoglutethimide and the cAMP analog $(Bt)_2cAMP$ showed greater rates of side-chain cleavage than mitochondria from cells incubated with aminoglutethimide alone *(78)*. After 6 h incubation with $(Bt)_2cAMP$, a significant increase was observed that increased over time to twofold at 24 h. A dose-response curve for $(Bt)_2cAMP$ showed a significant increase using concentrations higher that 0.1 mM. Another cAMP analog (8-Br-cAMP) and agents known to increase cAMP levels, such as cholera toxin (an activator of the Gsα protein), forskolin, an activator of the catalytic subunit of adenylyl cyclase, and isoproterenol (a β-adrenergic receptor agonist), were found to stimulate the rate of side-chain cleavage in mitochondria *(78)*. All these data demonstrate that cAMP stimulates C6 glial cell PREG formation. Because all the stimuli used increase cAMP synthesis or mimic cAMP, the amount of PREG formed in their presence represents the maximal rate of cholesterol transport and metabolism under the conditions used. Using the Rp diastereoisomer of adenosine 3',5'-cyclic phosphorothioate (Rp-cAMPS), an antagonist of the activation of cAMP-dependent protein kinase, an inhibition of the isoproterenol-stimulated rate of mitochondrial side-chain cleavage was observed, indicating that isoproterenol is acting via cAMP and cAMP-dependent protein kinase to stimulate C6-2B glial cell PREG formation. These results demonstrated that neurosteroid synthesis is regulated by β-adrenergic receptor agonists and intracellular second messenger systems (cAMP). Considering the time of the response (>12 h) these data suggest that the effects seen may be owing to a direct effect of cAMP on the expression of steroidogenic enzymes or other components of the steroidogenic machinery, including cholesterol de-esterification and use for steroidogenesis. These findings were recently extended by Zhang and colleagues *(79)*, who demonstrated that cAMP stimulates P450scc transcription in C6 glioma cells.

Considering that the amount of steroids synthesized depends on the amount of the substrate cholesterol available, we performed a series of experiments in the presence of the early precursor of cholesterol, mevalonolactone. As expected, following 10 min of incubation with mevalonolactone, steroidogenesis increased, indicating that glia cells have limited sources of endogenous cholesterol required to support a continuous steroid production. Addition of isoproterenol further increased (doubled) the amount of steroids synthesized, suggesting that an acute stimulation of the adenylyl cyclase by isoproterenol increased glial cell steroid formation by controlling an early step of the pathway *(78)*. This control may be localized either at the level of the StAR protein, a hormone-dependent protein found in steroid synthesizing tissues *(80)*, or at the level of the mitochondrial PBR *(6)*. Because StAR has not been found in brain *(80)*, and hormones and cAMP were found to induce rapid biochemical and morphological changes in the mitochondrial PBR *(39,57)*, this receptor is, at present, the only candidate to mediate the neurosteroidogenic effect of cAMP.

PBR in Neurosteroid Biosynthesis

We have examined PBR in brain tissue, primary glial cultures, and C6-2B glioma cells. Subcellular fractionation indicated that the majority of PBR is localized in the mitochondrial fraction *(14,81)*. Ligand-binding studies indicated that rat brain mitochondria contain approximately 1 pmol/mg protein PK 11195 binding sites. In contrast, mitochondria from primary glial cells and C6-2B glioma cells exhibited a very high density for PBR (25–50 pmol/mg protein). This single class of binding sites had an apparent Kd of 4 nM. Photolabeling with the radiolabeled isoquinoline PK 14105 confirmed that brain, primary glial, and C6-2B glioma cell PBR is characterized by the 18 kDa protein, similar to that identified in peripheral tissues *(14,81)*, recognized by an anti-PBR peptide antisera that we developed *(64*; Fig. 1). In addition, the glioma receptor expressed identical pharmacological profile to the adrenocortical and testicular Leydig-cell PBR. These findings demonstrated that within the CNS, PBR is found primarily in glial cells. In addition, the mitochondrial localization and density of PBR in glial cells suggest that it may serve a function similar to that seen in peripheral steroidogenic tissues. Interestingly, the PBR immunolocalization in C6-2B glioma cells was similar to that seen for P450scc (Fig. 1).

We then investigated whether PBR ligands affect PREG formation in C6-2B glial cell mitochondria. At nanomolar concentrations, PK 11195 and Ro5-4864 induced a twofold stimulation of mitochondrial steroid production *(55)*. A similar increase was obtained with anxiolytic benzodiazepines that bind to both class of benzodiazepine recognition sites, whereas clonazepam, a ligand selective for GABA$_A$ receptors, was ineffective at all concentrations tested *(55)*. In these studies, exogenous cholesterol was not supplied to the mitochondria, suggesting that PBR facilitates the transport of cholesterol from the outer mitochondrial membrane to the inner membrane, which is then metabolized by the P-450scc to form pregnenolone. Table 1 shows a summary of the data obtained using mitochondria from C6-2B glioma cells *(55)* compared to Leydig and adrenal cell mitochondria *(49,50)* and to rat brain mitochondria from two separate studies *(82,83)*. It is obvious that, in our hands and using the same methods, glial cell mitochondria have a rate of PREG production 10 times slower than adrenocortical or Leydig cell mitochondria. However, in all three models, PBR drug ligands stimulated the rate of pregnenolone formation by two- to threefold. In two separate studies, rat brain mitochondria had a greater rate of PREG formation *(82,83)*, although in another report the rate of PREG formation by rat brain mitochondria was found identical to that seen in C6-2B glial mitochondria (Table 2, *84*). In these studies, PBR drug ligands stimulated PREG formation by three to fivefold.

Biosynthesis of [^{3}H]cholesterol and [^{3}H]PREG was demonstrated in C6-2B glial cell cultures to occur within seconds upon addition of the precursor [^{3}H]mevalonolactone *(69)*. Addition of 100 nM Ro5-4864 resulted in 141 and 205% increases in cholesterol and PREG formation, respectively *(69)*. This effect of Ro5-4864 was dose- and time-dependent and demonstrated that PBR ligands also stimulate steroid formation in cultured glial cells.

Table 1
Rate of Pregnenolone Formation in Response to PBR Drug Ligands

Mitochondria		Pregnenolone, pmol/mg protein/min				
		Treatment (1 µM)				
	Ref.	Vehicle	Clonazepam	PK 11195	Ro5-4864	FGIN
MA-10 Leydig cell	(49)	15	13	40	38	42
Y-1 Adrenal cell	(50)	8.1	8.0	21	20	18
C6-2B glioma cells	(55)	1.0	1.1	2.3	2.0	2.2
Rat brain	(82)	21	29	175	84	ND
Rat brain	(83)	27	27	ND	145	150

Ro5-4864, 4'-chlorodiazepam; PK 11195, 1-(2-chlorophenyl)-N-methyl-N-(1-methyl-propyl)-3-isoquinolinecarboxamide; FGIN (FGIN-1-27), 2-hexyl-indole-3-acetamide. ND, not determined.

Table 2
Rate of Pregnenolone Formation in Response to Endogenous PBR Ligands

Mitochondria		Pregnenolone, pmol/mg protein/min		
		Treatment (1 µM)		
	Ref.	Vehicle	DBI	Protoporhyrin IX
MA-10 Leydig cell	(94)	15	40	16
Y-1 Adrenal cell	(94)	8.1	18	8.4
C6-2B glioma cells	(55)	1.0	2.2	1.3
Rat brain	(82)	21	40	ND
Rat brain	(84)	1.0	2.2	ND

ND, not determined.

In addition to the in vitro and in situ studies previously presented, PBR drug ligands were found to increase rat forebrain pregnenolone synthesis in vivo (85) and to elicit antineophobic and anticonflict actions, presumably via their PBR-mediated steroidogenic effect and the subsequent action of the synthesized neurosteroids on the $GABA_A$ receptor.

ENDOGENOUS LIGANDS OF PBR

In addition to the well-characterized drug ligands of PBR two other entities were identified as endogenous PBR ligands, porphyrins (86) and the polypeptide diazepam binding inhibitor (DBI) (6,87). Because in our model system porphyrins were found to have very low affinity for PBR and no effect on mitochondrial steroid formation (Table 2), we focused our studies on the role of DBI. DBI is a 10 kDa protein originally purified from brain by monitoring its ability to displace diazepam from the allosteric modulatory sites for GABA action on $GABA_A$ receptors (88,89). DBI was also independently purified and characterized for its ability to bind long-chain acyl-CoA-esters (90) and modulate insulin secretion (91). DBI was found to be present in a variety of tissues and to be highly expressed in steroidogenic cells (6).

DBI Acts via PBR

Binding of DBI to PBR was initially determined by examining the ability of DBI to displace high-affinity radiolabeled PBR drug ligands *(18,92,93)*. Competition studies for specific binding indicated that DBI displaced radiolabeled benzodiazepines with an inhibitory constant of 1–2 μM. In subsequent studies, we analyzed the binding of DBI to PBR under conditions identical to those used to examine DBI effects on mitochondrial steroid synthesis *(55)*. We found that the inhibitory constant of DBI for PBR binding inhibition was 100 nM, a value that correlates well with the EC_{50} of DBI for mitochondrial steroid synthesis induction. In addition, the stimulatory effect of DBI on steroid synthesis (*see* the following section) was specifically blocked by flunitrazepam, the PBR ligand shown to inhibit hormone-stimulated steroidogenesis *(94)*. To further demonstrate that DBI specifically binds to PBR, we performed crosslinking studies on Leydig cell mitochondria using metabolically labeled bioactive [^{35}S]DBI *(61)*. Two protein complexes were specifically labeled with in R2C Leydig cell mitochondria. A protein complex with an apparent molecular size of 27 kDa, recognized by an antiserum against PBR, suggesting that the 10 kDa DBI formed a specific complex with the 18 kD PBR protein. A second complex, migrating at 65 kDa, with an unidentified 55 kDa protein crosslinked to radiolabeled 10 kDa DBI was also formed.

DBI in Steroid/Neurosteroid Synthesis

In search of a cytoplasmic steroidogenesis-stimulating factor(s), a protein of 8,2 kDa molecular size was isolated from bovine adrenals shown to stimulate transport of cholesterol into mitochondria and transport from the outer to the inner membrane *(95)*. This 8,2 kDa protein was shown to be identical to DBI, except the loss of two amino acids (Gly-Ile) from the carboxy terminus *(96)*, and to have a long-half life *(97)*. We examined the effect of isolated 10 kDa DBI on mitochondria from adrenocortical and Leydig cells *(94)*. Dose-response curves indicated that a threefold stimulation is obtained with low concentrations (0.1–1 μM) of DBI, whereas higher concentrations have lower stimulatory effect on PREG formation. The stimulation obtained was similar to those reported for the 8.2 kDa des-(Gly-Ile)-DBI on bovine adrenocortical mitochondria *(95,98)*. Moreover, similar results were obtained using purified rat and bovine testis DBI *(18)*. In order to exclude the possibility that the stimulatory effect of DBI was owing to the α-helical structure of the protein, we used as control β-endorphin, which also possesses α-helical structures. β-endorphin did not affect the mitochondrial steroid synthesis *(94)*.

As previously noted, high concentrations of DBI (10 μM) gave lower stimulation of steroid synthesis than 100 nM DBI. When DBI was added in combination with a maximally stimulating concentration of Ro5-4864 (100 nM), the stimulatory effect of Ro5-4864 was abolished, suggesting that in C6-2B glial cells DBI may act as a partial agonist of PBR *(99)*.

We then showed that the amino-acid sequence 17–50 of the DBI bears the biological activity because the triacontatetraneuropeptide (TTN, DBI[17–50]) specifically stimulated mitochondrial steroidogenesis with a potency and efficacy similar to that of DBI *(94)*. TTN, together with other DBI peptide fragments were also found in adrenal and testis extracts, and we noted that DBI could be processed in vitro by mitochondria. Binding studies on mitochondria also indicated that TTN binds specifically to PBR *(93)*.

DBI and DBI processing products were also found to be present in brain and C6-2B glioma cell extract. DBI stimulated PREG formation by twofold in mitochondrial fractions from C6-2B glioma cells and rat brain (55; Table 2). In addition to DBI, the DBI peptide fragments DBI[17–50] and DBI[39–75] were found to be biological active in in vitro assays (55,82,84), whereas conflicting data has been presented for the fragment octadecaneuropeptide DBI[33-50] (55,82).

Taking into account the findings that

1. hCG increases PBR ligand binding (57);
2. DBI stimulates mitochondrial steroid formation acting via PBR (61,94); and
3. DBI is preferentially localized in the periphery of mitochondria (100), the possibility is raised that trophic hormones, by altering PBR, increase PBR interaction with DBI; PBR-DBI interaction triggers steroidogenesis.

In order to determine the *in situ* role of DBI in steroidogenesis, we suppressed cell DBI levels using antisense oligodeoxynucleotides. In order to overcome the commonly encountered oligodeoxynucleotide-uptake problems, we took advantage of the ability of steroidogenic cells to utilize exogenous cholesterol via the lipoprotein endocytotic pathway (101). Thus, we constructed cholesterol-linked phosphorothioate oligodeoxynucleotides (CHOL-ODNs) complementary to either the sense or the antisense strand of the 24 nucleotides encoding mouse DBI, 9 bases immediately 5' to the initiation codon ATG and 12 downstream the ATG codon. Treating MA-10 cells with CHOL-ODN antisense to DBI resulted in a dose-dependent reduction of DBI levels. In contrast, CHOL-ODN sense to DBI did not affect its expression. Saturating amounts of hCG increased MA-10 progesterone production by 150-fold. The addition of increasing concentrations of CHOL-ODNs sense to DBI or of a nonrelated sequence did not reduce the MA-10 response to hCG. In contrast, a twofold increase in the amount of steroids produced was observed owing to the cholesterol linked to the ODN, liberated in the cells and used as substrate for steroid synthesis. However, in the presence of CHOL-ODN antisense to DBI, in amounts shown to reduce DBI levels, MA-10 cells lost their ability to respond to hCG. In these studies the hCG-stimulated cAMP levels and P-450scc activity were not affected by the CHOL-ODNs used (101).

Using similar technology we also decreased DBI levels in the R2C Leydig cells (61). DBI-depleted R2C cells did not produce steroids, suggesting that DBI plays a vital role both in the acute stimulation of steroidogenesis by trophic hormones and in the constitutive steroid synthesis. Because we showed that DBI is not the long-sought labile factor, and that the site of hormone action is in the mitochondrion, we propose that hormones, by altering PBR, increase its interaction with DBI, which, in turn, triggers steroidogenesis.

Although PBR drug ligands did not have any direct effect on P450scc activity examined in mitoplasts, DBI induced a twofold stimulation of PREG synthesis. Evidence has been previously discussed that indicates that the outer mitochondrial membrane PBR mediates the effects of PBR ligands and DBI on intact mitochondria. However, the observation that DBI stimulates PREG production by inner mitochondrial membranes implies that this protein can also act via an additional PBR-independent mechanism. Further evidence which indicates the DBI acts directly on P450scc was then provided by observations in an in vitro reconstituted enzyme system (102,103), where DBI stimulated the production of PREG, suggesting that the non-PBR mechanism involved in steroidogenesis may result from direct activation of P450scc, or alternatively an indirect mechanism that may act via increasing the availability of cholesterol or by altering the rate of reduction of P450scc.

CONCLUSIONS

Considering the data presented in this review, we propose that the steroidogenic pool of cholesterol enters the channel formed by the 18 kD PBR protein and transfers from the outer leaflet of the outer mitochondrial membrane to the inner leaflet of the outer membrane. This activity may be directly stimulated by hormones via modulation of the PBR affinity for the endogenous ligand DBI, which is continuously present around the mitochondria *(100)*. Hormone or cAMP-induced changes in PBR affinity will lead to changes in PBR topography and the rapid formation of contact sites between the outer and inner mitochondrial membranes. Thus, cholesterol will be transported "passively" from the outer to the inner membrane. On the mitochondrial membrane contact-site formation, we should also consider here the role of DBI as an acyl-CoA binding protein *(90)*. DBI was shown to mediate intermembrane transport of long-chain acyl-CoA esters *(104)* and fatty acylation has been proposed as a mechanism employed in transport processes that require fusion of lipid bilayers *(105)*. Thus, DBI may induce the formation of additional contact sites.

It is evident that the presence of tissue-specific PBR-associated proteins may provide selectivity and sensitivity to the PBR function. In addition, it should be noted that the model proposed here does not exclude the presence of additional mechanisms, such as guanosine triphosphate (GTP) and calcium, involved in the process of the acute regulation of steroidogenesis *(46,106,107)*. Identifying and understanding the role of each component of the mitochondrial cholesterol transport apparatus and then their interaction and relationship should allow us to put together the puzzle of the acute regulation of steroidogenesis by hormones. This puzzle is even more complex in the brain because we have no information on the extracellular signal(s) regulating brain neurosteroid synthesis.

ACKNOWLEDGMENTS

This work was supported by Grant # IBN-9728261 from the National Science Foundation, ES-07747 from the National Institute of Environmental Health Sciences, NIH, and a grant from the Institut Henri Beaufour-IPSEN. V.P. was supported by a Research Career Development Award (HD-01031) from the National Institute of Child Health and Human Development, NIH.

REFERENCES

1. Haefely W, Kulcsar A, Mohler H, Pieri L, Polc P, Schaffner R. Possible involvement of GABA in the central actions of benzodiazepine derivatives. In: Costa E, Greengard P, eds. Advances in Biochemical Psychopharmacology, vol 14. Raven, New York, NY, 1975, pp. 131–151.
2. Costa E, Guidotti A. Molecular mechanism in the receptor actions of benzodiazepines. Annu Rev Pharmacol Toxicol 1979;19:531–545.
3. Braestrup C, Squires RF. Specific benzodiazepine receptors in rat brain characterized by high-affinity [^{3}H]diazepam binding. Proc Natl Acad Sci USA 1977;74:3805–3809.
4. Verma A, Snyder SH. Peripheral type benzodiazepine receptors. Annu Rev Pharmacol Toxicol 1989;29:307–322.

5. Gavish M, Katz Y, Bar-Ami S, Weizman R. Biochemical, physiological, and pathological aspects of the peripheral benzodiazepine receptor. J Neurochem 1992;58:1589–1601.

6. Papadopoulos V. Peripheral-type benzodiazepine/diazepam binding inhibitor receptor: biological role in steroidogenic cell function. Endocr Rev 1993;14:222–240.

7. Parola AL, Yamamura HI, Laird HE. Peripheral-type benzodiazepine receptors. Life Sci 1993; 52:1329–1342.

8. Krueger KE, Papadopoulos V. Cellular role and pharmacological implications of mitochondrial p-sites recognizing diazepam binding inhibitor as a putative endogenous ligand. In: Bartholini G, Garreau M, Morselli PL, Zivkovic B, eds. Imidazopyridines in anxiety disorders: a novel experimental and therapeutic approach. Raven, New York, NY, 1993, pp. 39–48.

9. Le Fur G, Perrier ML, Vaucher N, Imbault F, Flamier A, Uzan A, Renault C, Dubroeucq MC, Gueremy C. Peripheral benzodiazepine binding sites: effects of PK 11195, 1-(2-chlorophenyl)-N-(1-methyl-propyl)-3-isoquinolinecarboxamide. I. In vitro studies. Life Sci 1983;32:1839–1847.

10. Romeo E, Auta J, Kozikowski A P, Ma A, Papadopoulos V, Puia G, Costa E, Guidotti A. 2-Aryl-3-indoleacetamides (FGIN-1): a new class of potent and specific ligands for the mitochondrial DBI receptor. J Pharmacol Exper Ther 1992;262:971–978.

11. Campiani G, Nacci V, Fiorini I, De Filippis MP, Garofalo A, Ciani SM, Greco G, Novellino E, Williams D C, Zisterer DM, Woods MJ, Mihai C, Manzoni C, Mennini T. Synthesis, biological activity, and SARs of pyrrolobenzoxazepine derivatives, a new class of specific "peripheral-type" benzodiazepine receptor ligands. J Med Chem 1996;39:3435–3450.

12. Anholt RRH, DeSouza EB, Oster-Granite ML, Snyder SH 1985 Peripheral-type benzodiazepine receptors: autoradiograpic localization in whole-body sections of neonatal rats. J Pharmacol Exp Ther 1985;233:517–526.

13. Basile AS, Skolnick P. Subcellular localization of "peripheral-type" binding sites for benzodiazepines in rat brain. J Neurochem 1986;46:305–308.

14. Krueger KE, Papadopoulos V. Molecular and functional characterization of peripheral-type benzodiazepine receptors in glial cells. In: Racagni G, ed. Biological Psychiatry, vol 1. Elsevier Science, New York, 1991, pp. 744–746.

15. Anholt RRH, Pedersen PL, DeSouza EB, Snyder SH. The peripheral-type benzodiazepine receptor: localization to the mitochondrial outer membrane. J Biol Chem 1986;261:576–583.

16. Oke BO, Suarez-Quian CA, Riond J, Ferrara P, Papadopoulos V 1992 Cell surface localization of the peripheral-type benzodiazepine receptor in adrenal cortex. Mol Cell Endocr 1992;87:R1–R6.

17. Garnier M, Boujrad N, Oke BO, Brown AS, Riond J, Ferrara P, Suarez-Quian CA, Papadopoulos V. Diazepam binding inhibitor is a paracrine/autocrine regulator of Leydig cell proliferation and steroidogenesis. Action via peripheral-type benzodiazepine receptor and independent mechanisms. Endocrinology 1993;132:444–458.

18. Woods MJ, Williams DC. Multiple forms and locations for the peripheral-type benzodiazepine receptor. Biochem Pharm 1996;52:1805–1814.

19. Doble A, Ferris O, Burgevin MC, Menager J, Uzan A, Dubroeucq MC, Renault C, Gueremy C, Le Fur G. Photoaffinity labeling of peripheral-type benzodiazepine binding sites. Mol Pharm 1987;31:42–49.

20. Antkiewicz-Michaluk L, Mukhin AG, Guidotti A, Krueger KE. Purification and characterization of a protein associated with peripheral-type benzodiazepine binding sites. J Biol Chem 1988;263:17317–17321.

21. Riond J, Vita N, Le Fur G, Ferrara P. Characterization of a peripheral-type benzodiazepine binding site in the mitochondria of Chinese hamster ovary cells FEBS Lett 1989;245:238–244.

22. Sprengel R, Werner P, Seeburg PH, Mukhin AG, Santi MR, Grayson DR, Guidotti A, Krueger KE. Molecular cloning and expression of cDNA encoding a peripheral-type benzodiazepine receptor. J Biol Chem 1989;264:20415–20421.

23. Riond J, Mattei MG, Kaghad M, Dumont X, Guillemot JC, Le Fur G, Caput D, Ferrara P. Molecular cloning and chromosomal localization of a human peripheral-type benzodiazepine receptor. Eur J Biochem 1991;195:305–311.

24. Chang YJ, McCabe RT, Rennert H, Budarf ML, Sayegh R, Emanuel BS, Skolnick P, Srauss JF. The human "peripheral-type" benzodiazepine receptor: regional mapping of the gene and characterization of the receptor expressed from cDNA. DNA and Cell Biol 1992;11:471–480.

25. Parola AL, Stump DG, Pepperl DJ, Krueger KE, Regan JW, Laird II HE. Cloning and expression of a pharmacologically unique bovine peripheral-type benzodiazepine receptor isoquinoline binding protein. J Biol Chem 1991;266:14,082–14,087.

26. Garnier M, Dimchev AB, Boujrad N, Price MJ, Musto NA, Papadopoulos V. In vitro reconstitution of a functional peripheral-type benzodiazepine receptor from mouse Leydig tumor cells. Mol Pharm 1994;45:201–211.

27. Baker ME, Fanestil DD. Mammalian peripheral-type benzodiazepine receptor is homologous to CrtK protein of Rhodobacter capsulatus, a photosynthetic bacterium. Cell 1991;65:1–2.

28. Yeliseev AA, Kaplan S. A sensory transducer homologous to the mammalian peripheral-type benzodiazepine receptor regulates photosynthetic membrane complex formation in Rhodobacter sphaeroides 2.4.1. J Biol Chem 1995;270:21167–21175.

29. Casalotti SO, Pelaia G, Yakovlev AG, Csikos T, Grayson DR, Krueger KE. Structure of the rat gene encoding the mitochondrial benzodiazepine receptor. Gene 1992;121:377–382.

30. Papadopoulos V, Nowzari FB, Krueger KE. Hormone-stimulated steroidogenesis is coupled to mitochondrial benzodiazepine receptors. J Biol Chem 1991;266:3682–3687.

31. McEnery MW, Snowman AM, Trifiletti RR, Snyder SH. Isolation of the mitochondrial benzodiazepine receptor: association with the voltage-dependent anion channel and the adenine nucleotide carrier. Proc Natl Acad Sci USA 1992;89:3170–3174.

32. Farges R, Joseph-Liausun E, Shire D, Caput D, Le Fur G, Loison G, Ferrara P. Molecular basis for the different binding properties of benzodiazepines to human and bovine peripheral-type benzodiazepine receptors. FEBS Lett 1993;335:305–308.

33. Levitt, D. Gramicidin, VDAC, porin and perforin channels. Curr Opin Cell Biol 1990;2:689–694.

34. Mannella CA, Forte M, Colombini M. Toward the molecular structure of the mitochondrial channel, VDAC. J Bioenerg Biomembr 1992;24:7–19.

35. Szabo I, Zoratti M. The giant channel of the inner mitochondrial membrane is inhibited by cyclosporin A. J Biol Chem 1991;266:3376–3379.

36. Petronilli V, Constantini P, Scorrano L, Colonna R, Passamonti S, Bernardi P. The voltage sensor of the mitochondrial permeability transition pore is tuned by the oxidation-reduction state of vicinal thiols. J Biol Chem 1994;269:16638–16642.

37. Kinnally KW, Zorov DB, Antonenko YN, Snyder SH, McEnenery MW, Tedeshi H. Mitochondrial benzodiazepine receptor linked to inner membrane ion channel by nanomolar actions of ligands. Proc Natl Acad Sci USA 1993;90:1374–1378.

38. Papadopoulos V, Boujrad N, Ikonomovic MD, Ferrara P, Vidic B. Topography of the Leydig cell mitochondrial peripheral-type benzodiazepine receptor. Mol Cell Endocr 1994; 104:R5–R9.

39. Boujrad N, Vidic B, Papadopoulos V. Acute action of choriogonadotropin on Leydig tumor cells: Changes in the topography of the mitochondrial peripheral-type benzodiazepine receptor. Endocrinology 1996;137:5727–5730.

40. Stevens VL, Tribble DL, Lambeth JD. Regulation of mitochondrial compartment volumes in rat adrenal cortex by ether stress. Arch Biochem Biophys 1985;242:324–327.

41. Simbeni R, Pon L, Zinser E, Paltauf F, Daum G. Mitochondrial membrane contact sites of yeast. Characterization of lipid components and possible involvement in intramitochondrial translocation of phospholipids. J Biol Chem 1991;266:10047–10049.

42. Bernassau JM, Reversat JL, Ferrara P, Caput D, Lefur G. A 3D model of the peripheral benzodiazepine receptor and its implication in intra mitochondrial cholesterol transport. J Mol Graphics 1993;11:236–245.

43. Papadopoulos V. Pharmacologic influence on androgen biosynthesis. In: Russell LD, Hardy MP, Payne AH, eds. The Leydig Cell. Cashe River, Vienna, IL, 1996, pp. 597–628.

44. Simpson ER, Waterman MR. Regulation by ACTH of steroid hormone biosynthesis in the adrenal cortex. Can J Biochem Cell Biol 1983;61:692–707.

45. Hall PF. Trophic stimulation of steroidogenesis: In search of the elusive trigger. Rec Prog Horm Res 1985;41:1–39.

46. Kimura T. Transduction of ACTH signal from plasma membrane to mitochondria in adrenocortical steroidogenesis. Effects of peptide, phospholipid, and calcium. J Steroid Biochem 1986;25:711–716.

47. Jefcoate CR, McNamara BC, Artemenko I, Yamazaki T. Regulation of cholesterol movement to mitochondrial cytochrome P450scc in steroid hormone synthesis. J Steroid Biochem Molec Biol 1992;43:751–767.

48. Mukhin AG, Papadopoulos V, Costa E, Krueger KE. Mitochondrial benzodiazepine receptors regulate steroid biosynthesis. Proc Natl Acad Sci USA 1989;86:9813–9816.

49. Papadopoulos V, Mukhin AG, Costa E, Krueger KE. The peripheral-type benzodiazepine receptor is functionally linked to Leydig cell steroidogenesis. J Biol Chem 1990;265:3772–3779.

50. Krueger KE, Papadopoulos V. Peripheral-type benzodiazepine receptors mediate translocation of cholesterol from outer to inner mitochondrial membranes in adrenocortical cells. J Biol Chem 1990;265:15015–15022.

51. Ritta MN, Calandra RS. Testicular interstitial cells as targets for peripheral benzodiazepines. Neuroendocrinology 1989;49:262–266.

52. Thompson I, Fraser R, Kenyon CJ. Regulation of adrenocortical steroidogenesis by benzodiazepines. J Steroid Biochem Mol Biol 1994;53:75–80.

53. Barnea ER, Fares F, Gavish M. Modulatory action of benzodiazepines on human term placental steroidogenesis in vitro. Mol Cell Endocr 1989;64:155–159.

54. Amsterdam A, Suh BS. An inducible functional peripheral benzodiazepine receptor in mitochondria of steroidogenic granulosa cells. Endocrinology 1991;128:503–510.

55. Papadopoulos V, Guarneri P, Krueger KE, Guidotti A, Costa E. Pregnenolone biosynthesis in C6 glioma cell mitochondria: regulation by a Diazepam Binding Inhibitor mitochondrial receptor. Proc Natl Acad Sci USA 1992;89:5113–5117.

56. Tsankova V, Magistrelli A, Cantoni L, Tacconi MT. Peripheral benzodiazepine receptor ligands in rat liver mitochondria: effect on cholesterol translocation. Eur J Pharm 1995;294:601–607.

57. Boujrad N, Gaillard J-L, Garnier M, Papadopoulos V. Acute action of choriogonadotropin in Leydig tumor cells. Induction of a higher affinity benzodiazepine receptor related to steroid biosynthesis. Endocrinology 1994;135:1576–1583.

58. Whalin ME, Boujrad N, Papadopoulos V, Krueger KE. Studies on the phosphorylation of the 18 KDa mitochondrial benzodiazepine receptor protein. J Rec Res 1994;14:217–228.

59. Ward JA, Krantz S, Mendeloff J, Haltiwanger E. Interstital cell tumor of the testes: report of two cases. J Clin Endocrinol Metab 1960;22:1622–1629.

60. Freeman, DA. Constitutive steroidogenesis in the R2C Leydig tumor cell line is maintained by the adenosine 3':5'-cyclic monophosphate-independent production of a cycloheximide-sensitive factor that enhances mitochondrial pregnenolone biosynthesis. Endocrinology 1987; 120:124–132.

61. Garnier M, Boujrad N, Ogwuegbu SO, Hudson JR, Papadopoulos V. The polypeptide diazepam binding inhibitor and a higher affinity peripheral-type benzodiazepine receptor sustain constitutive steroidogenesis in the R2C Leydig tumor cell line. J Biol Chem 1994;269:22105–22112.

61a. Li H, Papadopoulos V. Peripheral-type benzodiazepine receptor function in cholesterol transport. Identification of a putative cholestrol recognition/interaction amino acid sequence and consensus pattern. Endocrinology 1998;139;4991–4997.

61b. Papadopoulos V, Amri H, Li H, Boujrad N, Vidic B, Garnier M. Targeted disruption of the peripheral-type benzodiazepine receptor gene inhibits steroidogenesis in the R2C leydig tumor cell line. J Biol Chem 1997;272:32,129–32,135.

62. Sedivy JM, Joyner AL. Gene targetting. WH. Freeman, New York, NY, 1992.

63. DeFeudis FV. 1991 Ginkgo biloba extract (EGb 761): pharmacological activities and clinical applications. Elsevier, Paris, 1991, p. 187.

64. Amri H, Ogwuegbu SO, Boujrad N, Drieu K, Papadopoulos V. In vivo regulation of the peripheral-type benzodiazepine receptor and glucocorticoid synthesis by the Ginkgo biloba extract EGb 761 and isolated ginkgolides. Endocrinology 1996;137:5707–5718.

65. Baulieu EE, Robel P. Neurosteroids: a new brain function? J Steroid Biochem Mol Biol 1990;37:395–403.

66. Corpechot C, Robel P, Axelson M, Sjövall J, Baulieu EE. Characterization and measurement of dehydroepiandrosterone sulfate in rat brain. Proc Natl Acad Sci USA 1981;78:4704–4707.

67. Corpechot C, Synguelakis M, Talha S, Axelson M, Sjövall J, Vihko R, Baulieu EE, Robel P. Pregnenolone and its sulfate ester in the rat brain. Brain Res 1983;270:119–125.

68. Paul SM, Purdy RH. Neuroactive steroids. FASEB J 1992;6:2311–2322.

69. Guarneri P, Papadopoulos V, Pan B, Costa E. Regulation of pregnenolone synthesis in C6 glioma cells by 4'-chlorodiazepam. Proc Natl Acad Sci USA 1992;89:5118–5122.

70. Prasad VVK, Vegesna SR, Welch M, Lieberman S. Precursors of the neurosteroids. Proc Natl Acad Sci USA 1994;91:3220–3223.

71. Cascio C, Prasad VVK, Lin YY, Lieberman S, Papadopoulos V. Detection of P450c17-independent pathways for dehydroepiandrosterone (DHEA) biosynthesis in brain glial tumor cells. Proc Natl Acad Sci USA 1998;95:2862–2867.

72. Jung-Testas I, Hu ZY, Baulieu EE, Robel P. Neurosteroids: biosynthesis of pregnenolone and progesterone in primary cultures of rat glial cells. Endocrinology 1989;125:2083–2091.

73. Shah SN. Cholesterol metabolism in brain. Adv Structural Biology 1993;2:171–189.
74. Norton WT, Poduslo SE. Myelinization in rat brain: changes in myelin composition during brain maturation. J Neurochem 1973;21:759–773.
75. Le Goascogne C, Robel P, Gouezou M, Sananes N, Baulieu EE, Waterman M. Neurosteroids: cytochrome P450scc in rat brain. Science 1987;237:1212–1215.
76. Sanne JL, Krueger KE. Expression of cytochrome P450 side-chain cleavage enzyme and 3β-hydroxysteroid dehydrogenase in the rat central nervous system: a study by polymerase chain reaction and in situ hybridization. J Neurochem 1995;65:528–536.
77. Guarneri P, Guarneri R, Cascio C, Pavasant P, Piccoli F, Papadopoulos V. Neurosteroidogenesis in rat retinas. J Neurochem 1994;63:86–96.
78. Papadopoulos V, Guarneri P. Regulation of C6 glioma cell steroidogenesis by adenosine 3',5'-cyclic monophosphate. Glia 1994;10:75–78.
79. Zhang P, Rodriguez H, Mellon SH. Transcriptional regulation of P450scc gene expression in neural and steroidogenic cells: implications for the regulation of neurosteroidogenesis. Mol Endocr 1995;9:1571–1582.
80. Clark BJ, Stocco DM. StAR- A tissue specific acute mediator of steroidogenesis. Trends Endocr Metab 1996;7:227–233.
81. Krueger KE, Papadopoulos V. The peripheral-type benzodiazepine receptor: cell biological role and pharmacological significance. In: Transmitter amino acid receptors: structures, transduction and models for drug development, FIDIA Research Foundation Symposium Series. Thieme, New York, NY, 1991;6:153–166.
82. McCauley LD, Park CH, Lan NC, Tomich JM, Shively JE, Gee KW. Benzodiazepines and peptides stimulate pregnenolone synthesis in brain mitochondria. Eur J Pharm 1995;276:145–153.
83. Romeo E, Cavallaro S, Korneyev A, Kozikowski AP, Ma D, Polo A, Costa E, Guidotti A. Stimulation of brain steroidogenesis by 2-aryl-indole–3-acetamide derivatives acting at the mitochondrial diazepam binding inhibitor receptor complex. J Pharm Exp Therapeut 1993;267:462–471.
84. Slobodyansky E, Antiekiewicz-Michaluk L, Martin B. Purification of a novel DBI processing product, DBI$_{39–75}$, and characterization of its binding site in rat brain. Reg Pept 1994;50:29–35.
85. Costa E, Cheney DL, Grayson DR, Korneyev A, Longone P, Pani L, Romeo E, Zivkovich E, Guidotti A. Pharmacology of neurosteroid biosynthesis. Ann N Y Acad Sci 1994;746:223–242.
86. Snyder S H, Verma A, Trifiletti R R The Peripheral-type benzodiazepine receptor: a protein of mitochondrial outer membranes utilizing porphyrins as endogenous ligands. FASEB J 1987;1:282–288.
87. Papadopoulos V, Brown AS. The peripheral-type benzodiazepine receptor, diazepam binding inhibitor, and steroidogenesis. J Steroid Biochem Mol Biol 1995;53:103–110.
88. Guidotti A, Forchetti CM, Corda MG, Konkel D, Bennet CD, Costa E. Isolation, characterization, and purification to homogeneity of an endogenous polypeptide with agonist action on benzodiazepine receptors. Proc Natl Acad Sci USA 1983;80:3531–3533.
89. Shoyab M, Gentry LE, Marquardt H, Todaro G. Isolation and characterization of a putative endogenous benzodiazepinoid (Endozepine) from bovine and human brain. J Biol Chem 1986;261:11968–11973.
90. Knudsen J, Hojrup P, Hansen HO, Hansen HF, Roepstorff P. Acyl-CoA-binding protein in the rat. Biochem J 1989;262:513–519.
91. Chen Z, Agerbeth B, Gell K, Andersson M, Mutt V, Ostenson C-G, et al. Isolation and characterization of porcine diazepam binding inhibitor, a polypeptide not only of cerebral occurence but also common in intestinal tissues and with effects on regulation of insulin release. Eur J Biochem 1988;174:239–245.
92. Bovolin P, Schlichting J, Miyata J, Ferrarese C, Guidotti A, Alho H. Distribution and characterization of diazepam binding inhibitor (DBI) in peripheral tissues of rat. Regul Pept 1990;29:267–281.
93. Guidotti A, Berkovich A, Mukhin A, Costa E. Diazepam binding inhibitor: response to Knudsen and Nielsen. Biochem J 1990;265:928–929.
94. Papadopoulos V, Berkovich A, Krueger KE, Costa E, Guidotti A. Diazepam Binding Inhibitor (DBI) and its processing products stimulate mitochondrial steroid biosynthesis via an interaction with mitochondrial benzodiazepine receptors. Endocrinology 1991;129:1481–1488.
95. Yanagibashi K, Ohno Y, Kawamura M, Hall PF. The regulation of intracellular transport of cholesterol in bovine adrenal cells: purification of a novel protein. Endocrinology 1988;123:2075–2082.
96. Besman MJ, Yanagibashi K, Lee TD, Kawamura M, Hall PF, Shively JE. Identification of des-(Gly-Ile)-endozepine as an effector of corticotropin-dependent adrenal steroidogenesis: Stimulation of cholesterol delivery is mediated by the peripheral benzodiazepine receptor. Proc Natl Acad Sci USA 1989;86:4897–4901.

97. Brown AS, Hall PF, Shoyab M, Papadopoulos V. Endozepine/Diazepam Binding Inhibitor in adreno-cortical and Leydig cell lines: absence of hormonal regulation. Mol Cell Endocr 1992; 83:1–9.
98. Yanagibashi K, Ohno Y, Nakamichi N, Matsui T, Hayashida K, Takamura M, Yamada K, Tou S, Kawamura M. Peripheral-type benzodiazepine receptors are involved in the regulation of cholesterol side chain cleavage in adrenocortical mitochondria. J Biochem 1989;106:1026–1029.
99. Papadopoulos V, Guarneri P, Pan B, Krueger KE, Costa E Steroid synthesis by glial cells. In: Neurosteroids. FIDIA Research Foundation Symposium Series. Thieme, New York, 1991;8:165–170.
100. Schultz R, Pelto-Huikko M, Alho H. Expression of diazepam binding inhibitor-like immunoreactivity in rat testis is dependent on pituitary hormones. Endocrinology 1992;130:3200–3206.
101. Boujrad N, Hudson JR, Papadopoulos V. Inhibition of hormone-stimulated steroidogenesis in cultured Leydig tumor cells by a cholesterol-linked phosphorothioate oligodeoxynucleotide antisense to diaz-epam binding inhibitor. Proc Natl Acad Sci USA 1993;90:5728–5731.
102. Brown AS, Hall PF. Stimulation by endozepine of the side-shain cleavage of cholesterol in a recon-stituted enzyme system. Biochem Biophys Res Commun 1991 180:609–614.
103. Boujrad N, Hudson JR, Papadopoulos V. Mediation of the hormonal stimulation of steroidogenesis by the polypeptide diazepam binding inhibitor. In: Bartke A., ed. Function of somatic cells of the testis. Springer-Verlag, New York, 1994, pp. 186–194.
104. Rasmussen JT, Faergeman NJ, Kristiansen K, Knudsen J. Acyl-CoA-binding protein can mediate intermembrane acyl-CoA transport and donate acyl-CoA for β-oxidation and glycerolipid synthesis. Biochem J 1994;299:165–170.
105. Pfanner N, Glick BS, Arden SR, Rothman JE. Fatty acylation promotes fusion of transport vesicles with Golgi cisternae. J Cell Biol 1990;110:955–961.
106. Xu X, Xu T, Robertson DG, Lambeth DJ. GTP stimulates pregnenolone generation in isolated rat adrenal mitochondria. J Biol Chem 1989;264:17674–17680.
107. Kowluru R, Yamazaki T, McNamara BC, Jefcoate CR. Metabolism of exogenous cholesterol by rat adrenal mitochondria is stimulated by physiological levels of free calcium and by GTP. Mol Cell Endocr 1995;107:181–188.

6

Aspects of Hormonal Steroid Metabolism in the Nervous System

Angelo Poletti, MD, Fabio Celotti, MD, Roberto Maggi, MD, Roberto C. Melcangi, MD, Luciano Martini, MD, and Paola Negri-Cesi

CONTENTS

INTRODUCTION
AROMATASE
5α-REDUCTASE
OTHER STEROID-METABOLIZING ENZYMES
REFERENCES

INTRODUCTION

It is known that hormonal steroids intervene in the control of a large number of brain functions both during the fetal and neonatal period, in which they act as "organizers," as well as during adulthood, when they act as "activators" or "inhibitors" of several physiological functions. Hormonal steroids may also participate in the process of aging of the central nervous system (CNS), especially in some specific structures (e.g., the hippocampus).

Classical intracellular receptors for each family of hormonal steroids have been shown to be present in many CNS structures. Some receptors may be preponderant in particular brain areas. For instance, glucocorticosteroid receptors (GR) and mineralocorticosteroid receptors (MR) appear to prevail in the limbic system, whereas the receptors for sex hormones (androgen receptors [AR], estrogen receptors [ER], progesterone receptors [PR]) have a more generalized distribution, even if they show peak concentrations in the hypothalamus and in the amygdala *(1,2)*. There is little information on the presence of the recently discovered ER type β *(3–5)*. It is still discussed whether GR, MR, AR, ERα, ERβ, and PR are present also in the specialized neurons, which, in the hypothalamus, synthesize luteinizing hormone-releasing hormone (LHRH) *(6–12)*. Recent data obtained using cultures of immortalized hypothalamic neurons (the

From: *Contemporary Endocrinology: Neurosteroids: A New Regulatory Function
in the Nervous System* Edited by: E.-E. Baulieu, P. Robel, and M. Schumacher
© Humana Press Inc., Totowa, NJ

GT1 cells) provide a positive answer to the question of the co-localization of LHRH with some steroid hormone receptors *(13,14)*.

It is interesting to note that the presence of receptors for hormonal steroids is not limited to neurons, but that these are also found, in similar concentrations, in glial elements (e.g., astrocytes and oligodendrocytes) *(15–19)*. This observation may have important physiological implications, because of the close cross-talk existing between neurons and glial cells.

Some hormonal steroids, and especially some of their metabolites, may act in the brain utilizing binding sites different from the classical intracellular steroid receptors. The interactions of some derivatives of hormonal steroids with binding sites on brain cell membranes *(20)*, with the opioid receptors *(21,22)* and with the receptors for recognized neurotransmitters (e.g., the $GABA_A$ receptor) has recently received great attention. The interaction with the appropriate subunit of the $GABA_A$ receptor appears to be a characteristic of the 5α-reduced steroids deriving from progesterone (PROG) and deoxycorticosterone (DOC), and possessing an hydroxyl group in the 3α position (e.g., 3α-hydroxy-5α-pregnan-20-one [allopregnanolone, 3α,5α-THPROG] and 3α,21-dihydroxy-5α-pregnan-20-one [tetrahydro deoxycorticosterone, 3α,5α-THDOC]) *(23)*.

One important aspect that has emerged in the last 30 years is that the brain in general, and some specialized CNS structures in particular, may metabolize hormonal steroids. Several enzymatic systems have been described and some of them have been fully characterized. Among these, some have the peculiarity of totally changing the endocrine profile of a given steroid (e.g., the aromatization of testosterone [T] to estradiol [E]), whereas others have the property of enhancing its activity (e.g., the 5α-reductase which converts T to dihydrotestosterone [5α-DHT]); moreover, some enzymes modify steroids so that their metabolites might interact with receptors other than the classical intracellular steroid receptors. Finally, other enzymes may decrease the damaging activity as, for example, the PROG and DOC metabolites of steroids on peculiar neuronal systems (e.g., the 11β-hydroxy steroid oxidoreductase).

This chapter describes in some detail the most important metabolic pathways involved in mediating the effects of steroid hormones in the CNS. The chapter deals in particular with the following enzymatic systems:

1. Aromatase (P450aro);
2. The isoforms of the 5α-Reductase (5α-R) and of the 3α-hydroxy steroid oxidoreductase (3α-HOR);
3. The isoforms of the 17β-hydroxy steroid oxidoreductase *(17β-HOR)* and of the 11β-hydroxy steroid oxidoreductase *(11β-HOR)*, and the steroid sulfotransferases (ST) and sulfatases.

No information will be provided on steroid synthesizing enzymes since this topic will be dealt with in other chapters.

AROMATASE

General Consideration on the P450aro

It is now generally accepted that, at least in rodents, androgens are necessary, during the fetal and/or early neonatal life, to masculinize the hypothalamic centers that control the male-type patterns of gonadotropin and growth hormone secretion *(24)*, as well as

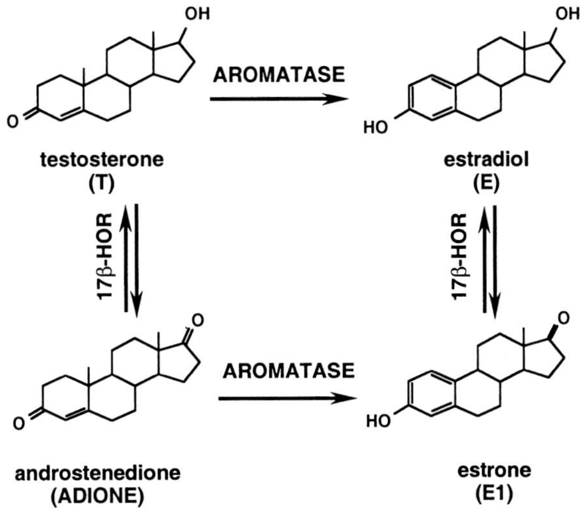

Fig. 1. The aromatase/17β-hydroxysteroid oxidoreductase (17β-HOR) pathways.

those that supervise the expression of male sexual behavior *(25,27)*. Recent data show that this "organizational" effect of androgens may also be present in other species (*see* ref. *28*). A theory, which is now universally accepted holds that the masculinizing effect of androgens is linked to their aromatization to estrogens *(1)*, a process that occurs in several regions of the brain, and especially in the hypothalamus and in the limbic system. In line with this theory, a high aromatizing activity has been found in the medial preoptic area (MPOA) of the hypothalamus, in the sexually dimorphic hypothalamic nucleus, in the limbic system and in the amygdala of fetal and/or neonatal rats and mice *(29–33)*. Estrogens may "masculinize" the brain because of their properties to influence neuronal survival and plasticity, to promote neuronal growth and dendrite arborization, and to facilitate the formation of synapses among hypothalamic neurons *(34,35)*. The conversion of T and androstenedione (ADIONE) into estrogens is also important in some species for inducing some aspects of sexual behavior in adulthood *(27)*.

Mechanism of Reaction

The P450aro is an enzymatic complex that interacts with T and ADIONE, two physiological substrates, with high affinity (n*M* range for both steroids), and that converts these Δ4-3 keto-androgens into estrogens (E and estrone [E1], respectively) (*see* Fig. 1). The process is linked to a still incompletely characterized series of reactions, which are known to occur in a single catalytic site. The final step of these reactions is the aromatization of the A ring of androgens to form the phenolic ring typical of estrogens *(36)*. The full reaction involves three hydroxylations, each requiring a mole of oxygen and a mole of nicotinamide-adenine-dinucleotide phosphate (NADPH) *(37)*. The last step appears to be nonenzymatic, and results in the concomitant loss of the C19 methyl group, in the stereospecific transfer of the 1β-hydrogen to the aqueous medium, and in the formation of the phenolic A-ring *(38)*. This property is now generally used to measure the activity of the enzyme in biological samples (e.g., tissue homogenates, subcellular fractions, cell cultures, and so forth), and it is referred to as the tritiated water method *(13,37,39,40)*;

this because the amounts of tritiated water released are equimolar to those of the estrogens formed from the [^{3}H]-labeled precursor used (normally, [1β-^{3}H]ADIONE).

Structural and Biochemical Properties of the P450aro

The P450aro is a membrane-bound enzyme localized in the endoplasmic reticulum; it is present in the brain, in the gonads (both in the ovary and in the testis), as well as in several extragonadal tissues (e.g., the human placenta, the adipose tissue, the skin) (*see* ref. *41*).

The enzyme is the product of the CYP19 gene, and is a member of the P450 cytochrome superfamily. In humans, it consists of a protein of 503 amino acids with an apparent molecular weight of about 58 kDa *(42)*. Associated to the enzyme, is the flavoprotein NADPH-cytochrome P450 reductase, which is responsible for transferring the reducing equivalents from NADPH to the P450aro *(43)*.

Studies on the amino-acid sequence of the P450aro, derived from the corresponding cDNA, revealed that the catalytic site is located towards the carboxy terminal of the protein, in a region rich in cysteine residues able to bind the heme iron. Near the heme-binding region, there is a portion (I-helix) which is believed to form the substrate-binding pocket. The putative membrane-spanning domain, characterized by a region of high hydrophobic amino acids, is located towards the amino-terminus of the protein. Site-directed mutagenesis experiments have revealed that the region between the amino acids 10 and 20 is critical for the conformational integrity of the enzyme *(42,44)*.

The CYP19 gene is located on the long arm of the chromosome 15, spans at least 70 kb, and is composed of 10 exons, the first of which (exon I) is untranslated *(45)*. The translation start site (ATG) is located in exon II, and the sequence encoding the open reading frame is identical in all tissues. Because of this, the aromatase proteins expressed in the various tissues have the same amino acid sequence. Owing to the high conservation of the protein during phylogenesis, there is a high degree of homology among the different species: for instance, 77, 81, and 73% between the human P450aro on one side and the rat, the mouse and the chicken enzymes on the other *(46,47)*. The possible existence of two different P450aro isoforms has been described only in pigs *(48)*.

The identity of the structure of the P450aro in the different tissues does not correspond to an analogous identity of the mRNAs coding for the protein. In some tissues (e.g., the human placenta, mouse and rat ovaries) the use of alternative splicing during the mRNA processing gives rise to P450aro transcripts of different length. In particular, three different mRNA species have been demonstrated in the rat ovary *(49)*; among these, only the largest one seems to be able to produce a functional protein, because the two smaller species lack the heme-binding domain coding region, and contain an unspliced intron. However, these two transcripts have not been identified in brain structures *(31)*. A high degree of heterogeneity has been demonstrated in the 5'-untranslated region of exon I. Exon I presents several subtypes (named exon I.a, I.b, and so forth, or, alternatively, I.1, I.2, and so forth) *(47,50–52)* which can be alternatively utilized for the synthesis of the different mRNA species in the various tissues. Moreover, the expression of tissue-specific P450aro transcripts occurs through the alternative utilization of multiple and distinct promoters located upstream to each exon subtype. Studies on the human, monkey, and rat brains have revealed that the major P450aro transcript of the hypothalamus and of the amygdala possesses an unique exon I (exon I-f), which is now considered the brain-specific one *(50–52)*. In the human brain, it has been found that the promoter region of exon I.f contains putative TATA and CAAT boxes (which participate in the initiation of the transcription), as well as a consensus sequence for Ad4, a factor involved in the regulation of the genes of all steroidogenic enzymes. Moreover, the analysis of the DNA sequence of this promoter region revealed the presence of a potential androgen/glucocorticoid binding site at about 300 bp upstream from exon I.f *(50)*. It is noteworthy that, both in humans and in rodents, the same promoter seems to be used for the transcription of the P450aro gene in the hypothalamus as well as in the amygdala. Because it is known that the expression of the enzyme is regulated in a different fashion by sex steroids in these two structures (*see* refs. *26* and *52*; also next section), it might be hypothesized that these brain regions possess structural and functional peculiarities (e.g., neuronal inputs, cell-specific transacting factors, and so forth), which could explain this phenomenon. Yamada-Mouri and coworkers *(52)* have recently confirmed that, in the CNS, the amount of P450aro mRNA derived from the "brain-specific" exon I-f predominates over other types of P450aro mRNA carrying the information of other types of exons I *(51)*. They have also shown that the ratio of the P450aro mRNA derived from exon I.f over the total P450aro mRNA is higher in the amygdala than in the hypothalamus. This observation further strengthens the region-specific regulation of the expression of this enzyme.

Distribution in the Brain

The regional distribution within the brain of the P450aro has been extensively investigated in different animal species by enzymatic activity assays, immunohistochemistry, and *in situ* hybridization techniques *(26,53,54)*. It has been demonstrated clearly that the enzyme has a discrete distribution, being mainly localized in brain areas (like the hypothalamus, the preoptic area, and the limbic system) involved in the control of reproductive functions. In particular, Jakab and coworkers *(55)*, using a purified polyclonal antiserum raised against the human placental P450aro, have identified, in the rat brain, two anatomically separate P450aro-immunoreactive areas: a "limbic-telencephalic system" including the lateral septal area, the bed nucleus of the stria terminalis, and the amygdaloid nuclei; and an "hypothalamic system," containing the paraventricular, lateral, and dorsomedial hypothalamic nuclei, as well as the MPOA and the ventral striatum. Interestingly, the same authors *(55)* have shown that the limbic-telencephalic system is apparently unresponsive to changes of the sex steroid "milieu," whereas the hypothalamic system is sensitive to steroid hormones. The exact physiological role of E formed in the limbic area is unknown, but it might be important for the control of synaptogenesis, of neuronal sprouting, and related phenomena *(56)*. On the contrary, the presence of P450aro-containing neurons in the septal area of adult rats *(57)* and birds *(58)* underlines the possibility that estrogens locally formed in this area might be involved in the activation of sexual and aggressive behavior in adult animals. Sanghera and coworkers *(29)* have detected an elevated P450aro immunoreactivity also in the reticular thalamic nucleus, the olfactory tract, and the piriform cortex; the significance of the presence of the P450aro in these regions is unclear, but it cannot be excluded that the enzyme might be involved in the modulation of some neuroendocrine functions, owing to the strict links between olfactory cues and reproductive phenomena.

The cellular and subcellular localization of the P450aro and of its expression has been extensively studied in the CNS and in cell cultures derived from the brain of different animal species, using radioenzymatic assays, immunohistochemical *(29,56,58–62)*, and *in situ* hybridization techniques *(54)*, as well as the reverse transcription-polymerase chain reaction (RT-PCR) technology *(63)*. In particular, studies performed in our laboratory using a radio-enzymatic assay on well-characterized primary cultures of different rat brain cell populations have demonstrated that only neurons are able to aromatize androgens, whereas astrocytes and oligodendrocytes (two components of the glia) are completely devoid of such an activity *(40)*. Experiments performed more recently using RT-PCR on the same types of cultures have confirmed that neurons are the only cells expressing the enzyme *(63)*. However, it is interesting to note that the P450aro does not appear to be present in the hypothalamic neurons synthetizing LHRH, as shown by studies in the GT1-1 cells *(13)*.

The absence of the aromatizing enzyme in glial cell might appear surprising, in view of the fact that the estrogen receptor and its messenger have been shown to be present in these cells *(17,64)*. An observation performed on enriched glial cell cultures of the developing Zebra Finch telencephalon, indicates that the P450aro might be present also in non-neuronal cells *(65)*; differences among species may explain the discrepancy. Within neurons, P450aro immunoreactivity has been localized mainly in the perikarya and in the cytoplasm of neuronal processes; the enzyme appears to be strictly associated with the membrane of the endoplasmic reticulum *(53,58,61)*. In the quail, P450aro activity and immunoreactivity have been recently found to be present in presynaptic endings *(66)*. This could suggest a possible role of locally formed estrogens in modulating neurotransmission at least in avian species; however, in the rat brain, P450aro activity is significantly lower in synaptosomal preparations than in total brain homogenates *(61)*.

The co-localization of P450aro and estrogen receptors has been studied immunohistochemically with dual-labeling techniques both in mice *(67)* and in quails *(30,68)*. The two proteins appear to be co-localized in the majority of fetal and neonatal neurons of the mouse, whereas conflicting results have been obtained in the quail. Moreover, estrogen receptors are found not only in neurons, but also in ependymal and in glial cells *(17)*, which do not express the P450aro. Therefore, estrogens appears to be able to exert in the brain both autocrine and paracrine effects.

PRE- AND POSTNATAL DEVELOPMENT

Because aromatization of androgens appears to be mandatory not only for the sexual differentiation of the brain towards male patterns, but also for the control of male sexual behavior in adulthood, many studies have been devoted to identify possible sex-specific differences in the expression and in the activity of the P450aro during development and in adult animals. It is generally agreed that, in the perinatal period, the levels of the enzyme are more elevated in the male than in the female brain *(60,69,70)*, apparently because the number of neurons expressing the P450aro is higher in males *(60)*. It is also agreed that, in general, the expression of the P450aro is higher in the perinatal rather than in the adult brain *(31,71,72)*. This appears to be true also in human beings, as shown by Honda and coworkers *(50)* using a quantitative RT-PCR analysis.

It must be noted, however, that the developmental time course of the P450aro (expression and bioactivity) is different in the various regions of the brain. In the preoptic/hypothalamic area of the fetal rat, both P450aro activity and mRNA appear on gestational days (GD)15/16, peak on GD 19/20, and gradually decrease during the perinatal period (GD21-22) to reach the low levels observed in adult animals *(31,54,55)*. By contrast, P450aro mRNA in the bed nucleus of the stria terminalis and in the amygdala does not decrease in the perinatal period, but remains high throughout development and in adulthood (*see* ref. *73*).

REGULATION OF THE P450ARO BY SEX STEROIDS

During Embryogenesis. The aforementioned patterns of P450aro activity and expression during embryogenesis suggest that, in the brain, this enzyme should be highly regulated. However, the factors involved in such regulation are still poorly understood. Because of the close temporal relationships between the secretion of T from the fetal testes and the expression of the P450aro in the CNS, many studies have been performed to assess the possible androgenic dependence of the central enzyme. The data present in the literature are conflicting. Lephart and coworkers *(74)*, using rat fetal hypothalamic explants maintained in vitro for 48 h, showed that T and 5α-DHT induce a significant and dose-dependent decrease in the P450aro activity; this effect seems to be linked to androgens acting as such, because under identical incubation conditions and steroid concentrations, E, PROG, and corticosterone were ineffective. On the contrary, Beyer and coworkers *(75)*, studying the P450aro activity in cultured mouse hypothalamic neurons, found that the addition of T was able to increase the formation of estrogens, an effect that could be blocked by flutamide, a potent androgen-receptor antagonist. Finally, in our *(73)* and other *(62)* laboratories, it has been shown that T and 5α-DHT, added at different doses and for different periods of time to rat hypothalamic or mouse diencephalic neuronal cultures, do not exert any significant influence on the P450aro (measured as biological activity or as mRNA expression). These conflicting results are probably due to differences in the animal species used, in the sex of the animals, in the experimental approaches, in the methodologies used, and so forth.

Nonsteroidal factors released by neurons, or by glial elements, may also modulate the expression of the P450aro, possibly in conjunction with androgens. In this context, it is interesting to recall that, in the brain, the P450aro can be modulated by factors causing either an increase of the formation of cAMP *(31)*, or the activation of the protein kinase C pathway *(73)*. Aromatization appears to be inhibited by 8-Br-cAMP or by β-receptor stimulation (known to be functionally coupled with the formation of cAMP *[31,76]*), suggesting that the increase of the noradrenergic activity observed in the perinatal period may induce the suppression of the P450aro occurring in the preoptic/hypothalamic area immediately after birth. This hypothesis, however, deserves further investigation, because cAMP has also been shown to enhance *(77)*, or not to modify *(73)* the neonatal brain P450aro.

Beyer and Hutchison *(78)* have investigated whether androgens could influence the morphological differentiation of hypothalamic P450aro-positive neurons in the mouse. Androgen treatment, unlike estrogen, stimulated the morphological differentiation of cultured embryonic hypothalamic P450aro-positive cells by increasing neurite outgrowth and branching, soma size, and the number of stem processes. This effect appeared to be brain region- and transmitter phenotype-specific: neither cortical P450aro-positive neurons nor hypothalamic GABAergic neurons responded to androgens. Moreover, the morphogenetic effects exerted by T appeared to depend on the activation of the AR, because these were completely inhibited by flutamide. Estrogen formation apparently is not involved in this phenomenon, because the antiestrogen tamoxifen was totally inefficient. Surprisingly, these studies *(78)* have not considered whether 5α-reduced steroids (e.g., 5α-DHT) might be more potent than T in inducing such an effect. In fact, it is known that the enzyme 5α-R is present in the hypothalamic neurons (*see* the section "5α-R Distribution in the Brain"). Moreover, double-labeling of hypothalamic P450aro-positive neurons revealed a considerable number of cells co-expressing AR and ER; on the contrary, cortical P450aro-positive cells did not label for AR *(78)*. These data clearly suggest that androgens may function as direct morphogenetic signals for the developing hypothalamic P450aro-positive cells.

In Adulthood. The influence of androgens on brain P450aro in pubertal *(72)* and adult animals has been extensively studied in different animal species *(79,80)*. These studies have been mainly performed evaluating the effect of androgen deprivation and of the subsequent androgen replacement on the activity and/or the expression of the enzyme. There is a general agreement on the dependence of the P450aro on the androgenic status of the animal. Castration is able to decrease, in the CNS, both P450aro activity and mRNA levels, whereas the treatment of castrated animals with T is able to bring back the enzyme to normal titers. T probably acts at transcriptional level, because it increases both the P450aro mRNA *(81,82)* and the number of cells showing positive immunoreactivity *(83)*. Moreover, the action of T is receptor-mediated, because male rats genetically insensitive to androgens, because of an AR mutation, possess very low P450aro activity in the brain despite normal circulating T levels.

At present, it has not been fully elucidated whether these effects of T in the brain of adult animals are linked to an action of the native form of the hormone or whether they need its conversion into 5α-reduced metabolites or into estrogens. Roselli *(84)* has found that the treatment of castrated rats with 5α-DHT results in an increased P450aro activity in the preoptic area, which, however, remains lower than that obtained after T administration; an enzymatic activity similar to that measured after T treatment has been obtained by the simultaneous administration of 5α-DHT plus E, even if E alone has no effect on either P450aro activity *(84)* or expression *(82)*. The possible synergistic effect of androgenic and estrogenic T metabolites has been confirmed also in the avian brain by immunocytochemistry and quantitative RT-PCR *(83)*. The results obtained both in rats and birds suggest that, at least in some brain areas, the local formation of both series of active metabolites of T is needed for the regulation of the transcription of brain P450aro. The synergistic effect of E and 5α-DHT on P450aro expression might be explained by the fact that estrogens are able to increase not only the concentration of AR in the brain *(83)*, but also the duration of receptor occupancy *(85)*. The effect of estrogens appears to be different in the mouse diencephalon; in fact, the administration of E to gonadectomized mice decreases the amount of P450aro mRNA in the structures considered *(86)*.

5α- AND 3α-HOR

A large body of data has shown that the enzymatic complex formed by the 5α-R and the 3α-HOR is present in the CNS (*see* refs. *28* and *87*). This system is very versatile, in the sense that every steroid possessing the Δ4-3keto configuration may be first 5α-reduced and subsequently 3α-hydroxylated (Fig. 2). In this chapter, the discussion will be limited only to the metabolism of those steroids that have been studied in some detail. These include T which can be converted into 5α-DHT and subsequently into 5α-andros-tane-3α,17β-diol (3α,5α-diol); PROG, which is metabolized into dihydroprogesterone (5α-DHPROG) and subsequently into 3α,5α-THPROG, and DOC, which can be transformed into 5α-dihydrodeoxycorticosterone (5α-DHDOC) and finally into 3α,5α-

THDOC (*see* Fig. 2). For clarity's sake, the data on the two families of enzyme (5α-R and 3α-HOR) will be presented and discussed separately, even if in many physiological conditions, they work jointly or in sequence.

General Consideration on the 5α-Reductases

It is well known that the transformation of T into 5α-DHT by the NADPH-dependent enzyme, 5α-R, has an established physiological role in peripheral androgen-dependent structures, and especially in the control of the development and function of the prostate. The intracellular formation of 5α-DHT precedes the binding of this 5α-reduced steroid to the AR, allowing the receptor-mediated activation of target genes. In the prostate, this metabolic transformation is a mechanism of amplification of the androgenic signal, since 5α-DHT possesses an affinity for the AR about four times higher than that of T *(88-91)*. Moreover, the activated AR appears to be more stable when 5α-DHT is bound *(90,91)*, because this compound exhibits a fivefold slower dissociation rate from the AR than T. 5α-DHT is consequently able to activate transcription at concentrations significantly lower than those of its precursor.

As previously mentioned, all steroids possessing a Δ4-3keto structure (androgens, PROG, and adrenal steroids) are substrates for the 5α-R, although with different affinities. For both isozymes (*see* next section), in the rat and in humans, the Kms for the main circulating representatives of the different classes of hormonal steroids rank in the following order: P > T > corticosterone = cortisol.

The reduction of the substrates to their dihydro forms is achieved by the stereospecific hydride transfer from the β-position of NADPH to the αC5 position of the steroid, yielding the enolate, which is then protonated by the medium, giving the saturated 3-ketone *(92,93)*. The 5α-reduction of the A ring is an irreversible process, and allows the subsequent 3α- or 3β-reduction of the 3-oxo group by the 3α-HOR or 3β-HOR; whereas the 3α-hydroxylation may give active steroids, the 3β-hydroxylation brings to the formation of inactive compounds *(28)*. In general, the reduction of the 3 position decreases the binding affinity to the intracellular receptors. In cooperation with other enzymes (*see* section "Other Steroid Metabolizing Enzymes"), the 5α-R/3α-HOR system may then participate in the catabolism of high concentrations of potentially neurotoxic steroids (e.g., the glucocorticosteroids, which may induce apoptotic processes on selected neuronal populations of the hippocampus). However, some 5α-reduced-3α-hydroxysteroids may exert important biological effects different from those of the parent steroids (*see* section "General Consideration on the 3α-HOR). The process of 5α-reduction in itself may play an important role for protecting the brain and several other structures (e.g., the blood vessels) from the damaging effects of an excess of estrogens *(94–96)*, this by utilizing and consequently eliminating the substrates (T and DIONE) of the P450aro. (*See* refs. *97* and *98* for further details.)

Structure and Biochemical Properties of the 5α-Reductase Isozymes

The existence of more than one 5α-R isozymes had been postulated years ago on the basis of studies utilizing various inhibitors *(99,100)*, and different substrates *(99)*. More recently, two isoforms of the 5α-R (called type 1 and type 2) have been cloned in humans, rat, and monkey *(101–106)*. In humans, the type 1 5α-R gene is composed of five exons and four introns and produces a protein of 259 amino acids. The type 2 5α-R gene has a similar structure, but the resulting protein is composed of 254 aminoacids. The structures of the enzymatic proteins, determined from their respective cDNAs, show a limited degree of homology (about 47%), and a predicted molecular weight of 28–29 kDa. The homology between the human and rat enzymes is 60% for the type 1, and 77% for the type 2 isozyme. The monkey isoforms are structurally and functionally more similar to their respective human counterparts. In terms of primary structures, both isozymes are composed of a high number of hydrophobic aminoacid residues, distributed throughout the molecule; this strongly imposes the localization of the enzymes in cell membranes (*see* this section). Consensus sequences for the binding of substrates similar to those present in other reducing enzymes have not been found in either isozyme, but mutational analysis has permitted to localize the region of substrate binding in the N-terminal portion of the protein, which is encoded by the first exon; the binding site for NADPH, the cofactor of the 5α-R, appears to be located in the C-terminal portion of the protein, a region encoded by the 4th and 5th exon. However, the exact location of both domains has not been defined, because amino acids relevant for the maintenance of a correct affinity for the substrate have been identified also in the C-terminal region of the molecule (*105*). Heterogeneity of the rat type 1 enzyme has been recently described and a cDNA coding for a 5α-R type 1b with four additional amino acids in the amino terminal region has been cloned (*107*). This protein shows a higher affinity for the various substrates than the shorter one, particularly in the case of cortisol for which the Km is decreased 7.5 fold; the decrease observed in the case of T and PROG is only 4.5-fold.

Despite the fact that the two major isoforms of the 5α-R (types 1 and 2) catalyze the same reaction (e.g., T to 5α-DHT, PROG to 5α-DHT, and so forth), they possess different biochemical and possibly functional properties.

In rats, the affinity of T for the type 1 isoform is about 15–20-fold lower than that determined for the type 2 isoform. The difference in affinity is still evident in the case of the human enzymes, but is less marked. Both in rat and in humans, the capability of reducing the substrate is much higher in the case of the type 1 isoform.

The two isoforms have a different pH optimum: the type 1 isoform is active in a wide range of pH (from 5–8), whereas the type 2 5α-R possesses a narrow pH optimum around 5, with a very low activity at pH 7.5. The two isozymes show also a differential sensitivity to synthetic inhibitors designed, like finasteride, to block the human type 2 isozyme (*108*), as well as to those not specifically designed for this isozyme (*109*). Finasteride interacts with four amino acid residues present in the N-terminal region of the protein (*108*). Little is known on the efficacy of "selective" 5α-R type 1 inhibitors on the rat and human type 2 isozymes.

The human type 1 gene (gene symbol SRD5A1) is located at the extreme tip of the short arm (p15) of chromosome 5. An apparently nonfunctional pseudogene, lacking introns and containing a premature translation termination codon, is present on the long arm of the X chromosome. The human type 2 gene (gene symbol SRD5A2) is present on the short arm of chromosome 2. The exon-intron structures of the two functional genes is identical, indicating an ancient gene duplication. In humans, the type 1 gene appears to be expressed at high levels in the liver and in the nongenital skin, and at low levels in the androgen target tissues (*105*). In the rat, the expression of this isoform is widely distributed throughout the various genital and nongenital tissues, with the highest levels in the liver. Both in rat and in humans, the type 2 isoform is concentrated especially in androgen-dependent structures, such as the epididymis (especially in the basal cells), the seminal vesicles, the genital skin, and the prostate, where it is mostly present in the stromal component. Only small amounts of 5α-R type 2 have been detected in other tissues. On the contrary, the type 1 isoform appears to be mainly located in the prostatic epithelial cells *(105,110)*.

There is no doubt that, in the prostate, a structure that contains both the type 1 and type 2 isozymes, the most relevant isozyme is represented by the type 2 isoform. The presence in human of a genetically determined ineffective type 2 isoform produces a syndrome of male pseudohermaphroditism (named after Imperato-McGinley) characterized by aplasia of the prostate and ambiguity of the external genitalia *(111,112)*. It is obvious that, in this pathological condition, the presence of a normal type 1 isozyme is unable to counteract the consequences of the abnormality of the type 2 isoform. No genetic deficiency syndromes of the type 1 isozyme have been described up to now in humans. In transgenic mice showing a 5α-R type 1 deficiency, a significant decrease in the number of live fetuses has been observed; this is apparently owing to an increased formation of estrogens, because the phenomenon can be reversed by antiestrogens administered to the mothers *(97,98)*.

Several studies have been performed to determine the subcellular localization of the 5α-Rs, but the results are not very consistent. However, in all cases, the enzyme appears to be strongly associated to cellular membranes (cytoplasmic or nuclear). A possible different subcellular localization of the two isozymes has been proposed by fractionation studies performed, in the authors' laboratory, on yeast cells genetically transformed to specifically produce the two rat isozymes. The data have shown that the type 1 isozyme is associated to the nuclei, whereas the type 2 isozyme is present in the microsomal fractions *(113)*.

Distribution in the Brain

Several studies indicate that an active 5α-R/3α-HOR system is present in the brain of several animal species. The majority of these studies have been performed before the existence of the two isozymes was known, and the data have been mainly obtained by measuring the activity of the 5α-R in the various tissue samples at pH 7.5. As previously mentioned, at this pH only the type 1 isozyme is fully functional, because the type 2 isoform has a pH preference in the acidic region. Because of this, the "old" information may be taken as indicative of the existence in the brain of the type 1 enzyme. This has been confirmed, after the cloning of the gene coding for the type 1 isoform, by demonstrating that the kinetic constants for the enzymes localized in the hypothalamus *(114)*, in the cerebral cortex, in the subcortical white matter, and in purified myelin membranes of adult male rats *(115)* are very similar to those of the recombinant type 1 isoform expressed in mammalian cells or in yeast cells, independently on whether T or PROG was used as the substrate *(113,116)*. However, these data do not exclude that the type 2 enzyme also might be present in the brain since its activity might have been masked by the higher capability of conversion typical of the type 1 isoform. It is also possible that the type 2 isozyme could be expressed only in some specific brain structure(s), or during some particular phases of life *(see* this section).

Because the majority of the data on the 5α-R present in the brain (evaluated as biological activity) have been reviewed in previous publications from this laboratory *(28,87,116,122)*, only the most relevant findings and the more recent developments will be discussed.

The formation of 5α-DHT from T has been reported to be several times higher in brain structures mainly composed of white matter (corpus callosum, midbrain tegumentum, and so forth) than in the cerebral cortex *(115,117–122)*. Further studies have linked this activity to the presence of myelin, and purified myelin shows a 5α-R activity about eight times higher than that of brain homogenates *(123)*. As previously mentioned, this activity may be attributed to the type 1 isozyme *(115)*, a finding that as been recently demonstrated using a specific polyclonal antibody raised against a synthetic peptide reproducing an antigenic/hydrophilic sequence of the type 1 isoform *(117)*. A strong specific immunostaining of the myelin sheaths of axons present in the optic chiasm has been demonstrated. The physiological meaning of the presence of the 5α-R in the myelin is still obscure at the moment, but the hypothesis that 5α-reduced steroids locally formed in the myelin might play a role in the process of myelination is certainly attractive. Such an hypothesis is indirectly supported by the data showing that there are peaks of 5α-R activity in the rat CNS *(124,125)* and in the purified CNS myelin in the first weeks of life *(115,123)*, at the time of the initiation of the process of myelinization *(126)*. Moreover, the cells that manufacture the myelin, the oligodendrocytes, possess some 5α-R activity.

The distribution of the 5α-R activity in the different cell types from the rat brain has already been analyzed *(63,127)* and it was observed that fetal rat neurons possess significantly higher amounts of 5α-R activity than neonatal oligodendrocytes and astrocytes, in the order *(28,128)*. Among glial cells, the type-2 astrocytes possess a considerable 5α-R activity, whereas type-1 astrocytes are almost devoid of activity. The enzyme 3α-HOR appears to be mainly localized in type 1 astrocytes *(128)*. The compartmentalization of two strictly correlated enzymes, the 5α-R and the 3α-HOR, in separate CNS cell populations suggests the simultaneous participation of neurons and glial cells in the 5α-reductive metabolism of T and other Δ4-3 keto steroids. Therefore, neurons are the cell population in which both the 5α-R and the P450aro *(40,63)* are present, indicating that probably the most important effects of androgens take place in neurons. Moreover, studies performed on undifferentiated stem cells originating from the mouse striatum demonstrated the presence of relevant 5α-R/3α-HOR activity *(129)*. During differentiation of these cells, the 5α-R activity increases significantly as time progresses, but at different time intervals for T and PROG conversion. The 5α-DHPROG formation peaks on day 7, whereas that of 5α-DHT increases only after 14 days of differentiation. Several explanation for this divergence are possible, like the presence of a third 5α-R with a high substrate specificity for PROG *(130)*.

Very few studies have been specifically dedicated thus far to analyze the distribution in the brain of the two 5α-R isozymes. In adult humans (postmortem samples of the cerebellum, hypothalamus, pons, and medulla oblongata), the combined results of immunoblotting with 5α-R polyclonal antisera, and of RNA blot hybridization, has indicated that apparently only the type 1 enzyme is present *(131,132; see* also *122* for review). However, in another study, the immunostaining of autopsy specimens has shown the presence of the type 2 enzyme in the pyramidal cells of the cerebral cortex *(132)*. Unpublished results of the authors' laboratory indicate the presence of the RNA coding for both isoforms in the human gray and white matters in samples of the temporal lobe obtained at surgery (Poletti A., Negri-Cesi P., Celotti F., Oppizzi G., Martini L., unpublished observations).

The expression/production of the two isoforms has also recently been studied on the whole brain of the rat. Some authors have shown that specific mRNAs coding for both isoforms *(104)* are detectable using Northern analysis on total RNA obtained from the whole brain of adult male rats; however, other authors have demonstrated that in the whole adult rat brain, the type 1 isoform is largely preponderant *(130)*. A recent study performed in the authors' laboratory using RT-PCR suggests that only the 5α-R type 1 might be present in the brain, because the mRNA coding for this isozyme has been found in cultured rat brain cells exclusively *(63)*. Obviously, data obtained in vitro are not fully demonstrative because of the absence of local and systemic influences. In line with this comment, a recent study performed in the authors' laboratory on the whole rat brain obtained at different stages of development (including adulthood) has shown the presence of high levels of type 1 mRNA at all ages examined, with an increase just before the time of birth *(133)*; this finding agrees with previous observations *(28,130)*. On the contrary, the expression of the type 2 isoform appears to be linked to specific times, being maximal in the perinatal period and almost undetectable in adulthood *(133)*. In a separate study, the type 2 mRNA has been found present in the hypothalamus and in the hippocampus *(134)* of adult animals. The observation that the type 2 isoform is transiently expressed in the whole brain during the late fetal and early postnatal life suggests that the enzyme may play some role in the process of sexual differentiation of the brain. During the sexual organization of the brain, a phenomenon mainly dominated by aromatization (*see* section "General Consideration on the P450aro") some regulatory role may be exerted also by 5α-DHT. The organizational effects of 5α-DHT appear limited, however, to some selected neuronal populations. For instance, 5α-DHT has been shown to induce, in male rat, a decrease of the volume of the sexually dimorphic nucleus of the accessory olfactory tract *(135)* to dimensions usually found in females. Conversely, the early postnatal administration to female rats of androgen receptor antagonists produces an increment of this nucleus to volumes not dissimilar to those found in males *(135)*. Moreover, in male rats, 5α-DHT is needed, together with estrogens, for a full development in the masculine direction of the sexually dimorphic spinal nucleus of the bulbocavernosus *(136–139)*. In amphibians (e.g., the bullfrog, *Rana catesbeiana*), 5α-DHT is responsible for the maintenance of the sexual dimorphism of the pretrigeminal nucleus *(140)*. The direct participation of androgens in the sexual differentiation of the brain is also supported by the fact that the number of AR is higher in the perinatal brain of male rats than in that of females *(141–143)*, and act as important morphogenetic signals for the development of the hypothalamic neurons which express the P450aro *(78)*. These androgenic effects are mediated through the activation of the AR, because they are suppressed by the antiandrogen flutamide, and are not influenced by antiestrogens *(78)*.

REGULATION OF THE 5α-REDUCTASE

The physiological control of the 5α-R in the brain is an issue that has not been answered to date. The data available were obtained mainly when the existence of the two isozymes was unknown. It is generally accepted that, in the brain, the enzymatic system formed by the 5α-R/3α-HOR is not sexually dimorphic. Moreover, several data indicate that this system is not regulated by sex steroids, because castration or substitution therapies are unable to influence its activity *(28)*. This has been shown both in the whole rat brain, and in specific CNS areas. Only a few studies appear to disagree with this conclusion. An increase in the 5α-R activity has been observed after orchidectomy in the basolateral amygdala of the rhesus monkey *(144)*, but not in several other brain structures (suprachiasmatic nucleus, supraoptic nucleus, lateral hypothalamus, basolateral nuclei of the septum, and caudate nucleus) *(28)*.

Also neural imputs seem to be ineffective in regulating the activity of the 5α-R at least at hypothalamic level. This was shown in the rat by abolishing, with appropriate pharmacological manipulations, inputs reaching the hypothalamus from other brain centers. The use of reserpine, atropine, p-chlorophenylalanine, morphine, and naloxone has excluded the participation of adrenergic, serotoninergic, cholinergic, and opioid mediators, respectively. The final demonstration of the lack of participation of input transported from extrahypothalamic neurons in the control of the hypothalamic levels of the 5α-R was obtained performing total hypothalamic deafferentations. The 5α-R activity remained unchanged in the isolated hypothalamus *(145)*.

The problem of possible differences in the control of the two 5α-R isoforms has been recently approached in the authors' laboratory as a consequence of the work previously cited, which had indicated a differentiated timing of the expression of the two isoforms during the rat life. The possible androgenic control on the gene expression of the two isozymes has been analyzed in vitro on cultured hypothalamic neurons, as well as in vivo exposing the animals *in utero* to the androgen antagonist flutamide *(133)*. T treatment greatly induced the expression of the 5α-R type 2 gene in cultured hypothalamic neurons, which normally do not express this isozyme. In vivo treatment with flutamide counteracted the expression of the type 2 gene occurring, at time of birth, in the whole brains of male neonates, whose genotype was determined by evaluating the expression of SRY, a male specific gene *(133)*. When the same phenomenon was analyzed in the neonatal female brain the effect of flutamide was not present, suggesting, for the first time, a sexual dimorphism in the formation of 5α-DHT in the brain. The data also bring one to hypothesize that factors other than androgens might control the expression of the 5α-R type 2 in females. There was no effect of T or flutamide on the expression of the type 1 gene in either sex.

General Consideration on the 3α-HOR

The enzyme(s) 3α-HOR may be considered the second element of the 5α-R/3α-HOR system; as previously mentioned, the enzyme may transform 5α-DHT into 3α,5α-diol, 5α-DHPROG into 3α,5α-THPROG, and the gluco- and mineralo-corticosteroids into their corresponding tetrahydroderivatives (Fig. 2). The formation of these 3α-hydroxylated derivatives is a process that may subserve different physiological roles; this reaction may be of importance: 1. for decreasing the amounts of intracellular 5α-reduced compounds available for binding to the corresponding intracellular steroid receptors; or 2. for producing steroid derivatives that may act through nongenomic mechanisms (e.g., via the GABA$_A$ receptor). At variance with the two isoforms of the 5α-R, the enzymes involved, appear to be able to catalyze the reaction both in the oxidative and in the reductive direction. The amounts of 5α-reduced/3α-hydroxylated compounds present at any given moment in a cell are therefore dependent on the equilibrium of this reaction.

The first 3α-HOR enzyme to be purified and then cloned has been that present in the rat liver cytosol *(146–148)*. The cDNA of this enzyme codes for a protein of 322 amino acids with an estimated molecular weight of 37 kDa and catalyzes the oxidoreduction of steroids using either NADP$^+$/NADPH or NAD$^+$/NADH as cofactors.

The analysis of the kinetic mechanisms of the reaction supports the obligatory binding of the cofactor before that of the substrate. The enzyme can work both in the oxidative and in the reductive directions, but oxidation appears to be the preferential function.

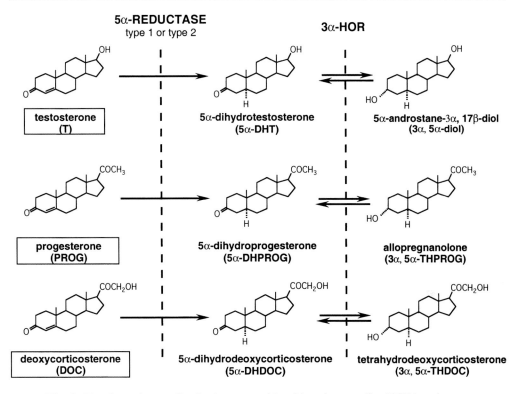

Fig. 2. The 5α-reductase/3α-hydroxysteroid oxidoreductase (3α-HOR) pathways.

The three-dimensional structure and relevant features of the rat liver cytosolic enzyme have been recently reported *(149–151)*. This enzyme shares 84% sequence similarity with the human liver dihydrodiol dehydrogenase (DD2), which is considered the human counterpart of the rat 3α-HOR *(152,153)*. The human enzyme has been defined dihydrodiol dehydrogenase because it is able to oxidize benzo(a)pyrene 7,8 epoxide to benzo(a)pyrene dihydrodiol. Also the rat enzyme possesses a similar metabolic activity on aromatic hydrocarbons. Multiple DDZ isoforms exist in the human liver, and at least three of them—DD1, DD2, and DD4—exhibit 3α-HOR activity *(153)*. The human gene is more than 47 kb in length, and contains, in the 5'-flanking region, consensus sequences for AP-1, and Oct-1 as well as multiple copies of perfect and imperfect steroid responsive elements (SRE) for the ER, and the GR/PR *(150,153)*. The rat liver enzyme has a low substrate specificity, acting both on C19 and C21 steroids and as previously mentioned, on nonsteroidal substrates.

Several metabolic studies suggest that the rat CNS possesses at least two 3α-HOR. It has indeed been shown that there are one cytosolic and one microsomal enzyme. Both types of enzymes appear to be endowed with oxidoreductase capabilities, but they might act in opposite directions *(148,154,155)*. The cytosolic form has been purified from the rat brain to apparent homogeneity *(156)* and preliminary attempts to clone it produced clones very similar to that of the liver enzyme *(153)*. The purified brain enzyme is a monomer, with an apparent molecular weight of about 31 kDa which shows a preference for NADPH, and high affinity for 5α-DHT; the enzyme shows a specific activity about 100-fold higher than that of the 5α-R type 1, indicating that in vivo it could rapidly transform the 5α-reduced compounds formed by the 5α-R *(156)*. Karavolas et al. *(155)* have isolated a cytosolic enzyme from the hypothalamus which shows an affinity for 3α,5α-THPROG much lower than that for 5α-DHPROG, indicating that the reductive activity might be its prevailing function. The brain cytosolic enzyme(s), like that of liver, is/are inhibited by all the major classes of nonsteroidal anti-inflammatory drugs *(153,156)*. Much less information is available on the microsomal 3α-HOR. This enzyme has not been purified so far; it appears to be NADH-linked with 300-fold lower affinity for 5α-DHPROG than for 3α,5α-THPROG, suggesting that the reaction may proceed in the oxidative direction *(155)*.

The distribution of the 3α-HOR(s) in the rat brain has been studied evaluating either the enzymatic activity or by immunocytochemistry (using a monoclonal antibody raised against the liver enzyme) in different brain regions *(148,153,154)*. All the data have consistently shown that the highest activities are in the olfactory bulb and in the olfactory tubercle. It has been shown that 3α-HOR is localized in astrocytes, particularly of the type 1 subfamily *(128)*. The formation of 3α,5α-diol from 5α-DHT is usually considered a mechanism of steroid catabolism, because 3α,5α-diol does not bind to the androgen receptor.

As already mentioned, some physiological metabolites formed through the 5α-R/3α-HOR pathway may interact with the GABA$_A$ receptor, and consequently may exert anxiolytic and anesthetic properties. This is particularly true for the 5α-reduced-3α-hydroxylated derivatives of PROG and DOC *(157–160)*, 3α,5α-THPROG and 3α,5α-THDOC, respectively. These two steroids are the most potent natural ligands of the GABA$_A$ receptor *(159)*, and do have potent sleep-inducing properties in rats *(161)*. Also some synthetic steroids (e.g., alphaxalone) possessing a 5α-reduced/3α-hydroxylated structure have been shown to be anxiolytic and/or hypnotic.

The role of the 5α-R in providing the 3α-HOR system with possible precursors for the final transformation into hypnotic compounds has been recently investigated using PROG as the test compound. It has been found that PROG induces a deep anesthetic effect both in male and female rats, which can be counteracted by 5α-R inhibitors (e.g., 4-MA and finasteride). These were totally ineffective when alphaxalone, nembutal, or diazepam, (agents known to interact with the GABA$_A$ receptor) were used. These results support the concept that PROG induces its anxyolytic/anesthetic effect through the formation of 5α-reduced/3α-hydroxylated compounds. These results are also supported by the recent observation that the anxiolytic effect of PROG is highly correlated with increased levels of 3α,5α-THPROG in the blood and in the brain *(162)*. It is possible that the process of 5α-reduction/3α-hydroxylation may acquire a particular physiological relevance in conditions in which the secretion of PROG and/or corticosteroids is particularly elevated (e.g., during pregnancy, in the second phase of the menstrual cycle, during stress, and so forth).

OTHER STEROID METABOLIZING ENZYMES

17β-Hydroxysteroid Oxidoreductase

The 17β-HOR intervenes bidirectionally in interconverting T and ADIONE, E and E1 (Fig. 1), and dehydroepiandrosterone and androst-5-ene-3β, 17β-diol.

At least five 17β-HOR isoenzymes, with different substrate specificity, regulation mechanisms, and individual cell-specific expression have been found in humans and

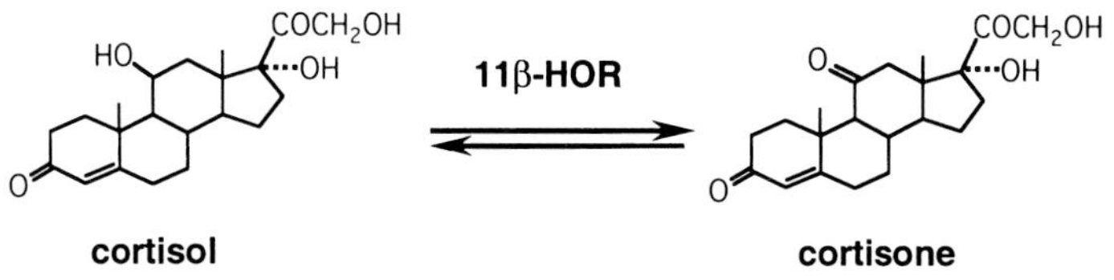

Fig. 3. The 11b-hydroxysteroid oxidoreductase (11b-HOR) pathway.

other animal species. These isozymes also differ in their reductive vs oxidative catalytic activities. 17β-HOR types 1, 3, and 5 are reductive enzymes, whereas the types 2 and 4 catalyze the reaction towards the oxidation of the substrates. High levels of 17β-HOR activity have been detected in the brain; this appears to be mainly owing to the presence of the type 1 isoform. In the rat brain, the enzyme has been detected immunocytochemically in the hypothalamus, thalamus, hippocampus, cerebral cortex, caudate-putamen, and in the pineal gland *(163)*. The enzyme seems to be present in the cytoplasm, and is active mainly in the reductive direction. Therefore, the main roles of this enzyme in the brain may be: 1. that of providing a preferential substrate (T) to the 5α-R and P450aro pathways; and 2. that to transform the E1 into the more effective E. Moreover, because both ADIONE and E1 are less potent than their precursors, this family of enzymes, acting in the oxidative direction, may decrease the androgenic and/or estrogenic exposure of the brain. It is interesting that, at variance with the P450aro and the 11β-HOR (*see* next section), the distribution of this enzyme is limited to the glia, to ependymal cells, and the tanycytes *(163)*. The parallelism with the higher presence of 3α-HOR in the glia (*see* "General Consideration on the 3α-HOR" section) reinforces the concept of an integrated function of neurons and glial cells in sex steroid metabolism.

11β-HOR

The 11β-HOR catalyzes the reaction converting the hydroxy-group in position 11 of the glucocorticosteroids (e.g., cortisol) into a ketone group (Fig. 3); by this mechanism, cortisol will be transformed into cortisone, a compound unable to bind either to the GR or to the MR. Because of this, the MR will be left free for the interaction with aldosterone, which otherwise would be prevented from reaching the MR *(164)* because the glucocorticosteroids are present in the circulation in much higher amounts. Therefore, the enzyme confers mineralocorticosteroids specificity to the MR, which, in reality, is nonselective, because it is sensitive to both glucocorticosteroids and mineralocorticosteroids. In humans, in the absence of the enzyme, the so-called "apparent mineralocortical excess syndrome," would appear *(165)*.

Two isoforms *(11β-HOR type 1 and type 2)* and some subforms of the enzyme have been described and found to be differentially expressed throughout the body. In the brain, the 11β-HOR type 1 appears to be widely expressed, with the highest levels in the cerebellum, in the hippocampus, in the hypothalamus *(166)*, and in the cerebral cortex. Detectable amounts are present also in the pituitary *(166)*. Like the P450aro, in all nervous structures considered, the enzyme 11β-HOR type 1 appears to be confined to neurons *(167)*. Its predominant role in the CNS-pituitary complex has been generally related to the control of glucocorticoid feedback effects. During the late fetal and early postnatal life, the 11β-HOR type 1 appears to be regulated by stress and glucocorticosteroids *(168)*.

The role of this isozyme in the inactivation of deleterious doses of glucocorticosteroids in the brain (*see* below this section) is controversial, because this isoform apparently exerts a predominant reductive function *(169)* facilitating the activation of inactive corticosteroids, rather than their inactivation.

The presence in the brain of the 11β-HOR type 2 has also been reported. Its distribution appears to be very limited, being apparently confined to the ventrolateral and ventromedial hypothalamus, the hippocampus, and the midbrain *(170)*. The expression of this isoform has also been found in the commissural portion of the nucleus tractus solitarius, in the subcommissural organ and in the medial vestibular nucleus. It appears, then, that the distribution in the brain of this isoform is more correlated to the major sites of action of aldosterone than that of the type 1 isoform. The midgestational fetal brain expresses high levels of 11β-HOR type 2, which therefore might modulate the effects of the gluco- and mineralocorticosteroids during brain development *(171)*. Owing to its exclusive capability of oxidation of cortisol and other glucocorticosteroids through one irreversible reaction, this enzyme is mainly viewed as protecting not only the binding of aldosterone, but also brain cells from the damage induced by excess of glucocorticosteroids owing to endogenous production (e.g., Cushings' syndrome), exogenous administration, or increased levels during stress and aging. The deleterious effects of stress and of glucocorticosteroids in the hippocampus of rats and other species are well known. Magnetic resonance imaging (MRI) technique has revealed that the hippocampal formation, a center for the organization of cognitive functions, undergoes a selective atrophy in various conditions characterized by glucocorticoid excess (*see 172*), even if those results are still debated *(173)*. Moreover, glucocorticosteroids exacerbate the effects of pathological insults (e.g., seizures, hypoxia-ischemia, and so forth) as well as those of the exposure to oxidative stress, free radicals, excitatory amino acids, and Alzheimer's disease-associated amyloid β-protein (Abeta) *(2,23,174–177)*. The direct damaging effects of glucocorticosteroids, as well as their potentiating effects on other insults, may be blocked by the specific GR antagonist RU486 *(178)*.

STs and Sulfatases

STs

STs are important especially because they increase the solubility of circulating hormonal steroids. The *sulfonation* of steroids transfers a sulfonate radical (SO_3-) to an hydroxyl-group acceptor site. Steroids in the conjugated form are usually inactive; however, they represent a "reservoir" for their ability to rapidly revert to the original hormones, through the action of STs. Some of these enzymes may also be active on drugs, xenobiotics, monoamines, neuropeptides, sphingolipids, and so forth. Several different types of ST have been described (*see* for review *179*). The most important species appear to be the following:

1. an hydroxysteroid-ST, which acts on alcohols, ascorbic acid, chloramphenicol, ephedrine, hydroxysteroids, but not on phenolic steroids (e.g., E);
2. an E1-ST, also called phenolic steroid-ST, responsible for sulfonation of the 3-hydroxyl-group of E1;
3. a steroid-ST which combines the activities of the hydroxysteroid and of the E1-ST because it acts both on E1 and E;

4. a cortisol (glucocorticosteroid)-ST, which acts on the 21-hydroxyl-group of cortisol and other glucocorticosteroids;
5. dehydroepiandrosterone-ST (DHEA-ST), which catalyzes the sulfonation of DHEA, the most abundant steroid in the circulation of humans and other primates; and
6. a chiral-specific pregnenolone-ST (PREG-ST), which acts on pregnenolone *(180)*. The E1-ST has been cloned from the human brain *(181)*.

Recently, Rajkowski et al. *(182)* have reported the presence of a DHEA-ST in the rat brain. The enzyme, however, seems to be poorly active, because it shows a Km for DHEA in the mmol range. The DHEA-ST, which is also active on PREG, is more effective in the brain of fetal animals, presenting a decreases at time of birth. A major peak of activity appears at time of puberty in both sexes, being, however, higher in females than in males.

STEROID SULFATASES (SSs)

The steroid sulfatases (SSs) catalyze the conversion of steroid sulfates into their corresponding active nonconjugated forms. Only few data are available on the action of SSs in the CNS. However, the enzymes are expressed and fully active in the brain, and their activity is maximal around birth. Moreover, in the brain of female rats the levels of SS increase dramatically after delivery and during lactation *(183)*. Recently, it has also been shown that the reduction of the metabolism of brain steroids via the blockade of the SSs activity (using the inhibitor p-*O*-(sulfamoyl)-N-tetradecanoyl tyramine), brings about an increase of memory retention. The potency of DHEAS in the scopolamine-induced amnesia test is increased by the same SS inhibitor *(184)*.

Catecholestrogens

E1 and E may be transformed into catecholestrogens through the hydroxylation of position 2 and/or 4 of the A ring (estrogen-2-hydroxylase and estrogen-2/4-hydroxylase) *(185)*. Catecholestrogens possess only a weak hormonal activity. Their major interest resides in the fact that they may be substrates of the enzyme catechol-*O*-methyl-transferase (COMT); because of this, they may interfere with the turnover of the catecholamines, and may consequently alter adrenergic transmission. This creates an additional interaction between steroids and neurotransmitters *(186,187)*.

REFERENCES

1. McEwen BS. Steroid homones are multifactorial messengers to the brain. Trends Endocrinol Metab 1991;2:62–67.
2. McEwen BS. Steroid hormone action in the brain: when is the genome involved? Horm Behav 1994;28:396–405.
3. Kuiper GGJM, Enmark E, Pelto-Huikko M, Nilsson S, Gustafsson J-A. Cloning of a novel estrogen receptor expressed in rat prostate and ovary. Proc Natl Acad Sci USA 1996;93:5925–5930.
4. Mosselman S, Polman J, Dijkema R. ERβ: identification and characterization of a novel human estrogen receptor. FEBS Lett 1996;392:49–53.
5. Tremblay GB, Tremblay A, Copeland NG, Gilbert DJ, Jenkins NA, Labrie F, Giguère V. Cloning, chromosomal localization, and functional analysis of the murine estrogen receptor β. Mol Endocrinol 1997;11:353–365.
6. Shivers BD, Harlan RE, Morrel JI, Pfaff DW. Absence of oestradiol concentration in cell nuclei of LHRH-immunoreactive neurons. Nature 1983;304:345–347.
7. Herbison AE, Theodosis DT. Localization of oestrogen receptors in preoptic neurons containing neurotensin but not tyrosine hydroxylase, cholecystokinin or luteinizing hormone-releasing hormone in the male and female rat. Neurosci 1992;50:283–298.

8. Watson RE, Langub MC, Landis JW. Further evidence that most luteinizing hormone-releasing hormone neurons are not directly estrogen-responsive: simultaneous localisation of luteinizing hormone-releasing hormone and estrogen receptor immunoreactivity in the guinea-pig brain. J Neuroendocrinol 1992;4:311–318.

9. Ahina RS, Harlan RE. Glucocorticoid receptors in LHRH neurons. Neuroendocrinol 1992; 56:845–850.

10. Huang X, Harlan RE. Absence of androgen receptors in LHRH immunoreactive neurons. Brain Res 1993;624:309–311.

11. Herbison AE, Robinson JE, Skinner DC. Distribution of Estrogen receptor-immunoreactive cells in the preoptic area of the ewe: co-localization with glutamic acid decarboxylase but not luteinizing hormone-releasing hormone. Neuroendocrinol 1993;57:751–759.

12. Lemhan MN, Karsch FJ. Do gonadotropin-releasing hormone, tyrosine hydroxylase-, and β-endorphin-immunoreactive neurons contain estrogen receptors? A double-label immunocytochemical study in the suffolk ewe. Endocrinology 1993;133:887–895.

13. Poletti A, Melcangi CR, Negri-Cesi P, Maggi R, Martini L. Steroid binding and metabolism in the luteinizing hormone-releasing hormone-producing neuronal cell line GT1-1. Endocrinology 1994;135:2623–2628.

14. Chandran UR, Attardi B, Friedman R, Dong K-W, Roberts JL, DeFranco DB. Glucocorticoid receptor-mediated repression of gonadotropin-releasing hormone promoter activity in GT1 hypothalamic cell lines. Endocrinology 1994;134:1467–1474.

15. Vielkind U, Walencewicz A, Levine JM, Bohn MC. Type II glucocorticoid receptors are expressed in oligodendrocytes and astrocytes. J Neurosci Res 1990;27:360–373.

16. Jung-Testas I, Renoir M, Bugnard H, Greene GL, Baulieu EE. Demonstration of steroid hormone receptors and steroid action in primary cultures of rat glial cells. J Steroid Biochem Mol Biol 1992;41:621–31.

17. Langub MC, Watson RE Jr. Estrogen receptor-immunoreactive glia, endothelia, and ependyma in guinea pig preoptic area and median eminence: electron microscopy. Endocrinology 1992;130:364–372.

18. Wolff JE, Laterra J, Goldstein GW. Steroid inhibition of neural microvessel morphogenesis in vitro: receptor mediation and astroglial dependence. J Neurochem 1992;58:1023–1032.

19. Jung-Testas I, Schumacher M, Robel P, Baulieu EE. Actions of steroid hormones and growth factors on glial cells of the central and peripheral nervous system. J Steroid Biochem Mol Biol 1994;48:145–154.

20. Ramirez VD, Zheng J. Membrane sex-steroid receptors in the brain. Frontiers Neuroendocrinol 1996;17:402–439.

21. Maggi R, Pimpinelli F, Casulari LA, Piva F, Martini L. Antiprogestins inhibit the binding of opioids to μ receptors in nervous membrane preparations Eur J Pharmacol 1996;301:169–177.

22. Su TP, London ED, Jaffe JH. Steroid binding at σ receptors suggests a link between endocrine, nervous and immune system. Science 1988;240: 219–221.

23. Paul SM, Purdy RH. Neuroactive steroids. FASEB J 1992;6:2311–2322.

24. Ho KY, Evans WS, Blizzard RM, Veldhuis JD, Merriam GR, Samojlik E, Furlanetto R, Rogol AD, Kaiser DL, Thorner MO. Effects of sex and age on the 24-hour profile of growth hormone secretion in man: importance of endogenous estradiol concentrations. J Clin Endocrinol Metab 1987;64:51–58.

25. Parson B, Rainbow T, McEwen BS. Organizational effects of testosterone via aromatization on feminine reproductive behavior and neural progestin receptors in rat brain. Endocrinology 1984;115:1412–1417.

26. Roselli CE, Resko JA. Aromatase activity in the rat brain: hormonal regulation and sex differences. J Steroid Biochem Mol Biol 1993;44:499–508.

27. Vagell ME, McGinnis MW. The role of aromatization in the restoration of male rat reproductive behvior. J Neuroendocrinol 1997;9:415–421.

28. Celotti F, Melcangi RC, Martini L. The 5α-reductase in the brain: molecular aspects and relation to brain function. Frontiers Neuroendocrinol 1992;13:163–215.

29. Sanghera MK, Simpson ER, McPhaul MJ, Kozlowski G, Conley AJ, Lephard ED. Immunocytochemical distribution of aromatase cytochrome P450 in the rat brain using peptide-generated polyclonal antibodies. Endocrinology 1991;129:2834–2844.

30. Balthazart J, Foidart A, Surlemont C, Harada N Distribution of aromatase immunoreactive cells in the mouse forebrain. Cell Tissue Res 1991;263: 71–79.

31. Lephart ED, Simpson ER, McPhaul MJ, Kilgore MW, Wilson JD, Ojeda SR. Brain aromatase cytochrome P-450 messenger RNA levels and enzyme activity during prenatal and perinatal development in the rat. Mol Brain Res 1992;16:187–192.

32. Wozniak A, Hutchison RE, Hutchison JB. Localisation of aromatase activity in androgen target areas of the mouse brain. Neurosci Lett 1992;146:191–194.

33. Harada N, Yamada K. Ontogeny of aromatase messenger ribonucleic acid in mouse brain: fluorimetrical quantitation by polymerase chain reaction. Endocrinology 1992;131:2306–2312.

34. Matsumoto A, Arai Y. Effect of estrogens on early postnatal development of synaptic formation in the hypothalamic arcuate nucleus of female rats. Neurosci Lett 1976;2:76–83.

35. Toran-Allerand CD. Gonadal hormones and brain development: implications for the genesis of sexual differentiation. Ann NY Acad Sci 1985;435:97–111.

36. Cole A, Robinson CH. Conversion of 19-oxo[2β-^{3}H]androgens into oestrogens by human placental aromatase. Biochem J 1990;268:553–561.

37. Thompson EA Jr , Siiteri PK. Utilization of oxygen and reduced nicotinamide adenine dinucleotide phosphate by human placental microsomes during aromatization of androstenedione. J Biol Chem 1974;249:5364–5372.

38. Fishman J, Raju MS. Mechanism of estrogen biosynthesis. J Biol Chem 1981;256:4472–4477.

39. Negri-Cesi P, Celotti F, Martini L. Androgen metabolism in the male hamster: 2. Aromatization of androstenedione in the hypothalamus and in the cerebral cortex: kinetic parameters and effect of exposure to different photoperiods. J Steroid Biochem 1989;32:65–70.

40. Negri-Cesi P, Melcangi RC, Celotti F, Martini L. Aromatase activity in cultured brain cells: difference between neurons and glia. Brain Res 1992;589:327–332.

41. Simpson ER, Merrill JC, Hollub AJ, Graham-Lorence S, Mendelson CR. Regulation of estrogen biosynthesis by human adipose cells. Endocrine Rev 1989;10:136–148.

42. Graham-Lorence S, Khalil MW, Lorence MC, Mendelson CR, Simpson ER. Structure-function relationships of human aromatase cytochrome P-450 using molecular modeling and site-directed mutagenesis. J Biol Chem 1991;266:11939–11946.

43. Simmons DL, Lalley PA, Kasper CB Chromosomal assignments of genes coding for components of mixed function oxidase system in mice. J Biol Chem 1985;260:515–521.

44. Amarneh B, Corbin CJ, Peterson JA, Simpson ER, Graham-Lorence S. Functional domains of human aromatase cytochrome P450 characterized by linear alignment and site-directed mutagenesis. Mol Endocrinol 1993;7:1617–1624.

45. Corbin JC, Graham-Lorence S, McPhaul M, Mason JI, Mendelson CR, Simpson ER. Isolation of a full-length cDNA insert encoding human aromatase system cytochrome P-450 and its expression in nonsteroidogenic cells. Proc Natl Acad Sci USA 1988;85:8948–8952.

46. Hickey GJ, Krasnow JS, Beattie WG, Richards JA. Aromatase cytochrome P450 in rat ovarian granulosa cells before and after luteinization: adenosine 3', 5'-monophosphate-dependent and independent regulation. Cloning and sequencing of rat aromatase cDNA and 5' genomic DNA. Mol Endocrinol 1990;4:3–12.

47. Simpson ER, Mahendroo MS, Means GD, Kilgore MW, Hinshelwood MM, Graham-Lorence S, Amarneh B, Ito Y, Fisher CR, Dodson MM, Mendelson CR, Bulun SE. Aromatase cytochrome P450, the enzyme responsible for estrogen biosynthesis. Endocrine Rev 1994;15:342–355.

48. Corbin CJ, Khalil MW, Conley AJ. Functional ovarian and placental isoforms of porcine aromatase. Mol Cell Endocrinol 1995;113:29–37.

49. Lephart ED, Peterson KG, Noble JF, George FW, McPhaul MJ. The structure of cDNA clones encoding the aromatase P-450 isolated from a rat Leydig cell tumor line demonstrates differential processing of aromatase mRNA in rat ovary and a neoplastic cell line. Mol Cell Endocrinol 1990;70:31–40.

50. Honda S, Harada N, Takagi Y. Novel exon 1 of the aromatase gene specific for aromatase transcripts in human brain. Biochem. Biophys Res Commun 1994;198:1153–1160.

51. Yamada-Mouri N, Hirata S, Hayashi M, Kato J. Analysis of the expression and the first exon of aromatase mRNA in monkey brain. J Steroid Biochem Mol Biol 1995;55:17–23.

52. Yamada-Mouri N, Hirata S, Kato J. Existence and expression of the untranslated first exon of aromatase mRNA in the rat brain. J Steroid Biochem. Mol Biol 1996;58:163–166.

53. Shinoda K. Brain aromatization and its associated structures. Endocrine J 1994;41:115–138.

54. Lauber ME, Lichtensteiger W. Pre- and postnatal ontogeny of aromatase cytochrome P450 messenger ribonucleic acid expression in the male rat brain studied by in situ hybridization. Endocrinology 1994;135:1661–1668.

55. Jakab RL, Horvath TL, Leranth C, Harada N, Naftolin F. Aromatase immunoreactivity in the rat brain: gonadectomy-sensitive hypothalamic neurons and an unresponsive "limbic ring" of the lateral septumbed nucleus- amygdala complex. J Steroid Biochem Molec Biol 1993;44:481–498.

56. Tsuruo Y, Ishimura K, Fujita H, Osawa Y. Immunocytochemical localization of aromatase-containing neurons in the rat brain during pre- and postnatal development. Cell Tiss Res 1994;278:29–39.

57. Jakab RL, Harada N, Naftolin F. Aromatase-(estrogen synthetase) immunoreactive neurons in the rat septal area. A light and electron microscopic study. Brain Res 1994;664:85–93.

58. Balthazart J, Foidart A, Surlemont C, Vockel A, Harada N. Distribution of aromatase in the brain of the Japanese quail, ring dove and zebra finch: an immunocytochemical study. J Comp Neurol 1990;301:276–288.

59. Balthazart J, Foidart A, Harada N. Immunocytochemical localization of aromatase in the brain. Brain Res 1990;514:327–333.

60. Beyer C, Green SJ, Barker PJ, Huskisson NS, Hutchison JB. Aromatase-immunoreactivity is localised specifically in neurones in the developing mouse hypothalamus and cortex. Brain Res 1994;638:203–210.

61. Roselli CE. Subcellular localization and kinetic properties of aromatase activity in rat brain. J Steroid Biochem Molec Biol 1995;52:469–477.

62. Abe-Dohmae S, Tanaka R, Harada N. Cell-type and region-specific expression of aromatase mRNA in cultured brain cell. Mol Brain Res 1994;24 153–158.

63. Poletti A, Negri-Cesi P, Melcangi RC, Colciago A, Martini L, Celotti F. Expression of androgen activating enzymes in cultured cells of developing rat brain. J Neurochem 1997;68:1298–1303.

64. Santagati S, Melcangi RC, Celotti F, Martini L, Maggi A. Estrogen receptor is expressed in different types of glial cells in culture. J Neurochem 1994;63:2058–2064.

65. Schlinger BA, Amur-Umarjee S, Shen P, Campagnoni T, Arnold AP. Neuronal and non-neuronal aromatase in primary cultures of developing zebra finch telencephalon. J Neurosci 1994; 14:7541–7552.

66. Balthazart J, Foidart A, Absil P, Harada N. Effects of testosterone and its metabolites on aromatase-immunoreactive cells in the quail brain: relationship with the activation of male reproductive behavior. J Steroid Biochem Mol Biol 1996;56:185–200.

67. Tsuruo Y, Ishimura K, Osawa Y. Presence of estrogen receptors in aromatase-immunoreactive neurons in the mouse brain. Neurosci Lett 1995;195:49–52.

68. Dellovade TL, Rissman EF, Thompson N, Harada N, Ottinger MA. Co-localization of aromatase enzyme and estrogen receptor immunoreactivity in the preoptic area during reproductive aging. Brain Res 1995;674:181–187.

69. Paden CM, Roselli CE. Modulation of aromatase activity by testosterone in transplants of fetal rat hypothalamus-preoptic area. Dev Brain Res 1987;33:127–133.

70. Sholl SA, Kim KL. Aromatase, 5α-reductase, and androgen receptor levels in the fetal monkey brain during early development. Neuroendocrinology 1994;52:94–98.

71. George FW, Ojeda SR. Changes in aromatase activity in the rat brain during embryonic, neonatal, and infantile development. Endocrinology 1982;111:522–529.

72. Lephart ED, Ojeda SR. Hypothalamic aromatase activity in male and female during juvenile-prepubertal development. Neuroendocrinology 1990;51:385–393.

73. Negri-Cesi P, Colciago A, Celotti F. The role of aromatase in the brain. In: Gennazzani AR, Petraglia F, Purdy RH, eds. The brain: source and target for sex steroid hormones. Parthenon, London, UK, 1996, pp. 135–149.

74. Lephart ED, Simpson ER, Ojeda SR. Effect of cyclic AMP and androgens on "in vitro" brain aromatase enzyme activity during development in the rat. J Neuroendocrinol 1992;4:29–36.

75. Beyer C, Green SJ, Hutchison JB. Androgen influence sexual differentiation of embrionic mouse hypothalamic aromatase neurons "in vitro". Endocrinology 1994;135:1220–1226.

76. Raum WJ, Marcano M, Swerdloff RS. Nuclear accumulation of estradiol derived from the aromatization of testosterone is inhibited by hypothalamic beta-receptor stimulation in neonatal female rat. Biol Reprod 1984;30:388–396.

77. Callard GV. Aromatization is cyclic AMP-dependent in cultured brain cells. Brain Res 1981;204:461–464.

78. Beyer C, Hutchison JB. Androgens stimulate the morphological maturation of embryonic hypothalamic aromatase immuno-reactive neurons in the mouse. Develop Brain Res 1997;98:74–81.

79. Resko JA, Connolly PB, Roselli CE, Abdelgadir SE, Choate JV. Selective activation of androgen receptors in the subcortical brain of male cynomolgus macaques by physiological hormone levels and its relationship to androgen-dependent aromatase activity. J Clin Endocrinol Metab 1993;76:1588–1593.

80. Fadem BH, Walters M, MacLusky NJ. Neuronal aromatase activity in a marsupial, the gray-tailed opossum (Monodelphis domestica): ontogeny during postnatal development and androgen regulation in adulthood. Dev Brain Res 1993;74:199–205.

81. Harada N, Yamada K, Foidart A, Balthazart J. Regulation of aromatase cytochrome P-450 (estrogen synthetase) transcripts in the quail brain by testosterone. Mol Brain Res 1992;15:19–26.

82. Abdelgadir SE, Resko JA, Ojeda SR, Lephart ED, McPhaul MJ, Roselli CE. Androgens regulate aromatase cytochrome P450 messenger ribonucleic acid in rat brain. Endocrinology 1994; 135:395–401.

83. Harada NH, Abe-Dohmae S, Loeffen R, Foidart A, Balthazart J. Synergism between androgens and estrogens in the induction of aromatase and its messenger RNA in the brain. Brain Res 1993;622:243–256.

84. Roselli CE. Synergistic induction of aromatase activity in the rat brain by estradiol and 5α-dihydrotestosterone. Neuroendocrinology 1991;53:79–84.

85. Roselli CE, Fasasi TE. Estradiol increases the duration of nuclear androgen receptor occupation in the preoptic area of the male rat treated with dihydrotestosterone. J Steroid Biochem Molec Biol 1992;42:161–168.

86. Yamada K, Harada N, Tamaru M, Takagi Y. Effects of changes in gonadal hormones on the amount of aromatase messenger RNA in mouse brain diencephalon. Biochem Biophys Res Commun 1993;195:462–468.

87. Poletti A, Martini L. Androgen-activating enzymes in the central nervous system. J Steroid Biochem Mol Biol 1999, in press.

88. Trapman J, Klaassen P, Kuiper GGJM, van der Korput JAGM, Faber PW, van Rooij HCJ, Van Kessel AG, Voorhorst MM, Mulder E, Brinkmann AO. Cloning, structure and expression of a cDNA encoding the human androgen receptor. Biochem Biophys Res Comm 1988;153:241–248.

89. Lubahn DB, Joseph DR, Sullivan PM, Willard HF, French FS, Wilson EM. Cloning of human androgen receptor complementary DNA and localization to the X chromosome. Science 1988;240:327–330.

90. Kovacs WJ, Griffin JE, Weaver DD, Carlson BR, Wilson, JD. A mutation that causes lability of the androgen receptor under conditions that normally promote transformation to the DNA binding state. J Clin Invest 1984;73:1095–1104.

91. Grino PB, Griffin JE, Wilson JD. Testosterone at high concentration interacts with the human androgen receptor similarly to dihydrotestosterone. Endocrinology 1990;126:1165–1172.

92. Abul-Hajj YJ. Stereospecificity of hydrogen transfer from NADPH by delta4–5α and delta4–5β reductase. Steroid 1972;20:215–222.

93. Levy MA, Brandt M, Greway AT. Mechanistic studies with solublized rat liver steroid 5α-reductase. Biochemistry 1990;29:2808–2815.

94. Brawer JR, Naftolin F, Martin J, Sonnenschein C. Effects of a single injection of estradiol valerate on the hypothalamic arcuate nucleus and on reproductive function in the female rat. Endocrinology 1978;103:501–512.

95. Brawer JR, Schipper H, Naftolin F. Ovary-dependent degeneration in the hypothalamic arcuate nucleus. Endocrinology 1980;107:274–279.

96. Naftolin F, Garcia-Segura LM, Keefe D, Leranth C, MacLusky NJ, Brawer JR. Estrogen effects on the synaptology and neural membranes of the rat hypothalamic arcuate nucleus. Biol Reprod 1990;42:21–28.

97. Mahendroo MS, Cala KM, Russell DW 5α-reduced androgens play a key role in murine parturition. Mol Endocrinol 1996;10:380–392.

98. Mahendroo MS, Cala KM, Landrum CP, Russell DW. Fetal death in mice lacking 5α-reductase type 1 caused by estrogen excess. Mol Endocrinol 1997;11:917–927.

99. Motta M, Zoppi S, Brodie AM, Martini L. Effect of 1,4,6-androstatriene–3,17-dione (ATD),4-hydroxy-4-androstene-3,17-dione (4-OH-A) and 4-acetoxy-4-androstene-3,17-dione (4-Ac-A) on the 5α-reduction of androgens in the rat prostate. J Steroid Biochem 1986;25:593–600.

100. Zoppi S, Lechuga M, Motta M. Selective inhibition of the 5α-reductase of the rat epididymis. J Steroid Biochem Mol Biol 1992;42:509–514.

101. Andersson S, Bishop RW, Russell DW. Expression and regulation of steroid 5α-reductase, an enzyme essential for male sexual differentiation. J Biol Chem 1989;264:16249–16255.

102. Andersson S, Berman DM, Jenkins EP, Russell DW. Deletion of steroid 5α-reductase 2 gene in male pseudohermaphroditism. Nature 1991;354:159–161.

103. Labrie F, Sugimoto Y, Luu-The V, Simard J, Lachance Y, Bachvarov D, Leblanc G, Durocher F, Paquet N. Structure of human type 2 5α-reductase gene. Endocrinology 1992;131:1571–1573.

104. Normington K, Russell DW. Tissue distribution and kinetic characteristics of rat steroid 5α-reductase isozymes: evidence for distinct physiological functions. J Biol Chem 1992;267:19548–19554.

105. Russell DW, Wilson JD. Steroid 5α-reductase: two genes/two enzymes. Ann Rev Biochem 1994;63:25–61.

106. Levy MA, Brandt M, Sheedy KM, Holt DA, Heaslip JI, Trill JJ, Ryan PJ, Morris RA, Garrison LM, Bergsma DJ. Cloning, expression and functional characterization of type 1 and type 2 steroid 5α-reductases from Cynomolgus monkey: comparison with human and rat isoenzymes. J Steroid Biochem Mol Biol 1995;52:307–319.

107. Lopez-Solache I, Luu-The V, Séralini G-E, Labrie F. Heterogeneity of rat type I 5α-reductase cDNA: cloning, expression and regulation by pituitary implants and dihydrotestosterone. Biochim Biophys Acta 1996;1305:139–144.

108. Thigpen AE, Russell DW. Four-amino acid segment in steroid 5α-reductase 1 confers sensitivity to finasteride, a competitive inhibitor. J Biol Chem 1992;267:8577–8583.

109. Poletti A, Rabuffetti M, Martini L. Effect of suramin on the biological activity of the two isoforms of the rat 5α-reductase. Steroids 1996;61:504–505.

110. Negri-Cesi P, Poletti A, Colciago A, Magni P, Martini P, Motta M. Presence of androgen-activating enzyme in the human prostatic cancer cell line LNCaP and in benign prostatic hyperplasia. The Prostate 1998;34:283–291.

111. Imperato-McGinley J, Guerrero L, Gautier T, Peterson RE. Steroid 5α-reductase deficiency in man: an inherited form of male pseudohermaphroditism. Science 1974;186:1213–1215.

112. Katz MD, Cai L, Zhu Y, Herrera C, DeFillo-Ricart M, Shackleton CHL, Imperato-McGinley J. The biochemical and phenotypic characterization of females homozygous for 5α-reductase-2 deficiency. J Clin Endocrinol Metab 1995;80:3160–3167.

113. Poletti A, Celotti F, Motta M, Martini L. Characterization and subcellular localization of rat 5α-reductases type 1 and type 2 expressed in yeast Saccharomyces cerevisiae. Biochem J 1996;314:1047–1052.

114. Campell JS, Karavolas HJ. The kinetic mechanism of the hypothalamic progesterone 5α-reductase. J Steroid Biochem 1989;32:283–289.

115. Poletti A, Celotti F, Melcangi RC, Ballabio M, Martini L. Kinetics properties of the 5αlpha-reductase of testosterone in the purified myelin, in the sub-cortical white matter, and in the cerebral cortex of the male rat brain. J Steroid Biochem 1990;35:97–101.

116. Poletti A, Rabuffetti M, Celotti F. The 5α-reductase in the rat brain. In: Gennazzani AR, Petraglia F, Purdy RH, eds. The brain: source and target for sex steroid hormones. Parthenon, London, UK, 1996, pp. 123–133.

117. Poletti A, Celotti F, Rumio C, Rabuffetti M, Martini L. Identification of type 1 5α-reductase in myelin membranes of male and female rat brain. Mol Cell Endocrinol 1997;129:181–190.

118. Snipes CA, Shore LS. Metabolism of testosterone in vitro by hypothalamus and other areas of rat brain. Andrologia 1982;14:81–85.

119. Krieger NR, Scott RG, Jurman ME. Testosterone 5α-reductase in rat brain. J Neurochem 1983;40:1460–1464.

120. MacLusky NJ, Clark CR, Shanabrough M, Naftolin F. Metabolism and binding of androgen in the spinal cord of the rat. Brain Res 1987;422:83–91.

121. Sholl SA, Goy RW, Kim KL. 5α-reductase, aromatase, and androgen receptor levels in the monkey brain during fetal development. Endocrinology 1989;124:627–634.

122. Celotti F, Negri-Cesi P, Poletti A. Testosterone metabolism in the mammalian brain. Brain Res Bull 1997;44:365–375.

123. Melcangi RC, Celotti F, Ballabio M, Castano P, Poletti A, Milani S, Martini L. Ontogenetic development of the 5α-reductase in the rat brain: cerebral cortex, hypothalamus, purified myelin and isolated oligodendrocytes. Dev Brain Res 1988;44:181–188.

124. Massa R, Justo S, Martini L. Conversion of testosterone into 5α-reduced metabolites in the anterior pituitary and in the brain of maturing rats. J. Steroid Biochem 1975;6:567–571.

125. Degtiar VG, Loseva B, Isatchenkov P. In vitro metabolism of androgens in hypothalamus and pituitary from infantile and adolescent rats of both sexes. Endocrinologia Experimentalis 1981;15:181–190.

126. Norton WT, Poduslo SE. Myelination in the rat brain: changes in myelin composition during brain maturation. J Neurochem 1973;21:759–773.

127. Melcangi CR, Celotti F, Ballabio M, Castano P, Massarelli R, Poletti A, Martini L. 5α-reductase activity in isolated and cultured neuronal and glial cells of the rat. Brain Res 1990;516:229–236.

128. Melcangi RC, Celotti F, Martini L. Progesterone 5α-reduction in neuronal and in different types of glial cell cultures: type 1 and 2 astrocytes and oligodentrocytes. Brain Res 1994;639:202–206.

129. Melcangi RC, Froelichsthal P, Martini L, Vescovi L. Steroid metabolizing enzymes in pluripotential progenitor central nervous system cells: effect of differentiation and maturation. Neurosci 1996;2:467–475.

130. Lephart ED. Brain 5α-reductase: cellular, enzymatic, and molecular perspectives and implications for biological function. Mol Cell Neurosci 1993;4:473–484.

131. Thigpen AE, Silver RI, Guileyardo JM, Casey ML, McConnel JD, Russell DW. Tissue distribution and ontogenity of steroid 5α-reductase isozyme expression. J Clin Invest 1993;92:903–910.

132. Eicheler W, Tuohimaa P, Vilja P, Adermann, K, Forssmann, WG, Aumüller G. Immunocytochemical localization of human 5α-reductase 2 with polyclonal antibodies in androgen target and non-target human tissues. J Histochem Cytochem 1994;42:664–675.

133. Poletti A, Negri-Cesi P, Rabuffetti M, Colciago A, Celotti F, Martini L. Transient expression of the type 2 5alpha-reductase isozyme in the brain of the late fetal and early post-natal life. Endocrinology 1998;139:2171–2178.

134. Poletti A, Coscarella A, Negri-Cesi P, Colciago A, Celotti F, Martini L. The 5alpha-reductase isozymes in the Central Central Nervous System. Steroids 1998;63:246–251.

135. Valencia A, Collado P, Cales JM, Segovia S, Perez Laso C, Rodriguez Zafra M, Guillamon A. Postnatal administration of dihydrotestosterone to the male rat abolishes sexual dimorphism in the accessory olfactory bulb: a volumetric study. Brain Res 1992;68:132–135.

136. Jurman ME, Erulkar SD, Krieger NR Testosterone 5α-reductase in spinal cord of *Xenopus laevis*. J Neurochem 1982;38:657–661.

137. Hauser KF, McLusky NJ, Toran-Allerand CD. Androgen action in fetal spinal cultures: metabolic and morphologic aspects. Brain Res 1987;406:62–72.

138. Matsumoto A, Micevych PE, Arnold P. Androgen regulates synaptic input to motoneurones of the adult rat spinal cord. J Neurosci 1988;8:4168–4176.

139. Goldstain LA, Sengelaub DR. Timing and duration of dihydrotestosterone treatment affect the development of motoneuron number and morphology in a sexually dimorphic rat spinal nucleus. J Compar Neurol 1992;326:147–157.

140. Boyd SK, Tyler CJ, DeVries GJ. Sexual dimorphism in the vasotocin system of the bullfrog (*Rana catesbeiana*). J Compar Neurol 1992;325:313–325.

141. Weisz J, Ward IL. Plasma testosterone and progesterone titers of pregnant rats, their male and female fetuses and neonatal offspring. Endocrinology 1980;106:306–316.

142. Meaney MJ, Aitken DH, Jensen LK, McGinnis MY, McEwen BS. Nuclear and cytosolic androgen receptor levels in the limbic brain of neonatal male and female rats. Dev Brain Res 1985;23:179–185.

143. Takani K, Kawashima S. Culture of rat brain preoptic area neurons: effects of sex steroids Int J Dev Neurosci 1993;11:63–70.

144. Roselli CE, Stadelman H, Horton LE, Resko JA. Regulation of androgen metabolism and luteinizing hormone-releasing hormone content in discrete hypothalamic and limbic areas of male rhesus macaques. Endocrinology 1987;120:97–106.

145. Celotti F, Negri-Cesi P, Limonta P, Melcangi C. Is the 5α-reductase of the hypothalamus and of the anterior pituitary neurally regulated? Effects of hypothalamic deafferentations and of centrally acting drugs. J Steroid Biochem 1983;19:229–234.

146. Cheng KC, White PC, Quin KN. Molecular cloning and expression of rat liver 3α-hydroxysteroid dehydrogenase. Mol Endocrinol 1991;5: 823–828.

147. Pawlovski JE, Huizinga M, Penning TM. Cloning and sequencing of the cDNA for rat liver 3α-hydroxysteroid/dihydrodiol dehydrogenase. J Biol Chem 1991;266: 8820–8825.

148. Cheng KC, Lee J, Khanna M, Quin KN. Distribution and ontogeny of 3α-hydroxysteroid dehydrogenase in the rat brain. J Steroid Biochem Molec Biol 1994;50: 85–89.

149. Bennett MJ, Schlegel BP, Lez JM, Penning TM, Lewis M. Structure of 3α-hydroxysteroid/dihydrodiol dehydrogenase complexed with NADP+. Biochemistry 1996;33:10702–10711.

150. Penning TM. 3α-hydroxysteroid dehydrogenase: three dimensional structure and gene regulation. J Endocrinol 1996;150:175–187.

151. Penning TM, Bennett ML, Smith-Hoog S, Schlegel BP, Jez JM, Lewis M. Structure and function of 3α-hydroxysteroid dehydrogenase Steroids 1997;62:101–111.
152. Cheng KC. Molecular cloning of rat liver 3α-hydroxysteroid dehydrogenase and identification of structure related proteins from rat lung and kidney. J Steroid Biochem Molec Biol 1992;43: 1083–1088.
153. Penning T, Pawlowski JE, Schlegel BP, Jez JM, Lin H-K, Hoog SS, Bennett MJ, Lewis M. Mammalian 3α-hydroxysteroid dehydrogenases. Steroids 1996;61:508–523.
154. Krieger NR, Scott RG. 3α-hydroxysteroid dehydrogenase in rat brain. J Neurochem 1984;42:887–890.
155. Karavolas HJ, Hodges D Neuroendocrine metabolism of progesterone and related progestins. In: Chadwick D., Widdows K., eds. Steroids and Neuronal Activity. Ciba Foundation Symposium, vol 153. Wiley, Chichester, 1990, pp. 22–55.
156. Penning T, Sharp RB, Krieger NR. Purification properties of 3α-hydroxysteroid dehydrogenase from rat brain cytosol: inhibition by nonsteroidal anti-inflammatory drugs and progestins. J Biol Chem 1985;260:15266–15272.
157. Selye H. Anaesthetic effect of steroid hormones. Proc Soc Exp Biol Med 1941,46: 116–121.
158. Selye H. Correlation between the chemical structure and the pharmacological actions of the steroids. Endocrinology 1942;30: 437–453.
159. Majewska MD, Harrison NL, Schwartz RD, Barker JL, Paul SM. Steroid hormone metabolites are barbiturate-like modulators of the GABA receptor. Science 1986;232:1004–1007.
160. Harrison NL, Majewska MD, Harrington JW, Barker JL. Structure-activity relationships for steroid interaction with the gamma-aminobutyric acid$_A$ receptor complex. J Pharmacol Exp Therap 1987;241:346–353.
161. Mendelson WB, Martin JV, Perlis M, Wagner R, Majewska MD, Paul SM. Sleep induction by an adrenal steroid in the rat. Psychopharmacol 1987;93:226–229.
162. Bitran D, Shiekh M, McLeod M. Anxiolytic effect of progesterone is mediated by neurosteroid allopregnanolone at brain GABAA receptors. J Neurochem 1995;7:171–177.
163. Pelletier G, Luu-The V, Labrie F. Immunocytochemical localization of type 1 17β-HSD in the rat brain. Brain Res 1995;704:233–239.
164. Krozowski Z, Obeyesekere V, Smith R, Mercer W Tissue-specific expression of an 11β-hydroxysteroid dehydrogenase with a truncated N-terminal domain. A potential mechanism for differential intracellular localization within mineralocorticoid target cells. J Biol Chem 1992;267:2569–2574.
165. White PC, Mune T, Rogerson F, Kayes KM, Agarwal AK. Molecular analysis of 11β-hydroxysteroid dehydrogenase and its role in the syndrome of apparent mineralocorticoid excess. Steroids 1997;62:83–88.
166. Seckl JR. 11β-Hydroxysteroid dehydrogenase in the brain: a novel regulator of glucocorticoid action? Frontiers Neuroendocrinol 1997;18:49–99.
167. Moisan M-P, Seckl JR, Edwards CRW. 11β-hydroxysteroid dehydrogenase bioactivity and messenger RNA expression in rat forebrain: localization in hypothalamus, hippocampus, and cortex. Endocrinology 1990;127:1450–1455.
168. Low SC, Moisan MP, Noble JM, Edwards CR, Seckl JR. Glucocorticoids regulate hippocampal 11β-hydroxysteroid dehydrogenase activity and gene expression in vivo in the rat. J Neuroendocrinol 1994;6:285–290.
169. Low SC, Chapman KE, Edwards CR, Seckl JR. 'Liver-type' 11β-hydroxysteroid dehydrogenase cDNA encodes reductase but not dehydrogenase activity in intact mammalian COS–7 cells. J Mol Endocrinol 1994;13:167–174.
170. Zhou MY, Gomez-Sanchez EP, Cox DL, Cosby D, Gomez-Sanchez CE. Cloning, expression, and tissue distribution of the rat nicotinamide adenine dinucleotide-dependent 11β-hydroxysteroid dehydrogenase. Endocrinology 1995;136:3729–3734.
171. Stewart PM, Murry BA, Mason JI. Type 2 11β-hydroxysteroid dehydrogenase in human fetal tissues. J Clin Endocrinol Metab 1994;78:1529–1532.
172. Sapolsky RM. Why stress is bad for your brain. Science 1996;273:749–750.
173. Yehuda R. Stress and glucocorticoid. Science 1997;275:1662–1663.
174. Sapolsky RM, Pulsinelli WA. Glucocorticoids potentiate ischemic injury to neurons: therapeutic implications. Science 1985;229:1397–1400.
175. Sapolsky RM, Packan DR, Vale WW. Glucocorticoid toxicity in the hippocampus: in vitro demonstration. Brain Res 1988;453:369–371.

176. Hatzinger M, Z'Brun A, Hemmeter U, Seifritz E, Baumann F, Holsboer-Trachsler E, Heuser IJ. Hypothalamic-pituitary-adrenal (HAP) system function in patients with Alzheimer's disease. Neurobiol Aging 1995;16:205–209.
177. Behl C, Widmann M, Trapp T, Holsboer F. 17b-estradiol protects neurons from oxidative stress-induced cell death in vitro. Biochem Biophys Res Commun 1995;216:473–482.
178. Behl C, Lezoualc'h F, Trapp T, Widmann M, Skutella T, Holsboer F. Glucocorticoids enhance oxidative Strees-Induced cell death in hippocampal neurons In Vitro, Endocrinology 1997;138:101–106.
179. Strott CA. Steroid sulfotransferases.Endocrine Rev 1996;17:670–697.
180. Luu-The V, Bernier F, Dufort I. Steroid sulfotransferases. J Endocrinol 1996;150:87–97.
181. Bernier F, Leblanc G, Labrie F, Luu-The V. Structure of human estrogen and aryl sulfotransferase gene. Two mRNA species issued from a single gene. J Biol Chem 1994;269:28200–28205.
182. Rajkowski KM, Robel P, Baulieu EE. Hydroxysteroid sulfotransferase activity in the rat brain and liver as a function of age and sex. Steroids 1997;62:427–436.
183. Mortaud S, Donsez-Darcel E, Roubertoux PL, Degrelle H. Murine steroid sulfatase gene expression in the brain during postnatal development and adulthood. Neurosci Lett 1996;215:145–148.
184. Li PK, Rhodes ME, Burke AM, Johnson DA. Memory enhancement mediated by the steroid sulfatase inhibitor(p-O-sulfamoyl)-N-tetradecanoyl tyramine. Life Sci 1997;60:45–51.
185. Bui QD, Weisz J, Wrighton SA. Hepatic catecholestrogen synthesis: differential effect of sex, inducers of cytochrome P-450 and of antibody to the glucocorticoid inducible cytochrome P-450 on NADPH-dependent estrogen-2-hydroxylase and on organic hydroperoxide dependent estrogen-2/4-hydroxylase activity of rat hepatic microsomes. J Steroid Biochem 1990;37:285–293.
186. Nicoletti F, Speciale C, Sortino MA, Panetta MS, Di Giorgio RM, Canonico PL. Estrogen effects on nigral glutammic acid decarboxylase activity: a possible role for catecholestrogens. Eur J Pharm 1985;115:297–300.
187. Komura S, Ohishi N, Yagi K. Catecholestrogen as a natural antioxidant. Ann NY Acad Sci USA 1996;786:419–429.

7

The Selective Interaction of Neurosteroids with the GABA$_A$ Receptor

Jeremy J. Lambert, MD, Delia Belelli, MD, Susan E. Shepherd, MD, Marco Pistis, MD and John A. Peters, MD

CONTENTS

INTRODUCTION
MOLECULAR MECHANISM OF NEUROSTEROID ACTION
HETEROGENEITY OF NEUROSTEROID BINDING SITES
STRUCTURE ACTIVITY RELATIONSHIP FOR STEROID
    AT THE GABA$_A$ RECEPTOR
CONCLUDING REMARKS
REFERENCES

INTRODUCTION

Some endogenous pregnane steroids have long been known to produce rapid sedative and anesthetic effects *(1)*. The speed of onset of these behavioral effects precludes a genomic mechanism of action for such steroids, but it was not until Harrison and Simmonds *(2)* demonstrated that a synthetic steroidal anesthetic, alphaxalone (3α-hydroxy-5α-pregnane-11,20-dione), selectively enhanced the interaction of GABA with the GABA$_A$ receptor, that a logical mechanism to explain the behavioral effects of these compounds emerged. GABA acting via the GABA$_A$ receptor mediates much of the "fast" inhibitory synaptic transmission in the mammalian brain *(3)*. The GABA$_A$ receptor is a member of the cysteine-cysteine loop transmitter-gated ion channel family that includes glycine, nicotinic, and 5-HT$_3$ receptors *(4)*. Upon activation by GABA, the associated chloride selective ion channel is opened that increases neuronal membrane conductance and effectively shunts the influence of excitatory transmitters such as glutamate *(3)*.

Interestingly, the function of this receptor can be allosterically enhanced by a wide range of structurally diverse compounds, which include a number of intravenous anesthetic agents, barbiturates, and benzodiazepines *(5)*. Behaviorally, like the pregnane

From: *Contemporary Endocrinology: Neurosteroids: A New Regulatory Function in the Nervous System* Edited by: E.-E. Baulieu, P. Robel, and M. Schumacher
© Humana Press Inc., Totowa, NJ

steroids, such compounds are anxiolytic, anticonvulsant, sedative, and at high doses, anesthetic *(5)*. The receptor is a heteropentamer constructed from a number of distinct subunits (e.g., α_{1-6}, β_{1-3}, γ_{1-3}, δ, ϵ) *(6)*. These subunits have a discrete distribution within the central nervous system (CNS) *(7,8)* and the subunit composition of the receptor influences both the physiological and pharmacological properties of the receptor *(6)*.

The potent interaction of alphaxalone with the $GABA_A$ receptor inferred from extracellular recording techniques was confirmed utilizing voltage-clamp techniques *(9,10)*. Subsequent experiments extended these observations to include a number of endogenous pregnane steroids and some of these, including allopregnanolone ($3\alpha,5\alpha$-THPROG), pregnenolone ($3\alpha,5\beta$-THPROG), and tetrahydrodeoxycorticosterone ($3\alpha,5\alpha$-THDOC) were found to be more potent than alphaxalone (reviewed in ref. *11*). Indeed, concentrations of these steroids as low as 1 nM are active at the $GABA_A$ receptor *(12)*. These steroids were known to be produced by peripheral endocrine glands such as the adrenal and ovary. However, the observation that the CNS can synthesize these steroids has heightened interest in the field, because it provides a mechanism whereby the major inhibitory circuitry of the brain may be regulated by locally produced modulators *(13)*.

MOLECULAR MECHANISM OF NEUROSTEROID ACTION

An analysis of the effect of alphaxalone on the power spectra produced by GABA-induced current fluctuations, recorded from spinal neurones, provided an initial indication that one effect of the steroid was to prolong the open time of the $GABA_A$ receptor ion channel *(9)*. Consistent with these observations, single-channel recordings made from membrane patches excised from bovine chromaffin cells demonstrated GABA-modulatory concentrations of the endogenous steroid $3\alpha,5\alpha$-THPROG to dramatically prolong the GABA mean channel open time, but to have no effect on the single-channel conductance *(14–16)*. In those studies, multiple interconverting conductance states prevented a quantitative kinetic analysis of the neurosteroid effect. By contrast, the $GABA_A$ receptors of mouse spinal neurones exhibit long epochs where a single main conductance state predominates *(17,18)*. Kinetic analysis of such data segments reveals three kinetically distinct open states, and the neurosteroids appear to act primarily by increasing the relative frequency of occurrence of two open states of intermediate and long duration *(18,19)*. The depressant barbiturates produce a similar effect on GABA channel kinetics. However, unlike barbiturates, the neurosteroids also increase the frequency of single-channel openings. At concentrations generally greater (>300 nM) than those required for GABA modulation, the pregnane steroids have a second effect to directly activate the $GABA_A$ receptor channel complex *(10,14,20)*. Compared to the GABA-mimetic actions of propofol and pentobarbitone, the magnitude of the direct effects exerted by the steroids are small, but they occur at much lower concentrations *(21,22)*. Furthermore, the steroid-induced conductance is of a sufficient magnitude to shunt the neuronal input resistance, such that the depolarization evoked by glutamate receptor activation falls below the threshold for action potential discharge *(23)*. Hence, this modest, but potent, direct effect of the neurosteroids could contribute to their behavioral actions.

Many of the electrophysiological studies that have investigated the GABA-modulatory actions of the pregnane steroids have been performed at relatively low GABA concentrations, under conditions approaching steady state. However, recent studies suggest that at least for some GABA-ergic synapses within the CNS, the concentration of synaptically released GABA is sufficient to saturate a small number of postsynaptic GABA$_A$ receptors *(3)*. Therefore, it may be of greater physiological relevance to determine the effects of neurosteroids on GABA-evoked currents produced by rapidly applied saturating concentrations of GABA. Utilizing nucleated patches isolated from cerebellar granule cells, Zhu and Vicini *(24)* demonstrated that the current elicited by a rapid (rise time 200 μs), but brief (1 ms), application of a saturating concentration of GABA, decayed with a fast and slow time course. The miniature inhibitory postsynaptic current (mIPSC), which is a consequence of the activation of postsynaptic GABA$_A$ receptors by synaptically released GABA, can exhibit a similar time course *(24)*. For both the synaptic event and the current produced by rapid agonist application, the fast decay is thought to result from a population of channels oscillating between agonist bound open and closed configurations, whereas the slower phase is a reflection of receptors entering and exiting various desensitized states *(25)*. Hence, for the GABA$_A$ receptor, desensitization is paradoxically proposed to prolong, rather than curtail, the synaptic event.

3α,5α-THDOC prolonged the slow time constant of decay of the GABA-evoked current recorded from nucleated patches by slowing the recovery of the receptors from desensitization *(24)*. Consistent with this proposal, on isolated outside out patches, 3α,5α-THDOC increased the channel open probability (produced by a saturating concentration of GABA) by increasing the number of late channel openings *(24)*. Hence, the prolongation of synaptic currents reported for hippocampal neurones in culture *(26,27)* and neurones of rat hippocampal and cerebellar slices *(28)* may result from an action of the pregnane steroid to alter receptor desensitization.

Finally, in a recent report on the effects of a low concentration (10 n*M*) of 3α,5α-THPROG on inhibitory synaptic transmission in a co-culture model of hypothalamic neurones and intermediate lobe cells of the rat pituitary, the steroid had no effect on the amplitude or time course of mIPSCs, but greatly increased their frequency by interacting with presynaptic GABA$_A$ receptors *(29)*.

HETEROGENEITY OF NEUROSTEROID BINDING SITES

A number of studies indirectly suggest that the neurosteroids differentiate between GABA$_A$ receptor isoforms. The evidence includes: multiphasic concentration-response curves for some steroids in both ligand binding and functional assays; the demonstration that the influence of neurosteroids in both radioligand binding and Cl⁻ flux assays is brain region-dependent and the effect of binary combinations of certain steroids on the binding of [^{35}S]TBPS and [^{3}H] flunitrazepam to rat brain membranes *(30–32)*. However, studies investigating the interaction of neurosteroids with recombinant receptors have provided a somewhat confusing picture. In the interests of clarity, the following discussion will be restricted mainly to functional (electrophysiological) assays.

Role of the β Subunit

Whole-cell voltage-clamp and single channel recording techniques applied to human embryonic kidney cells (HEK-293) demonstrated both the GABA-modulatory and GABA-mimetic actions of 3α,5α-THPROG and 3α,5α-THDOC to be preserved in cells transfected with $\alpha_1\beta_1\gamma_{2L}, \alpha_1\beta_1$, or β_1 subunits *(33)*. Hence, the steroid site is even represented on the homo-oligomeric (β$_1$ subunit). The GABA-modulatory and GABA-mimetic actions of the anticonvulsant loreclezole *(34)* and the general anesthetic etomidate

Table 1
The Influence of the Subunit Composition
of the GABA$_A$ Receptor on the GABA-Modulatory Effects
of 3α-Hydroxy-5α-Pregnan-20-One and 5α-Pregnan-3α,20α-Diol

Subunit combination	EC_{50} 3α-hydroxy-5α- pregnan-20-one (nM)	E_{max} (% of GABA maximum)	EC_{50} 5α-pregnan- 3α,20α-diol (nM)	E_{max} (% of GABA maximum)
Rat brain mRNA	123 ± 6	66 ± 2	ND	ND
$α_1β_2γ_{2L}$	177 ± 2	75 ± 4	ND	ND
$α_1β_1γ_{2L}$	89 ± 6	69 ± 4	179 ± 9	40 ± 4
$α_2β_1γ_{2L}$	145 ± 11	66 ± 6	1200 ± 30	48 ± 3
$α_3β_1γ_{2L}$	74 ± 1	67 ± 7	224 ± 30	37 ± 2
$α_6β_1γ_{2L}$	220 ± 12	132 ± 6	803 ± 95	44 ± 5
$α_6β_3γ_{2L}$	264 ± 33	90 ± 9	ND	ND

[a]All parameters are calculated from steroid concentration-effect relationships obtained from a minimum of four oocytes expressing human recombinant GABA$_A$ receptors, or those receptors resulting from rat brain mRNA. The EC_{50} is defined as the concentration of steroid which produces an enhancement of the GABA (EC_{10})-evoked current to 50% of the maximum potentiation produced by that steroid. The E_{max} is the maximum potentiation of the GABA (EC_{10})-evoked current produced by the steroid expressed as a percentage of the GABA maximum. ND, not determined.

(35–37) are greatly influenced by the isoform of the β subunit expressed, with β$_2$ and β$_3$ subunit-containing receptors being favored over those incorporating a β$_1$ subunit. However, for hetero-oligomeric receptors (α$_1$β$_X$γ; where x = 1, 2, or 3) the neurosteroids 3α,5α-THPROG, 3α,5β-THPROG and alphaxalone do not discriminate between β subunit isoforms (37,38) (see Table 1).

Role of the α Subunit

The isoform of the α subunit (α$_{1–6}$) exhibits a profound influence on the benzodiazepine pharmacology of the GABA$_A$ receptor (6,39). To date, a consensus has not emerged from studies investigating the role of the α subunit in the actions of steroids at the GABA$_A$ receptor. Electrophysiological studies performed with HEK 293 cells transfected with α$_1$β$_1$γ$_2$, α$_3$β$_1$γ$_2$ and α$_5$β$_1$γ$_2$ subunits demonstrated the steroids to act similarly across these receptors (40). These findings are in agreement with our own studies, utilizing the oocyte expression system, where the EC_{50} for 3α,5α-THPROG and the maximal potentiation of the GABA-evoked current (Emax) produced by the steroid was little influenced by the (subtype (α$_X$ β$_1$ γ$_{2L}$; where x = 1,2,3; see Table 1) incorporated into the receptor complex. Similarly, the actions of ganaxolone (3α-hydroxy-3β-methyl-5α-pregnan-20-one), currently under going clinical trials as an anticonvulsant, see in section "C3 Substitution") and 5α-pregnan-3α,20α-diol were only modestly influenced by the α subunit-subtype (41,42) (see Table 1). However, in another study performed on oocytes, the maximal GABA potentiating effect of 3α,5α-THPROG was found to be greater for α$_1$ vs α$_2$ or α$_3$ subunit-containing receptors (43). In addition, discord exists concerning the role of the α$_6$ subunit. When tested against GABA$_A$ receptors composed of the α$_6$β$_1$γ$_2$ subunits expressed in HEK 293 cells, steroid enhancement of the effect of GABA is reduced when compared to receptors containing α$_1$, α$_3$, or α$_5$ subunits in combination with β and γ$_2$ (40).

However, when studied in oocytes, the maximal enhancement of the GABA-evoked current by 3α,5α-THPROG at the $\alpha_6\beta_1\gamma_{2L}$ subunit combination was approximately twice that of the other combinations tested, although the EC$_{50}$ for the steroid was little affected by subunit composition (see Table 1). Interestingly, the magnitude of the maximal enhancement is reduced for $\alpha_6\beta_3\gamma_{2L}$ vs $\alpha_6\beta_1\gamma_{2L}$ subunit-containing receptors (Table 1). The geometry of the oocyte prevents the rapid application of the agonist to the receptor plane (the maximal rise time of the inward current response is several hundred milliseconds), and hence receptor desensitization would be anticipated to reduce the true peak amplitude of the inward current response to GABA. We observed 3α,5α-THPROG to increase by threefold the response evoked by a saturating concentration of GABA (3 mM) at receptors composed from $\alpha_6\beta_1$ and γ_{2L} subunits, whereas the steroid produced little or no potentiation of the maximal response to GABA mediated by receptors containing α_1, α_2, or α_3 subunits in association with β_1 and γ_{2L}. These results may hint at a selective action of the steroid to retard desensitization at α_6 subunit containing receptors. However, more detailed studies utilizing single channel analysis and rapid agonist application are required to better understand the effects of the neurosteroid on α_6 subunit-containing receptors. An α_6 selective interaction of 3α,5α-THPROG is consistent with the results of both radioligand binding (44) and autoradiographic experiments (23). These observations may be important for the behavioral actions of the neurosteroids, given the exclusive localization of the α_6 subunit within the granule cells of the cerebellum (7). At all recombinant GABA$_A$ receptor isoforms examined, 5α-pregnane-3α,20α-diol produces a reduced maximal potentiation compared with 3α,5α-THPROG (41). However, unlike 3α,5α-THPROG, the maximal enhancement of GABA produced by the 20-keto reduced compound (see section "C20 Substitution") was little influenced by the α subtype (α_1, α_2, α_3, and α_6; see Table 1) present within the receptor complex.

Role of the γ Subunit

The isoform of the γ subunit (γ_{1-3}) present within the GABA$_A$ receptor complex influences the benzodiazepine pharmacology: indeed the presence of a γ subunit is obligatory for reproducible allosteric modulation by these agents (6). Electrophysiological experiments conducted on transiently transfected HEK-293 cells demonstrated that the magnitude of the enhancement of GABA-evoked currents by pregnane steroids was much greater for the $\alpha_1\beta_1\gamma_1$ subunit combination than for receptors composed of $\alpha_1\beta_1\gamma_{2L}$ or $\alpha_1\beta_1\gamma_3$ subunits (40). This observation has potential physiological importance because glial cells, which are a major site of neurosteroid synthesis in the brain, possess steroid sensitive GABA$_A$ receptors and are known to express the γ_1 subunit (13,45,46). Hence, it is possible that such locally produced steroids act as endogenous modulators of the GABA$_A$ receptors of glial cells.

Role of δ and ε Subunits

In some brain regions, native GABA$_A$ receptors may contain an δ subunit or perhaps the newly discovered ε subunit (47–49). Expression of the δ subunit, in combination with α and β subunits, greatly reduced the GABA-modulatory actions of 3α,5α-THDOC, but had little effect on the GABA-mimetic actions of the steroid (50). By a combination electrophysiological recording and single cell PCR, the investigators demonstrated a temporal correlation between a reduction in the GABA modulatory effects 3α,5α-

THDOC in cerebellar granule cells and the appearance of the δ subunit *(50)*, suggesting that these observations may be of physiological relevance.

Recently, the properties of a novel GABA$_A$ receptor subunit (ε) have been described *(48)*. The incorporation of this subunit into α and β subunit-containing receptors dramatically reduced the GABA modulatory effects of 3α,5α-THPROG, but had little effect on the GABA-mimetic actions of this neurosteroid *(48)*. The GABA modulatory actions of the anesthetics propofol and pentobarbitone were similarly affected *(48)*. In contrast to these data, an independent study reported little influence of the ε subunit on the GABA modulatory properties of 3α,5α-THPROG *(49)*. Whether these contradictory observations are owing to a single amino acid difference between the ε clones (i.e., Ala102, ref. *48*; Ser102, ref. *49*) remains to be determined.

STRUCTURE ACTIVITY RELATIONSHIP
FOR STEROIDS AT THE GABA$_A$ RECEPTOR

Initial studies of the structural requirements for steroid interaction with the GABA$_A$ receptor emphasized active compounds to possess a 5α- or 5β-reduced pregnane (or androstane) skeleton with an α-hydroxyl at C3 of the steroid A ring and a keto group at either C20 of the pregnane steroid side chain or C17 of the androstane ring system *(2,14,26,30,51,52)*. The compounds 3α,5α-THPROG, 3α,5β-THPROG, 3α,5α-THDOC, and androsterone (3α-hydroxy-5α-androstan-17-one) are prototypical in this respect. Subsequent investigations, which have probed the steroid structure activity relationship (SAR) in greater detail, have led to considerable refinement and extension of this scheme. In particular, it is probably inappropriate to refer simplistically to a single SAR. Complications arise first from GABA$_A$ receptor heterogeneity, which may provide for binding sites at which steroids display differing affinities and/or efficacies (*see* Heterogeneity of Neurosteroid Binding Sites), and second, from the fact that the GABA-modulatory and GABA-mimetic activities of the steroids can be differentially influenced by the subunit composition of the receptor (*see* Role of δ and ε Subunits). The following summary of the SAR for steroid interaction with the GABA$_A$ receptor should thus be read with the caveat that it may not be universally applicable.

The Ring System

A saturated ring system no longer appears to be an absolute requirement for activity. The compound 4-pregnen-3α-ol-20-one, for example, exhibits a potency and efficacy similar to that of 3α,5α-THPROG in a variety of assays *(53)*. Similarly, 5α-preg-9(11)-en-3-ol-20-one retains some activity *(53)*. Furthermore, the steroid A ring per se is not essential for activity as judged by the effectiveness of certain benz[e]indene 3(R)-carbonitriles as steroid analogs *(54)*.

C3 Substitution

The first reports of steroid modulation of the GABA$_A$ receptor clearly identified the nature and configuration of the substituent at the C3 position of the steroid A ring as a primary determinant of steroid action. This is exemplified by the epimerization of the 3-hydroxyl group of the anesthetic steroid alphaxalone to the β-configuration, yielding betaxalone (3β-hydroxy-5α-pregnane-11,20-dione), which acts neither as an anesthetic, nor as a positive allosteric modulator of the GABA$_A$ receptor *(2,10)*. The 3β-hydroxy epimers of the naturally occurring compounds 3α,5α-THPROG, 3α,5β-THPROG and 3α,5α-THDOC, are similarly ineffective in potentiating GABA *(26,30,52,55)*. However, 3α,5α-THPROG and epiallopregnanolone (3β,5α-THPROG), when utilized at relatively high concentrations, do share the ability to enhance the rate of desensitization of GABA$_A$ receptor mediated current responses, indicating that this aspect of their action is not stereoselective *(12)*. Oxidation of the 3-hydroxyl group to the ketone *(14,26,53,56)*, greatly reduces, or abolishes, allosteric modulation by 5α-and 5β-pregnanes. Similarly, the introduction of oxime, acetate, or methyl groups at the C3 position essentially abolishes activity *(53,56,57)*. It seems likely that the free hydroxyl group at C3, via hydrogen bond donatation, is an important determinant of the primary docking of the steroid molecule to the GABA$_A$ receptor *(57)*.

A serious limitation to the potential use of pregnane steroids as therapeutic agents (other than as short-acting intravenous general anesthetics) is their susceptibility to rapid metabolism via conjugation or oxidation of the crucial 3-hydroxyl group. Such reactions can be retarded to some extent by substitution at the 3β-position. An example is provided by ganaxolone, the 3β-methyl substituted analogue of 3α,5α-THPROG, which largely retains the potency and efficacy of the parent compound *(42)*. Importantly, orally administered ganaxolone, unlike 3α,5α-THPROG, demonstrates anticonvulsant activity against chemically induced seizures in rats *(42)*. Within the 5α-pregnane series, the introduction of simple alkyl 3β-substituents larger than a methyl group results in a reduction in both potency and efficacy (the latter being inferred from incomplete displacement of the binding of [^{35}S]TBPS to the receptor complex in radioligand binding assays). Similar effects are observed on the introduction of a certain alkene, alkyne and alkyl halide substituents *(58)*. Specifically, in assays of the allosteric regulation of the GABA$_A$ receptor that include the displacement of [^{35}S]TBPS binding, enhancement of [^{3}H]muscimol and [^{3}H] flunitrazepam binding, and the potentiation of GABA-evoked chloride currents, 3α-hydroxy-3β-trifluoromethyl-5α-pregnan-20-one consistently displays the properties of partial agonist: the compound displays reduced efficacy in comparison to 3α,5α-THPROG and antagonizes positive allosteric regulation by the latter *(59)*. Steroids with limited efficacy could, in principle, offer advantages over full-agonists in certain clinical settings. Interestingly, within the 5β-pregnane series, 3β-substitution apparently does not result in a reduction in efficacy *(58)*. Indeed, certain 3β-phenylethynyl analogues of 3α,5β-THPROG retain not only the full agonist character of the parent steroid, but in addition demonstrate a marked increased in potency *(57)*. Optimal activity is associated with the ethynyl spacer unit, which places the phenyl ring at an appropriate distance from the steroid nucleus, and the presence of electron withdrawing groups (e.g., 4-acetyl; 4-carbethoxy) at the 4-position of the phenyl ring. The latter are postulated to act as hydrogen bond acceptors that participate in secondary docking of the steroid at the receptor complex *(57)*.

The C17 Side Chain

The side chain at C17 in the pregnane steroids examined to date must be in the β configuration for activity *(53,56)*. Similarly, although substitution of the acetyl side chain with a carbonitrile moiety produces a compound with an activity rivaling that of 3α,5α-THPROG, the β orientation of the substituent is once again crucial.

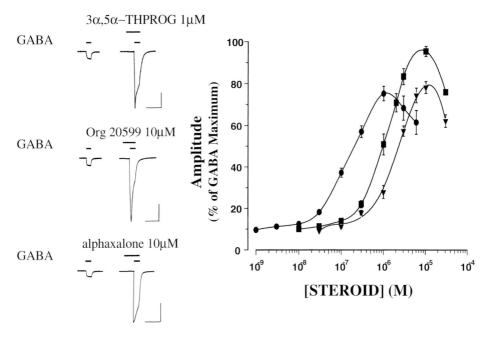

Fig. 1. The water soluble steroid Org 20599 potently enhances GABA-evoked currents mediated by human GABA$_A$ receptors with the subunit composition $\alpha_1\beta_1\gamma_{2L}$ expressed in *Xenopus* oocytes. Left, Each pair of traces illustrates the augmentation of inward current responses evoked by the bath application of GABA (at a concentration that gives a response 10% of the maximum (EC$_{10}$) by 1 μM 3α-hydroxy-5α-pregnan-20-one (3α,5α-THPROG), 10 μM Org 20599, and 10 μM alphaxalone. The increases in current amplitude illustrated are examples of those evoked by maximally effective concentrations of the steroids. The periods of drug application are denoted by the horizontal lines above each trace. The recordings for each steroid were made from different oocytes voltage-clamped at a holding potent of –60 mV. Calibration bars: vertical 200 nA; Horizontal 1 min. Right: Graphical depiction of the concentration-dependent potentiation of GABA-evoked currents by 3α,5α-THPROG: (●); Org 20599, (■); and alphaxalone, (▼). Currents are expressed as a percentage of the maximal GABA current. Each point represents the mean data obtained from four oocytes. Error bars indicate the S.E.M.

C20 SUBSTITUTION

The presence of a carbonyl group at C20 of the acetyl side chain was initially deemed essential to the activity of pregnane steroids at the GABA$_A$ receptor *(26)*. However, subsequent studies have revealed 20-keto reduced analogues of 3α,5α-THPROG and 3α,5β-THPROG (i.e., pregnanediols) to modulate GABA$_A$ receptor activity in a manner consistent with partial agonism *(see* Fig. 1). The potency and efficacy of such pregnanediols are dependent on structural determinants that include cis or trans fusion of the A and B rings and the orientation (α or β) or the 20-hydroxyl moiety *(41,60)*.

C21 SUBSTITUTION

The presence of a hydroxyl group at C21 (as the in naturally occurring 3α,5α-THDOC) or its esterification to the acetate or mesylate produces only modest reductions in activity *(53)*. Similarly, from studies conducted with a series of water-soluble morpholinyl steroids *(see* section "Water Soluble Steroids"), it appears that the steroid binding site of the

Table 2
The Selectivity of Action
of the Anesthetic Steroids Alphaxalone and Minaxolone

Receptor	Alphaxalone	Minaxolone
GABA$_A$	2.2 ± 0.3 µM	0.5 ± 0.1 µM
($\alpha_1\beta_2\gamma_{2L}$: EC$_{50}$)	(78 ± 3%)	(93 ± 5%)
Glycine	60 µM	11 ± 1 µM
(Rat spinal cord/$\alpha_1\beta$: EC$_{50}$)	No effect	(89 ± 4%)
AMPA/kainate	60 µM	100 µM
(Rat cerebellum: IC$_{50}$)	No effect	No effect
NMDA	30 µM	30 µM
(Rat cerebellum: IC$_{50}$)	No effect	No effect
Nicotinic	5 ± 1 µM[b]	19 ± 3 µM
(Rat $\alpha_4\beta_2$: IC$_{50}$)		
Nicotinic	13 ± 2 µM[b]	11 ± 1 µM
(Chick α_7: IC$_{50}$)		
5-HT$_3$	~50 µM[b]	8 ± 1 µM
(h5-HT$_{3A}$: IC$_{50}$)		

[a]All experiments were performed on oocytes voltage-clamped at a holding potential of –60 mV. The sources of receptor were: GABA$_A$, human $\alpha_1\beta_2\gamma_{2L}$; glycine, human α_1 rat β for alphaxalone, and rat spinal cord mRNA for minaxolone; kainate and NMDA, rat cerebellar mRNA; neuronal nicotinic, rat $\alpha_4\beta_2$ and chick α_7; 5-HT$_3$, human 5-HT$_{3A}$. All experiments upon GABA$_A$ and glycine receptors utilized the EC$_{10}$ concentration of the natural agonist. For the other receptors, the appropriate agonist EC$_{50}$ was used. For GABA$_A$ and glycine receptors, the steroid EC$_{50}$ and the maximum potentiation produced in parenthesis are given. For kainate, NMDA, nicotinic, and 5-HT$_{3A}$ receptors, the IC$_{50}$ values are given where appropriate.

[b]Denotes betaxalone to be equieffective with alphaxalone. Where quantified, all data are the mean ± S.E.M. of observations made from 3–5 oocytes.

GABA$_A$ receptor can accept a range of functional groups, including hydroxyl, chloride, acetate, thioacetate, thiocyanate, and azide moieties *(61)*.

Water Soluble Steroids

It is possible to confer water solubility on pregnane steroids without substantial loss of activity at the GABA$_A$ receptor. An example is provided by minaxolone (2β-ethoxy-3α-hydroxy-11α-dimethylamino-5α-pregnan-20-one), studied clinically as a general anesthetic in humans approximately 15 years ago, wherein the incorporation of the 11α-dimethyl amino group results in water solubility *(62)*. Interestingly, in addition to retaining activity at the GABA$_A$ receptor *(61,63)*, minaxolone (unlike alphaxalone) acts as a positive allosteric modulator of strychnine-sensitive glycine receptors, albeit with reduced potency vis à vis the effect of the anesthetic on GABA$_A$ receptors *(64)* (*see* Table 2). Whether this feature can be attributed to only one, or both, of the structural elements (2β-ethoxy and 11α-dimethylamino substituents) that distinguish minaxolone from alphaxalone remains to be determined.

Modulation of GABA$_A$ receptor activity by pregnane steroids rendered water soluble by the introduction of a 2β-morpholinyl group has recently been described in detail *(22,61)* (*see* Fig. 2). It is clear that the steroid binding site of the GABA$_A$ receptor can

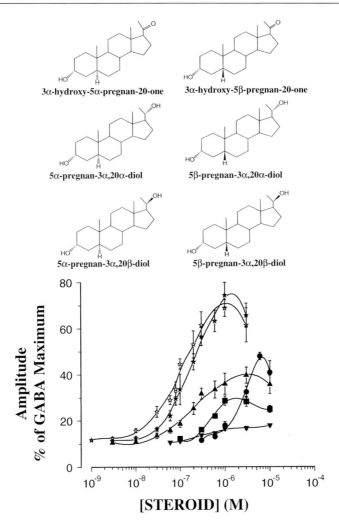

Fig. 2. Reduction at C20 decreases the GABA modulatory effects of the pregnane steroids. Top, The chemical structures of six progesterone metabolites tested for GABA-modulatory effects. Bottom, Graphical representation of the relationship between the concentration of bath applied steroid and the current produced by GABA (expressed relative to the current produced by a saturating concentration of GABA). All experiments were performed at a holding potential of –60 mV on *Xenopus* oocytes expressing human $\alpha_1\beta_1\gamma_{2L}$ receptors. The steroids investigated were 3α,5α-THPROG, (☆); 3α,5β-THPROG, (★); 5α-pregnan-3α,20α-diol, (▲); 5β-pregnan-3α,20α-diol, (■); 5α-pregnan-3α,20β-diol, (●); and 5β-pregnan-3α,20β-diol, (▼). Each point is the mean of data obtained from four to seven oocytes. Vertical lines give the S.E.M.

tolerate rather bulky substituents at the 2β-position, because even a 2,6 dibutyl morpholinyl derivative of alphaxalone is accommodated without loss of potency *(61)*. Within a series of 2β-morpholinyl steroids, 11-keto derivatives are generally more potent allosteric modulators of GABA$_A$ receptor activity than their 11-desoxy analogues *(61)*. This accords with previous studies of pregnanes lacking water solubility, where introduction of a keto group at C11 resulted in some loss of activity. The introduction of a hydroxyl moiety at this position, or C12, produces compounds that are essentially inactive *(53)*.

Enantioselectivity of Steroid Action

Compelling evidence for a direct interaction between certain pregnane steroids and the GABA$_A$ receptor has recently been adduced from studies with enantiomeric pairs of steroids and benz[e]indenes. The endogenous neurosteroid (+)-3α,5α-THPROG (which differs from alphaxalone in that C11 is unsubstituted) is an anesthetic and acts as a positive allosteric modulator of the GABA$_A$ receptor *(26,51,52)*. Significantly, the enantiomer (–)-3α,5α-THPROG demonstrates greatly reduced GABA-modulatory and anesthetic potency in tadpoles and mice *(65,66)*. Enantiomers act dissimilarly only in a chiral (e.g., protein) environment. A similar correlation between GABA-modulatory and anesthetic potency has been established for androstane enantiomers bearing a 17β-carbonitrile substituent *(65)* and for the enantiomers of the benz[e]indene BI-1 *(66)*. These observations provide a cogent argument for direct interactions between pregnane steroid anesthetics and the GABA$_A$ receptor and reinforce earlier observations suggesting alphaxalone to be an effective modulator of GABA only when applied extracellularly *(23)*.

NEUROSTEROID SELECTIVITY
ACROSS THE TRANSMITTER-GATED ION CHANNEL FAMILY

Given the clear behavioral effects of those neurosteroids that modulate the GABA$_A$ receptor, the question arises as to whether those effects are purely determined by an action at the GABA$_A$ receptor, or if additional ion channels or receptors may contribute. Here, we consider the selectivity of steroid action across some members of the transmitter-gated ion channel family of receptors *(4,67)* (*see* Table 2).

Glycine Receptors

Although GABA is recognized as the major inhibitory neurotransmitter in the mammalian brain in the brain stem and spinal cord, the majority of inhibitory neuronal pathways utilize the neurotransmitter glycine, which mediates neuronal depression by activating anion-selective, strychnine-sensitive glycine receptors. GABA$_A$ and glycine receptor proteins are composed of subunits that exhibit significant sequence homology and a predicted common transmembrane topology *(67)*. Indeed, it has been suggested that glycine receptors evolved from GABA$_A$ receptors *(67)*. The glycine receptor is proposed to exist as a pentameric arrangement of subunits drawn from two families, α and β. Four isoforms of the α subunit (α$_{1-4}$) have been identified. Like the GABA$_A$ receptor, these subunits exhibit distinctive expression patterns within the CNS *(68,69)* and hence the pharmacological and functional properties of the inhibitory receptors that they form are unlikely to be homogeneous, but may be region-, and indeed, neurone-specific.

Although GABA$_A$ and glycine receptors exhibit sequence homology and common functional properties, the majority of GABA-modulatory neurosteroids are quite inert at the glycine receptor. Hence, alphaxalone is reported to have no effect on glycine-evoked responses recorded from the rat cuneate nucleus slice preparation *(2)* or spinal neurones *(9,70)*. Similarly, high concentrations of alphaxalone (*see* Table 2), and 3α,5α-THPROG, are without effect at recombinant glycine receptors (α$_1$β or α$_1$) expressed in *Xenopus laevis* oocytes *(71,72)*.

Not all steroids are ineffective at the glycine receptor. The water soluble steroid minaxolone (*see* Water Soluble Steroids) produced a large enhancement of glycine-evoked currents recorded from oocytes preinjected with rat spinal cord mRNA, albeit at concentrations approximately 20-fold greater than those required to produce a comparable enhancement of $GABA_A$-mediated currents (64) (Table 2). Arguably, of most interest is the observation that 20α-dihydrocortisone ($17\alpha,20\alpha,21$-trihydroxy-pregn-4-ene-3,20-dione) α-cortol (5α-prenane-$3\alpha,11\beta,17\alpha,20\alpha,21$-pentol) and hydrocortisone ($11\beta,17\alpha,21$-trihydropregn-4-ene-3,20-dione) enhance the glycine receptor-mediated depolarization of rat optic nerve, but have no effect on $GABA_A$ receptor-mediated responses (73). However, hydrocortisone is reported to be inactive at the glycine receptor of chick spinal neurones (70). Finally, pregnenolone sulfate; (PREGS; 3β-hydroxy-pregn-5-en-20-one sulfate) is equipotent as an antagonist at $GABA_A$ and glycine receptors (70).

Ionotropic Glutamate Receptors

Glutamate is the dominant, fast, excitatory neurotransmitter in the mammalian CNS. The ionotropic glutamate receptors function as transmitter-gated cation selective ion channels and have been classified on the basis of structural, pharmacological, and electrophysiological criteria into three main subtypes: N-methyl-D-aspartate (NMDA) receptors, DL-α-amino-3-hydroxy-5-methyl-4-isopropionic acid (AMPA) receptors, and kainate receptors (4,74–76). These receptors are composed of multiple subunits, and for each of the three receptor classes (NMDA, kainate, and AMPA), subtypes exist as a consequence of the combination of distinct subunit isoforms (74,76). Although initially described as having a membrane topology similar to that of the nicotinic, glycine, and $GABA_A$ receptors, the ionotropic glutamate receptors are now thought to be distinct from the cysteine-loop receptors and instead constitute a separate family (4,75).

The interaction of the GABA-modulatory neurosteroids with ionotropic glutamate receptors has not been investigated, but the synthetic anesthetics alphaxalone and minaxolone appear inert at these receptors. Hence, kainate-evoked whole cell currents recorded from rat hippocampal neurones are unaffected by alphaxalone (23). Similarly, kainate-evoked currents recorded from oocytes preinjected with a preparation of rat cerebellar mRNA are not influenced by relatively high concentrations of alphaxalone or minaxolone (see Table 2). To place these observations in perspective, much lower concentrations of these steroids are effective at the $GABA_A$ receptor (64,72) (Table 2). In addition, alphaxalone has no effect on NMDA-evoked currents recorded from rat hippocampal neurones (23), or on NMDA-induced currents recorded from oocytes (Table 2). Similarly, minaxolone was ineffective at the NMDA receptor (Table 2). In apparent contradiction to these observations, alphaxalone is reported to suppress the depolarizing response of hippocampal neurones to ionophoretically applied glutamate (23). However, at the relatively high concentration necessary for the latter effect, alphaxalone directly activates the $GABA_A$ receptor (10). Hence, the dissimilar influence of this anesthetic on glutamate-evoked currents and depolarizations recorded under voltage- and current-clamp respectively, is due to the GABA-mimetic action of the steroid, which decreases the neuronal input resistance and shunts the glutamate-evoked depolarization.

Finally, at concentrations greater than those producing inhibition at glycine and $GABA_A$ receptors, PREGS allosterically enhances the actions of NMDA at the NMDA receptor, but has little or no effect at AMPA and kainate receptors (77).

Nicotinic Receptors

Neuronal nicotinic receptor subtypes in the CNS and peripheral nervous system exhibit diverse pharmacological and biophysical properties *(78)*. This heterogeneity is probably based on the isoforms of the α and β subunits (α_2–α_9, β_{2-4}) which can combine to form hetero-oligomeric and homo-oligomeric (α_{7-9}) nicotinic receptors *(78)*. Although distributed throughout the CNS, the role of nicotinic receptors is not well understood, because there are few clear examples of synaptic transmission mediated by nicotinic receptors. However, clear effects of exogenously applied nicotinic agonists on neurotransmitter release (e.g., increases in the frequency of spontaneous postsynaptic currents mediated by GABA and glutamate) have been reported *(78–80)*. Furthermore, neuronal nicotinic receptors are implicated in memory acquisition, anxiety, analgesia, synaptic plasticity, and excitotoxicity. Recently, certain isoforms of nicotinic receptor have been shown to be exceptionally sensitive to certain general anesthetics *(81)*. Early studies with alphaxalone demonstrated both muscle nicotinic receptors and "neuronal-type" nicotinic receptor of bovine chromaffin cells to be inhibited by high micromolar concentrations of the anesthetic *(10,82)*. Similarly, we have found alphaxalone to inhibit recombinant neuronal nicotinic receptors ($\alpha_4\beta_2$ and α_7) at such concentrations (Table 2). The water-soluble anesthetic minaxolone is similarly effective at these receptors (Table 2). To place these observations in context, the aqueous concentration of alphaxalone achieved during surgical anaesthesia is approximately 3.6 μM *(72)*. Hence, it is conceivable that an action at neuronal nicotinic receptors may contribute to the behavioral action of alphaxalone. However, for the nicotinic receptors of bovine chromaffin cells *(10)*, and for $\alpha_4\beta_2$ and α_7 recombinant receptors expressed in oocytes, we found the behaviorally inert 3β-ol diastereomer of alphaxalone, betaxalone, to be equipotent in blocking the current evoked by nicotine or acetylcholine. Hence, it is unlikely that neuronal nicotinic receptors constitute an important locus of action for this steroid.

Progesterone (PROG) and testosterone (T), at high micromolar concentrations, also produce a rapid concentration-dependent inhibition of neuronal $\alpha_4\beta_2$ nicotinic receptors expressed in oocytes *(83)*. Interestingly PROG coupled to bovine serum albumin (BSA; a water soluble compound that does not partition into the plasma membrane) was equieffective with the parent steroid, suggesting the PROG site to be located extracellularly. In the same study, cholesterol and 3α,5β-THPROG were found to be inert *(83)*.

5-HT$_3$ Receptors

5-HT$_3$ receptors are ligand-gated cation selective channels with a discrete distribution within the CNS and peripheral nervous systems *(84)*. Only one 5-HT$_3$ receptor subunit (5-HT$_{3A}$) has been isolated to date, but pharmacological heterogeneity between species results from small differences in primary amino-acid sequence of the receptor cloned, for example, from humans and mice *(85)*. The 5-HT$_3$ receptor functions efficiently as a homo-oligomeric complex. Behavioral studies with 5-HT$_3$ receptor selective antagonists have implicated the receptor in anxiety, cognition and addictive behaviors, but the sole clinical use of such compounds is at present in the prevention of emesis and nausea triggered by cytotoxic drugs, radiation and surgical procedures involving the use of a general anesthetic. In the present study, blockade of currents mediated by human 5-HT$_3$ receptors expressed in oocytes was observed only with high concentrations of alphaxalone. The diastereomer, betaxalone, was equieffective in this respect (Table 2).

Minaxolone, although demonstrating greater antagonist potency than alphaxalone, blocked the 5-HT$_3$ receptor only at concentrations much higher than those effective in modulating GABA$_A$ receptor activity.

CONCLUDING REMARKS

The selectivity of the neurosteroids for the GABA$_A$ receptor, their impressive potency, together with the demonstration that the CNS can synthesize such agents, strongly suggests this steroid-neurotransmitter interaction may subserve an important physiological or pathophysiological role. However, to clarify such an endogenous role, there is a urgent requirement for a potent, and selective, neurosteroid antagonist, analogous to the benzodiazepine receptor antagonist, flumazenil (6). Furthermore, the development of a selective radioligand, used in conjunction with appropriate genetically modified recombinant GABA$_A$ receptors, may permit the identification of the neurosteroid binding domain(s) on the receptor protein. Whether or not the steroids play a physiological role, they have clear behavioral effects and these may in the future be exploited for therapeutic benefit.

Finally, some of the GABA-active steroids described here are metabolites of hormones that do exert genomic effects in the CNS. Hence, steroids may influence brain activity, and therefore behavior, by a complex interaction of transcriptional and nongenomic actions.

ACKNOWLEDGMENTS

D. B. and M. P. are supported by the MRC, and SES by Glaxo-Wellcome, Stevenage, UK. This work was partly supported by an equipment grant from the Royal College of Anaesthetists, London, UK, and EC Biomedicine and Health grant BMH4-CT97-2359. We are grateful to Dr. Paul Whiting and Prof. Heinrich Betz for providing the GABA$_A$ and glycine receptor cDNAs, and to Dr. Jim Boulter and Prof. Jean-Pierre Changeux for the neuronal nicotinic cDNAs.

REFERENCES

1. Selye H. Anaesthetic effects of steroid hormones. Proc Soc Exp Biol Med 1941;46:116–121.
2. Harrison NL, Simmonds MA. Modulation of the GABA$_A$ receptor complex by a steroid anaesthetic. Brain Res 1984;323:287–292.
3. Mody I, DeKoninck Y, Otis TS, Soltesz I. Bridging the cleft at GABA synapses in the brain. Trends Neurosci 1994;17:517–525.
4. Barnard EA. The transmitter-gated channel: a range of receptor types and structures. Trends Pharmacol Sci 1996;17:305–309.
5. Sieghart W. Structure and pharmacology of γ-aminobutyric acid$_A$ receptor subtypes. Pharmacol Rev 1995;47:182–234.
6. Smith GB, Olsen RW. Functional domains of GABA$_A$ receptors. Trends Pharmacol Sci 1995;16:162–168.
7. Laurie DJ, Seeburg PH, Wisden W. The distribution of 13 GABA$_A$ receptor subunit mRNAs in the rat brain. II. Olfactory bulb and cerebellum. J Neurosci 1992;12:1063–1076.
8. Wisden W, Laurie DJ, Monyer H, Seeburg PH. The distribution of 13 GABA$_A$ receptor subunit mRNAs in the rat brain. I. Telencephalon, diencephalon, mesencephalon. J Neurosci 1992;12: 1040–1062.
9. Barker JL, Harrison NL, Lange GD, Owen, DG. Potentiation of γ-aminobutyric-acid-activated chloride conductance by a steroid anaesthetic in cultured rat spinal neurones. J Physiol 1987;386:485–501.
10. Cottrell GA, Lambert JJ, Peters, JA. 1987 Modulation of GABA$_A$receptor activity by alphaxalone. Br J Pharmacol 1987;90:491–500.

11. Lambert JJ, Belelli D, Hill-Venning C, Peters JA. Neurosteroids and GABA$_A$ receptor function. Trends Pharmacol Sci 1995;16:295–303.

12. Woodward RM, Polenzani L, Miledi R. Effects of steroids on γ-aminobutyric acid receptors expressed in *Xenopus* oocytes by poly (A)$^+$RNA from mammalian brain and retina. Mol Pharmacol 1992;41:89–103.

13. Robel P, Baulieu E-E. Neurosteroids: biosynthesis and function. In: de Kloet R, Sutanto W, eds. Neurobiology of Steroids. Methods in Neurosciences, vol 22. Academic, San Diego, CA, 1994, pp. 36–50.

14. Callachan H, Cottrell GA, Hather NY, Nooney JM, Peters JA. Modulation of the GABA$_A$ receptor by progesterone metabolites. Proc Royal Soc Lond 1987;B231:359–369.

15. Lambert JJ, Peters JA, Cottrell GA. Actions of synthetic and endogenous steroids on the GABA$_A$ receptor. Trends Pharmacol Sci 1987;8:224–227.

16. Hill-Venning C, Belelli D, Peters JA, Lambert JJ. Electrophysiological studies of the neurosteroid modulation of the GABA$_A$ receptor. In: de Kloet, E.R. & Sutanto, W, eds. Neurobiology of Steroids, Methods in Neurosciences, vol 22. Academic, San Diego, CA, 1994, pp. 446–467.

17. MacDonald RL, Rogers CJ, Twyman RE. Barbiturate modulation of kinetic properties of the GABA$_A$ receptor channel of mouse spinal neurones in culture. J Physiol 1989;417:483–500.

18. MacDonald RL, Olsen RW. GABA$_A$ receptor channels. Ann Rev Neurosci 1994;17:569–602.

19. Twyman RE, MacDonald RL. Neurosteroid regulation of GABA$_A$ receptor single channel kinetic properties of mouse spinal cord neurones in culture. J Physiol 1992;456:215–24.

20. Robertson B. Actions of anaesthetics and avermectin on GABA$_A$ chloride channels in mammalian dorsal root ganglion neurones. Br J Pharmacol 1989;98:167–176.

21. Belelli D, Callachan H, Hill-Venning C, Peters JA, Lambert JJ. Interaction of positive allosteric modulators with human and *Drosophila* recombinant GABA receptors expressed in *Xenopus laevis* oocytes. Br J Pharmacol 1996;118:563–576.

22. Hill-Venning C, Peters JA, Callachan H, Lambert JJ, Gemmell DK, Anderson A, Byford A, Hamilton N, Hill DR, Marshall RJ, Campbell AC. The anaesthetic action and modulation of GABA$_A$ receptor activity by the novel water soluble aminosteroid Org 20599. Neuropharmacology 1996;35:1209–1222.

23. Lambert JJ, Peters JA, Sturgess, NC, Hales TG. Steroid modulation of the GABA$_A$ receptor complex: electrophysiological studies. In: Chadwick D, Widdows K, eds. Steroids and Neuronal Activity, CIBA Foundation Symposium, vol 153. Wiley, Chichester, 1990, pp. 56–82.

24. Zhu WJ, Vicini S. Neurosteroid prolongs GABA$_A$ channel deactivation by altering kinetics of desensitized states. J Neurosci 1997;17:4032–4036.

25. Jones MV, Westbrook GL. The impact of receptor desensitization on fast synaptic transmission Trends Neurosci 1996;19:96–101.

26. Harrison NL, Majewska MD, Harrington JW, Barker JL. Structure activity relationships for steroid interaction with the γ-amino-butyric acid$_A$ receptor complex. J Pharmacol Exp Ther 1987;241:346–353.

27. Harrison NL, Vicini S, Barker JL. A steroid anesthetic prolongs inhibitory postsynaptic currents in cultured rat hippocampal neurons. J Neurosci 1987;7:604–609.

Cooper EJ, Johnston, GAR, Edwards FA. Developmental differences in synaptic GABA-ergic currents in hippocampal and cerebellar cells of male rats. Soc Neurosci Abs 1996;22:810.

29. Poisbeau P, Feltz P, Schlichter R. Modulation of GABA$_A$ receptor-mediated IPSCs by neuroactive steroids in a rat hypothalamo-hypophyseal co-culture model. J Physiol 1997;500.2:475–485.

30. Gee KW, Bolger MB, Brinton RE, Coirini H, McEwen BS. Steroid regulation of the chloride ionophore in rat brain: structure activity requirements, regional dependence and mechanism of action. J Pharmacol Exp Ther 1988;241:346–353.

31. Prince RJ, Simmonds MA. Differential antagonism by epipregnanolone of alphaxalone and pregnanolone potentiation of [^{3}H] flunitrazepam binding suggests more than one class of binding site for steroids at GABA$_A$ receptors. Neuropharmacology 1993;32:59–63.

32. Olsen RW, Sapp DW. Neuroactive Steroid Modulation of GABA$_A$ receptors. In: Biggio G, Sanna E, Serra M, Costa E, eds. GABA$_A$ Receptors and Anxiety: From Neurobiology to Treatment. Advances in Biochemical Psychopharmacology, vol 48. Raven, New York, NY, 1995, pp. 57–74.

33. Puia G, Santi MR, Vicini S, Pritchett DB, Purdy RH, Paul SM, Seeburg PH, Costa E. Neurosteroids act on recombinant human GABA$_A$ receptors. Neuron 1990;4:759–765.

34. Wingrove PB, Wafford KA, Bain C, Whiting PJ. The modulatory action of loreclezole at the γ-aminobutyric acid type A receptor is determined by a single amino acid in the β$_2$ and β$_3$ subunit. Proc Natl Acad Sci USA 1994;91:4569–4573.

35. Belelli D, Lambert JJ, Peters JA, Wafford KA, Whiting PJ. The interaction of the general anesthetic etomidate with the γ-aminobutyric acid type A receptor is influenced by a single amino acid. Proc Natl Acad Sci USA 1997;94:11,031–11,036.
36. Hill-Venning C, Belelli D, Peters JA Lambert JJ. Subunit dependent interaction of the general anaesthetic etomidate with the γ-aminobutyric acid type A receptor. Br J Pharmacol 1997;120:749–756.
37. Sanna E, Murgia A, Casula A, Biggio G. Differential subunit dependence of the actions of the general anesthetics alphaxalone and etomidate at γ-aminobutyric acid type A receptors expressed in *Xenopus laevis* oocytes. Mol Pharmacol 1997;51:484–490.
38. Hadingham KL, Wingrove PB, Wafford KA, Bain C, Kemp J.A, Palmer KJ, Wilson AW, Wilcox AS, Sikela JM, Ragan CI, Whiting PJ. Role of the β subunit in determining the pharmacology of human γ-aminobutyric acid type A receptors. Mol Pharmacol 1993;44:1211–1218.
39. Lüddens H, Korpi ER, Seeburg PH. GABA$_A$/benzodiazepine receptor heterogeneity: neurophysiological implications. Neuropharmacology 1995;34:245–254.
40. Puia G, Ducic I, Vicini S, Costa E. Does neurosteroid modulatory efficacy depend on GABA$_A$ receptor subunit composition? Receptors-Channels 1993;1:135–142.
41. Belelli D, Lambert JJ, Peters JA, Gee KW, Lan, NC. Modulation of human GABA$_A$ receptor by pregnanediols. Neuropharmacology 1996;35:1223–1231.
42. Carter RB, Wood PL, Weiland S, Hawkinson JE, Belelli D, Lambert JJ, White HS, Wolf HF, Mirsadeghi S, Tahir SH, Bolger MB, Lan NC, Gee KW. Characterization of the anticonvulsant properties of ganaxolone (CCD 1042;3α-hydroxy-3β-methyl-5α-pregnan-20-one), a selective, high-affinity, steroid modulator of the γ-aminobutyric acid$_A$ receptor. J Pharmacol Exp Ther 1997;280:1284–1295.
43. Shingai R, Sutherland ML, Barnard EA. Effects of subunit types of cloned GABA$_A$ receptor on the response to a neurosteroid. Eur J Pharmacol 1991;206:77–80.
44. Korpi ER, Lüddens H. Regional γ-aminobutyric acid sensitivity of t-butylbicyclophosphoro[^{35}S]thionate binding depends upon γ-aminobutyric acid$_A$ receptor α subunit. Mol Pharmacol 1993;44:87–92.
45. Chvátal A, Kettenman H. Effects of steroids on γ-aminobutyrate-induced currents in cultured rat astrocytes. Pflügers Arch 1991;419:263–266.
46. Melcangi RC, Celotti F, Martini L. Progesterone 5-α reduction in neuronal and in different types of glial cell cultures: type 1 and 2 astrocytes and oligodendrocytes. Brain Res 1994;639:202–206.
47. McKernan RM, Whiting PJ. Which GABA$_A$ receptor subunits really occur in the brain? Trends Neurosci 1996;19:139–143.
48. Davies PA, Hannah MC, Hales TG, Kirkness EF. Insensitivity to anaesthetic agents conferred by a class of GABA$_A$ receptor subunit. Nature 1997;385:820–823.
49. Whiting PJ, McAllister G, Vasilatis D, Bonnert TP, Heavens RP, Smith DW, Hewson L, O'Donnell R, Rigby MR, Sirinathsinghji DJS, Marshall G, Thompson SA, Wafford KA. Neuronally restricted RNA splicing regulates the expression of a novel GABA$_A$ receptor subunit conferring atypical functional properties. J Neurosci 1997;17:5027–5037.
50. Zhu WJ, Wang JF, Krueger KE, Vicini S. δ Subunit inhibits neurosteroid modulators of GABA$_A$ receptors. J Neurosci 1996;16:6648–6656.
51. Majewska MD, Harrison NL, Schwartz RD, Barker, JL, Paul SM. Steroid hormones are barbiturate-like modulators of the GABA receptor. Science 1986;323:1004–1007.
52. Peters JA, Kirkness EF, Callachan H, Lambert JJ, Turner AJ. Modulation of the GABA$_A$ receptor by depressant barbiturates and pregnane steroids. Br J Pharmacol 1988;94:1257–1269.
53. Hawkinson JE, Kimbrough CL, Belelli D, Lambert JJ, Purdy RH, Lan NC. Correlation of neuroactive steroid modulation of [^{35}S]t-butylbicyclophosphorothionate and [^{3}H]flunitrazepam binding and γ-aminobutyric acid$_A$ receptor function. Mol Pharmacol 1994;46:977–985.
54. Rodgers-Neame NT, Covey DF, Hu Y, Isenberg KE, Zorumski CF. Effects of a benz[e]indene on GABA-gated chloride currents in cultured post-natal rat hippocampal neurons. Mol Pharmacol 1992;42:952–957.
55. Kokate G, Svensson BE, Rogawski MA. Anticonvulsant activity of neurosteroids: correlation with γ-aminobutyric acid-evoked chloride current potentiation. J Pharmacol Exp Ther 1994; 270:1223–1229.
56. Purdy RH, Morrow AL, Blinn JR, Paul SM. Synthesis, metabolism and pharmacological activity of 3α-hydroxy steroids which potentiate GABA-receptor mediated chloride ion uptake in rat cerebral cortical synaptosomes. J Med Chem 1990;33:1572–1581.
57. Upasani RB, Yang KC, Acosta-Burruel M, Konkoy CS, McLellan JA, Woodward RM, Lan NC, Carter RB, Hawkinson JE. 3α-hydroxy-3β-(phenylethynyl)-5β-pregnan-20-ones: synthesis and

pharmacological activity of neuroactive steroids with high affinty for GABA$_A$ receptors. J Med Chem 1997;40:73–84.

58. Hogenkamp DJ, Tahir SH, Hawkinson JE, Upasani RB, Alauddin M, Kimbrough CL, Acosta-Burreul M, Whittemore ER, Woodward RM, Lan NC, Gee KW, Bolger MB. Synthesis and *in vitro* activity of 3β-substituted-3α-hydroxypregnan-20-ones: allosteric modulators of the GABA$_A$ receptor. J Med Chem 1997;40:61–72

59. Hawkinson JE, Drew JA, Kimbrough CL, Chen J-S, Hogenkamp DJ, Lan NC, Gee KW, Shen K-Z, Whittemore ER, Woodward RM. 3α-hydroxy-3β-trifluoromethyl-5α-pregnan-20-one (Co 2-1970): a partial agonist at the neuroactive steroid site of the γ-aminobutyric acid$_A$ receptor. Mol Pharmacol 1996;49:897–906.

60. McCauley LD, Liu V, Chen J.-S, Hawkinson JE, Lan NC, Gee KW. Selective actions of certain neuro-active pregnanediols at the γ-aminobutyric acid type A receptor complex in rat brain. Mol Pharmacol 1995;47:354–362.

61. Anderson A, Boyd AC, Byford A, Campbell AC, Gemmell DK, Hamilton NM, Hill DR, Hill-Venning C, Lambert JJ, Maidment MS, May V, Marshall RJ, Peters JA, Rees DC, Stevenson D, Sundaram H. Anaesthetic activity of novel water-soluble 2β-morpholinyl steroids and their modulatory effects at GABA$_A$ receptors. J Med Chem 1997;40:1668–1681.

62. Phillips GH, Ayres BE, Bailey EJ, Ewan GB, Looker BE, May PJ. Water-soluble steroidal anaesthetics. J. Steroid Biochem 1979;11:79–86.

63. Lambert JJ, Hill-Venning C, Peters JA, Sturgess NC, Hales TG. The actions of anesthetic steroids on inhibitory and excitatory amino acid receptors. In: Barnard EA, Costa E, eds. Transmitter Amino Acid Receptors: Structure: Transduction and Models for Drug Development. Fidia Research Foundation Symposium Series, vol 6. Thieme, New York, 1991, pp. 219–236.

64. Shepherd SE, Peters JA, Lambert JJ. The interaction of intravenous anaesthetics with rat inhibitory and excitatory amino acid receptors expressed in *Xenopus laevis* oocytes. Br J Pharmacol 1996;119:364P.

65. Wittmer LL, Hu Y, Kalkbrenner M, Evers AS, Zorumski CF, Covey DF. Enantioselectivity of steroid-induced γ-aminobutyric acid$_A$ receptor modulation and anesthesia. Mol Pharmacol 1996;50:1581–1586.

66. Zorumski CF, Wittmer LL, Isenberg KE, Hu Y, Covey DF. Effects of neurosteroid and benz[e]indene enantiomers on GABA$_A$ receptors in cultured hippocampal neurones and transfected HEK–293 cells. Neuropharmacology 1996;35:1161–1168.

67. Ortells MO, Lunt GG. Evolutionary history of the ligand-gated ion- channel superfamily of receptors. Trends Neurosci 1995;18:121–127.

68. Malosio ML, Marqueze-Pouey B, Kuhse J, Betz H. Widespread expression of glycine receptor subunit mRNAs in the adult and developing rat brain. EMBO J 1991;90:2401–2409.

69. Kuhse J, Betz H, Kirsch J. The inhibitory glycine receptor: architecture, synaptic localization and molecular pathology of a post-synaptic ion-channel complex. Curr Opin Neurobiol 1995;5:318–323.

70. Wu FS, Gibbs TT, Farb DH. Inverse modulation of gamma-aminobutyric acid- and glycine-induced currents by progesterone. Mol Pharmacol 1990;37:597–602.

71 Pistis M, Belelli D, Peters JA, Lambert JJ. Positive allosteric modulation of recombinant glycine and GABA$_A$ receptors by general anaesthetics: a comparative study. Br J Pharmacol 1996;119:362P.

72 Lambert JJ, Belelli D, Shepherd S, Muntoni A-L, Pistis M, Peters JA. The GABA$_A$ receptor: an important locus for intravenous anaesthetic action. In: Gases in Medicine: Anaesthesia (Smith EB, Daniels S, eds.). 8th BOC Priestley Conference. Royal Society of Chemistry, London, 1998, pp. 121–137.

73 Prince RJ, Simmonds MA. Steroid modulation of the strychnine-sensitive glycine receptor. Neuropharmacology 1992;31:201–205.

74. Bettler B, Mulle C. Neurotransmitter receptors. 2. AMPA and Kainate receptors. Neuropharmacology 1995;34:123–138.

75. Wo ZG, Oswald RE. Unravelling the modular design of glutamate-gated ion channels. Trends Neurosci 1995;18:161–167.

76. Sucher NJ, Awobuluyi M, Choi Y-B, Lipton SA. NMDA receptors: from genes to channels. Trends Pharmacol Sci 1996;17:348–355.

77. Wu FS, Gibbs TT, Farb DH. Pregnenolone sulphate: a positive allosteric modulator at the N-methy-D-aspartate receptor. Mol Pharmacol 1991;40:333–336.

78. Albuquerque EX, Alkondon M, Pereira EFR, Castro NG, Schrattenholz, A, Barbosa CTF, Bonfante-Cabarcas R, Aracava, Y, Eisenberg HM, Maelicke A. Properties of neuronal nicotinic acetylcholine receptors: pharmacological characterization and modulation of synaptic function. J Pharmacol Exp Ther 1997;280:1117–1136.

79. McGee DS, Heath MJS, Gelber S, Devay P, Role LW. Nicotine enhancement of fast excitatory synaptic transmission in CNS by presynaptic receptors. Science 1995;269:1692–1696.
80. Gray R, Rajan AS, Radcliffe K, Yakehiro M, Dani J. Hippocampal synaptic transmission enhanced by low concentrations of nicotine. Nature 1996;383:713–716.
81. Evers AS, Steinbach JH. Super sensitive sites in the central nervous sytsem: anesthetics block brain nicotinic receptors Anesthesiology 1997;86:760–762.
82. Gillo B, Lass Y. The mechanism of steroid anaesthetic (alphaxalone) block of acetylcholine-induced ionic currents. Br J Pharmacol 1984;82:783–789.
83. Valera S, Ballivet M, Bertrand D. Progesterone modulates a neuronal nicotinic acetylcholine receptor. Proc Natl Acad Sci USA 1992;89:9949–9953.
84. Peters JA, Malone HM, Lambert JJ. Recent advances in the electrophysiological characterization of $5\text{-}HT_3$ receptors. Trends Pharmacol Sci 1992;13:391–397.
85. Belelli D, Balcarek JM, Hope AG, Peters JA, Lambert JJ, Blackburn TP. Cloning and functional expression of a human 5-hydroxytryptamine type 3AS receptor ($5\text{-}HT_3R\text{-}A_S$) subunit. Mol Pharmacol 1995;48:1054–1062.

8 Potentiation of GABAergic Neurotransmission by Steroids

Robert H. Purdy, PhD and Steven M. Paul, MD

CONTENTS

INTRODUCTION
DIASTEREOMERIC SELECTIVITY OF GABAERGIC STEROIDS
ENANTIOMERIC SELECTIVITY OF GABAERGIC STEROIDS
NEUROACTIVE STEROIDS IN ALCOHOL DEPENDENCE
   AND WITHDRAWAL
NEUROACTIVE STEROIDS IN AFFECTIVE DISORDERS
CONCLUSIONS
ACKNOWLEDGMENTS
REFERENCES

INTRODUCTION

The endogenous 3α-hydroxy ring A-reduced steroids allopregnanolone and pregnanolone are among the most active ligands of gamma amino butric acid A ($GABA_A$) receptors, with affinities equal to or greater than those of other known ligands such as barbiturates, and even benzodiazepines *(1,2)*. It is, therefore, not surprising that numerous 3α-hydroxy steroids have anxiolytic, hypnotic, anticonvulsant, and anesthetic effects when administered to laboratory animals *(2)*. These pharmacological actions, together with their low intrinsic toxicity and lack of hormonal activity, have led an expanding number of laboratories to investigate their physiological and pharmacological properties in both laboratory animals and humans. Efforts are also underway to develop novel synthetic anxiolytic, hypnotic, and anticonvulsant steroids as therapeutic agents. In this chapter, we discuss a few selected areas related to the pharmacology, physiology, and chemistry of GABAergic neuroactive steroids, including their potential roles in alcohol dependence and withdrawal, as well as in affective disorders.

Diastereomeric Selectivity of GABAergic Steroids

Structure-activity studies in several laboratories have established a marked diastereomeric selectivity of 3-hydroxysteroids for $GABA_A$ receptors *(1–3)*. Thus,

From: *Contemporary Endocrinology: Neurosteroids: A New Regulatory Function in the Nervous System* Edited by: E.-E. Baulieu, P. Robel, and M. Schumacher
© Humana Press Inc., Totowa, NJ

many 3α-hydroxysteroids in the pregnane (5β) or allopregnane (5α) series are positive allosteric modulators of $GABA_A$ receptors, whereas the diastereomeric 3β-hydroxy-steroids are essentially inactive in this respect. (A diasteriomer has the opposite configuration at one of the chiral centers, e.g., at C-3 in this case.) This generalization is not intended to imply that epiallopregnanolone (3β,5α-TH PROG) is devoid of biological activity. For example, Yu and Ticku (4) reported that 5-d treatment of cultured cortical neurons with 3β,5α-TH PROG reversed the effect of 3α,5α-TH PROG at the same concentration (2 μM).

Esterification and oxidation of the 3α-hydroxyl group greatly reduces activity. There are other notable exceptions, such as 3α-hydroxy derivatives in the 5α-pregn-9(11)-ene series, 11α- and 12α-hydroxylated metabolites, and a C-17 diastereomer with the 17α-acetyl side chain, all of which have negligible activity as allosteric modulators of $GABA_A$ receptors (5). In the case of the potent synthetic steroid 3α-hydroxy-5α-androstane-17β-carbonitrile (ACN), its 17α-diastereomer is also inactive (5). However, when there is a ketone group at C-17 rather than the 17β-acetyl group, 3α-hydroxy-5α-androstan-17-one (androsterone) is as active as allopregnanolone or pregnanolone in potentiating $GABA_A$ receptors (6). The effect of these structural alterations at C-17 highlight the importance of a hydrogen bond acceptor in the region of the steroid side chain (5–7).

There is also evidence for the presence of multiple steroid-binding sites on $GABA_A$-receptors, initially described by Morrow et al. (8), which limits the interpretation of the results of structure-activity studies. Moreover, because these receptors exist as hetero-oligomers with different subunits, the results of studies employing neuronal membranes from brain tissue provide only an average response from multiple forms of $GABA_A$-receptors from the particular tissue. With these caveats in mind, it is of some interest to examine a few other diastereomeric distinctions.

Hawkinson et al. (9) demonstrated that pregnanolone (but not allopregnanolone) showed two-component allosteric modulation of radioactive flunitrazepam and tert-butylbicyclophosphorothionate (TBPS) binding to neuronal membranes from specific regions of bovine brain. Evidence for both high- and low-affinity binding sites for pregnanolone was also found in membranes from the rat brain. Their results were interpreted to mean that this 5β-reduced steroid, which is a major neuroactive steroid in humans, shows selective binding to different types of $GABA_A$ receptors. Furthermore, McCauley et al. (10) have found that 5β-pregnane-3α,20β-diol, which has limited efficacy as an allosteric modulator, is a selective ligand for the high-affinity binding site of pregnanolone. They concluded that partial agonist activity and receptor subtype selectivity are not mutually exclusive, which could explain why certain neuroactive steroids have limited efficacy.

There is accumulating evidence for the ability of other steroids to act as antagonists (or negative allosteric modulators) of $GABA_A$ receptors. Among endogenous steroids, epipregnanolone (3β,5β-TH PROG) antagonized the potentiation of flunitrazepam binding produced by 3α,5β-TH PROG, 3α,5α-TH PROG, and alfaxalone (11,12). Through an extensive investigation of the synthesis and in vitro activity of 3β-substituted derivatives of allopregnanolone, Hogenkamp et al. (13) prepared the 3β-trifluoromethyl derivative Co 2-1970, shown in Fig. 1. Hawkinson et al. (14) demonstrated that Co 2-1970 (10 μM) produced a concentration-dependent antagonism of $GABA_A$ receptors, which resulted in an 11-fold reduction in the apparent binding affinity of allopreg-

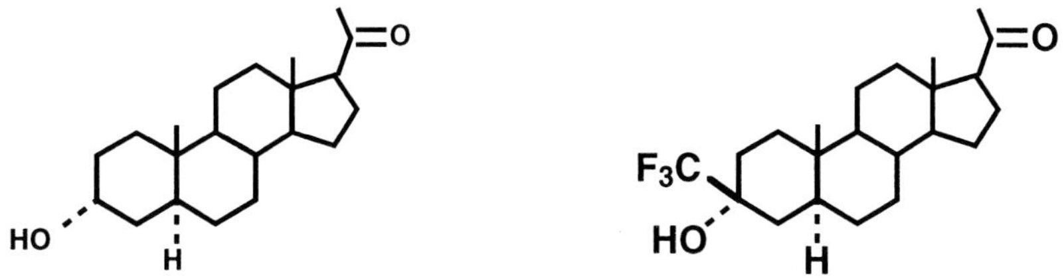

3α-hydroxy-5α-pregnan-20-one
3α,5α-TH PROG

3α-hydroxy-3β-trifluoromethyl-5α-pregnan-20-one
Co 2-1970

Fig. 1. Structures of allopregnanolone (3α,5α-TH PROG) and 3α-hydroxy-3β-trifluoromethyl-5α-pregnan-20-one (Co 2-1970).

nanolone. In this extensive pharmacological study, the authors also demonstrated the effective partial agonist activity of Co 2-1970.

ENANTIOMERIC SELECTIVITY OF GABAERGIC STEROIDS

Studies of the binding and electrophysiological activity of neuroactive steroids have demonstrated that the effects of these steroids do not result from steroid binding at the benzodiazepine, barbiturate, picrotoxin or GABA recognition sites associated with $GABA_A$ receptor complexes. These results have led to the concept of unique binding site(s) for a group of neuroactive steroids on GABA receptors *(1–3, 5–7)*. Although there has been no satisfactory demonstration of the specific binding of radioactive steroid ligands to such sites, a significant correlation has been obtained between physiological and behavioral effects and in vitro structure-activity relationships of GABAergic neuroactive steroids *(7)*.

Nevertheless, because of the lipophilic nature of these steroids, it was important to determine whether their effects on ion channels (such as the GABA-gated chloride ion channel) were simply due to nonspecific perturbation of lipid bilayers *(15)*. In a series of elegant studies, Covey and colleagues, have synthesized a series of steroid and benz[*e*]indene enantiomers, in order to provide a test of the hypothesis that these compounds exert their effects on chiral region(s) of protein recognition sites in the ion channels *(16–18)*. The six compounds initially chosen for study are shown in Fig. 2.

As isolated in pure form from women's pregnancy urine by Marker et al. in 1937 *(19)*, an ethanol solution of 3α,5α-TH PROG rotated plane-polarized light in a positive direction, indicated as (+). This steroid has eight chiral centers, six at the ring fusions of the four rings, and two more at C-3 and C-17. This leads to a possible $2^8 = 256$ different stereoisomers. One of these stereoisomers is (–)3α,5α-TH PROG, shown on the upper right of Fig. 2, where all eight of the eight chiral centers of natural (+)3α,5α-TH PROG have been inverted in the rigorous total chemical synthesis of the (–) enantiomer. It is an absolute mirror image of the natural (+) enantiomer, as seen in the two-dimensional drawing where solid lines (β configuration) are used for bonds above the plane of the drawing in Fig. 2, and dotted lines (α configuration) for bonds below the plane. These enantiomers (as opposed to diastereomers) have identical physical properties except for their rotation of plane-polarized light and would be expected to perturb the lipid bilayer in a similar manner, as contrasted with their expected dissimilar binding to protein

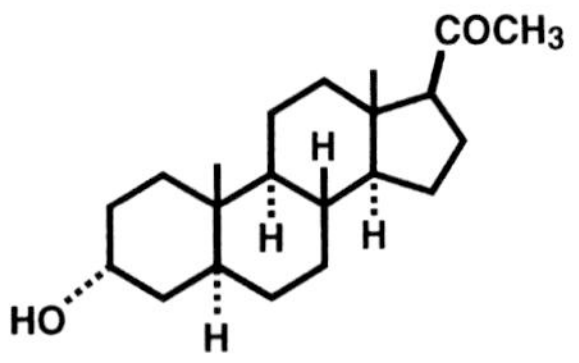

Fig. 2. Structures of the enantiomeric pairs of compounds prepared by Hu et al. *(20)*.

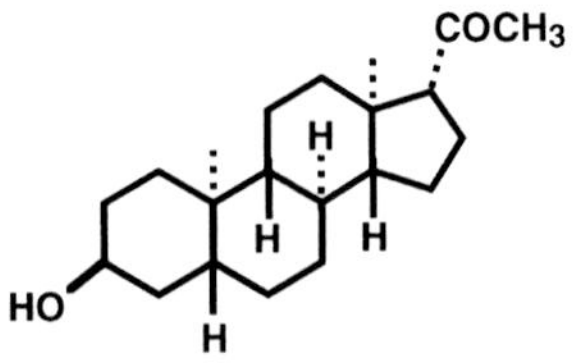

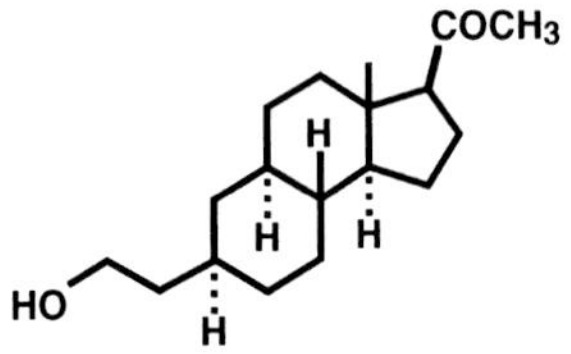

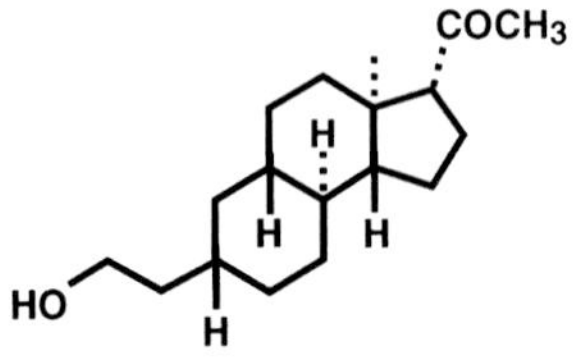

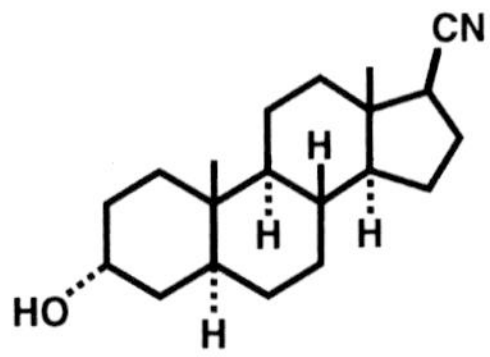

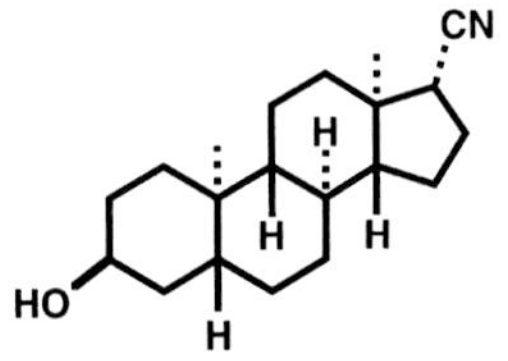

receptor site(s). Similarly, the total synthesis of the benz[*e*]indene enantiomer (–)-BI-1 was performed *(20)*, as well as the multi-step preparation of the enantiomer (–)-ACN of the synthetic GABA$_A$ potentiator (+)-ACN (3α-hydroxy-5α-androstane-17β-cya-nonitrile).

The two pairs of steroidal enantiomers (Fig. 2) were compared for their ability to potentiate GABA-mediated chloride ion currents in rat hippocampal neurons *(16)*. The unnatural synthetics (–)3α,5α-TH PROG and (–)-ACN, were essentially inactive, com-pared with (+)3α,5α-TH PROG and (+)-ACN, respectively. This was also the case for direct activation of GABA$_A$ receptors seen at concentrations up to 100 μ*M* in these hippocampal neurons. The (+) enantiomers of 3α,5α-TH PROG and ACN also produced anesthesia in tadpoles at considerably lower concentrations than the respective (–) enan-tiomers *(16)*. This was also the case for (+)-BI-1 compared to (–)-BI-1 *(20)*.

Surprisingly, the (–) enantiomers of 3α,5α-TH PROG and ACN did have significant anesthetic activity in tadpoles even though their maximal electrophysiological effect was a doubling of the GABA current. Conversely, the (+) enantiomers of 3α,5α-TH PROG and ACN caused anesthesia in tadpoles at concentrations much lower than those that produced maximal electrophysiological effects. Additionally, these enantiomers showed synergistic effects both electrophysiologically and as anesthetics, where thresh-old doses of the enantiomers gave an augmented effect when they were administered together. The authors concluded from these results that (1) neuroactive steroid-induced anesthesia probably results from potentiation of GABA currents, rather than from direct activation of chloride currents; and (2) the (+) and (−) enantiomers probably bind to different sites on GABA receptors *(16)*.

In a further report, Zorumski et al. *(17)* demonstrated that the three (+) enantiomers shown in Fig. 2 were more potent and effective than their respective unnatural (−) enantiomers in the enhancement of $GABA_A$-receptor-mediated evoked synaptic currents in microcultures of rat hippocampal neurons. Together, these results strongly support the action of these steroids and benz[*e*]indenes at unique chiral binding sites on protein regions of $GABA_A$ receptors, rather than through perturbation of membrane lipids.

In a further extension of this approach, the unnatural enantiomers of pregnanolone sulfate ($3\alpha,5\beta$-TH PROGS), pregnenolone sulfate (PREGS), and dehydroepiandrosterone sulfate (DHEAS) were prepared by total synthesis *(21)*. The natural (+) enantiomers of these sulfate esters have been established by electrophysiological methods to be negative allosteric modulators of $GABA_A$-receptors in cultured rat hippocampal neurons *(6)*. The inhibitory effect of natural (+)-DHEAS was about sevenfold greater than that of the synthetic (−)-DHEAS *(21)*. However, negligible enantioselectivity was found for $3\alpha,5\beta$-TH PROGS or PREGS compared to their unnatural enantiomers. These results suggest that different mechanisms and/or sites of action may be operating for the effect of DHEAS, compared with the pregnane sulfate esters, on GABA-mediated chloride ion currents *(21)*. The data also provide novel evidence for a direct binding interaction of DHEAS with a chiral recognition site of these receptor(s). The extension of this approach, exploring the enantioselectivity of neuroactive steroids, to other neurotransmitter systems will be invaluable.

NEUROACTIVE STEROIDS IN ALCOHOL DEPENDENCE AND WITHDRAWAL

Neurosteroids that potentiate $GABA_A$-receptor activity have characteristic behavioral effects resembling those of ethanol in many respects, including anxiolytic, anticonvulsant, and sedative-hypnotic activity *(22–25)*. The neurosteroids of greatest current interest in alcohol research are allopregnanolone and its 21-hydroxy analog allotetrahydrodeoxycorticosterone ($3\alpha,5\alpha$-THDOC). Allopregnanolone and $3\alpha,5\alpha$-THDOC increase responding in the conflict portion of the Geller-Seifter test (anticonflict activity), and produce similar anxiolytic-like effects in the elevated plus-maze test *(26,27)*. Ethanol itself has similar effects at $GABA_A$ receptors, causing a potentiation of the inhibitory effects of GABA at these chloride ion channels *(28)*. There is accumulating evidence that ethanol and neuroactive steroids have interactive effects. For example, in neonatal rats, Zimmerberg et al. *(25)* showed that prenatal exposure to ethanol decreased the sensitivity to the anxiolytic effects of allopregnanolone. Furthermore, chronic exposure of adult rats and mice to ethanol led to an increased sensitivity to the anticonvulsant effects of allopregnanolone *(29,30)*.

Drug discrimination procedures have been used effectively to determine similarities amongst $GABA_A$-receptor ligands *(31)*. Allopregnanolone and $3\alpha,5\alpha$-THDOC produced complete generalization in those rats previously trained to discriminate pentobarbital and ethanol *(32)*. However, Ator et al. also found that rats previously trained to discriminate lorazepam did not generalize to these neuroactive steroids *(32)*. These results also suggest that the discriminative stimulus effects of these steroids are not mediated through the benzodiazepine binding sites of these $GABA_A$ receptors. In a subsequent investigation, Grant et al. *(33)* demonstrated that in female *Macaca fascicularis* monkeys allopregnanolone produced subjective behavioral effects similar to those of ethanol. It is to be emphasized here that allopregnanolone is an endogenous steroid alcohol in nonhuman primates.

A universal consequence of chronic alcohol consumption in humans and rodents is the activation of the hypothalamic-pituitary-adrenal (HPA) axis, with resulting elevations of circulating CRF, ACTH, and glucocorticoids, similar to other stressors *(34–36)*. In human alcoholics, Romeo et al. *(37)* have also found markedly decreased levels of allopregnanolone during early withdrawal from alcohol. The chronic stressor effect of alcohol withdrawal is supported by the demonstration by Spencer and McEwen *(38)* of adrenal atrophy and thymus involution following several weeks of ethanol exposure.

Allopregnanolone has been shown to protect against bicuculline-induced seizures in alcohol-dependent rats *(29)*. Furthermore, these alcohol-withdrawn rats are sensitized to the anticonvulsant effects of allopregnanolone, where they show a 5 to 15-fold increase in the maximal anticonvulsant effect of allopregnanolone on bicuculline-induced seizures, compared to controls *(39)*. These results suggest that chronic alcohol consumption causes sensitization to allopregnanolone, in contrast to the tolerance and cross-tolerance that develops to alcohol and benzodiazepines. Although sensitization to the anticonvulsant effects of allopregnanolone was found in both sexes of rats following chronic alcohol treatment, female rats in estrus, (when allopregnanolone levels are elevated), show lower seizure susceptibility than males during alcohol withdrawal. Females also show enhanced sensitivity to the protective effects of allopregnanolone.

It has been proposed by Devaud et al. *(39)* that GABAergic neuroactive steroids like allopregnanolone, 3α,5α-TH DOC, pregnanolone, and 3α,5β-THDOC may protect against the negative symptoms of alcohol dependence, including the anxiety, agitation, and dysphoria of alcohol withdrawal. These symptoms can promote continued alcohol consumption in rats and humans *(40)*. Thus, the foregoing GABAergic neuroactive steroids may contribute to the lower incidence of alcoholism in women versus men during the years of normal menstruation *(41–43)*, as brain levels of neuroactive steroids are markedly increased during human menstrual cycles *(44)*, as was observed in the estrous cycles of female rats *(2)*. When the estrous cycles of rats were synchronized, Roberts et al. *(45)* found that ethanol is more rewarding during diestrus than during proestrus and estrus phases where allopregnanolone levels are elevated.

It has been difficult to quantify the effects of menstrual cycle phase on sensitivity to the subjective effects of ethanol in women. In a recent study of fertile women ($n = 189$), the plasma levels of allopregnanolone in the follicular phase were similar to those in age-matched men ($n = 48$), whereas allopregnanolone in the luteal phase peaked at about a 10-fold higher level in plasma (4.5 nM; *46*). In the early follicular phase, ethanol consumption has been related to the relief of dysphoria in alcoholic or moderate drinkers *(47)*, although other reports are at variance with this result. Nevertheless, the fluctuations of allopregnanolone concentrations during the menstrual cycle probably alter sensitivity to the stimulus effects of ethanol. This conclusion is supported by the findings of Grant et al. *(48)*, that monkeys showed an order of magnitude more sensitivity to the discriminative stimulus effects of ethanol and the ethanol-like effects of allopregnanolone during the luteal phase of the menstrual cycle. In this context, Smith et al. *(49)* have provided evidence suggesting that fluctuations in allopregnanolone levels can result in alterations in the expression of $GABA_A$ receptors in the brain; in their study a decreased transcription of the gene encoding the $\alpha4$ subunit of the $GABA_A$ receptor in the hippocampus was found. The work of Smith and colleagues (49) suggest that progesterone metabolism to allopregnanolone (and thus increased brain levels of this GABAergic neuroactive steroid) may underline an endogenous "progesterone withdrawal" syndrome similar, perhaps, to alcohol/barbiturate withdrawal. This mechanism may also underlie premenstrual syndrome and/or postpartal anxiety/depression (2).

NEUROACTIVE STEROIDS IN AFFECTIVE DISORDERS

Major depression and alcohol dependence are among the most common psychiatric disorders. Comorbidity between these disorders is also common (50), but little is known also about the dual-diagnosis population of depressed alcoholics. In an initial double-blind, placebo-controlled study of such comorbid patients, Cornelius et al. (51), using fluoxetine, a selective serotonin reuptake inhibitor (SSRI), found efficacy for fluoxetine in reducing the depressive symptoms and the alcohol consumption of these patients. The authors suggested that "the anti-drinking effect of fluoxetine was not entirely due to its antidepressant effect," but that the pharmacology was "unclear."

Interestingly, a possible role for allopregnanolone and pregnanolone in major depression has been suggested by Uzunova et al. (52) who have recently found that the concentration of these steroids in CSF of depressed patients is low compared with normal control individuals and is restored to normal after successful treatment with the antidepressants fluoxetine or fluvoxamine. Furthermore, the circulating levels of these two neurosteroids have been found to be decreased in depressed patients by Romeo et al. (53) and restored after treatment with fluoxetine and other antidepressants. Because these neurosteroids also decrease the activity of the HPA axis (54), which is markedly altered in depression (55), it would appear that allopregnanolone and pregnanolone may play a role in the pathophysiology of depression. It is significant to note that "stress" and depression share a variety of neuroendocrine abnormalities (56), and an increase in brain and plasma levels of allopregnanolone has been described following stress in experimental animals (57). Also, Uzunov et al. (58) have shown that the administration of fluoxetine and paroxetine (but not imipramine) to rats increases the brain level of allopregnanolone without increasing the levels of several other neurosteroids. This is presently presumed to be the result of a decreased rate of oxidative metabolism of 3α-5α-TH PROG to 5α-dihydroprogesterone that, as shown in Fig. 3, is a reversible reaction catalyzed by 3α-hydroxy steroid oxidoreductase. It is to be noted that Romeo et al. (53) found a concomitant decrease in $3\beta,5\alpha$-TH PROG in eight patients treated with fluoxetine as plasma levels of $3\alpha,5\alpha$-TH PROG were restored. In these patients the plasma levels of 5α-dihydroprogesterone did not change significantly. This is consistent with a shift in the direction of reduction of the 3-keto group of 5α-dihydroprogesterone.

CONCLUSIONS

This chapter has summarized some key advances in the chemistry and pharmacology of natural and synthetic steroids (neuroactive steroids) that modulate the action of GABA, a major inhibitory neurotransmitter in the brain. Attention has also been focused on the potential role of GABAergic neurosteroids in alcohol dependence and withdrawal, as well as in affective disorders. These are two areas where a growing body of evidence

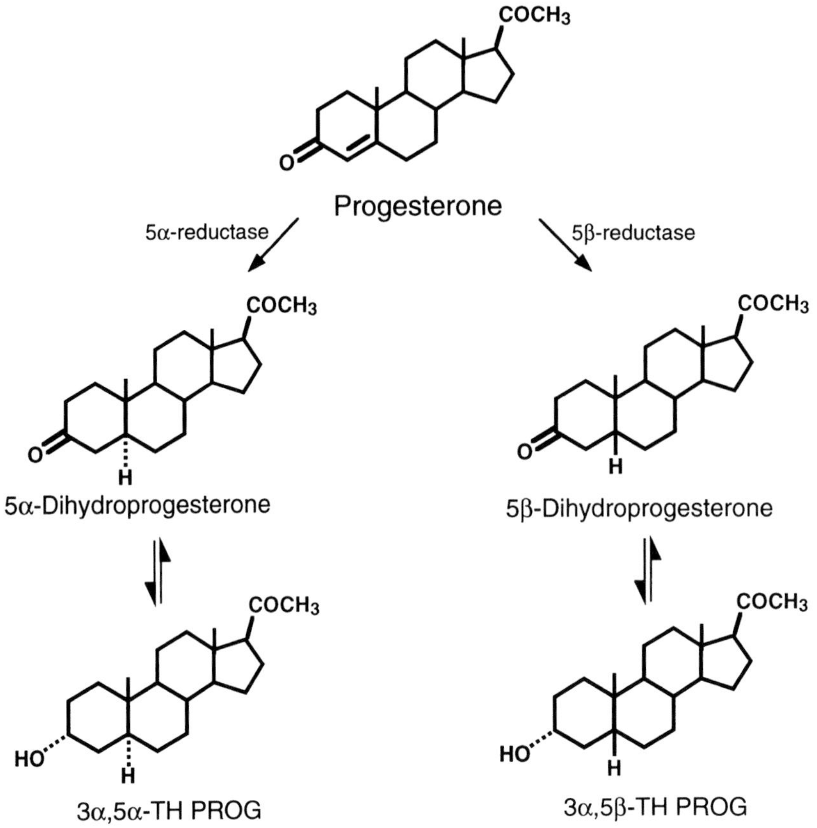

Fig. 3. Metabolic pathway for the formation of allopregnanolone (3α,5α-TH PROG) and pregnanolone (3α,5β-TH PROG).

suggests that these steroids may play a role in the behavioral and neuroendocrine consequences of stress-induced disorders. The now well-characterized interaction of neuroactive steroids with $GABA_A$ receptors will continue to prompt further efforts to delineate the mechanism of action of steroids on neuronal membranes, with emphasis on the rapid alteration of neuronal excitability.

ACKNOWLEDGMENTS

This work was supported in part by National Institutes of Health Grant NIAA AA06420 to The Scripps Research Institute. We are indebted to Elizabeth P. Gordon and Pamela J. Edmonds for their excellent editorial assistance.

REFERENCES

1. Paul SM, Purdy RH. Neuroactive steroids. FASEB J 1992;6:2311–2322.
2. Lambert JJ, Belelli D, Hill-Venning C, Peters JA. Neurosteroids and $GABA_A$ receptor function. Trends Pharmacol Sci 1995;16:295–303.
3. Olsen RW, Sapp DW. Neuroactive steroid modulation of $GABA_A$ receptors. Adv Biochem Psychopharmacol 1995;48:57–74.

4. Yu R, Ticku MK. Chronic neurosteroid treatment produces functional heterologous uncoupling at the γ-aminobutyric acid type A/benzodiazepine receptor complex in mammalian cortical neurons. Mol Pharmacol 1995;47:603–610.

5. Purdy RH, Morrow AL, Blinn JR, Paul SM. Synthesis, metabolism, and pharmacological activity of 3α-hydroxy steroids which potentiate GABA$_A$ receptor-mediated chloride uptake in rat cerebral cortical synaptoneurosomes. J Med Chem 1990;33:1572–1581.

6. Park-Chung M, Purdy RH, Gibbs TT, Farb DH. Inverse modulation of the GABA$_A$ receptor at distinct sites by steroids. Brain Res, submitted.

7. Hawkinson JE, Kimbrough CL, Belelli D, Lambert JL, Purdy RH, Lan NC. Correlation of neuroactive steroid modulation of [^{35}S]t-butylbicyclophosphoro-thionate and [^{3}H]flunitrazepam binding and γ-aminobutyric acid$_A$ receptor function. Mol Pharmacol 1994;46:977–985.

8. Morrow AL, Pace JR, Purdy RH, Paul SM. Characterization of steroid interactions with γ-aminobutyric acid receptor-gated chloride ion channels: Evidence for multiple steroid recognition sites. Mol Pharmacol 1990;37:263–270.

9. Hawkinson JE, Kimbrough CL, McCauley LD, Bolger MB, Lan NC, Gee KW. The neuroactive steroid 3α-hydroxy-5β-pregnan-20-one is a two-component modulator of ligand binding to the GABA$_A$ receptor. Eur J Pharmacol 1994;269:157–163.

10. McCauley LD, Liu V, Chen JS,. Hawkinson JE, Lan NC, Gee KW. Selective actions of certain neuroactive pregnanediols at the γ-aminobutyric acid type A receptor complex in rat brain. Mol Pharmacol 1995;47:354–362.

11. Prince RJ, MA Simmonds. Differential antagonism by epipregnanolone of alfaxalone and pregnanolone potentiation of [^{3}H]flunitrazepam binding suggests more than one class of binding sites at GABA$_A$ receptors. Neuropharmacology 1993;32:59–63.

12. Pignataro L, Fizer de Plazas S. Epipregnanolone acts as a partial agonist on a common neurosteroid modulatory site of the GABA$_A$ receptor complex in avian CNS. Neurochem Res 1997;22:221–225.

13. Hogenkamp DJ, Hasan Tahir SH, Hawkinson JE, Upasani RB, Alauddin M, Kimbrough C.L, Acosta-Burruel M, Whittemore ER, Woodward RM, Lan NC, Gee KW, Bolger MB. Synthesis and *in vitro* activity of 3β-substituted-3α-hydroxypregnan-20-ones: allosteric modulators of the GABA$_A$ receptor. J Med Chem 1997;40:61–72.

14. Hawkinson JE, Drewe JA, Kimbrough CL, Chen JS, Hogenkamp DJ, Lan NC, Gee KW, Shen KZ, Whittemore ER, Woodward RM. 3α-hydroxy-3β-trifluoromethyl-5α-pregnan-20-one (Co 2-1970): A partial agonist at the neuroactive steroid site of the γ-aminobutyric acid$_A$ receptor. Mol Pharmacol 1996;49:897–906.

15. Makriyannis A, DiMeglio CM, Fesik SW. Anesthetic steroid mobility in model membrane preparations as examined by high-resolution ^{1}H and ^{2}H NMR spectroscopy. J. Med. Chem. 1991;34:1700–1703.

16. Wittmer LL, Hu Y, Kalkbrenner M, Evers AS, Zorumski CF, Covey DF. Enantioselectivity of steroid-induced γ-aminobutyric acid$_A$ receptor modulation and anesthesia. Mol Pharmacol 1996;50:1581–1586.

17. Zorumski CF, Wittmer LL, Isenberg KE, Hu Y, Covey DF. Effects of neurosteroid and benz[e]indene enantiomers on GABA$_A$ receptors in cultured hippocampal neurons and transfected HEK-293 cells. Neuropharmacology 1996;35:1161–1168.

18. Zorumski CF, Mennerick SJ, Covey DJ. Enantioselective modulation of GABAergic synaptic transmission by steroids and benz[e]indenes in hippocampal microcultures. Synapse 1998;29:162–171.

19. Marker RE, Kamm O, McGrew RV. Sterols. IX. Isolation of *epi*-pregnanol-3-one-20 from human pregnancy urine. J Am Chem Soc 1937;59:616–618.

20. Hu Y, Wittmer LL, Kalkbrenner M, Evers AS, Zorumski CF, Covey DF. Neurosteroid analogs. 5. Enantiomers of neuroactive steroids and benz[e]indenes: total synthesis, electrophysiological effects on GABA$_A$ receptor function and anesthetic action in tadpoles. J Chem Soc Perkin Trans I 1997;3665–3671.

21. Nilsson KR, Zorumski CF, Covey DF. Neurosteroid analogues. 6. The synthesis and GABA$_A$ receptor pharmacology of enantiomers of dehydroepiandrosterone sulfate, pregnenolone sulfate, and (3α)-3-hydroxypregnan-20-one sulfate. J Med Chem 1998;41:2604–2613.

22. Britton KT, Page M, Baldwin H, Koob GF. Anxiolytic activity of steroid anesthetic alphaxalone. J Pharmacol Exp Ther 1991;258:124–129.

23. Melchior CL, Ritzmann RF. Dehydroepiandrosterone is an anxiolytic in mice on the plus-maze. Pharmacol Biochem Behav 1994;47:437–441.

24. Melchior CL, Ritzmann RF. Pregnenolone and pregnenolone sulfate, alone and with ethanol, in mice on the plus-maze. Pharmacol Biochem Behav 1994;48:893–897.

25. Zimmerberg B, Drucker PC, Weider JM. Differential behavioral effects of the neuroactive steroid allopregnanolone on neonatal rats prenatally exposed to alcohol. Pharmacol Biochem Behav 1995;51:463–468.

26. Wieland S, Belluzzi JD, Stein L, Lan NC. Comparative behavioral characterization of the neuroactive steroids 3α-OH-5α-pregnan-20-one and 3α-OH-3β-pregnan-20-one in rodents. Psychopharmacology 1995;118:65–71.

27. Brot MD, Akwa Y, Purdy RH, Koob GF, Britton KT. The anxiolytic-like effects of the neurosteroid allopregnanolone: Interactions with GABA$_A$ receptors. Eur J Pharmacol 1997;325:1–7.

28. Suzdak PD, Schwartz RD, Skolnick P, Paul SM. Ethanol stimulates γ-aminobutyric acid receptor-mediated chloride transport in rat brain synaptoneurosomes. Proc Natl Acad Sci USA 1986;83:4071–4075.

29. Devaud LL, Purdy RH, Morrow AL. The neurosteroid, 3α-hydroxy-5α-pregnan-20-one, protects against bicuculline-induced seizures during ethanol withdrawal in rats. Alcohol Clin Exp Res 1995;19:350–355.

30. Finn DA, Roberts AJ, Crabbe JC. Neuroactive steroid sensitivity in withdrawal seizure-prone and -resistant mice. Alcohol Clin Exp Res 1995;19:410–415.

31. Ator NA. Drug discrimination and drug stimulus generalization with anxiolytics. Drug Dev Res 1990;20:189–204.

32. Ator NA, Grant KA, Purdy RH, Paul SM, Griffiths RR. Drug discrimination analysis of endogenous neuroactive steroids in rats. Eur J Pharmacol 1993;241:237–243.

33. Grant KA, Azarov A, Bowen CA, Mirkis S, Purdy RH. Ethanol-like discriminative stimulus effects of the neurosteroid 3α-hydroxy-5α-pregnan-20-one in female Macaca fascicularis monkeys. Psychopharmacology 1996;124:340–346.

34. Pohorecky LA. The interaction of alcohol and stress: a review. Neurosci Biobehav Rev 1981;5:209–229.

35. Roberts AJ, Chu HP, Crabbe JC, Keith LD. Differential modulation by the stress axis of ethanol withdrawal seizure expression in WSP and WSR mice. Alcohol Clin Exp Res 1991;15:412–417.

36. Keith LD, Crabbe JC. Specific and nonspecific effects of ethanol vapor on plasma corticosterone in mice. Alcohol 1992;9:529–533.

37. Romeo E, Brancati A, De Lorenzo A, Fucci P, Furnari C, Pompili E, Sasso GF, Spalletta G, Troisi A, Pasini A. Marked decrease of plasma neuroactive steroids during alcohol withdrawal. Clin Neuropharmacol 1996;19:366–369.

38. Spencer RL, McEwen BS. Adaptation of the hypothalamic-pituitary-adrenal axis to chronic ethanol stress. Neuroendocrinology 1990;52:481–489.

39. Devaud LL, Purdy RH, Finn FA, Morrow AL. Sensitization of γ-aminobutyric acid-A receptors to neurosteroids in rats during ethanol withdrawal. J Pharmacol Exp Ther 1996;278:510–517.

40. Gordis E. Critical issues in alcoholism research. Int J Addict 1995;30:497–505.

41. Calahan D. Quantifying alcohol consumption: Patterns and problems. Circulation 1981;64:7–14.

42. Hilton ME. Drinking patterns and drinking problems in 1984: Results from a general population survey. Alcohol Clin Exp Res 1987;11:167–175.

43. Hilton ME, Clark WB. Society, culture and drinking patterns reexamined. Rutgers Center of Alcohol Studies, New Brunswick, NJ 1991.

44. Bixo M, Anderson A, Winblad B, Purdy RH, Bäckström T. Progesterone, 5α-pregane-3, 20-dione and 3α:-hydroxy-3α-pregnan-20-one in specific regions of the human female brain in different endocrine states. Brain Res 1997;764:173–178.

45. Roberts AJ, Smith AD, Weiss F, Rivier C, Koob GF. Estrous cycle effects on operant responding for ethanol in female rats. Alcohol Clin Exp Res 1998;22:1564–1569.

46. Genazzani AR, Petraglia F, Bernardi F, Casarosa E, Salvestroni C, Tonetti A, Nappi RE, Luisi S, Palumbo M, Purdy RH, Luisi M. Circulating levels of allopregnanolone in humans: Gender, age, and endocrine influences. J Clin Endocrinol Metab 1998;83:2099–2103.

47. Mello NK, Mendelson JH, Lex BW. Alcohol use and premenstrual symptoms in social drinkers. Psychopharmacology 1990;101:448–455.

48. Grant KA, Azarov A, Shively CA, Purdy RH. Discriminative stimulus effects of ethanol and 3α-hydroxy-5α-pregnan-20-one in relation to menstrual cycle phase in cynomolgus monkeys (*Macaca fascicularis*). Psychopharmacology 1997;130:59–68.

49. Smith SS, Gong QH, Hsu FC, Markowitz RS, ffrench-Mullen JMH, Li X. GABA$_A$ receptor α4 subunit suppression prevents withdrawal properties of an endogenous steroid. Nature 1998;392:926–930.

50. Kessler RC, McGonagle K.A, Nelson CB,. Hughes M, Swartz M, Blazer DG. Sex and depression in the National Comorbidity Survey: II. Cohort effects, J Affect Disord 1994;30:15–26.

51. Cornelius JR, Salloum IM, Ehler JG, Jarrett PJ, Cornelius MD, Perel JM, Thase ME, Black A. Fluoxetine in depressed alcoholics: A double-blind, placebo-controlled trial. Arch Gen Psychiatry 1997;54:700–705.

52. Uzunova V, Sheline Y, David JM, Rasmusson A, Uzunov DP, Costa E, Guidotti A. Increase in the cerebrospinal fluid content of neurosteroids in patients with unipolar major depression who are receiving fluoxetine or fluvoxamine. Proc Natl Acad Sci USA 1998;95:14,865–14,870.

53. Romeo E, Strohle A, Spaletta G, Di Michele F, Hermann B, Holsboer F. Effects of antidepressant treatment on neuroactive steroids in major depression. Am J Psychiatry 1998;155:910–913.

54. Patchev VK, Shoaib M, Holsboer F, Almeida OFX. The neurosteroid tetrahydroprogesterone counteracts corticotropin-releasing hormone-induced anxiety and alters the release and gene expression of corticotropin-releasing hormone in the rat hypothalamus. Neuroscience 1994;62:265–271.

55. Holsboer F, Lauer CJ, Schreiber W, Krieg JC. Altered hypothalamic-pituitary-adrenocortical regulation in healthy subjects at high familial risk for affective disorders. Neuroendocrinology 1995;62:340–347.

56. Holsboer F, Spengler D, Heuser I. The role of corticotropin-releasing hormone in the pathogenesis of Cushing's disease, anorexia nervosa, alcoholism, affective disorders and dementia. Prog Brain Res 1992;93:385–417.

57. Purdy RH, Morrow AL, Moore PH Jr, Paul SM. Stress-induced elevations of GABA$_A$ receptor-active steroids in the rat brain. Proc Natl Acad Sci USA 1991;88:4553–4557.

58. Uzunov DP, Cooper TB, Costa E, Guidotti A. Fluoxetine-elicited changes in brain neurosteroid content measured by negative ion mass fragmentography. Proc Natl Acad Sci USA 1996;93:12,599–12,604.

9

Neurosteroid Antagonists of the GABA$_A$ Receptors

Maria Dorota Majewska, MD

CONTENTS

INTRODUCTION
NEUROSTEROIDS AS AN ANTAGONIST OF GABA$_A$ RECEPTORS
PHYSIOLOGICAL ROLE OF GABA-ANTAGONISTIC STEROIDS
REFERENCES

INTRODUCTION

During the past 15 years it became evident that the brain is capable of the *de novo* synthesis of steroids called "neurosteroids," which have been recognized as important regulators of neuronal activities *(1,2).* The definition of "neurosteroids" encompasses the steroids synthesized in nervous tissues as well as some adrenal and gonadal steroids that directly affect neurotransmission. Although estrogens, androgens and glucocorticoids are also neuroactive, they are generally not considered as neurosteroids, because their genomic actions generalize to their activities in other tissues. The synthesis of neurosteroids is discussed in other chapters of this monograph and will not be addressed here. This chapter describes biochemical, physiological, and behavioral aspects of the GABA$_A$ receptor antagonistic actions of neurosteroids, primarily pregnenolone sulfate (PREGS) and dehydroepiandrosterone sulfate (DHEAS), and discusses their psycho-physio-pathological significance (for comprehensive review, *see* ref. *2*). PREGS and DHEAS are present in significant amounts in brains of different species, ranging from rodents to primates, including humans *(3–6).*

NEUROSTEROIDS AS ANTAGONIST OF GABA$_A$ RECEPTORS

The ubiquitous GABA$_A$ receptor complex is a protein pentamer *(7)* whose activation by GABA opens the associated chloride channel, leading to increased chloride conductance and resulting usually in hyperpolarization of neuronal membrane. In the brain, heterogenous forms of GABA$_A$ receptors exist with different combinations of polypeptide subunits, which change during development *(8,9).* Activity of the GABA$_A$ receptors is enhanced by hypnotic-anesthetic drugs such as benzodiazepines

From: *Contemporary Endocrinology: Neurosteroids: A New Regulatory Function in the Nervous System* Edited by: E.-E. Baulieu, P. Robel, and M. Schumacher
© Humana Press Inc., Totowa, NJ

and barbiturates and is inhibited by the convulsants such as picrotoxin, bicuculline, and pentylenetetrazol.

An early finding of a modulatory effect of cholesterol on $GABA_A$ receptors (M. D. Majewska, 1992, unpublished observation), led me to explore the GABA-ergic activity of other steroids. In several collaborative studies we observed that certain steroids act as GABA-agonists, whereas others act as antagonists (2). My early investigations concerned mostly the activity of PREGS, whose presence in the brain was discovered at that time (3,4). In mammals, pregnenolone, and PREGS are precursors of all steroids produced in the brain and peripheral tissues. Initially we described bimodal effect of PREGS on binding of GABA agonist muscimol to $GABA_A$ receptors in rat synaptosomal membranes and brain slices (10). PREGS increased muscimol binding at nanomolar concentrations and decreased it at micromolar concentrations. Subsequent studies revealed mixed $GABA_A$ agonistic/antagonistic features of PREGS, because although this steroid potentiated benzodiazepine binding, it also inhibited barbiturate-induced enhancement of benzodiazepine binding (11). GABA-antagonistic properties of PREGS were also inferred from its competitive inhibition of binding of the convulsant TBPS. The final proof of $GABA_A$ antagonistic actions of PREGS was furnished by functional assays that demonstrated that this steroid at micromolar concentrations and in a dose-dependent manner inhibited GABA-induced chloride transport or current in synaptoneurosomes and neurons, respectively (11–13). Binding studies revealed that radiolabeled PREGS interacts with several recognition sites in synaptosomal membranes and that it's micromolar affinity site corresponds with the site of convulsant binding to the $GABA_A$ receptor (14).

Experiments performed with cloned receptors revealed that subunit composition of the $GABA_A$ receptors determines their sensitivity to neurosteroids (15). For example, the agonistic actions of nanomolar concentrations of PREGS, which were observed in binding experiments (10), could not be detected in electrophysiological recordings in neurons isolated from neonatal rat cerebral cortex (12), but were seen in recombinant receptors containing combinations of α-2 and α-3 subunits (15). This suggests that the neurosteroids may have distinct actions in different neurons which contain distinct subtypes of $GABA_A$ receptors.

DHEAS, which is a major adrenal hormone in humans, behaves as a $GABA_A$ receptor antagonist similar to PREGS. At low micromolar concentrations, it blocks GABA-induced currents in isolated neurons and appears to interact with the site close to that of barbiturate actions (16,17). DHEAS and PREGS accelerate fast desensitization of $GABA_A$ receptors (15,18) and we showed that presence of sulfate group at 3β position of the steroid A-ring enhances their antagonistic potency (16,17). The hypothetical models proposed that the neurosteroids most likely interact with hydrophobic domains of protein subunits of $GABA_A$ receptors (1,19), but the structure-specific interactions of steroids with phospholipids in neuronal and glial cells (20) may also contribute to their complex binding patterns (14,17) and their synaptic actions.

Predominantly GABA-antagonistic features of PREGS and DHEAS contrast with purely GABA-agonistic actions of other naturally occurring steroids, such as allopregnanolone (3α,5α-THPROG; 3α-hydroxy-5α-pregnan-20-one), tetrahydro-deoxycorticosterone (3α,5α-THDOC; 3α,21α-dihydroxy-5α-pregnan-20-one), or androsterone (3α-hydroxy-5α-androstan-17-one), which we (21,22) and others (23) have described.

The GABA-ergic steroids modulate the synaptic events and may play a critical role in neuronal plasticity. GABA-agonistic steroids prolong inhibitory postsynaptic potentials (IPSP) *(22)* and depress depolarizing responses to glutamate and glutamate-induced action potentials *(24)*, whereas GABA antagonistic DHEAS and PREGS reduce the amplitudes of IPSP (18), thus enhancing neuronal depolarization. Consistently, excitatory effects of PREGS and DHEAS on neurons were reported *(25)*, along with their convulsant actions in animals *(26)*. Additional dimension of central actions of neurosteroids stems from their analogous modulatory activity at $GABA_A$ receptors in astrocytes *(27)*. Because the astrocytic receptors are believed to participate in the regulation of Cl$^-$ homeostasis *(28)*, the synaptic activity of neurosteroids may be magnified by their cooperative actions at both neuronal and glial receptors. Allosteric agonistic actions of these neurosteroids on the N-methyl-D-aspartate (NMDA) receptors *(29)* may synergistically potentiate their neuroexcitatory effects. As different neurosteroids modulate $GABA_A$ (and NMDA) receptors in opposite directions, a ratio between the excitatory and inhibitory steroids may shape synaptic activity.

PHYSIOLOGICAL ROLE OF GABA-ANTAGONISTIC STEROIDS

The neuroactive effects of certain steroids were recognized in 1920s by Cashin and Moravek *(30)*, who described the anesthetic action of intravenously injected cholesterol. Next, Selye *(31)* showed hypnotic actions of progesterone and deoxycorticosterone (DOC), and his studies led to the development of steroidal anesthetics, structurally similar to 3α,5α-THPROG and 3α,5α-THDOC *(22,32)*. The anesthetic effects of progesterone and those of 3α,5α-THPROG and 3α,5α-THDOC *(33,34)* as well as their anxiolytic *(35)* and antiaggressive *(36)* features can now be explained by their potentiation of $GABA_A$ receptor function *(21)*.

Hypnotic/anxiolytic actions of 3α,5α-THPROG and 3α,5α-THDOC contrast with the behavioral effects of GABA-antagonistic neurosteroids. DHEA injected intraperitoneally in doses 100–150 mg/kg produced tonic-clonic seizures in mice, but in lower doses it caused sedation *(26)*. The convulsant effects of DHEA most likely resulted from its GABA-antagonistic activity *(16,17)*, whereas the sedative effects could be mediated by the GABA-agonistic DHEA metabolite, androsterone. Also PREGS, injected intracerebroventricularly (8 μg/10 μL) reduced the barbiturate-induced sleep in rats *(37)*, but at lower doses it tended to prolong the sleep. Ubiquitous distribution of $GABA_A$ receptors in the central nervous system (CNS) and their vital role in control of neuronal excitability suggest that bimodal regulation of these receptors by the neurosteroids determines many brain functions and behaviors. Increase in synaptic concentrations of DHEAS or PREGS should augment neuronal excitability, and CNS arousal, and have analeptic effects, whereas elevation in concentrations of 3α,5α-THPROG or 3α,5α-THDOC should enhance neuronal inhibition, facilitating sleep and reducing anxiety *(35)*. A fine interplay may exist between the hypnotic/anxiolytic steroids and the excitatory ones, which not only counteract each other actions, but are also metabolically linked, as the antagonistic steroids PREGS and DHEAS, can be converted in the brain and in the periphery to the agonistic ones, 3α,5α-THPROG and androsterone *(2)*. Hence, metabolic activity of enzymes responsible to these conversions may to some degree determine neuronal activity.

Neurosteroids and CNS Development

Plasma levels of adrenal DHEA and DHEAS undergo dramatic developmental changes *(38,39)*, suggesting that they may be involved in ontogeny. Ther role in brain development is implied by the experiments that showed that DHEA and DHEAS enhance neuronal and glial survival and differentiations in cultures from embryonic brains *(40)*. Neurodevelopmental actions of DHEA(S) may be, in part, mediated via their actions at the GABA$_A$ receptors, whose subunit composition changes during fetal and neonatal development *(8,9)*. In early embryonic and postnatal life, GABA acting via GABA$_A$ receptors depolarizes neurons from rat cortex, cerebellum, or spinal cord *(41)* and in immature neurons GABA stimulates chemokinesis *(42)*, thereby facilitating neuronal migration. Because the "immature" GABA$_A$ receptors are modulated by the neurosteroids *(15,44)*, an interplay between expression of distinct receptor subtypes manifesting different sensitivity to neurosteroids *(15,44)*, and changing concentrations of neurosteroids in brains of the fetuses and neonates may sculpt neurodevelopmental processes. A role of DHEA in the development deserves special attention. This steroid appears to be synthesized in the CNS, because it was present in brains of adult rats even after adrenalectomy and gonadectomy *(3)*, but the efforts to find the cytochrome P450c17, which has 17-hydroxylase-17,20-lyase activity (and which converts PREG to DHEA) in brains of adult rats were unsuccessful *(45)*. Nonetheless, mRNA for P450c17 was detected in brains of rat embryos *(46)*. The transient developmental presence of DHEA synthesizing enzyme in the embryonic brain, combined with striking developmental changes of DHEA levels in plasma, strongly suggest an important role of this hormone in CNS development. For example, the very high plasma concentration of DHEAS at birth in humans *(39)* may have an essential analeptic role during birth both for fetus and mother.

Neurosteroids and Sex Differentiation of the Brain

It has been now firmly established that morphological, neurochemical and functional differences exist between female and male brains (reviewed in ref. *47*). In most sexually dimorphic animals, including mammals, the intrinsic pattern of sexual development is female. The male pattern of development is determined by a switching mechanism located in mammals in specific gene(s) on the Y chromosome *(48)*, resulting in the formation of testes from the indifferent genital ridge early in embryonic development. Further diversion from the default female pathway of development to the male path depends on organizational and activational actions of fetal testosterone and other androgens.

GABA system is intimately involved in brain development and it participates in sex differentiation of the brain. This is convincingly illustrated by the experiments performed by Segovia et al. *(49)* showing that the perinatal exposure of rats to the GABA agonist, diazepam, alters sexual dimorphism in the rat accessory olfactory bulb. It is very likely therefore that the GABAergic steroids, whose concentrations change during fetal, neonatal, and peripubertal life, may also participate in sex differentiation of the brain. One can surmise that relative concentrations of the GABA-antagonistic steroids (DHEAS, DHEA, and PREGS), vs those of GABA-agonistic steroids (3α,5α-THPROG, 3α,5α-THDOC, and androsterone) at critical periods of development may chisel certain aspects of sexual brain development.

Neurosteroids in Learning, Memory and Brain Aging

In mature neurons, stimulation of $GABA_A$ receptors produces mainly hyperpolarization, hence GABAergic steroids there may have opposite actions than in immature neurons (where GABA is depolarizing). Brinton *(50)* showed the GABA agonistic steroid $3\alpha,5\alpha$-THPROG increased chloride influx in hippocampal neuronal cultures and induced reversible structural regression of these neurons. This implies that GABAergic steroids play a dynamic role in shaping neuronal architecture, and as such, may have critical function in learning, memory, and neuron survival during aging or stress. In this aspect, PREGS and DHEAS, as GABA antagonists, should facilitate neuronal structural growth. Such effect of DHEAS was indeed observed in vitro in neuronal and glial cultures *(40)*.

Deterioration of cognitive functions typically accompanies aging. The role of GABA in learning and memory is evidenced by the fact that GABA antagonists facilitate the hippocampal long-term potentiation (LTP) *(51)*; LTP is a synaptic process mediated via excitatory neurotransmitters, believed to be fundamental for long-term memory. Because an inhibitory input provided by the GABAergic interneurons sets a threshold for postsynaptic modification of excitatory inputs *(52)*, the GABAergic steroids are likely to influence memory. In this context, DHEAS, DHEA, and PREGS, as GABA-antagonists, are expected to enhance learning and memory, and the GABA-agonistic steroids are expected to impair memory, in an analogous manner, as barbiturates and benzodiazepines produce amnesia *(53)*, whereas GABA antagonists, picrotoxin and pentylenetetrazol, reverse amnesia and improve memory *(54,55)*. Pentylenetetrazol was even used with some success in treatment of geriatric patients with impaired memory *(56)*. Indeed, PREGS and DHEAS/DHEA were shown to improve memory in aging mice *(57,58)* and to prevent pharmacologically induced amnesia *(59)*. Potentiating effects of DHEA on automatized memory have been also recently documented in humans *(60)*. DHEA(S) acting at the $GABA_A$ receptors may additionally enhance memory by augmenting the rapid eye movement (REM) sleep *(61)*, which is believed to be involved in consolidation of memory. In contrast, the GABA-agonistic progesterone metabolites seem to impair automatized memory tasks *(62)*.

Excessive GABAergic tone may accelerate neuronal degeneration and brain aging. This concept is consistent with marked cognitive impairments associated with cerebral atrophy observed in chronic users of benzodiazepines *(63)*. Marczynski reported that chronic administration of the benzodiazepine antagonist, flumazenil, improved memory and prolonged the life-span of rats, and he proposed a GABA/benzodiazepine hypothesis of brain aging *(64)*. Augmentation of GABAergic tone during aging and in brain degeneration is suggested by increased activity of glutamic acid decarboxylase found in brains of humans who died from Alzheimer disease *(64)*, and by the enhanced GABA-activated currents measured in neurons from aged rats *(65)*. Globally, these effects would reduce neuronal excitability and possibly accelerate neuronal aging. In this context, PREGS and DHEAS, being antagonists of $GABA_A$ receptors, may counteract some of the effects of aging in neurons, thus improving memory and promoting neuronal survival *(40,57,58)*. Concordantly, some studies showed lower than normal levels of DHEAS in serum of patients diagnosed with Alzheimer disease and multi-infarct dementia *(66,67)* and in men with organic brain syndrome *(68)*.

Although peripheral steroids can penetrate blood brain barrier, the brain and CSF levels of DHEA and DHEAS are better forecasters of their central actions than plasma levels. In fact, plasma DHEAS levels, although predictive of mortality, were not generally predictive of cognitive functions in elderly (69). Postmortem studies on individuals who died at age >60 yr, showed higher DHEA and DHEAS levels in cerebral cortices of women than men (5). This intriguing observation—which needs to be replicated—may be significant, despite a small sample size, because it was consistent in four cerebral cortical areas, whereas DHEA/DHEAS levels in other brain regions were not different between the two sexes and there were no gender differences in cerebral concentrations of other steroids (5). In CSF of patients (50–60 yr old) no gender difference was found in DHEA levels (about 120 pg/mL), but women had significantly lower levels of DHEAS (515 pg/mL) than men (872 pg/mL) (70). There was also a negative correlation between CSF levels of DHEAS and aging in men but not in women. The physiological significance of these observations is not known, but it is intriguing to find out if the higher concentrations of DHEAS in cerebral cortices in women combined with absence of decline of this steroid with age in women could be responsible in some way for their generally greater longevity. It is conceivable that higher CSF concentrations of DHEAS in men than in women may be indicative of greater loss of this steroid from men's brains, possibly as a result of their earlier aging-related brain degeneration (71), as elevated CSF concentrations of DHEAS were also found in patients with neuropathies (70). Collectively, the above observations, although still incomplete, appear to suggest that declining levels of DHEA/DHEAS and PREGS in the brain may accelerate brain aging and may be concordant with earlier death.

Neurosteroids in Biological Rhythms and Stress

Plasma levels of adrenal steroids typically undergo diurnal cyclical changes (72). Likewise, there are circadian variations in the brain concentrations of neurosteroids (73). In the brain of the nocturnal animal rat, DHEAS levels peak at the prenocturnal hours and remain high through the first half of the dark cycle (73), following the plasma pattern. In humans, DHEAS in plasma manifests modest circadian rhythms and its higher levels are generally found during day hours and lower at night (73,74). The brain levels of DHEAS in humans may undergo similar diurnal changes as the plasma levels. The elevated concentrations of DHEAS and other excitatory steroids may serve an analeptic role during periods of intense activity.

The pioneering work of Selye (75) delineated the essential role of adrenal steroids during stress. Concentrations of GABA antagonistic neurosteroids, PREGS, and DHEAS are also elevated in the brain during stress (1), thus increasing neuronal arousal. On the other hand, increased synthesis of the GABA-agonistic steroid 3α,5α-THDOC, may calm the brain during stress. Hence the relative ratios of excitatory to inhibitory neurosteroids may determine to some extend the individual's behavior during stress. Complex role of neurosteroids in stress was discussed in detail elsewhere (2).

Neurosteroids and Personality, Aggressivity, and Drug Dependence

Neuromodulatory actions of steroids at the $GABA_A$ receptors invite the speculation that their profile in plasma and the CNS contributes to different personality traits. The steroid profile is genetically determined; it changes during the development, aging, pregnancy, stress, and in some pathologies. Theoretically, a higher proportion of excitatory steroids to inhibitory ones would result in anxiety-prone, introvert type of personality, characterized by higher level of resting arousal, greater sensitivity accompanied by a tendency to augment the incoming stimuli, and a low threshold for positive hedonic tone *(76)*. Elevated concentrations of DHEAS and PREGS may contribute to this personality by increasing basal CNS arousal and may be responsible for their high sedation threshold *(77)*. In contrast, a higher ratio of inhibitory steroids to the excitatory ones could result in a personality with tendency for blunted reaction to stimuli, an extreme cases of which would be "sensation seekers," characterized by an atypically high threshold for arousal who require very strong stimuli to achieve positive hedonic tone. There is an empirical support to this thesis, because women characterized by highly expansive personalities and men manifesting type A behavior were shown to have markedly lower plasma levels of the excitatory steroid DHEAS, than women with low expansivity or men characterized as type B *(73,74,78)*. The type A personality was also marked by excessive secretion of cortisol. Lower levels of DHEA(S), and especially lower DHEA(S) to cortisol ratios in type A individuals may contribute to their greater cardiovascular morbidity and generally higher mortality.

Characteristic for type A personality is also a tendency for antisocial behaviors and substance abuse. We have recently demonstrated that the low plasma levels of DHEA(S) are highly predictive of propensity to relapse in detoxified cocaine addicts *(79)*. Lower than normal plasma levels of DHEA were also found in children and adolescents with attention deficit hyperactivity disorder (ADHD) *(80)*, and this disorder constitutes a major risk factor for stimulant dependence *(81)*. One can predict therefore that supplementation of some cocaine addicts with DHEA may compensate for the existing deficits of this steroid and might aid their treatment. We have initiated testing this hypothesis in a clinical trial.

Aggressivity is an element of personality that remains under strong hormonal control. Androgens typically induce intermale aggression in all species and they were shown to provoke infanticide by male rodents, whereas castration or treatment with anti-androgenic drugs results in gentling of males *(82)*. DHEA suppressed aggressivity of castrated males against lactating females *(83)*. The biological mechanism of this effect is not known and may be complex. Antiaggressive effect of DHEA, as an GABA antagonist, is inconsistent with general antiaggressive features of GABA-agonistic drugs *(84)*. Most benzodiazepines are antiaggressive, although sometimes they evoke paradoxical "rage reactions" and increased hostility in humans *(85)*. Also, the GABA-agonistic steroid $3\alpha,5\alpha$-THDOC reduces aggression *(36)*. In this context, antiaggressive effects of DHEA could be explained by its metabolism to the anxiolytic androsterone and/or by its ability to increase hypothalamic and possibly cortical levels of serotonin *(86)* that is inversely correlated with aggressivity *(87)*.

Neurosteroids and Mood

Steroid hormones are known for their the powerful effect on affect. Cyclical changes of gonadal steroid levels may influence the neurotransmission and may be responsible for premenstrual or posparturitional mood changes in some women *(2,47)*. DHEAS was recently shown to potentiate NMDA-induced noradrenaline release from hippocampal slices *(88)*. The latter mechanism, combined with DHEA proserotonergic actions *(86)*, may be accountable for the reported antidepressant effects of DHEA in humans *(60)* and it may contribute to potentiating effect of DHEA on memory, in which norepinephrine plays a pivotal role *(89,90)*. Recent placebo controlled study by the Yen et al. *(91)* documented positive mood effect of supplementation of middle-aged people with DHEA, along with other beneficial physiological effects. Also past and recent clinical studies with pregnenolone suggest that this neurosteroid may have mood improving and analeptic effects *(19)*.

Role of GABA-ergic Steroids in Parturition

In addition to their abundance in the CNS, the $GABA_A$ receptors are present in variety of peripheral tissues. We have discovered a novel mechanism of regulation of uterine motility by the steroids acting via $GABA_A$ receptors *(92)*. The GABA-agonistic steroid $3\alpha,5\alpha$-THPROG, decreased uterine contractions, whereas GABA-antagonistic PREGS, strongly potentiated them. Because the concentrations of $3\alpha,5\alpha$-THPROG, along with those of progesterone, increase greatly during pregnancy, this steroid, acting via $GABA_A$ receptors, may have a direct calming effect on the uterus. On the other hand, the GABA-antagonistic steroids, whose plasma and umbilical cord concentrations rise at time of birth, may contribute to rapid increase of uterine contractions during parturition.

REFERENCES

1. Baulieu EE, Robel P, Vatier O, Haug A, Le Goascogne C, Bourreau E. Neurosteroids: pregnenolone and dehydroepiandrosterone in the rat brain. In: Fuxe K, Agnati LF, eds. Receptor-Receptor Interactions: A New Intramembrane Integrative Mechanisms. MacMillan, Basingstoke, UK, 1987, pp. 89–104.
2. Majewska MD. Neurosteroids: endogenous bimodal modulators of the $GABA_A$ receptor. Mechanism of action and physiological significance. Prog Neurobiol 1992;38:279–295.
3. Corpechot C, Robel P, Axelson M, Sjovall J, Baulieu EE. Characterization and measurement of dehydroepiandrosterone sulfate in rat brain. Proc Natl Acad Sci USA 1981;78:4704–4707.
4. Corpechot C, Synguelakis M, Talha S, Axelson M, Sjovall J, Vihko R, Baulieu EE, Robel P. Pregnenolone and its sulfate ester in the rat brain. Brain Res 1983;270:119–125.
5. Lanthier A, Patwardhan VV. Sex steroids and 5-en–3β-hydroxysteroids in specific regions of the human brain and cranial nerves. J Steroid Biochem 1986;25:445–449.
6. Lacroix C, Fiet J, Benais JP, Gueux B, Bonete R, Villette JM, Gourmel B, Dreux C. Simultaneous radioimmunoassay of progesterone, androst-4-ene-dione, pregnenolone, dehydroepi-androsterone and 17-hydroxyprogesterone in specific regions of human brain. J Steroid Biochem 1987;28:317–325.
7. Schofield PR, Darlison MG, Fujita M, Burt DR, Stephenson FA, Rodriguez H, Rhee LM, Ramachandran J, Reale V, Glencorse TA, Seeburg PH, Barnard EA. Sequence and functional expression of the $GABA_A$ receptor shows a ligand-gated receptor super-family. Nature 1987;328:8221–227.
8. Laurie DJ, Wisden W, Seeburg PH. The distribution of thirteen GABA-A receptor subunit mRNAs in the rat brain. III. Embryonic and postnatal development. J Neurosci 1992;12:4151–4172.
9. Poulter MO, Barker JL, O'Carroll AM, Lolait SJ, Mahan LC. Differential and transient expression of GABA-A receptor alpha-subunit mRNAs in the developing rat CNS. J Neurosci 1992;12:2888–2900.
10. Majewska MD, Bisserbe JC, Eskay RE. Glucocorticoids are modulators of $GABA_A$ receptors in brain. Brain Res 1985;339:178–182.
11. Majewska MD, Schwartz RD. Pregnenolone-sulfate: an endogenous antagonist of the γ-aminobutyric acid receptor complex in brain? Brain Res 1987;404:355–360.
12. Majewska MD, Mienville JM, Vicini S. Neurosteroid pregnenolone sulfate antagonizes electrophysiological responses to GABA in neurons. Neurosci Lett 1988;90:279–284.
13. Mienville JM, Vicini S. Pregnenolone sulfate antagonizes $GABA_A$ receptor-mediated currents via a reduction of channel opening frequency. Brain Res 1989;489: 190–194.
14. Majewska MD, Demirgoren S, London ED. Binding of pregnenolone sulfate to rat brain membranes suggests multiple sites of steroid action at the $GABA_A$ receptor. Eur J Pharmacol Mol Pharmacol Sect 1990;189:307–315.

15. Zaman SH, Shingai R, Harvey RJ, Darlison MG, Barnard EA. Effects of subunit types of the recombinant GABA$_A$ receptor on the response to a neurosteroid. Eur J Pharmacol Mol Pharmacol Sect 1992;225:321–330.

16. Majewska MD, Demirgoren S, Spivak CE, London ED. The neurosteroid dehydroepiandrosterone sulfate is an antagonist of the GABA$_A$ receptor. Brain Res 1990;526:143–146.

17. Demirgoren S, Majewska MD, Spivak CE, London ED. Receptor binding and electrophysiological effects of dehydroepiandrosterone sulfate, an antagonist of the GABA$_A$ receptor. Neuroscience 1991;45:127–135.

18. Spivak CE. Desensitization and noncompetitive blockade of GABA$_A$ receptors in ventral midbrain neurons by a neurosteroid dehydroepiandrosterone sulfate. Synapse 1994 16:113–122.

19. Roberts E. Pregnenolone: from Selye to Alzheimer and a model of pregnenolone sulfate binding site to the GABA$_A$ receptor. Biochem Pharmacol 1995;1:1–16.

20. Ueda I, Tatara T, Chiou JS, Krishna PR. Structure-selective anesthetic action od steroids: anesthetic potency and effects on lipid and protein. Anesth Analg 1994;78:718–725.

21. Majewska MD, Harrison NL, Schwartz RD, Barker JL, Paul SM. Steroid hormone metabolites are barbiturate-like modulators of the GABA$_A$ receptor. Science 1986;232:1004–1007.

22. Harrison NL, Majewska MD, Harrington JW, Barker LL. Structure–activity relationships for steroid interaction with the γ-aminobutyric acid$_A$ receptor complex. J Pharm Exp Ther 1987; 241:346–353.

23. Peters JA, Kirkness EF, Callachan H, Lambert JJ, Turner AJ. Modulation of the GABA$_A$ receptor by depressant barbiturates and pregnane steroids. Brit J Pharmacol 1988;94:1257–1269.

24. Lambert JJ, Peters JA, Strugges NC, Hales TG. Steroid modulation of the GABA$_A$ receptor complex: electrophysiological studies. In: Chadwick D, Widdows K, eds. Steroids and Neuronal Activity, Ciba Foundation Symposium, vol 153, Wiley, Chichester, UK, 1990, pp. 56–70.

25. Carette B, Poulain P. Excitatory effect of dehydroepiandrosterone, its sulphate esther and pregnenolone sulphate, applied by iontophoresis and pressure, on single neurons in the septo-optic area of the guinea pig. Neurosci Lett 1984;45:205–210.

26. Heuser G, Eidelberg E. Steroid induced convulsions in experimental animals. Endocrinology 1961;69:915–924.

27. Chvatal A, Kettenmann H. Effect of steroids on gamma-aminobutyrate-induced currents in cultured rat astrocytes. Pflugers Arch 1991;419:263–266.

28. MacVicar BA, Tse FWY, Cracton SE, Kettenmann H. GABA activated chloride channels in astrocytes of hippocampal slices. J Neurosci 1989;9:3577–3583.

29. Wu F-S, Gibbs TT, Farb, DH. Pregnenolone sulfate: a positive allosteric modulator at the N-methyl-D-aspartate receptor. Mol Pharmacol 1991;40:333–336.

30. Cashin MF, Moravek V. The physiological actions of cholesterol. Am J Physiol 1927;82:294–298.

31. Selye H. Correlations between the chemical structure and the pharmacological actions of the steroids. Endocrinol 1942;30:437–452.

32. Gyermek L, Soyka LF. Steroid anesthetics. Anesthesiology 1975;42:331–344.

33. Holzbauer M. Physiological aspects of steroids with anaesthetic properties. Med Biol 1976;54:227–242.

34. Kraulis I, Foldes G, Tarikov H, Dubrovsky B, Birmingham MK. Distribution, metabolism and biological activity of deoxycorticosterone in ventral nervous system. Brain Res 1975;88:1–14.

35. Crawley JN, Glowa JR, Majewska MD, Paul SM. Anxiolytic activity of endogenous adrenal steroid. Brain Res 1986;339:382–386.

36. Kavaliers M. Inhibitory influences of adrenal steroid, 3α,5α-tetrahydrodeoxycorticosterone on aggression and defeat-induced analgesia in mice. Psychopharmacol. (Berlin) 1988;95:488–492.

37. Majewska MD, Bluet-Pajot MT, Robel P, Baulieu EE. Pregnenolone sulfate antagonizes barbiturate-induced sleep. Pharmacol Biochem Behav 1989;33:701–703.

38. Hopper BR, Yen SSC. Circulating concentrations of dehydroepiandrosterone and dehydroepiandrosterone sulfate during puberty. J Endocrinol Metab 1975;40:458–461.

39. De Peretti E, Forest MG. Unconjugated dehydroepiandrosterone plasma levels in normal subjects from birth to adolescence in human: the use of a sensitive radioimmunoassay. J Clin Endocrinol Metab 1976;43:982–991.

40. Roberts E, Bologa L, Flood JF, Smith GE. Effects of dehydroepiandrosterone and its sulfate on brain tissues in culture and on memory in mice. Brain Res 1987;406:357–362.

41. Cherubini E, Gaiarsa JL, Ben-Ari Y. GABA: an excitatory transmitter in early postnatal life. TINS 1991;14:515–519.

42. Behar TN, Schaffner AE, Colton CA, Samogyi R, Olah Z, Lehel C, Barker JL. GABA-induced chemokinesis and NGF-induced chemotaxis of embryonic spinal cord neurons. J Neurosci 1994;14:29–38.

43. Smith SV, Barker JL. Depolarizing responses to 3α-OH-reduced pregnane steroid metabolites and GABA occur in the majority of embryonic rat cortical cells. Soc Neurosci Abstr 1991;17, 749.

44. Shingai R, Sutherland ML, Barnard EA. Effects of subunit types of cloned $GABA_A$ receptor on the response to a neurosteroid. Eur J Pharmacol Mol Pharmacol Sect 1991;206:77–80.

45. Robel P, Akwa Y, Corpechot C, Hu ZY, Jung-Testas I, Kabbadj K, Le Goascogne CL, Morfin R, Vourc'h C, Young J, Baulieu EE. Neurosteroids: biosynthesis and function of pregnenolone and dehydroepiandrosterone in the brain. In: Motta M, ed. Brain Endocrinology. Raven, New York, 1991, pp. 105–132.

46. Campagnone NA, Bulfone A, Rubenstein JLR and Mellon CH. Steroid enzyme P450c-17 is expressed in the embryonic central nervous system. Endocrinology 1995;136:1–11.

47. Majewska MD. Sex differences in brain morphology and pharmacodynamics. In: Jensvold MF, Halbreich U, Hamilton JA, eds. Psychopharmacology and Women. American Psychiatric Association Press, Washington, DC, 1996, pp. 73–83.

48. Koopman P, Gubbay J, Vivian N, Goodfellow P, Lovell-Badge R. Male development of chromosomally female mice transgenic for Sry. Nature 1991;351:117–121.

49. Perez-Laso C, Valencia A, Rodriguez-Zafra M, Cales JM, Guillamon A, Segovia S. Perinatal adminstration of diazepam alters sexual dimorphism in the rat accessory olfactory bulb. Brain Res 1994;634:1–6.

50. Brinton RD. The neurosteroid 3α-hydroxy–5α-pregnane–20-one induces architectural regression in cultured fetal hippocampal neurons. J Neurosci 1994;14:2763–2774.

51. Wigstrom H, Gustaffson B. Facilitation of hippocampal long-lasting potentiation by GABA-antagonists. Acta Physiol Scand 1985;125:159–172.

52. Douglas RM, Goddard GV, Rives M. Inhibitory modulation of long-term potentiation: evidence for a postsynaptic control. Brain Res 1982;240:259–272.

53. Roehrs T, Zorick FJ, Sicklesteel JM, Wittig RM, Hartse KM, Roth T. Effects of hypnotics on memory. J Clin Psychopharmacol 1983;3:310–313.

54. Breen RA, McGaugh JL. Facilitation of maze learning with post-trial injections of picrotoxin. J Comp Physiol Psychol 1961;54:498–501.

55. Irwin S, Benuazizi A. Pentylenetetrazol enhances memory function. Science 1966;152:100–102.

56. Morrison BO. Oral metrazol in the care of the aged: a review of twenty eight cases. J Am Geriatr Soc 1958;8:895–898.

57. Flood JF, Roberts E. Dehydroepiandrosterone sulfate improves memory in aging mice. Brain Res 1988;448:178–181.

58. Flood J, Morley JE, Roberts E. Pregnenolone sulfate enhances post-training memory processes when injected in very low doses into limbic system structures: the amygdala is by ra the most sensitive. Proc Natl Acad Sci USA 1995;92:10810–10810.

59. Flood JF, Smith GE, Roberts E. Dehydroepiandrosterone and its sulfate enhance memory retention in mice. Brain Res 1988;447:269–278.

60. Wolkowitz OM, Reus VI, Roberts E, Manfredi F, Chan T, Ormitson S, Johnson R, Canick J, Brizendine L, Weingartner H. Antidepressant and cognition-enhancing effects of DHEA in major depression. New York Academy of Science Conferences, "Dehydroepiandrosterone (DHEA) and Aging," Abstract, 1995, p. 19.

61. Friess E, Trachsel L, Guldner J, Schier T, Steiger A. Holsbnoer F. DHEA administration increases rapid eye movement sleep and EEG power in the sigma frequency range. Am Physiol Soc 1995; E107–E113.

62. Sanders SA, Reinisch JM. Behavioral effects on humans of progesterone related compounds during development and in the adult. In: Ganten D, Pfaff D, eds. Actions of Progesterone on the Brain. Springer-Verlag, Berlin, 1985, pp. 175–206.

63. Moodley P, Golombok S, Shine P, Lader M. Computerized axial brain tomograms in long-term benzodiazepine users. Psychiatry Res 1993;48:135–144.

64. Marczynski TJ, Artwohl J, Marczynska B. Chronic administration of flumazenil increases life span and protects rats from age-related loss of cognitive functions: a benzodiazepine/GABAergic hypothesis of brain aging. Neurobiol Aging 1994;15:69–84.

65. Griffith WH, Murchison DA. Enhancement of GABA-activated membrane currents in aged Fisher 344 basal forebrain neurons. J Neurosci 1995;15:2407–2416.

66. Sunderland T, Merril CR, Harrington MG, Lawlor BA, Molchan SE, Martinez R, Murphy DL. Reduced plasma dehydroepiandrosterone concentrations in Alzheimer's disease. Lancet 1989;2:570.

67. Nassman B, Olsson T, Backstrom T, Eriksson S, Grakvist K, Viitanen M, Bucht G. Serum dehydroepiandrosterone sulfate in Alzheimer's disease and multi-infarct dementia. Biol Psychiatry 1991;30:684–690.

68. Rudman D, Shetty KR, Mattson DE. Plasma dehydroepiandrosterone sulfate in nursing home men. J Am Geriatr Soc 1990;38:421–427.

69. Barrett-Connor E, Edelstein S. A prospective study of dehydroepiandrosterone sulfate and cognitive function in an older population: the Rancho Bernardo study. J Am Geriatr Soc 1994;42:520–423.

70. Azuma T, Matsubara T, Shima Y, Haeno S, Fujimoto T, Tone K, Shibata N, Sakoda S. Neurosteroids in cerebrospinal fluid in neurologic disorders. J Neurol Sci 1993;120:87–92.

71. Cowell PE, Turetsky BI, Gur RC, Grossman RI, Shtasi DL, Gur RE. Sex difference in aging of the human frontal and temporal lobes. J Neurosci 1994;14:4748–4755.

72. Martin C. Hormone secretion cycles. In: Endocrine Physiology. Oxford University Press, New York, 1985, pp. 62–65.

73. Robel P, Baulieu EE, Synguelakis M, Halberg F. Chronobiologic dynamics of Δ5–3β-hydroxysteroids and glucocorticoids in rat brain and plasma and human plasma. In: Pauley JE, Scheving LE, eds. Advances in Chronobiology, part A. Liss, New York, 1987, pp. 451–465.

74. Hermida RC, Halberg F, Del Pozo F. Chronobiologic pattern discrimination of plasma hormone, notably DHEAS and TSH, classifies an expansive personality. Chronobiologia 1985;12:105–136.

75. Selye H. The evolution of the stress concept-stress and cardiovascular disease. In: Levi L, ed. The Psychosocial Environment and Psychosomatic Diseases. Oxford University Press, London, 1971, pp. 299–311

76. Eysenek HJ. Psychophysiology and personality: extraversion, neuroticism and psychoticism. In: Physiological Correlates of Human Behavior. London, Academic Press, 1983, pp 13–29.

77. Lader M. Anxiety and depression. In: Gale A, Edwards JA, eds. Physiological Correlates of Human Behavior. Academic, London, 1983, pp. 155–167.

78. Fava M, Littman A, Halperin P. Neuroendocrine correlates of the type A behavior pattern: a review and hypothesis. Int J Psychiatry Med 1987;17:289–308.

79. Wilkins J, Van Gorp W, Hinken C, Welch B, Wheatley S, Plotkin D, Moore L, Setoda D, Majewska MD. Relapse to cocaine use may be predicted in early abstinence by low plasma dehydroepiandrosterone-sulfate levels. In: Harris L, ed. NIDA Research Monograph Series, USDHHS, National Institutes of Health, 1997, vol. 174, p.277.

80. Nottelmann ED, Susman EJ, Inoff-Germain BA, Cutler GB, Loriaux DL, Chrousos GP. Developmental process on early adolescence: relationships between adolescent adjustment problems and chronologic age, pubertal stage, and puberty related serum hormone levels. J Pediatr 1987;110:473–480.

81. Majewska MD. Cocaine addiction as a neurological disorder: implications for treatment. In: Majewska MD, ed. Neurotoxicity and Neuropathology Associated with Cocaine Abuse. NIDA Research Monograph Series, vol 163, National Institutes of Health, Rockville, MD, 1996, pp. 1–26.

82. Carlson NR. Aggressive behavior. In: Physiology of Behavior. Allyn and Bacon, Boston, 1991, pp. 357–363.

83. Schlegel ML, Spetz JF, Robel P, Haug M. Studies on the effects of dehydroepiandrosterone and its metabolites on attack by castrated mine on lactating intruders. Physiol Behav 1985;34:867–870.

84. Molina V, Ciesielski L, Gobaille S, Mandel P. Effects of potentiation of the GABAergic neurotransmission in the olfactory bulbs on mouse-killing behavior. Pharmacol Biochem Behav 1986; 24:657–664.

85. Leventhal B, Brodie HK. The pharmacology of violence. In: Hamburg DA &Trudeau MB, eds. Biobehavioral Aspects of Aggression. Liss, New York, NY, 1981, pp. 85–106.

86. Abadie J, Wright B, Correa G, Browne ES, Porter JR, Swec F. Effect of dehydroepiandrosterone on neurotransmitter levels and appetite regulation of the obese Zucker rat. Diabetes, 1993;42:662–669.

87. Linnoila VM, Virkinnen M. Aggression, suicidality, and serotonin. J Clin Psychiatry, 1992; (Suppl)53:46–51.

88. Monnet FP, Mahe V, Robel P, Baulieu EE. Neurosteroids, via sigma receptors, modulate the [3H]norepinephrine release evoked by N-methyl-D-aspartate in the rat hippocampus. Proc Natl Acad Sci USA, 1995;92:3774–3778.

89. Stanton PK, Survey JM. Depletion of norepinephrine, but not serotonin, reduces long-term potentiation in dentae gyrus of rat hippocampal slices. J Neurosci 1985;5:2169–76.

90. Sara SJ, Vankov A, Herve A. Locus coeruleus-evoked responses in behaving rats: a clue to the role of noradrenaline in memory. Brain Res Bull 1994;35:457–65.
91. Morales A, Nolan JJ, Nelson JC, Yen SSC. Effects of replacement dose of dehydroepiandrosterone in men and women of advancing age. J Clin Endocrin Metab 1994;78:1360–1367.
92. Majewska MD, Vaupel B. Steroid regulation of uterine motility via $GABA_A$ receptor in the rabbit: a novel mechanism? J Endocrin 1991;131:427–434.

10

Modulation of Ionotropic Glutamate Receptors by Neuroactive Steroids

Terrell T. Gibbs, MD, Nader Yaghoubi, MD,
Charles E. Weaver, Jr., MD,
Mijeong Park-Chung, MD, Shelley J. Russek, MD,
and David H. Farb, MD

CONTENTS

INTRODUCTION
STEROID MODULATION OF NMDA RECEPTORS
STEROID MODULATION OF NON-NMDA RECEPTORS
DO NEUROSTEROIDS ACT AS ENDOGENOUS MODULATORS
    OF GLUTAMATE RECEPTOR FUNCTION?
MODULATION OF EXCITOTOXIC CELL DEATH
    BY NEUROACTIVE STEROIDS
CONCLUSION
REFERENCES

INTRODUCTION

Our laboratory has been investigating the modulatory role of a novel class of glutamate receptor modulators, the neuroactive steroids. Neuroactive steroids may be synthesized by nervous tissue *(1–4)*, in which case they are referred to as neurosteroids. Alternatively, neuroactive steroids may be synthesized in peripheral tissues or may be synthetic steroid compounds that are exogenously introduced into the central nervous system (CNS).

Although steroids are classically thought to act via intracellular steroid hormone receptors that bind to DNA sequences to modify gene expression, certain steroids have been shown to have direct effects on ligand-gated ion channels of neuronal membranes (Table 1). In particular, various steroids have been shown to modulate directly both native *(5–7)* and recombinant *(8–13)* $GABA_A$ receptors, as well as glycine receptors *(7,13a)*. Steroid effects on voltage-sensitive calcium channels have also been described *(14,15)*.

Glutamate receptors may be divided into two broad classes, metabotropic and ionotropic receptors. Metabotropic receptors ($mGluR_{1–8}$) are G-protein coupled *(16)*, and as with other G-protein coupled receptors, have seven putative transmembrane

From: *Contemporary Endocrinology: Neurosteroids: A New Regulatory Function
in the Nervous System* Edited by: E.-E. Baulieu, P. Robel, and M. Schumacher
© Humana Press Inc., Totowa, NJ

Table 1
Steroid Modulators of Neurotransmitter Receptors and Ion Channels

Steroid	Glutamate receptor			GABA$_A$	Gly	nAch	Voltage-sensitive calcium channels		
	NMDA	AMPA/kainate	Quisqualate				N	P	L
Pregnenolone	ne [μM] (19,24)						– G-p [nM] (124)	ne [nM] (124)	– G-p [nM] (124)
Pregnenolone sulfate	+ [μM] (19,24)	– [μM] (19)		– [μM] (7,19,125)	– [μM] (7)		– G-P [nM] (124)	– G-p [nM] (124)	– G-p [nM] (124)
Pregnenolone hemisuccinate	+ [μM] (21,59,126)								
Pregnenolone hemisuccinate methyl ester	ne [μM] (126)								
Pregnenolone-3β-D-glucosiduronate	ne [μM] (21)								
Pregnenolone 3-acetate							ne [nM] (124)	ne [nM] (124)	ne [nM] (124)
7-Keto pregnenolone sulfate	ne [μM] (58,59) – [μM] (21)			ne [μM] (58)					

Compound								
11β-OH-Pregnenolone sulfate	ne [μM] (21,126)	− [μM] (58,59)						− [μM] (58)
11-Keto-pregnenolone sulfate	ne [μM] (21,126)							ne [μM] (58)
17-Hydroxy-pregnenolone 3-sulfate	+ [μM] (21,126)							
20β-Dihydropregnenolone sulfate	+ [μM] (21,126)							
21-Acetoxy-pregnenolone sulfate	+ [μM] (21,126)							
3α-Hydroxypregn-5,16-dien-20-one sulfate	ne [μM] (21)							
3β-Hydroxyandrost-5-ene-17β-carboxylic acid methyl ester sulfate	+ [μM] (21)							
Progesterone	ne [μM] (58)	+ [μM] (7) − (9)	− [μM] (7)	− [μM] (127, 128)	ne [μM] (124)	ne [μM] (124)	ne [μM] (124)	

(continued)

Table 1 (*continued*)

Steroid	Glutamate receptor			GABA$_A$	Gly	nAch	Voltage-sensitive calcium channels		
	NMDA	AMPA/kainate	Quisqualate				N	P	L
17α-OH-progesterone				+ [μM] (7)	– [μM] (7)				
Deoxycorticosterone				+ [μM] (7)	– [μM] (7)				
Tetrahydrodeoxy-corti-costerone (THDOC)				+ [nM] (5,29,130)					
3α-Hydroxy-5α-pregnane-11,20-dione				+ [nM] (129)					
Corticosterone				+ [μM] (7)	– [μM] (7)				
5α-Pregnan-3α-11β,21-triol-20-one (allotetrahydro-corticosterone)				– [nM] (5)			– G-p [nM] (124)		
Aldosterone				+ [μM] (130)					
Hydrocortisone				ne [μM] (7)	ne [μM] (7)				

Compound							
3α-Hydroxy-5α-pregnan-20-one (allopregnanolone)					+ [μM] (5,7, 129,130)	ne [μM] (7)	
3α-Hydroxy-5β-pregnan-20-one (pregnanolone)		ne [μM] (58,59)			+ [nM] (129,130)		
3β-Hydroxy-5β-pregnan-20-one (epipregnanolone)					ne [μM] (129,130)		
3β-Hydroxy-5α-pregnan-20-one (epiallopregnanolone)		ne [μM] (21,60)			ne [μM] (129,130)		
3α-Hydroxy-5α-pregnane-11,20-dione (alfaxalone)			ne [μM] (131)	ne [μM] (131)	+ [μM] (132,133)		− [μM] (134)
3β-Hydroxy-5α-pregnane-11,20-dione (betaxalone)					ne [nN] (134)		− [μM] (134)
5β-Pregnan-3α-ol-11-keto, D-ring amidine (RU5135)					[nM] (135)	− [nM] (135)	
3α-Hydroxy-5β-pregnan-20-one sulfate (allopregnanolone sulfate)	− [μM] (58,59)	ne [μM] (21)					

171

(continued)

Table 1 (*continued*)

Steroid	Glutamate receptor			GABA$_A$	Gly	nAch	Voltage-sensitive calcium channels		
	NMDA	AMPA/kainate	Quisqualate				N	P	L
3α-Hydroxy-5β-pregnan-20-one sulfate (pregnanolone sulfate)	− [μM] (21,56)								
3α-Hydroxy-5β-pregnan-20-one hemisuccinate (pregnanolone hemisuccinate)	− [μM] (58,59)								
3β-Hydroxy-5β-pregnan-20-one sulfate (epipregnanolone sulfate)	− [μM] (21)								
3β-Hydroxy-5α-pregnan-20-one sulfate (epiallopregnanolone sulfate)	ne [μM] (21) + [μM] (58,59)								
Hydrocortisone	− [μM] (19)								
Hydrocortisone sulfate	ne [μM] (60)								
Testosterone				+ [μM] (58)					

Dehydroepiandrosterone				– [μM] *(58)*	
Dehydroepiandrosterone sulfate	ne [μM] *(21,24,56)*			– [μM] *(58,136)*	
Dehydroepiandrosterone methyl-thio-phosphonothioate				– [μM] *(58)*	
Androsterone				+ [μM] *(58,130)*	
Androsterone sulfate	– [μM] *(56)*			– [μM] *(58)*	
Epiandrosterone sulfate				– [μM] *(58)*	
5α-Androstan-3α,17β-diol				+ [μM] *(58)*	
Androstenedione			+ [nM] *(88)*	+ [μM] *(58)*	
Estradiol	– [μM] *(58,61)*	ne [nM] *(88,113,137)*	+ [nM] *(88,137)*	ne [nM] *(88)*	– G-p [pM] *(15)*

(continued)

Table 1 (*continued*)

Steroid	Glutamate receptor			$GABA_A$	Gly	nAch	Voltage-sensitive calcium channels		
	NMDA	AMPA/kainate	Quisqualate				N	P	L
17β-Estradiol 3-sulfate	ne [μM] (58)								
17β-Estradiol 3-benzoate	ne [μM] (56)								
17β-Estradiol 3-hemisuccinate	– [μM] (58,59)								
17β-Estradiol 17-hemisuccinate	– [μM] (58)								
17β-Estradiol 3,17-hemisuccinate	– [μM] (58)								
17α-Estradiol	ne [nM] (88)	ne [nM] (88)							ne [pM] (15)
17α-Estradiol 3-sulfate				ne [μM] (58)					

+, positive modulation; –, negative modulation; ne, no effect; [ ], concentration range tested; G-p, indirect effect through activation of G-proteins.

regions. Ionotropic glutamate receptors are directly coupled to cation channels and are responsible for the majority of the excitatory synaptic responses in the mammalian CNS. These receptors are divided into three pharmacologically distinct classes of ion channels distinguished by sensitivity to the selective agonists N-menthyl-D-aspartate (NMDA), α-amino-3-hydroxy-5-methyl-4-isoxazolepropionate (AMPA), and kainate. When activated, the NMDA receptor opens a pore permeable to Ca^{2+}, Na^+, and K^+. AMPA and kainate receptors, when activated, allow Na^+ and K^+ ions to pass through, although some AMPA receptors are also permeable to Ca^{2+} [17].

Since the isolation of the first functional recombinant glutamate-receptor clone in 1989 [18], at least 34 other glutamate-receptor subunits have been cloned. On the basis of *in situ* hybridization and immunocytochemistry, these subunits have been differentially localized to various brain regions. These findings imply a molecular basis for functional differences in glutamate receptor pharmacology depending on brain region and subunit composition. Our laboratory demonstrated that ionotropic glutamate receptors can be directly modulated in both positive and negative directions by certain neuroactive steroids. This was described in electrophysiological studies showing that pregnenolone sulfate (PREGS) acts as a positive allosteric modulator of the NMDA receptor in chick embryo spinal-cord neurons [19]. In these studies, 100 μM PREGS increased the 30 μM NMDA induced current by approximately 200%. In contrast, responses to AMPA and kainate application were inhibited by approximately 30% in the presence of 100 μM PREGS.

Calcium influx studies using microspectrofluorimetry in cultured rat hippocampal neurons subsequently confirmed and extended these electrophysiological findings by establishing that PREGS can also potentiate NMDA-activated calcium influx [20], and the results from a series of steroids showed that steroids can either potentiate or inhibit NMDA-activated calcium influx [21].

These studies are consistent with early studies of glutamate-receptor modulation using single-unit recordings from rat cerebellar neurons, which showed that systemic steroids can have profound effects on glutamate-receptor activity. Systemic administration of estradiol enhances neuronal excitation by iontophoretically applied glutamate [22], whereas systemic progesterone (PROG) rapidly attenuates the excitation produced by iontophoretic application of NMDA and non-NMDA agonists [23]. These studies, however, were done in intact animals with systemically administered steroids using relatively nonspecific recording techniques.

Other electrophysiological studies, this time on dissociated rat hippocampal neurons, reported approximately 70% potentiation of NMDA responses and 6% inhibition of AMPA and kainate responses by 50 μM PREGS [24]. Single-channel studies of the mechanism of pregnenolone sulfate potentiation reported that PREGS increased both the mean single-channel open time and channel opening frequency, with no effect on the single-channel conductance [24,25].

Recent work from our own laboratory has focused on further understanding the mechanisms by which neuroactive steroids can modulate glutamate receptors. This work has taken three different approaches:

1. Modulation of excitatory amino acid-induced currents in mammalian neurons maintained in culture;
2. Modulation of excitatory amino acid-induced currents in recombinant receptors expressed in *Xenopus* oocytes; and
3. Modulation of excitatory amino acid-induced excitotoxicity.

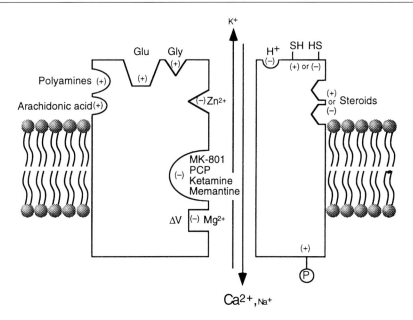

Fig. 1. Schematic model of NMDA receptor binding sites. Schematic model of the NMDA receptor shows hypothesized binding sites for agonist, glutamate (Glu), and modulators glycine (Gly), Zn^{2+}, Ca^{2+}, Mg^{2+}, phencyclidine (PCP), and other dissociative anesthetics, and H^+. Phosphorylation consensus sequences are present on the intracellular surface of the receptor. Thiol groups in close proximity on the receptor are thought to constitute the redox modulatory site. Steroids bind to at least two distinct sites and potentiate or inhibit NMDA receptor function.

STEROID MODULATION OF NMDA RECEPTORS

The NMDA receptor subtype is known to play a fundamentally important role in CNS function. Ongoing work from many laboratories has established the involvement of NMDA receptors in multiple aspects of brain development *(26–28)*, synaptic plasticity associated with long-term potentiation *(29,30)*, and pathology related to glutamate-mediated excitotoxicity *(31)*. In particular, neuropathological mechanisms mediated by NMDA receptors have been implicated in neurological disorders including ischemic stroke *(32,33)*, infection with HIV *(34)*, neurodegenerative diseases *(35–42)*, kindling epileptogenesis *(43)*, and schizophrenia *(44,45)*.

Electrophysiological investigation of the NMDA receptor has revealed a rich modulatory pharmacology (Fig. 1). The glutamate binding site binds naturally occurring excitatory amino acids (glutamate, aspartate, cysteate, and homocysteate), the selective synthetic agonist NMDA, as well as competitive antagonists. Binding of glycine at the glycine coagonist site is an absolute requirement for receptor activation *(46)*. The endogenous compounds spermine and spermidine bind to the polyamine site and potentiate NMDA receptor function *(47,48)*. At higher concentrations, polyamines produce a voltage-dependent inhibition, probably by binding within the channel *(49)*. There are multiple divalent cation binding sites: Binding of Mg^{2+} to a site within the channel pore is voltage-dependent. Depolarization relieves block by physiological levels of Mg^{2+} *(50–52)*, which allows the NMDA receptor to serve as a "coincidence detector;" i.e., the NMDA receptor channel only conducts ions when the cell is sufficiently depolarized via other receptors to relieve Mg^{2+} blockade. Phencyclidine (PCP)-like compounds, such as MK-801 (dizocilpine) bind to a dissociative anesthetic site located within the channel pore and cause use-dependent block *(53)*. Decreased pH leads to inhibition of receptor function, supporting the presence of a H^+ binding site *(54)*. Phosphorylation consensus sequences are present on the intracellular surface of the receptor. Thiol groups in close proximity on the receptor are also thought to constitute a modulatory site sensitive to redox reagents *(55)*. Reducing agents such as dithiothreitol (DTT) enhance activity of the receptor, whereas oxidizing agents are inhibitory.

To these well-characterized modulatory sites can now be added sites for steroid neuromodulators. Neuroactive steroids act rapidly, and with a high degree of structural specificity, consistent with direct action at specific modulatory sites on the NMDA receptor, rather than an indirect effect mediated by the lipid bilayer or other membrane proteins. Neuroactive steroid modulation is independent of the action of glycine *(19,56)*, spermine, arachidonic acid, or redox agents *(57–59)*, indicating that neurosteroids act through a distinct class of modulatory sites.

The interaction between the positive modulator PREGS and the negative modulator 3α-hydroxy-5α-pregnan-20-one sulfate (epipregnanolone sulfate) is not competitive, indicating that despite their structural similarity (Fig. 2), the effects of these two modulators on the NMDA receptor are mediated through separate sites. Thus, there must be at least two sites on the NMDA receptor for interaction with steroid modulators. The inhibitory effect of epipregnanolone sulfate is probably not owing to binding within the channel pore, because inhibition is voltage-independent. Sites for both positive and negative steroid modulators are most likely associated with the extracellular aspect of the NMDA receptor, because PREGS and epipregnanolone sulfate are both ineffective when applied intracellularly *(57–59)*.

Structure-Activity Studies
 of NMDA Receptor Modulation by Neuroactive Steroids

Structure-activity data for steroid modulation of NMDA receptor function indicate that, as is the case for GABA$_A$ receptors, small modifications in steroid structure can lead to profound changes in modulatory activity (Table 1). PREGS and all other highly efficacious positive modulators identified to date have a double bond between C-5 and C-6, suggesting that the pregnene structure is important for potentiation *(21,58,60)*. However, reduction of this double bond with the introduction of C-5α stereochemistry yields the pregnane steroid epiallopregnanolone sulfate, which retains moderate potentiating activity *(58,59)*, indicating that the requirement for a double bond is not absolute. In contrast, the sulfated C-5β isomers, pregnanolone sulfate and epipregnanolone sulfate, are strongly inhibitory, whereas the C-3α, C-5α isomer, allopregnanolone sulfate, shows reduced inhibition of NMDA-induced currents, suggesting that C-5β stereochemistry enhances inhibitory efficacy *(21,58–60)*.

Dehydroepiandrosterone sulfate (DHEAS) is only a weak potentiator, suggesting that the side chain at C-21 is important for potentiation. Similarly, introduction of a ketone or hydroxyl at C-11 or a ketone at C-7 eliminates potentiation *(21,58,60)*. In contrast, there appears to be latitude for modifications to the C-17 side chain, as 20β-dihydropregnenolone sulfate and 21-acetoxy-pregnenolone sulfate both retain potentiating activity *(21,58,60)*.

Pregnenolone Sulfate

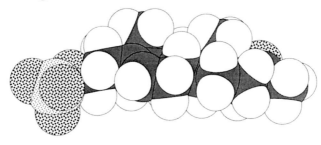

Epipregnanolone Sulfate

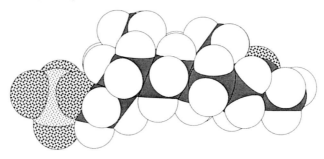

Fig. 2. Space-filling models of pregnenolone sulfate and epipregnanolone sulfate. Space-filling representations of pregnenolone sulfate and epipregnanolone sulfate serve to illustrate the similarity between these two molecules, which have opposite modulatory effects on NMDA receptor function.

The C-3 sulfate is not essential for interaction with the NMDA receptor, as pregnanolone hemisuccinate has inhibitory activity similar to pregnanolone sulfate, and pregnenolone hemisuccinate has potentiating activity similar to PREGS *(21,58,60)*. Nevertheless, a negatively charged group at C-3 appears to be important, as pregnanolone, pregnenolone (PREG), and pregnenolone hemisuccinate methyl ester are all inactive *(56,60)*. A notable exception to this rule is estradiol, which inhibits the NMDA receptor despite having only a hydroxyl group at C-3 *(61)*. It is possible that the reduction in the pK_a of the C-3 hydroxyl owing to the aromatic nature of the estradiol A ring allows sufficient ionization for it to function as a negatively charged group. Alternatively, it may be that estradiol derivatives inhibit the NMDA receptor by a different mechanism than pregnane steroids.

Interpretation of structure-activity data is complicated by the recent finding that positive and negative steroid modulators act at separate sites *(57–59)*. Thus, it is possible that a compound could be mistakenly classified as inactive because its positive and negative modulatory effects cancel out. It is possible that competition studies will help to resolve these questions. Alternatively, if the positive and negative steroid modulatory sites on the receptor can be identified, it may be possible to disable one or the other by site-directed mutagenesis to study structure-activity relations of each site separately.

Modulation of Recombinant NMDA Receptors by Neuroactive Steroids

The NMDA subtype of glutamate receptors is thought to be comprised of subunits from two distinct gene families, NMDAR1 and NMDAR2. The NMDAR1, or NR1, gene was originally isolated from rat brain using expression cloning *(62)*. Subsequent work has led to the isolation of at least seven additional isoforms that are generated by alternative splicing of the RNA transcript *(63–65)*. Isolation of the NMDAR2, or NR2, gene family has revealed a family of subunits including the NR2A, NR2B, NR2C, and NR2D genes *(66–69)*. Coassembly of different NR1 splice variants and NR2 subtypes results in receptors that vary from one another in response amplitude, agonist affinity, and antagonist sensitivity *(69)*, as well as modulation by glycine *(66)*, ethanol *(70)*, Mg^{2+} *(68)*, spermine *(71)*, and reducing agents *(72)*. Studies of the effects of subunit composition on steroid sensitivity are likely to yield insights into the nature and location of neuroactive steroid modulatory sites. To begin to investigate the subunit dependence of steroid modulation, we examined the effects of steroids on recombinant NMDA receptors expressed in *Xenopus* oocytes. PREGS potentiates NMDA induced currents in oocytes expressing heteromeric $NR1_{100}$:NR2A receptors, demonstrating that no other neuron-specific factors are required to confer steroid sensitivity. In these oocytes, 100 µM PREGS potentiates the 100 µM NMDA response by over 300% (Fig. 3). As in neurons, onset of potentiation is rapid, with clear potentiation evident even when PREGS and NMDA are simultaneously applied. Recovery from potentiation is also rapid, with responses returning almost to baseline after 30 s. Also consistent with our results from neuronal cultures *(56)*, the steroid pregnanolone sulfate inhibits NMDA responses in oocytes *(73)*. The ability to observe steroid modulation of recombinant NMDA receptors offers the prospect of using mutagenic approaches to identify specific regions of the NMDA receptor that contribute to steroid modulation.

STEROID MODULATION OF NON-NMDA RECEPTORS

The non-NMDA glutamate receptors may be subdivided into kainate and AMPA-preferring receptors, although in practice, kainate is typically used in physiological studies of AMPA receptors in spite of its lower potency than AMPA, because of its greater efficacy and slower desensitization of AMPA receptors. Molecular cloning has revealed that the AMPA receptors may be assembled from GluR1-4 subunits *(18,74–76)*, whereas expression of GluR5-7 yields kainate receptors. Although a clear delineation of their respective functions in vivo has been difficult to elucidate owing to their overlapping agonist sensitivities and the lack of highly selective antagonists, AMPA receptors are thought to play important roles in synaptic plasticity *(77)* and nervous system development *(78)*. AMPA receptors have been found clustered at postsynaptic sites *(79)*, consistent with the idea that they serve as the primary depolarizing receptors for mediation of fast excitatory neurotransmission. Although high-affinity kainate receptors are abundantly expressed in mammalian brain *(80)*, the role of kainate receptors in CNS synaptic transmission is unclear. In the peripheral nervous system, kainate receptors have been characterized in dorsal root ganglion neurons, and exhibit a rapidly desensitizing response to kainate *(81)*. In the CNS, kainate receptors have been postulated to be either located presynaptically *(82,83)* or localized to dendrites *(84,85)*. At presynaptic sites, a modulatory role in which kainate receptors regulate neurotransmitter release has been proposed *(86)*.

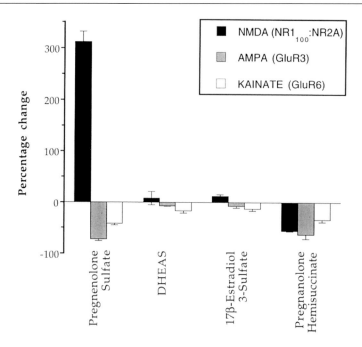

Fig. 3. Modulation of recombinant glutamate receptors by neuroactive steroids. A summary chart is shown that illustrates the effects of selected neuroactive steroids on recombinant NMDA, AMPA, and kainate receptors expressed in *Xenopus* oocytes. Oocytes were injected with cRNA encoding heteromeric NR1$_{100}$:NR2A NMDA, homomeric GluR3 (flop) AMPA, or homomeric GluR6 kainate receptor subunits. Following 3–5 d of incubation, two-electrode voltage clamp recording was used to measure steroid modulation of responses to 100 μM NMDA, 100 μM kainate, and 10 μM kainate responses, respectively, for the three glutamate receptor subtypes. Bars indicate the percentage change in the agonist induced current in the presence of the indicated steroid, as compared to the current in the absence of steroid. Steroids were applied at a concentration of 100 μM and oocytes were pre-equilibrated with steroid for 10 s prior to coapplication of steroid and agonist with all solutions containing 5% DMSO. V$_{H}$ = –100 mV.

Steroid modulation of non-NMDA receptors has been studied in less depth than NMDA receptors, but it is clear that many neuroactive steroids also affect this class of glutamate receptors. In contrast to NMDA receptors, almost all reported steroid effects on kainate and AMPA receptors have been inhibitory. In particular, PREGS, which greatly potentiates NMDA-induced currents, inhibits kainate- and AMPA-induced currents (19) of chick spinal cord neurons in culture. Similar results are obtained with recombinant kainate and AMPA receptors expressed in *Xenopus* oocytes. As shown in Fig. 3, PREGS potentiates the NMDA-induced current in oocytes expressing NR1$_{100}$ and NR2A subunits of the NMDA receptor, but inhibits kainate-induced currents in oocytes expressing GluR3 AMPA receptor or GluR6 kainate receptor subunits. On the other hand, DHEAS and 17β-estradiol-3-sulfate show little, if any, activity on all three glutamate receptor subtypes, whereas pregnanolone sulfate, which is inhibitory for NMDA receptors, is also inhibitory for kainate and AMPA receptors (73,87). In view of evidence that steroid positive and negative modulatory sites of the NMDA receptor are distinct, it is tempting to speculate that a negative modulatory site might be conserved in all glutamate gated ion channels, but that the positive modulatory site might be unique to NMDA receptors. On the other hand, electrophysiological studies on hippocampal slices from ovariectomized rats reported increases in excitatory postsynaptic potential (EPSP) amplitude and potentiation of AMPA and kainate responses by 10 nM estradiol (88)—a rather surprising finding, because modulatory effects of steroids on glutamate receptors have generally been found to occur in the micromolar concentration range. The same group, however, later reported no effect of either 100 nM estradiol or 100 μM PREGS on kainate-induced currents in outside-out patch recordings from hippocampal CA1 neurons (25). A potentiating effect of 17β-estradiol on some types of non-NMDA receptors could possibly account for the apparently paradoxical findings that 17β-estradiol inhibits NMDA responses of rat hippocampal neurons in culture (61), but acutely potentiates glutamate responses of rat cerebellar Purkinje cells (22,89).

DO NEUROSTEROIDS ACT AS ENDOGENOUS MODULATORS OF GLUTAMATE RECEPTOR FUNCTION?

Two important unresolved questions are whether neurosteroids play a modulatory role in the normal functioning of the nervous system, and whether neurosteroids contribute to CNS pathology. Neuromodulatory effects on GABA$_A$ or NMDA receptors have been reported for many neurosteroids. On the other hand, most of the reported modulatory effects of neurosteroids occur in the micromolar concentration range (except for potentiation of the GABA$_A$ receptor by allopregnanolone, which can be observed at submicromolar concentrations). Because bulk concentrations of steroids in the CNS are typically in the nanomolar range (2), some mechanism of concentration or focal release would seem to be required for steroids to play a role in the normal functioning of the nervous system. Primary cultures of glial cells containing astrocytes and oligodendrocytes synthesize cholesterol and PREG from mevalonalactone (90), and mitochondria derived from oligodendrocytes convert cholesterol to PREG (3). This suggests that PREGS may be synthesized and stored in oligodendrocytes. PREGS carries a full negative charge and should not readily diffuse across a lipid bilayer, raising the possibility that it may be concentrated and sequestered in glial cells. Focal release of PREGS from glia could then give rise to local concentrations sufficient to modulate ligand gated ion channels. Thus, PREGS and other sulfated steroids may represent a means of communication between glia and neurons.

Alternatively, it is possible that high CNS steroid levels might occur in particular circumstances. The concentrations of PREGS and other neurosteroids in brain tissue have been shown to increase in response to changes in physiological state. Neurosteroid levels increase in male rats following surgical stress (91,92), electroshock (93), and sexual encounters with female rats (94). In female rats, brain neurosteroid levels fluctuate during the estrous cycle and pregnancy (95). Pregnanolone sulfate, a negative modulator of the NMDA receptor, is the sulfated form of the neurosteroid pregnanolone, which is a potent positive modulator of the GABA$_A$ receptor. Pregnanolone sulfate and its stereoisomers allopregnanolone sulfate and epiallopregnanolone sulfate are major metabolites of PROG (96–98), whereas epipregnanolone sulfate appears to be a minor metabolite (99). The plasma concentrations of these sulfated steroids in women closely parallel the levels of PROG, peaking around the time of parturition. Concentrations of pregnanolone sulfate and allopregnanolone sulfate reach 1–2 μM in the peripheral circulation of woman during the late stages of pregnancy *(96–98)*. Because they exist as negatively charged species, sulfated steroids would not be expected to easily enter the brain from the periphery in the absence of an active transport system. However the enzymes required for the conversion of PROG to allopregnanolone and the addition of sulfate to neurosteroids are present in the brain *(100,101)*, and it is possible that sulfated steroids are produced either *de novo* or from circulating PROG. Systemic administration of PREGS to rats causes an increase in PREGS content within the brain. It has been proposed that PREGS in the circulation may have sulfate removed by the action of peripheral steroid sulfatases, cross the blood brain barrier as PREG, and then be resulfated by steroid neuronal sulfotransferases *(102)*. A similar mechanism may enable sulfated PROG metabolites to enter and accumulate in the CNS.

Sulfated steroids, including PREGS, have been measured in brain *(1,91,94,101)*, but the concentrations of sulfated pregnane steroids have not been determined. If present in the brain at sufficient concentration, PREGS may constitute an additional mechanism for modulation of neuronal activity. Elevation of PREGS levels during CNS damage could constitute an innate neuroprotective mechanism. PREG and pregnanolone do not modulate NMDA-induced currents *(19,56)*, and we have shown that neither of these steroids modulates NMDA-induced neuronal death (C. E. Weaver, Jr., unpublished data). Sulfation therefore converts an inactive neurosteroid to an active form, suggesting that steroid sulfotransferases and sulfatases may play an important role in the modulation of NMDA receptor function in the CNS. It is interesting to note that the apparent K_Ms for PREG sulfatase measured in adult hippocampus and hippocampal cultures are in the low micromolar range (10 and 14 μM respectively; C. E. Weaver, Jr., unpublished data). Under physiological conditions the substrate/K_m ratio for enzymes is typically between 0.01 and 1 *(103)*. This suggests that the physiological concentration of PREGS is between 0.1 and 10 μM. This is a concentration range at which PREGS would be expected to have modulatory effects on NMDA-induced currents and NMDA-induced cell death.

MODULATION OF EXCITOTOXIC CELL DEATH
BY NEUROACTIVE STEROIDS

Regardless of endogenous levels, steroids that inhibit NMDA receptor function might provide novel therapeutic treatments for CNS trauma, stroke, and neurodegenerative diseases. Prolonged exposure of neurons to glutamate induces delayed, Ca^{2+} dependent cell death. Specific blockade of NMDA receptors is sufficient to attenuate most of the neuronal death that develops after in vivo ischemia, hypoglycemia, in vitro hypoxia, or exposure to NMDA or glutamate *(104–108)*. NMDA-gated channels have been shown to be permeable to Ca^{2+} *(109)*. It has, therefore, been proposed that NMDA receptors play an important role in glutamate excitotoxicity by increasing Ca^{2+} influx. There is a strong correlation of the effects of neuroactive steroids on NMDA-induced Ca^{2+} accumulation by neurons *(20,21)* with modulation of the NMDA induced membrane current (Fig. 4), indicating that neuroactive steroids can be expected to be effective in modulating NMDA-induced neuronal death.

Exacerbation of NMDA-Induced Neuronal Death by PREGS

We have examined a number of steroids for their ability to modulate NMDA-induced neuronal death. Consistent with its ability to potentiate NMDA induced currents and increases in intracellular Ca^{2+}, PREGS exacerbates the toxic effects of NMDA exposure

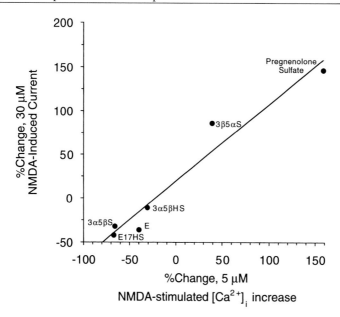

Fig. 4. Steroid modulation of NMDA-induced whole cell currents and NMDA-induced increases in intracellular calcium are correlated. Calcium influx experiments were carried out on cultures of rat hippocampal neurons. Whole cell currents were measured in chick spinal cord neurons at a holding potential of –70 mV. Values are means ± SEM of the percentage change, calculated as (response in presence of steroid/control response) – 1 × 100%. When the percentage change in NMDA-induced whole cell current are plotted against the percentage change in NMDA-induced calcium increase a strong positive correlation is observed ($r = 0.973$), suggesting that steroids are direct modulators of the NMDA receptor. $3\alpha5\beta S$ and $3\alpha5\beta S$ refer to pregnanolone sulfate and epiallopregnanolone sulfate, respectively, whereas $3\alpha5\beta HS$ is pregnanolone hemisuccinate. E and E17HS are estradiol and 17β-estradiol 17-hemisuccinate, respectively.

on rat hippocampal neurons when present during acute NMDA exposure, but does not increase neuronal death in the absence of NMDA or when added after NMDA washout *(110)*, suggesting that the exacerbation of neuronal death caused by PREGS requires the simultaneous activation of NMDA receptors. In addition, potentiation of chronic NMDA-induced neuronal death by PREGS is completely blocked by MK-801. Taken together, these results support a selective pharmacological interaction of pregnenolone sulfate with NMDA receptors.

Neuroprotective Effects
of Pregnanolone Hemisuccinate In Vitro and In Vivo

In contrast to the effects of PREGS, pregnanolone hemisuccinate, an inhibitor of the NMDA-induced current and intracellular Ca^{2+} accumulation, dose-dependently protects primary cultures of rat hippocampal neurons against NMDA-induced neuronal death, and exhibits potent neuroprotective properties in rats subjected to permanent middle cerebral artery occlusion. Pregnanolone hemisuccinate was administered either 5 or 30 min after MCA occlusion as a 7 mg/kg iv bolus followed by a continuous 7 mg/kg/hr iv infusion. When pregnanolone hemisuccinate was administered beginning 5 min after the onset of ischemia, the volume of cortical and subcortical infarct was reduced by 47% and

26%, respectively. When infusion was delayed until 30 min after the onset of ischemia, the volume of cortical infarct was reduced by 39%, with no reduction apparent in the subcortical region *(111)*. As a therapeutic for the treatment of stroke, it is extremely important that neuroprotective agents be effective when given after the onset of ischemia. The demonstration that pregnanolone hemisuccinate is neuroprotective even when administration is delayed until 30 min after the onset of ischemia indicates that pregnanolone hemisuccinate may be a clinically useful compound for the treatment of stroke.

In addition we have also demonstrated in mice that pregnanolone hemisuccinate prevents NMDA-induced convulsions, and is analgesic in the late phase of formalin-induced pain, an animal model for chronic neuropathic pain *(111)*. These results suggest that in addition to neuroprotection pregnanolone hemisuccinate may potentially be useful in the treatment of seizure and chronic pain.

Neuroprotective Effects of Estradiol

Although the primary effect of estradiol on the CNS is to promote neuronal excitation *(112)*, we have found that estradiol inhibits NMDA-induced whole cell currents and NMDA-stimulated increases in intracellular free calcium, and protects against NMDA-induced neuronal death *(61)*. Estradiol (10 nM) has been reported to potentiate neuronal responses in CA1 hippocampal neurons through an interaction with non-NMDA receptors with no effect on NMDA receptor-mediated responses *(25,88)*. Glutamate-stimulated increases in intracellular calcium were similarly unaffected by 100 nM estradiol *(113)*. In our experiments, micromolar concentrations of estradiol were required to inhibit NMDA-induced responses.

Estradiol and its metabolites are potent antioxidants *(114–116)*. Oxidative stress and specifically lipid peroxidation are thought to play a significant role in the neuronal death initiated by NMDA receptor activation *(117,118)*. Previously, the neuroprotective effects of estradiol have been attributed to its ability to inhibit lipid peroxidation *(115,119–121)*. The phenolic A ring of estrogens is critical for antioxidant potential. Non phenolic steroids, such as cholesterol and testosterone, show little antioxidant properties *(114)*. 17α-Estradiol, which also has a phenolic A-ring structure, did not inhibit NMDA-induced neuronal death, arguing that neuroprotection by estradiol is not owing to its antioxidant action, although there is evidence that antioxidant effects can contribute to protective effects of estradiol under other experimental circumstances *(121,122)*. Taken together, these results suggest that neuroprotection by estradiol is mediated by direct inhibition of NMDA-stimulated calcium entry. It has recently been reported that the risk of Alzheimer's disease and related dementia is decreased in women who have received estrogen therapy *(123)*. Our findings suggest that the neuroprotective effects of estrogen may in part be through direct negative modulation of NMDA receptors. The possible benefit of estrogen therapy to women who have already developed symptoms of Alzheimer's disease may be related to a slowing of the progression of disease by protecting neurons against excessive NMDA receptor activation. Alternatively, amelioration of symptoms may be through the ability of estrogen to potentiate AMPA and kainate receptors, thereby facilitating neurotransmission.

CONCLUSION

Abnormal activation of amino-acid receptors is hypothesized to play a role in the etiology of psychiatric disorders, and to contribute to brain damage associated with neurodegenerative diseases such as Alzheimer's and Parkinson's, seizures, and stroke. Neuroactive steroids can exert profound modulatory effects on glutamate receptors, raising the possibility that endogenous neurosteroids may play a role in regulating excitatory synaptic activity in the CNS, or that abnormal steroid levels could contribute to CNS pathology. Studies of steroid modulation of excitotoxicity raise the prospect that steroid negative modulators may be clinically useful as neuroprotective agents, and reveal that endogenous positive modulators may sensitize neurons to excitotoxic neurodegeneration. Understanding the mechanisms of steroid actions on the CNS may lead to new strategies for the treatment of such disorders. Regardless of their physiological role, neuroactive steroids offer a novel pharmacologic approach to regulating the activity of excitatory amino acid receptors in the CNS.

ACKNOWLEDGMENTS

Research support was provided by National Institute of Mental Health Grant MH-49469. N. Y. and C. E. W. were recipients of Pharmaceutical Manufacturer's Association Foundation Medical Student Fellowships in Pharmacology-Clinical Pharmacology. C. E. W. was the recipient of a fellowship from the American Heart Association.

REFERENCES

1. Corpéchot C, Synguelakis M, Talha S, Axelson M, Sjövall J, Vihko R, Baulieu E-E, Robel P. Pregnenolone and its sulfate ester in the rat brain. Brain Res 1983;270:119–125.
2. Lanthier A, Patwardhan VV. Sex steroids and 5-en-5β-hydroxysteroids in specific regions of the human brain and cranial nerves. J Steroid Biochem 1986;25:445–449.
3. Hu ZY, Bourreau E, Jung-Testas I, Robel P, Baulieu EE. Neurosteroids: oligodendrocyte mitochondria convert cholesterol to pregnenolone. Proc Natl Acad Sci USA 1987;84:8215–8219.
4. Robel P, Bourreau E, Corpéchot C, Dang DC, Halberg F, Clarke C, Haug M, Schlegel ML, Synguelakis M, Vourch C, Baulieu EE. Neuro-steroids: 3β-hydroxy-Δ5-derivatives in rat and monkey brain. J Steroid Biochem 1987;27:649–655.
5. Majewska MD, Harrison NL, Schwartz RD, Barker JL, Paul SM. Steroid hormone metabolites are barbiturate-like modulators of the GABA response. Science (Wash, DC) 1986;232:1004–1007.
6. Puia G, Santi M, Vicini S, Pritchett DB, Purdy RH, Paul SM, Seeburg PH, Costa E. Neurosteroids act on recombinant human GABA_A receptors. Neuron 1990;4:759–765.
7. Wu FS, Gibbs TT, Farb DH. Inverse modulation of γ-aminobutyric acid- and glycine-induced currents by progesterone. Mol Pharmacol 1990;37:597–602.
8. Shingai R, Sutherland ML, Barnard EA. Effects of subunit types of the cloned GABA_A receptor on the response to a neurosteroid. Eur J Pharmacol 1991;206:77–80.
9. Woodward RM, Polenzani L, Miledi R. Effects of steroids on GABA receptors expressed in *Xenopus* oocytes by poly(A)+ RNA from mammalian brain and retina. Mol Pharmacol 1991;41:89–103.
10. Zaman S, Shingai R, Harvey R, Darlison M, Barnard EA. Effects of subunit types of the recombinant GABA_A receptor on the response to a neurosteroid. Eur J Pharmacol 1992;225:321–330.
11. Hadingham KL, Wingrove PB, Wafford KA, Bain C, Kemp JA, Palmer KJ, Wilson AW, Wilcox AS, Sikela JM, Ragan CI, Whiting PJ. Role of the beta subunit in determining the pharmacology of human GABA_A receptors. Mol Pharmacol 1993;44:1211–1218.
12. Puia G, Ducic I, Vicini S, Costa E. Does neurosteroid modulatory efficacy depend on GABA_A receptor subunit composition? Receptors Chanels 1993;1:135–42.
13. Rabow L, Russek SJ, Farb DH. From ion currents to genomic analysis: recent advances in GABA_A receptor research. Synapse 1995;21:189–274.
13a. Prince, R J, M A Simmonds. Steroid modulation of the strychnine-sensitive glycine receptor. Neuropharmacology 1992;31:201–205.
14. ffrench-Mullen JMH, Tokutomi N, Akaike N. The effect of temperature on the GABA-induced chloride current in isolated sensory neurones of the frog. Br J Pharmacol 1988;95:753–762.

15. Mermelstein PG, Becker JB, Surmeier DJ. Estradiol reduces calcium currents in rat neostriatal neurons via a membrane receptor. J Neurosci 1996;16:595–604.

16. Pin J, Duvoisin R. Neurotransmitter receptors I: The metabotropic glutamate receptors: structure and functions. Neuropharmacology 1995;34:1–26.

17. Hollmann M, Hartley M, Heinemann S. Ca^{2+} permeability of KA-AMPA-gated glutamate receptor channels depends on subunit composition. Science (Washington, DC) 1991;252:851–853.

18. Hollmann M, O'Shea-Greenfield A, Rogers SW, Heinemann S. Cloning by functional expression of a member of the glutamate receptor family. Nature (London) 1989;342:643–648.

19. Wu FS, Gibbs TT, Farb DH. Pregnenolone sulfate: a positive allosteric modulator at the NMDA receptor. Mol Pharmacol 1991;40:333–336.

20. Irwin RP, Maragakis NJ, Rogawski MA, Purdy RH, Farb DH, Paul SM. Pregnenolone sulfate augments NMDA receptor mediated increases in intracellular Ca^{2+} in cultured rat hippocampal neurons. Neurosci Lett 1992;141:30–34.

21. Irwin RP, Lin SZ, Rogawski MA, Purdy RH, Paul SM. Steroid potentiation and inhibition of N-methyl-D-aspartate receptor-mediated intracellular Ca^{++} responses: structure activity studies. J Pharmacol Exp Ther 1994;271:677–682.

22. Smith S S, Waterhouse BD, Woodward DJ. Sex steroid effects on extrahypothalamic CNS I Estrogen augments neuronal responsiveness to iontophoretically applied glutamate in the cerebellum. Brain Res 1987;422:40–51.

23. Smith SS. Progesterone administration attenuates excitatory amino acid responses of cerebellar Purkinje cells. Neuroscience 1991;42:309–320.

24. Bowlby M. Pregnenolone sulfate potentiation of N-methyl-D-aspartate receptor channels in hippocampal neurons. Mol Pharmacol 1993;43:813–819.

25. Wong M, Moss RL. Patch-clamp analysis of direct steroidal modulation of glutamate receptor-channels. J Neuroendocrinol 1994;6:347–355.

26. Artola A, Singer W. NMDA receptors and developmental plasticity in visual neocortex. In: Watkins JC, Collingridge GL, eds. The NMDA Receptor. Oxford University Press, Oxford, UK, 1989, pp. 153–166.

27. McDonald JW, Johnston MV. Physiological and pathophysiological roles of excitatory amino acid during central nervous system development. Brain Res Rev 1990;15:41–70.

28. Komuro H, Rakic P. Modulation of neuronal migration by NMDA receptors. Science (Washington, DC) 1993;238:355–358.

29. Collingridge GL, Kehl SJ, McLennan H. Excitatory amino acids in synaptic transmission in the Schaffer collateral-commissural pathway of the rat hippocampus. J Physiol (London) 1983;334:33–46.

30. Bliss TVP, Collingridge GL. A synaptic model of memory: long-term potentiation in the hippocampus. Nature (London) 1993;361:31–39.

31. Choi, DW. Glutamate neurotoxicity and diseases of the nervous system. Neuron 1988;1:623–634.

32. Choi DW, Rothman SM. The role of glutamate neurotoxicity in hypoxic-ischemic neuronal death. Annu Rev Neurosci 1990;13:171–182.

33. Wahlestedt C, Golanov E, Yamamoto S, Yee F, Ericson H, Yoo H, Inturrisi CE, Reis DJ. Antisense oligodeoxynucleotides to NMDA-R1 receptor channel protect cortical neurons from excitotoxicity and reduce focal ischaemic infarctions. Nature (London) 1993;363:260–263.

34. Lipton S, Choi YB, Pan ZH, Lei S, Chen H, Sucher N, Loscalzo J, Singel D, Stamler J. A redox-based mechanism for the neuroprotective and neurodestructive effects of nitric oxide and related nitroso-compounds. Nature 1993;364:626–632.

35. Plaitakis A, Berl S, Yahr MD. Abnormal glutamate metabolism in adult-onset degenerative neurological disorder. Science 1982;216:193–196.

36. Beal MF, Kowall NW, Ellison DW, Mazurek MF, Swartz KJ, Martin JB. Replication of the neurochemical characteristics of Huntington's disease by quinolinic acid. Nature (London) 1986;321:168–172.

37. Young AB, Greenamyre JT, Hollingsworth Z, Albin R, D'Amato C, Shoulson I, Penney JB. NMDA receptor losses in putamen from patients with Huntington's disease. Science (Washington, DC) 1988;241:981–983.

38. Greenamyre JT, Young AB. Excitatory amino acids and Alzheimer's disease. Neurobiol Aging 1989;10:593–602.

39. Plaitakis A. Glutamate dysfunction and selective motor neuron degeneration in amyotrophic lateral sclerosis: a hypothesis. Ann Neurol 1990;28:3–8.

40. Greenamyre JT. Neuronal bioenergetic defects, excitotoxicity and Alzheimer's disease: 'use it and lose it'. Neurobiol Aging 1991;12:334–336.
41. Greenamyre JT, O'Brien FC. N-methyl-D-aspartate antagonists in the treatment of Parkinson's disease. Arch Neurol 1991;48:977–981.
42. Rothstein JD, Martin LJ, Kuncl RW. Decreased glutamate transport by the brain and spinal cord in amyotrophic lateral sclerosis. N Engl J Med 1992;326:1454–1468.
43. Pratt GD, Kokaia M, Bengzon J, Kokaia Z, Fritschy JM, Mohler H, Lindvall O. Differential regulation of NMDA receptor subunit mRNAs in kindling-induced epileptogenesis. Neuroscience 1993;57:307–318.
44. Olney JW, Farber NB. Glutamate receptor dysfunction and schizophrenia. Arch Gen Psychiatry 1995;52:998–1007.
45. Zylberman I, Javitt DC, Zukin SR. Pharmacological augmentation of NMDA receptor function for treatment of schizophrenia. Ann NY Acad Sci 1995;757:487–491.
46. Kleckner NW, Dingledine R. Requirement for glycine in activation of NMDA receptors expressed in Xenopus oocytes. Science (Washington, DC) 1988;241:835–837.
47. Ransom RW, Stec NL. Cooperative modulation of [^{3}H]MK-801 binding to the N-methyl-D-aspartate receptor-ion channel complex by L-glutamate, glycine, polyamines. J Neurochem. 1988;51:830–836.
48. Lehmann J, Colpaert F, Canton H. Glutamate and glycine co-activate while polyamines merely modulate the NMDA receptor complex. Prog Neuro-Psychopharmacol Biol Psychiatry 1991;15:183–190.
49. Williams K, Dawson VL, Romano C, Dichter MA, Molinoff PB. Characterization of polyamines having agonist, antagonist and inverse agonist effects at the polyamine recognition site of the NMDA receptor. Neuron 1990;5:199–208.
50. Ault B, Evans R, Francis A, Oaks D, Watkins J. Selective depression of excitatory amino acid induced depolarizations by magnesium ions in isolated spinal cord preparations. J Physiol 1980;307:413–428.
51. Mayer M, Westbrook G, Guthrie P. Voltage-dependent block by Mg^{2+} of NMDA responses in spinal cord neurones. Nature (London) 1984;309:261–263.
52. Nowak L, Bregestovski P, Ascher P, Herbet A, Prochiantz A. Magnesium gates glutamate-activated channels in mouse central neurones. Nature (London) 1984;307:462–465.
53. Muir K, Lees K. Clinical experience with excitotory amino acid antagonist drugs. Stroke 1995;26:503–513.
54. Kaku D, Giffard R, Choi D. Neuroprotective effects of glutamate antagonists and extracellular acidity. Science (Washington, DC) 1993;260:1516–1518.
55. Aizenman E, Lipton SA, Loring RH. Selective modulation of NMDA responses by reduction and oxidation. Neuron 1989;2:1257–1263.
56. Park-Chung M, Wu FS, Farb DH. 3α-Hydroxy–5β-pregnan-20-one sulfate: a negative modulator of the NMDA-induced current in cultured neurons. Mol Pharmacol 1994;46:146–150.
57. Park-Chung M, Wu FS, Purdy RH, Gibbs TT, Farb DH. Distinct sites for positive and negative modulation of NMDA receptors by sulfated steroids. Soc Neurosci Abst 1996;22:1280.
58. Park-Chung M. Steroids as Functional Modulators of Amino Acid Receptors. 1997; PhD Thesis, Dept. of Pharmacology and Experimental Therapeutics, Boston University, Boston.
59. Park-Chung M, Wu FS, Purdy RH, Malayev AA, Gibbs TT, Farb DH. Distinct sites for inverse modulation of NMDA receptors by sulfated steroids. Mol Pharmacol 1997;56:1113–1123.
60. Farb DH, Gibbs TT. Steroids as modulators of amino acid receptor function. In: Stone TW, ed. CNS Transmitters and Neuromodulators: Neuroactive Steroids. CRC, Boca Raton, FL, 1996, p. 23–36.
61. Weaver CE Jr, Park-Chung M, Gibbs TT, Farb DH. 17β-Estradiol protects against NMDA-induced excitotoxicity by direct inhibition of NMDA receptors. Brain Res 1997;761:338–341.
62. Moriyoshi K, Masu M, Ishii T, Shigemoto R, Mizuno N, Nakanishi S. Molecular cloning and characterization of the rat NMDA receptor. Nature (London) 1991;354:31–37.
63. Nakanishi N, Axel R, Shneider NA. Alternative splicing generates functionally distinct NMDA receptors. Proc Natl Acad Sci USA 1992;89:8552–8556.
64. Sugihara H, Moriyoshi K, Ishii T, Masu M, Nakanishi S. Structures and properties of seven isoforms of the NMDA receptor generated by alternative splicing. Biochem Biophys Res Commun 1992; 185:826–832.
65. Yamazaki M, Mori H, Araki K, Mori KJ, Mishina M. Cloning, expression and modulation of a mouse NMDA receptor subunit. FEBS Lett 1992;300:39–45.

66. Katsuwada T, Kashiwabuchi N, Mori H, Sakimura K, Kushiya E, Araki K, Meguro H, Masaki H, Kumanishi T, Arakawa M, Mishina M. Molecular diversity of the NMDA receptor channel. Nature (London) 1992;358:36–41.

67. Meguro H, Mori H, Araki K, Kushiya E, Kutsuwada T, Yamazaki M, Kumanishi T, Arakawa M, Sakimura K, Mishina M. Functional characterization of a heteromeric NMDA receptor channel expressed from cloned cDNAs. Nature (London) 1992;357:70–74.

68. Monyer H, Sprengel R, Schoepfer R, Herb A, Higuchi M, Lomeli H, Burnashev N, Sakman B, Seeburg PH. Heteromeric NMDA receptors: molecular and functional distinction of subtypes. Science (Washington, DC) 1992;256:1217–1221.

69. Ishii T, Moriyoshi K, Sugihara H, Kadotani H, Yokoi M, Akazawa C, Masu M, Shigemoto R, Mizuno N, Nakanishi S. Molecular characterization of the family of the N-methyl-D-aspartate receptor subunits. J Biol Chem 1993;268:2836–2843.

70. Chu B, Anantharam V, Treistman SN. Ethanol inhibition of recombinant heteromeric NMDA channels in the presence and absence of modulators. J Neurochem 1995;65:140–148.

71. Zheng X, Zhang L, Durand GM, Bennett MV, Zukin RS. Mutagenesis rescues spermine and Zn^{2+} potentiation of recombinant NMDA receptors. Neuron 1994;12:811–818.

72. Kohr G, Eckardt S, Luddens H, Moyer H, Seeburg PH. NMDA receptor channels: subunit-specific potentiation by reducing agents. Neuron 1994;12:1031–1040.

73. Yaghoubi N, Malayev A, Russek SJ, Gibbs TT, Farb DH. Neurateroid modulation of recombinant glutamate receptors. Brain Res 1998;803:153–160.

74. Boulter J, Hollmann M, O'Shea-Greenfield A, Hartley M, Deneris E, Maron C, Heinemann S. Molecular cloning and functional expression of glutamate receptor subunit genes. Science (Washington, DC) 1990;249:1033–1037.

75. Keinanen K, Wisden W, Sommer B, Werner P, Herb A, Verdoorn TA, Sakmann B, Seeburg PH. A family of AMPA-selective glutamate receptors. Science (Washington, DC) 1990;249: 556–560.

76. Nakanishi S, Shneider NA, Axel R. A family of glutamate receptor genes-evidence for the formation of heteromultimeric receptors with distinct channel properties. Neuron 1990;5:569–581.

77. Linden DJ, Dickinson MH, Smeyne M, Connor JA. A long-term depression of AMPA currents in cultured cerebellar Purkinje neurons. Neuron 1991;7:81–89.

78. Monyer H, Seeburg PH, Wisden W. Glutamate-operated channels-developmentally early and mature forms arise by alternative splicing. Neuron 1991;6:799–810.

79. Craig AM, Blackstone CD, Huganir RL, Banker G. The distribution of glutamate receptors in cultured rat hippocampal neurons: postsynaptic clustering of AMPA-selective subunits. Neuron 1993;10:1055–1068.

80. Wisden W, Seeburg PH. A complex mosaic of high-affinity kainate receptors in rat brain. J Neurosci 1993;13:3582–3598.

81. Huettner JE. Glutamate receptor channels in rat DRG neurons: activation by kainate and quisqualate and blockade of desensitization by ConA. Neuron 1990;5:255–266.

82. Ferkany JW, Zaczek R, Coyle JT. Kainic acid stimulates excitatory amino acid neurotransmitter release at presynaptic receptors. Nature (London) 1982;298:757–759.

83. Coyle, JT. Neurotoxic action of kainic acid. J Neurochem 1983;41:1–11.

84. Ulas J, Monaghan DT, Cotman CW. Kainate receptors in the rat hippocampus: a distribution and time course of changes in response to unilateral lesions of the entorhinal cortex. J Neurosci 1990;10:2352–2362.

85. Mondadori C, Ducret T, Häusler A. Elevated corticosteroid levels block the memory-improving effects of nootropics and cholinomimetics. Psychopharmacology 1992;108:11–15.

86. Represa A, Tremblay E, Ben-Ari Y. Kainate binding sites in the hippocampal mossy fibers: localization and plasticity. Neuroscience 1987;20:739–748.

87. Yaghoubi N, Gibbs TT, Farb DH. Evaluation of neurosteroid modulation of kainate receptors using an automated system for oocyte electrophysiology. Soc Neurosci Abst 1995;20:1109.

88. Wong M, Moss RL. Long-term and short-term electrophysiological effects of estrogen on the synaptic properties of hippocampal CA1 neurons. J Neurosci 1992;12:3217–3225.

89. Smith SS, Waterhouse BD, Woodward DJ. Locally applied estrogens potentiate glutamate-evoked excitation of cerebellar Purkinje cells. Brain Res 1988;475:272–282.

90. Jung-Testas I, Hu ZY, Baulieu EE, Robel P. Neurosteroids: biosynthesis of pregnenolone and progesterone in primary cultures of rat glial cells. Endocrinology 1989;125:2083–2091.

91. Corpéchot C, Robel P, Axelson M, Sjövall J, Baulieu EE. Characterization and measurement of dehydroepiandosterone sulfate in rat brain. Proc Natl Acad Sci USA 1981;78:4704–4707.

92. Purdy RH, Morrow AL, Moore PH Jr, Paul SM. Stress-induced elevations of GABA$_A$ receptor-active steroids in the rat brain. Proc Natl Acad Sci USA 1991;88:4553–4557.

93. Korneyev A, Guidotti A, Costa E. Regional and Interspecies differences in brain progesterone metabolism. J Neurochem 1993;61:2041–2047.

94. Corpéchot C, Leclerc P, Baulieu EE, Brazeau P. Neurosteroids: regulatory mechanisms in male rat brain during heterosexual exposure. Steroids 1985;45:229–234.

95. Paul SM, Purdy RH. Neuroactive steroids. FASEB J 1992;6:2311–2322.

96. Sjövall K. Sulfates of pregnanolones, pregnanediols and 16-hydroxysteroids in plasma from pregnant women. Ann Clin Res 1970;2:409–413.

97. Sjövall K. Gas chromatographic determination of steroid sulfates in plasma during pregnancy. Ann Clin Res 1970;2:393–408.

98. Axelson, M, B-L Sahlberg. Group separation and gas chromatography mass spectrometry of conjugated steroids in plasma. J Steroid Biochem 1982;18:313–321.

99. Karavolas HJ, Hodges DR. Neuroendocrine metabolism of progesterone and related progestins. Steroids and Neuronal Activity. Ciba Foundation Symposium. 1990;153:22–55.

100. Lambert JJ, Belelli D, Hill-Venning C, Peters JA. Neurosteroids and GABA$_A$ receptor function. Trends Pharmacol Sci 1995;16:295–303.

101. Robel P, Young J, Corpéchot C, Mayo W, Perché F, Haug M, Simon H, Baulieu EE. Biosynthesis and assay of neurosteroids in rats and mice: functional correlates. J Steroid Biochem Mol Biol 1995;53:355–360.

102. Romeo E, Cheney DL, Zivkovic I, Costa E, Guidotti A. Mitochondrial diazepam-binding inhibitor receptor complex agonists antagonize dizocilpine amnesia: putative role for allopregnanolone. J Pharmacol Exp Ther 1994;270:89–96.

103. Stryer L. Biochemistry. Freeman, New York, NY, 1988.

104. Simon R, Swan J, Griffiths T, Meldrum B. Blockade of N-methyl-D-aspartate receptors may protect against ischemic damage in the brain. Science (Washington, DC) 1984;226:850–852.

105. Wieloch T. Hypoglycemia-induced neuronal damage prevented by an N-methyl-D-aspartate antagonist. Science 1985;230:681–683.

106. Weiss J, Goldberg M, Choi D. Ketamine protects cultured neocortical neurons from hypoxic injury. Brain Res 1986;380:186–190.

107. Goldberg M, Weiss J, Pham P, Choi D. N-methyl-D-aspartate receptors mediate hypoxic neuronal injury in cortical culture. J Pharmacol Exp Ther 1987;243:784–791.

108. Choi D, Koh J, Peters S. Pharmacology of glutamate neurotoxicity in cortical cell culture: attenuation by NMDA antagonists. J Neurosci 1988;8:185–196.

109. Mac Dermott A, Mayer M, Westbrook G, Smith S, Barker J. NMDA-receptor activation increases cytoplasmic calcium concentration in cultured spinal cord neurones. Nature (London) 1986;361:65–90.

110. Weaver CE Jr, Wu FS, Gibbs TT, Farb DH. Pregnenolone sulfate exacerbates NMDA-induced death of hippocampal neurons. Brain Res 1998;803:129–136.

111. Weaver CE Jr, Marek P, Park-Chung M, Tam SW, Farb DH. Neuroprotective activity of a new class of steroidal inhibitors of the N-methyl-D-aspartate receptor. Proc Natl Acad Sci USA 1997;94:1045–1054.

112. Smith SS. Female sex steroid hormones: from receptors to networks to performance: actions on the sensorimotor system. Prog Neurobiol 1994;44:55–86.

113. Murphy DD, Segal M. Regulation of dendritic spine density in cultured rat hippocampal neurons by steroid hormones. J Neurosci 1996;16:4059–4068.

114. Nakano M, Sugioka K, Naito I, Takekoshi S, Niki E. Novel and potent biological antioxidants on membrane phospholipid peroxidation: 2-hydroxy estrone and 2-hydroxy estradiol. Biochem Biophys Res Comm 1987;142:919–924.

115. Niki E. Antioxidants in relation to lipid peroxidation. Chem Phys Lipid 1987;44:227–253.

116. Miura T, Muraoka S, Ogiso T. Inhibition of lipid peroxidation by estradiol and 2-hydroxyestradiol. Steroids 1996;61:379–383.

117. Beal M. Mechanisms of excitotoxicity in neurologic disease. FASEB J 1992;6:3338–3344.

118. Chan PH. Role of oxidants in ischemic brain damage. Stroke 1996;27:1124–1129.

119. Hall E, Pazara K, Linseman K. Sex differences in postischemic neuronal necrosis in gerbils. J Cereb Blood Flow Metab 1991;11:292–298.

120. Emerson CS, Headrick JP, Vink R. Estrogen improves biochemical and neurologic outcome following traumatic brain injury in male rats, but not in females. Brain Res 1993;608:95–100.

121. Behl, C, Widmann M, Trapp T, Holsboer F. 17-β estradiol protects neurons from oxidative stress-induced cell death in vitro. Biochem Biophys Res Commun 1995;216:473–482.

122. Green PS, Bishop J, Simpkins JW. 17α-Estradiol exerts neuroprotective effects on SK-N-SH cells. J Neurosci 1997;17:511–515.

123. Paganini-Hill A, Henderson VW. Estrogen deficiency and risk of Alzheimer's disease in women. Am J Epidem 1994;140:2560–261.

124. ffrench-Mullen JMH, Danks P, Spence KT. Neurosteroids modulate calcium currents in hippocampal CA1 neurons via a pertussis toxin-sensitive G-protein-coupled mechanism. J Neurosci 1994;14:1963–1977.

125. Majewska MD, Schwartz RD. Pregnenolone-sulfate: an endogenous antagonist of the γ-aminobutyric acid receptor complex in brain. Brain Res 1987;404:355–360.

126. Farb DH, Gibbs TT, Wu FS, Gyenes M, Friedman L, Russek SJ. Steroid modulation of amino acid neurotransmitter receptors. In: Biggio G, Concas A, Costa E, eds. GABAergic Synaptic Transmission: Molecular, Pharmacological, Clinical Aspects. Raven, New York, 1992, pp. 119–131.

127. Bertrand D, Valera S, Bertrand S, Ballivet M, Rungger D. Steroids inhibit nicotinic acetylcholine receptors. Neuroreport 1991;2:277–280.

128. Valera S, Ballivet M, Bertrand D. Progesterone modulates a neuronal nicotinic acetylcholine receptor. Proc Natl Acad Sci USA 1992;89:9949–9953.

129. Harrison NL, Majewska MD, Harrington JW, Barker JL. Structure-activity relationships for steroid interaction with the γ-aminobutyric acid$_A$ receptor complex. J Pharmacol Exp Ther 1987; 241:346–353.

130. Peters J, Kirkness E, Callachan H, Lambert J, Turner A. Modulation of the GABA$_A$ receptor by depressant barbiturates and pregnane steroids. Br J Pharmacol 1988;94:1257–1269.

131. Hill-Venning C, Peters JA, Lambert JJ. The interaction of steroids with inhibitory and excitatory amino acid receptors. Clin. Neuropharm. 1992;15(Suppl. Pt A):683A–684A.

132. Harrison NL, Simmonds MA. Modulation of the GABA receptor complex by a steroid anaesthetic. Brain Res 1984;323:287–292.

133. Barker JL, Harrison NL, Lange GD, Owen DG. Potentiation of γ-aminobutyric-acid-activated chloride conductance by a steroid anaesthetic in cultured rat neurons. J Physiol (London) 1987;386:485–501.

134. Cottrell GA, Lambert JJ, Peters JA. Modulation of GABA$_A$ receptor activity by alphaxalone. Br J Pharmacol 1987;90:491–500.

135. Simmonds MA., Turner JP. Antagonism of inhibitory amino acids by the steroid derivative RU5135. Br J Pharmacol 1985;84:631–635.

136. Majewska MD, Demirgören S, Spivak CE, London ED. The neurosteroid dehydroepiandrosterone sulfate is an allosteric antagonist of the GABA$_A$ receptor. Brain Res 1990;526:143–146.

137. Gu Q, Aguila MC, Moss RL. 17β-estradiol potentiation of inward kainate-induced currents in acutely dissociated hippocampal neurons. Soc Neurosci Abst 1995;21:54.

11

Steroidal Modulation of Sigma Receptor Function

Stéphane Bastianetto, MD, François Monnet, MD Jean-Louis Junien, MD, and Rémi Quirion, MD

CONTENTS

INTRODUCTION
RECEPTOR BINDING AND MOLECULAR STUDIES
FUNCTIONAL ASSAYS
SOURCE OF STEROIDS σ LIGANDS
CONCLUSIONS
REFERENCES

INTRODUCTION

The term "sigma" (σ) receptor was coined by Martin et al. *(1)*, who identified the unique psychotomimetic effects of N-allylnormetazocine (SKF-10047), a prototypic benzomorphan, and has initially been designated as a subtype of opioid receptors. σ ligands belong to diverse structural classes including (+)-benzomorphans ([+]-SKF 10047, [+]-pentazocine), morphinans (dextrometorphan), guanidines (1,3-di-o-tolyl-guanidine or DTG), phenothiazines (perphenazine, chlorpromazine), butyrophenones (haloperidol), tricyclic antidepressants (imipramine), monoamine oxydase inhibitors (clorgyline), serotonin uptake inhibitors (sertraline), piperazines (α-[4-fluorophenyl]-4-[5-fluoro-2-pyrimidinyl]-1-piperazine butanol or BMY-14802), phenylpiperidines ([+]3-[3-hydroxyphenyl]-N-[1-propyl]piperidine or [+]-3PPP), cytochrome P-450 inhibitors (proadifen), anticonvulsants (phenytoin), addictive drugs (cocaine, amphetamine), polyamines (ifenprodil), and certain steroids (progesterone [PROG], testosterone) (for reviews, *see* refs. *2* and *3*).

However, the denomination "σ" refers to drugs active in behavioral tests and pharma-cologically effective in human or rodents. It has thus constituted a functional concept rather than corresponded to a molecular entity. This notion was further strengthened by preclinical and clinical studies that have reported on the potential therapeutic usefulness of selective σ ligands in the treatment of certain disorders of the CNS, including cognitive and mnesic deficits *(4–12)*, psychosic disorders *(13–16)*, anxiety *(17–19)* and

From: *Contemporary Endocrinology: Neurosteroids: A New Regulatory Function in the Nervous System* Edited by: E.-E. Baulieu, P. Robel, and M. Schumacher
© Humana Press Inc., Totowa, NJ

Table 1
Summary of Some Features of σ_1 and σ_2 Receptor Subtypes

Subtype	σ_1	σ_2
Representative agonists[b]	(+)-pentazocine, SA-4503 JO-1784, PRE-084, DHEA/DHEAS PREGS[a]	Reduced haloperidol Ibogaine, CB64D (−)-deoxybenzomorphans
Representative antagonists[b]	Haloperidol NE-100, BD-1047, BD-1063, BMY 14802 PROGESTERONE	
Proposed functional assays[c]	Learning impairment induced by dizocilpine in mice Modulation of NMDA receptors in rat hippocampus (CA$_3$ subfield)	Dystonia and rotation behaviour in rats
Nature of the cloned receptor protein[d]	Δ_8–Δ_7 sterol isomerase (cholesterol biosynthesis)	?
Punative endogenous ligands[e]	Progesterone DHEA/DHEAS (?) PREGS (?)	Divalent cations (Zn^{2+})
Potential therapeutic applications[f]	Cognitive enhancement/brain repair Anti-ischemic Antidepressant Antipsychotic	Motor disorders Anxiety

[a]Considered an inverse agonist.
[b]Adapted with permission from refs. (1,2,12,39,63, and 108).
[c]Adapted with permission from refs. (2,5, and 35).
[d]Adapted with permission from refs. (5 and 56).
[e]Adapted with permission from refs. (39,68, and 108).
[f]Adapted with permission from refs. (4–23).

neuroprotection (20–23), as well as diseases affecting motor and posture controls (24). During the last two decades, this theoretical concept was partially clarified. Biochemical and behavioral studies in the 1980s, using various selective and nonselective σ ligands, indicated that σ receptors were distinct from any known receptors, including the phencyclidine/N-methyl-D-aspartate (NMDA) receptor complex (25–26), and represented a unique class of binding sites (27). Numerous biological effects were ascribed to σ ligands, such as the modulation of dopaminergic, NMDA-related glutamatergic, monoaminergic, and cholinergic neurotransmissions (4,28–43).

The variety of these pharmacological effects, as well as binding and drug discrimination studies, suggested the existence of at least two subtypes of σ receptors, termed sigma$_1$ (σ_1) and sigma$_2$ (σ_2) (44). These subtypes are currently differentiated on the basis of their respective biochemical and pharmacological properties (Table 1). The σ_1 subtype exhibits high affinity for DTG, haloperidol, and (+)-benzomorphans, binds preferentially to (+)-isomers and is proposed to be associated with pertussis toxin-sensitive G$_{i/o}$ proteins. Its possible neuroprotective and anti-amnesic effects may result from an indirect modulation of the NMDA receptor *(5,7,8,20,21,23,45)*. The σ_1 subtype may also modulate the antidepressant and antipsychotic activities of certain σ ligands *(13,17–18)*. Conversely, the σ_2 subtype exhibits no stereoselectivity and/or only low affinities for the (+)-benzomorphans and steroids, is not modulated by pertussis toxin-sensitive $G_{i/o}$ proteins, and is predominantly located in the motor system. Clinically, the σ_2 subtype may be involved in the motor and anxiolytic effects of σ ligands *(19,46–47)*.

As previously mentioned, a better understanding of the role of σ receptors in physiological and pathophysiological processes has been hampered by the lack of molecular insight, which rendered enigmatic the accurate relevance of σ receptors and favored some controversy regarding their functions. To solve the apparent "Sigma Enigma" *(48)*, several attempts have been made to identify the nature of σ receptors. Since 1986, two proteins labeled by a specific σ ligand [^{3}H]-azido-DTG, have been solubilized and partially purified from rodent tissues and pheochromocytoma (PC-12) cell membranes. It has been suggested that the upper and lower molecular weight proteins represent the σ_1 (25–29 kDa) and the σ_2 (18–21 kDa) subtype, respectively *(49–52)*. The most recent attempt has resulted in the purification from guinea pig liver of a [^{3}H]-(+)-pentazocine-binding protein with the pharmacological profile of the σ_1 subtype and the cloning of the corresponding cDNA *(53)*. This protein (25.3 kDa) is distinct from any known mammalian proteins and possesses at least one putative transmembrane domain. This protein and its corresponding cloned cDNA were found to have a respective 30% and 66% sequence homology with yeast-like Δ_8–Δ_7 sterol isomerases (these isomerases are involved in the biosynthesis of lanosterol, a polycyclic precursor of cholesterol), strengthening the notion that σ receptors, and evidently the σ_1 subtype, do not represent a classical transmitter receptor *(53)*. Although attempts to demonstrate a yeast sterol isomerase activity of the σ_1 cloned cDNA have not been successful yet *(53)*, the recent cloning of a murine Δ_8–Δ_7 sterol isomerase similar to human emopamil (an anti-ischemic drug)-binding protein supports this hypothesis, because emopamil has σ binding affinities *(54–55)*. Therefore, mammalian and yeast Δ_8–Δ_7 sterol isomerases may represent two new members of the sigma receptor family *(56)*.

The identification of putative endogenous ligands is also indispensable to establish better the relevance of σ receptors. However, the isolation of unique endogenous σ ligands has not been successful yet, despite the evidence of their existence in rodent *(57–58)*, porcine *(59)*, and human *(60)* brains. Apart from non-fully characterized polypeptides (denoted "sigmaphins" by Su et al. *[57]*), neuropeptide Y (NPY) has been proposed as a putative endogenous σ ligand because it competed, in vitro, for [^{3}H]-(+)-SKF-10047 binding sites *(61)*. However, the genuine affinity of NPY for σ receptors failed to be confirmed *(62–64)*, and purported in vivo interactions between NPY and σ receptors are likely being indirect and mediated by the Y_1 receptor subtype *(65–67)*.

In parallel, functional assays have provided evidence for direct interactions between certain steroids and σ receptors *(68–74)*. In this chapter, we summarize these recent results and address the key involvement of σ receptors in the modulation of some of the steroids.

RECEPTOR BINDING AND MOLECULAR STUDIES

An exhaustive study of representative steroids derived from cholesterol has been performed initially in rodent brain homogenates by Su et al. *(68)* and reproduced by other

Table 2
Apparent Affinities of Steroids for s Receptors in Guinea-Pig Brain and Spleen

Steroids	Brain [^{3}H}(+)-SKF10047 $K_i(nM)^a$	Brain [^{3}H}(+)-3PPP $IC_{50}(nM)^b$	Sleep [^{3}H]haloperidol IC50(nM)^c
Progesterone	268	260	310
11b-Hydroxyprogesterone	1535	–	1900
11a-Hydroxyprogesterone	10.000	–	–
17a-Hydroxyprogesterone	>10.000	5600	–
Testosterone	1014	450	770
5a-Dihydrotestosterone	–	430	525
5a-Androstane-3b,17b-diol	–	>10.000	–
5a-Androstane-3a,17b-diol	–	10.000	–
Pregnenolone	>10.000	7000	–
Pregnenolone sulfate	3196	–	–
5b-Pregnane-3,20-dione	–	–	270
5a-Pregnane-3,20-dione	–	–	620
17a-Hydroxypregnenolone	–	>10.000	–
Corticosterone	4074	8000	–
Deoxycorticosterone	938	680	–
Estriol	>10.000	–	–
Estradiolhemisuccinate	>10.000	–	–
Androstane	–	600	–
Dehydroepiandrosterone	–	3700	–
5a-Androstane-3,17-dione	–	700	–

^{a}Adapted with permission from ref. *(68)*.
^{b}Adapted with permission from ref. *(70)*.
^{c}Adapted with permission from ref. *(73)*.

groups *(69–74)* (Table 2). PROG ($K_i = 268$ nM) showed the highest affinity for σ_1 binding sites labeled by [^{3}H]-(+)-SKF-10047 followed by testosterone (T) ($K_i = 1014$ nM) in guinea pig brain membranes *(68)*. Similarly, in rat brain membranes, McCann et al. *(72)* demonstrated that PROG and T exhibited high selectivity for the σ_1 ($K_i = 25$ and 50 nM, respectively) over the σ_2 ($K_i > 15$ µM) subtype. Interestingly, the σ_1-like binding site in smooth endoplasmic reticulum of the rat liver is competed by several steroids including PROG, 5α-dihydrotestosterone (5α-DHT), T, corticosteroids and, to a lesser extent, 7β-estradiol *(73)*. In this latter study, the authors proposed that 85% of specific PROG-binding sites differed from steroid/drug-metabolizing enzymes and did not participate in the PROG-metabolizing processes and thus likely corresponded to σ-binding sites. Other reports confirmed the ability of PROG and T to bind to σ-binding sites in rodent spleen, liver, and brain membranes and indicated that, except for 5α-DHT and deoxycorticosterone (DOC), the other steroid hormones involved in steroidogenesis displayed only weak ($K_i > $ µM) or negligible ($K_i > 10$ µM) affinities for σ receptors *(68–71)*. Recently, Ramamoorthy et al. *(74)* have shown that selective σ ligands as well as PROG and T inhibited σ binding sites labeled by [^{3}H]-haloperidol to purified human placental brush border membranes of the syncytiotrophoblasts. According to the classification of σ receptors, the rank order of affinity of these drugs for σ receptors (haloperidol > clorgyline >> DTG = PROG > T > rimcazole) is distinctly characteristic of the σ_1 subtype. Interestingly, the potencies of PROG and T to inhibit the σ binding sites are similar to those reported by Su et al. *(68)* in rodent brain (310 vs 268 nM for PROG and 970 vs 1014 nM for testosterone). DOC, the free and the sulfated forms of pregnenolone (PREG) and 3α-pregnan-5α-ol-20-one (allopregnanolone; 3α, 5α = THPROG) were at least one order of magnitude less potent, whereas estradiol was 100-fold less potent than PROG and T. Scatchard analysis of binding data was indicative of a competitive interaction between PROG and the placental haloperidol binding sites. Using [^{3}H]-(+)-pentazocine and the arylazide (–)[^{3}H]-azidopamil as specific probes, Hanner et al. *(53)* demonstrated that peripheral σ_1 receptor binding sites were competed by PROG (K_i = 572 nM), and T (K_i = 2340 nM), but not corticosterone (K_i = 49.8 μM). The amino-acid sequence of this unique protein and the subsequent structure–activity relationship provided key information showing that σ_1 binding sites carry a lipophilic sterol/steroid-binding domain, which may explain the affinity of the σ_1 subtype for some steroids. Conversely, selective and high affinity σ ligands such as (+)-pentazocine and haloperidol showed high affinities (IC_{50} = 63.9 and 15.5 nM, respectively) for [^{3}H]-PROG binding sites in rat liver membrane extracts, further supporting the hypothesis that these steroids could constitute endogenous σ ligands, especially for the σ_1 subtype *(69)*. Table 2 summarizes the affinity of various steroid hormones for σ binding sites.

FUNCTIONAL ASSAYS

In the classical model of genomic steroid hormone action, steroids diffuse across plasma membranes and bind to cytosol or nuclear receptors. The binding of steroids to intracellular receptors modulates with a latency of minutes to hours the transcription and expression of genes and then promotes proteins, including those of neurotransmitter receptors *(75–76)*. However, all of the neuronal action of steroids cannot be accounted for by this model in the CNS. Some steroids, termed "neurosteroids" (because they are locally synthesized from PREG in neural and brain tissues), have been shown to affect briefly and suddenly neuronal firing pattern and activity. Rapid, nongenomic effects of steroids have been shown to modulate the activity of various neurotransmitter systems, suggesting the existence of additional specific binding sites on neuronal membranes. Indeed, steroids may simultaneously modulate excitatory and inhibitory neurotransmitters-gated ion channels or directly inhibit ion channels activity, indicating that at least acutely they regulate the balance between excitatory and inhibitory processes in the CNS (for reviews, *77–81*). For example, the existence of steroid recognition sites on the GABA$_A$/benzodiazepine receptor (associated) chloride ionophore is well-established *(82)*. Pregnenolone sulfate (PREGS) and dehydroepiandrosterone sulfate (DHEAS) inhibited the GABA$_A$ receptor complex at physiological concentrations, whereas the PROG metabolites tetrahydroprogesterone and tetrahydrodeoxycorticosterone potentiated GABAergic neurotransmission (for review, *see* ref. *83*). High μM concentrations of 3α-hydroxy-5β-pregnan-20-one sulfate inhibited ion currents and increased intracellular Ca^{2+} concentrations evoked by NMDA *(84–85)*. PREGS and DHEA/DHEAS were also able to inhibit voltage-activated Ca^{2+} channels in hippocampal neurons *(86–87)* or potentiated NMDA-sensitive glutamatergic neuronal response or NMDA-gated ion currents in spinal cord and hippocampal neurons while they inhibited non-NMDA glutamatergic response *(84,88–92)*. DHEA/DHEAS, PREG/PREGS as well as T and dihydrotestosterone facilitated learning processes and cognitive abilities in humans *(93–95)*, and enhanced or restored memory retention in rodents *(11–12,96–107)*. It has also been proposed that the neuromodulatory actions of neuroactive steroids on $GABA_A$ and NMDA receptors may explain, in part (along with σ sites), their ability to enhance or restore learning/memory processes in rodents *(99,103–106)*.

Interestingly, selective σ ligands shared with certain steroids the ability to modulate the NMDA responsiveness in the hippocampus in vivo and in vitro *(34–39,108,109)* and to reverse the amnesic effects induced by dizocilpine, a NMDA receptor antagonist *(5–8)*. The involvement of σ receptors in the modulation of the NMDA response by σ ligands is now established *(34–38,109)*. Using an in vivo electrophysiological paradigm of unitary extracellular recordings, we have shown that selective $σ_1$ ligands such as JO-1784 ([+]N-cyclopropylmethyl-N-methyl-1,4-diphenyl-1-ethyl-but-3-en-1-ylamine hydrochloride or igmesine), BD-737 (1S,2R (–)cis-N-[2-(3,4-dichlorophenyl)ethyl]-N-methyl-2-(1-pyrrolidinyl)cyclohexamine) or (+)-pentazocine potentiated NMDA-induced neuronal activity in the CA1 and CA3 regions of the rat hippocampus (34–38, 109). These putative σ-mediated effects were selectively reversed by σ antagonists such as BMY-14802 or haloperidol at doses that by themselves did not modify the NMDA-induced activation of pyramidal neurons. Spiperone, a selective D2 dopamine receptor antagonist which has no affinity for sigma receptors *(28)*, was ineffective in antagonizing the potentiating effects of DTG or (+)-pentazocine, suggesting that the activation of σ receptors may be responsible for the antagonistic effects of haloperidol. Using an in vitro model of NMDA-evoked [³H]noradrenaline release from preloaded rat hippocampal slices, we have also shown that JO-1784, BD-737 and (+)-pentazocine potentiated whereas DTG inhibited the NMDA response *(36,39)*. Both effects of σ drugs were prevented by the high affinity σ antagonists haloperidol and/or BD-1063 (1(2-(3,4-dichlorophenyl)ethyl)-4-methyl piperazine).

More recently, we have reported that several steroids might modulate in vitro NMDA responses by interacting with σ receptors *(39)*. Indeed, DHEAS potentiated (in the 30 nM to 3 μM concentration range), whereas PREGS inhibited (in the 100 nM to 3 μM concentration range) NMDA-evoked [³H]noradrenaline release. In contrast, PREG, DHEA, and 3α,5α-tetrahydroprogesterone remained inactive (up to 3 μM). The respective actions of both steroids (at 300 nM) were reversed by the σ antagonist BD-1063 (100 nM) and haloperidol (100 nM), but not by spiperone (100 nM), indicating that DHEAS and PREGS acted via σ receptors. It is noteworthy that the preferential effectiveness of PREGS over PREG is correlated with binding data obtained by Su et al. *(68)* (K_i values of 3.2 μM for PREGS, K_i values > 10 μM for PREG). The discrepancy between the in vitro affinity of PREGS and its effective concentration in this model might be owing to methodological procedures. Interestingly, PROG is inactive (at 100 nM) by itself on this NMDA-related response, but prevented the respective effects of DHEAS (300 nM), PREGS (300 nM), and DTG (300 nM), indicating that PROG acted as a σ antagonist. A pretreatment with pertussis toxin, a selective blocker of the Gi/o types of G proteins, abolished the potentiating effects of DHEAS and the inhibitory effects of PREGS on the NMDA-evoked [³H]noradrenaline release. These data suggested that the effects of DHEAS and PREGS involved the $σ_1$ subtype which, unlike the $σ_2$ subtype, may be modulated by Gi/o proteins *(38)*. Subsequently, Maurice et al. *(10)* reported that subcutaneous injections of DHEAS (from 5–20 mg/kg, sc) attenuated learning impairments induced by dizocilpine in passive avoidance task in mice. These effects were suppressed by a co-treatment with BMY-

14802 (5 mg/kg, ip) and by a chronic treatment with haloperidol (4 mg/kg/day, sc, 7 d), which possibly induced a down-regulation of the σ_1 subtype. Using the amnesia model induced by β-amyloid *(25–35)* in mice, Maurice et al. *(11)* showed that steroids like DHEA/DHEAS and PREG/PREGS shared with σ_1 agonists [(+)-pentazocine, PRE-084] the ability to reverse β-amyloid-induced amnesia. The effects of these steroids and σ_1 agonists were antagonized by haloperidol and PROG, respectively, confirming that some of the anti-amnesic effects of steroids may involved an interaction with the σ_1 subtype.

Using an in vivo extracellular electrophysiological model in the rat, Bergeron et al. *(110)* recently showed that the intravenous administration of DHEA (from 100 μg/kg to 2 mg/kg) or σ_1 agonists ([+]-pentazocine, JO-1784) selectively potentiated the excitatory response of pyramidal neurons to microiontophoretic applications of NMDA. The potentiating effects of DHEA were abolished by the σ_1 antagonist NE-100 (25 μg/kg, iv) and haloperidol (20 μg/kg, iv) (but not by spiperone), and also by a pertussis toxin-pretreatment, bringing further credence that steroids acted on the σ_1 subtype. Low doses of PROG (at 20 μg/kg, iv) reversed the potentiating effects of DHEA (250 μg/kg, iv) or those of σ agonists at doses that did not modify the neuronal response induced by NMDA. Despite the absence of σ-mediated effects of PREGS (which may be explained by the inability of ester sulfates to cross readily the blood brain barrier), the authors concluded on the involvement of σ receptors in the modulatory effects of the steroids. The discrepancy between the ineffectiveness of DHEA in vitro vs in vivo remains unexplained. The concentrations of DHEAS are higher than those of DHEA both in the human and rodent brain and blood *(111–115)*. The weak activities of sulfatases, sulfotransferases, or hydroxylases in the brain make it doubtful of the in vitro local conversion of DHEAS into DHEA or its metabolism *(115–117)*. Similarly, it is unlikely that DHEA is converted within few minutes in vivo into DHEAS in the brain owing to the weak activity of the sulfotransferase *(116)*. Rapid and extensive metabolism of DHEA by conversion to its metabolites, including T, 5α-DHT, and estradiol occurs peripherically in rodent *(115,117)*. Consistent with this hypothesis, Monnet et al. (unpublished data) have observed that both T and estradiol enhanced the NMDA-evoked [^{3}H]noradrenaline release from preloaded spayed rat hippocampal slices and speculated that DHEA could act per se and/or be converted in vivo into T and estradiol, which may bind to σ receptors.

Taken together, these results suggest that steroids may modulate glutamate/NMDA receptor neurotransmission via an interaction with the σ_1 subtype, which may explain their promnesic effects. DHEA/DHEAS and PREGS would act as σ_1 "agonist" and σ_1 inverse "agonist" respectively, whereas progesterone acts as a σ_1 "antagonist" (Table 1). Table 3 summarizes the features of the functional σ/steroid interactions.

SOURCE OF STEROIDS σ LIGANDS

It is now crucial to determine if the concentrations of PROG and its metabolites as well as those of DHEA/DHEAS and PREGS required to modulate the σ_1 subtype correspond to those found in vivo, depending or not on the endocrine status of the body. Human and rodent plasma levels of PROG most significantly rise (up to 0.5 μ*M*) during late pregnancy *(118–121)*. Therefore, the placental *(74)* and CNS *(68,70)* σ receptors may represent effective targets involved in the physiological action of several steroid hormones during pregnancy (particularly PROG with K_i values are from 260 to 572 n*M*). In contrast, the amount of free serum PROG during diestrus is only about 2%, making it an

Table 3
Summary of Features of Functional σ/Steroid Interactions

Functional Assays	Agonists	Antagonists
Attenuation of learning impairment induced by dizocilpine or β-amyloid$_{25-35}$ in mice[a]	(+)-Benzomorphans DTG, PRE-084 DHdEA/DHEAS PREG/PREGS	Haloperidol BMY-14802, NE-100 progesterone
In vivo potentiation of NMDA-induced hippocampal neuronal activity in rat[b]	(+)-pentazocine, DTG JO-1784, BD-737 DHEA	Haloperidol, (+)-3PPP NE-100, BMY 14802 progesterone, testosterone[c]
Potentiation of NMDA-induced [^{3}H]-noradrenaline release in rat hippocampal slices[d]	(+)-pentazocine JO-1784, BD-737 DHEAS, testosterone[e] estradiol, DTG[f], PREGS[f]	Haloperidol, BD-1063 progesterone

[a]Data used with permission from refs. (5,7,8,11,12).
[b]Data used with permission from refs. (34,35,108).
[c]Data Used with permission from ref. (108).
[d]Data used with permission from refs. (36,39).
[e]Data used with permission from ref. (39).
[f]Considered as inverse agonists.

unlikely candidate as a prominent functional endogenous σ ligand (121). Accordingly, Bergeron et al. (110) investigated the effects of hormonal changes on the neuromodulatory actions of σ agonists and steroids on hippocampal NMDA stimulatory response. Their results indicated that the potentiation of the NMDA response induced by DTG was significantly greater in ovariectomized females (in which the levels of PROG are low) than that seen in males or in nonovariectomized females at d one and 3 of the menstrual cycle (diestrus). Moreover, at d 18 of pregnancy (when PROG reached its highest levels; 118–120), the potentiating effects of σ agonists and DHEA on the NMDA response were abolished. In contrast, at d 5 of puerperium (at which time the plasma levels of PROG are at their lowest), the effects of these compounds on hippocampal NMDA stimulatory action were similar to those observed in ovariectomized females (110). The relevance of this observation is underlined by the reports indicating that the levels of PROG present in various brain areas (113,122–124) were similar to those found in the blood (119–121). High concentrations (μM) of DHEAS and PREG/PREGS have found in the rat brain, all largely independent of adrenal and gonadal sources. Their levels are much higher than those found in the blood and those of PROG in the rat and human brains (111–114,125–130). This would be consistent with the hypothesis that steroids, such as DHEAS and PREGS, and to a lesser extent DHEA, which is 10 times less abundant in rodent brain than its ester sulfate, might act as endogenous σ ligands. This has raised the possibility of autocrine and paracrine effects of these steroids, although their plasma levels were undetectable (117,131).

Taken together, these data indicated that DHEA/DHEAS and PREGS as well as PROG, depending on the menstrual cycle, can modulate both in vivo and in vitro σ receptor-mediated effects, and that peripheral levels of these steroids affect the CNS σ system-related events. It also suggested that σ receptors (most likely σ$_1$) may be associated with emotional behaviors, particularly during pregnancy and the post-partum period, at which time PROG levels are, respectively, high and low to modulate σ receptors. However, the precise mechanism(s) by which this modulation occurs remain(s) unknown. It is likely that the σ antagonist PROG might induce a down regulation of σ receptors since that repeated administration of haloperidol, a purported σ antagonist, induced a decrease of a density of σ binding sites in rat *(132)* and in human *(133)* brain whereas a specific D2 antagonist lacking σ properties did not affect the density of σ sites *(132)*.

CONCLUSIONS

The "σ enigma" has been a mystery for over two decades, with some raging debates occuring at times *(2,44,48)*. All these confusions have even raised doubts on the genuine existence of unique σ receptors *(134–135)*. The most recent cloning of the σ_1 receptor clearly and definitively resolves this issue *(53)*. However, the very nature of the cloned protein, an intracellular enzyme possibly involved in cholesterol/steroid biosynthesis, raises other questions, regarding putative endogenous modulators. Steroids such as PROG, DHEA, PREG, and their sulfate esters are particularly interesting in that context and may help to resolve this point. In fact, binding and functional data strongly suggest that these steroids, and in particular PROG, possess the necessary requirements to act and be considered as endogenous ligands for the σ_1 receptor subtype. Naturally, recent evidence for interactions between steroids and σ receptors do not exclude additional effects of steroids on other brain receptors such as $GABA_A$ *(83)* and NMDA *(84)* receptors. The very fact that steroids have been shown to modulate a very broad spectrum of CNS effects even suggests that steroids likely interact with multiple target sites, including σ receptors to induce their actions. However, they may behave uniquely as endogenous ligands for the σ_1 receptor subtype, other target sites such as GABA, and glutamate possessing well-characterized endogenous ligands.

ACKNOWLEDGMENTS

This work was supported by research grants from the Medical Research Council of Canada (MRCC) to R. Q., the Fondation de France and the Ministère de la Recherche to F. M. R. Q. holds "Chercheur Boursier" awards from le Fonds de la Recherche en Santé du Québec.

REFERENCES

1. Martin WR, Eades CG, Thompson JA, Huppler RE, Gilbert PE. The effects of morphine- and nalorphine-like drugs in the nondependent and morphine-dependent chronic spinal dog. J Pharmacol Exp Ther 1976;197:517–532.
2. Walker JM, Bowen WD, Walker FO, Matsumoto RR, De Costa B, Rice KC. Sigma receptors: biology and function. Pharmacol Rev 1990;42:355–402.
3. DeCosta BR, He XS. Structure-activity relationships and evolution of sigma receptor ligands (1976-present). In: Itzhak, Y., ed. Sigma Receptors. Academic, San Diego, CA, 1994, pp. 45–111.
4. Matsuno K, Senda T, Matsunaga K, Mita S. Ameliorating effects of σ receptor ligands on the impairment of passive avoidance tasks in mice: involvement in the central acetylcholinergic system. Eur J Pharmacol 1994;261:43–51.
5. Maurice T, Hiramatsu M, Itoh J, Kameyama T, Hasegawa T, Nabeshima T. Behavioral evidence for a modulating role of σ ligands in memory processes. I. Attenuation of dizocilpine (MK–801)-induced amnesia. Brain Res 1994;647:44–56.
6. Maurice T, Hiramatsu M, Kameyama T, Hasegawa T, Nabeshima T. Behavioral evidence for a modulating role of σ ligands in memory processes. II. Reversion of carbon monoxide-induced amnesia. Brain Res 1994;647:57–64.

7. Maurice T, Hiramatsu M, Itoh J, Kameyama T, Hasegawa T, Nabeshima T. Low dose of 1,3-di(2-tolyl)guanidine (DTG) attenuates MK-801-induced spatial working memory impairment in mice. Psychopharmacology 1994;114:520–522.

8. Maurice T, Su TP, Parish DW, Nabeshima T, Privat A. PRE-084, a selective PCP derivative, attenuates MK-801-induced impairment of learning in mice. Pharmacol Biochem Behav 1994;49:859–869.

9. Maurice T, Su T-P, Parish DW, Privat A. Prevention of nimodipine-induced impairment of learning by the selective σ ligand PRE-084. J Neural Transm 1995;102:1–18.

10. Maurice T, Roman F, Su T-P, Privat A. Beneficial effects of sigma agonists on the age-related learning impairment in the senescence-accelerated mouse (SAM). Brain Res 1996;733:219–230.

11. Maurice T, Junien JL, Privat A. Dehydroepiandrosterone sulfate attenuates dizocilpine-induced learning impairment in mice via σ$_1$-receptors. Behav Brain Res 1996;83:159–164.

12. Maurice T, Privat A. Sigma1 (sigma 1) receptor agonists and neurosteroids attenuate B25-35-amyloid peptide-induced amnesia in mice through a common mechanism. Neuroscience 1998;83: 413–428.

13. Ferris RM, White HL, Tang FLM, Russell A, Harfenist M. Rimcazole (BW 234U), a novel antipsychotic agent whose mechanism of action cannot be explained by a direct blockade of postsynaptic dopaminergic receptors in brain. Drug Dev Res 1986;9:171–188.

14. Munetz MR, Schulz SC, Bellin M, Harty I. Rimcazole (BW234U) in the maintenance treatment of outpatients with schizophrenia. Drug Dev Res 1989;16:79–83.

15. Snyder SH, Largent BL. Receptor mechanisms in antipsychotic drug action: focus on sigma receptors. J Neuropsychiatry 1989;1:7–15.

16. Gewirtz GR, Gorman JM, Volavka J, Macaluso J, Gribkoff G, Taylor DP, Borison R. BMY 14802, a sigma receptor ligand for the treatment of schizophrenia. Neuropsychopharmacology 1994;10:37–40.

17. Matheson GK, Guthrie D, Bauer C, Knowles A, White G, Ruston C. Sigma receptor ligands alter concentrations of corticosterone in plasma in the rat. Neuropharmacology 1991;30:79–87.

18. Junien J-L, Gue M, Bueno L. Neuropeptide Y and sigma ligand act through a G1 protein to block the psychological stress and corticotropin-releasing factor induced colonic motor activation in rats. Neuropharmacology1991;30:1119–1124.

19. Sanchez C, Arnt J, Perregaard. Lu–28179-a selective sigma ligand with potent anxiolytic effects. Soc Neurosci Abst 1995;21:385.

20. Kirk CJ, Reddy NL, Fisher JB, Wolcott TC, Knapp AG, McBurney RN. *In vitro* neuroprotection by substitued guanidines with varying affinities for the N-methyl-D-aspartate receptor ionophore and for sigma sites. J Pharmac Exp Ther 1994;271:1080–1085.

21. DeCoster MA, Klette KL, Knight ES, Tortella FC. σ receptor-mediated neuroprotection against glutamate toxicity in primary rat neuronal cultuRes Brain Res 1995;671:45–53.

22. Lesage AS, De Loore KL, Peeters L, Leysen JE. Neuroprotective sigma ligands interfere with the glutamate-activated NOS pathway in hippocampal cell culture. Synapse 1995;20:156–164.

23. Lockhart BP, Soulard P, Benicourt C, Privat A, Junien JL. Distinct neuroprotective profiles for σ ligands against N-methyl-D-aspartate (NMDA), and hypoxia-mediated neurotoxicity in neuronal culture toxicity studies. Brain Res 1995;675:110–120.

24. Matsumoto R, Bowen W, Tom M, Vo V, Truong D, De Costa B. Characterization of two novel σ receptor ligands: antidystonic effects in rats suggest σ receptor antagonism. Eur JPharmacol 1995;280:301–310.

25. Zukin SR, Brady KT, Slifer BL, Balster RL. Behavioral and biochemical stereoselectivity of sigma opiate/PCP receptors. Brain Res 1984;294: 174–177.

26. Mendelsohn LG, Kalra V, Johnson BG, Kercner GA. Sigma opioid receptor: characterization and co-identity with the phencyclidine receptor. J Pharmac Exp Ther 1985;33:597–602.

27. Quirion R, Chicheportiche R, Contreras PC, Johnson KM, Lodge D, Tam SW, Woods JH, Zukin SR. Classification and nomenclature of phencyclidine and sigma receptor sites. Trends Neurosci 1987;10:444–446.

28. Steinfels GF, Tam SW, Cook L. Electrophysiological effects of selective σ-receptor agonists, antagonists, and the selective phencyclidine receptor agonist MK–801 on midbrain dopamine neurons. Neuropsychopharmacology 1989;2: 201–208.

29. Iyengar S, Dilworth VM, Mick SJ, Monahan JB, Contreras PC, Rao TS, Wood PL. Sigma receptors modulate both A9 and A10 dopaminergic neurons in the rat brain: Functional interaction with NMDA receptors. Brain Res 1990;524:322–326.

30. Iyengar S, Mick S, Dilworth V, Michel J, Rao TS, Farah JM, Wood PL. Sigma receptors modulate the hypothalamic-pituitary-adrenal (HPA) axis centrally: evidence for a functional interaction with NMDA receptors, *in vivo*. Neuropharmacology 1990;29:299–303.

31. VanderMaelen CP, Braselton JP. Effects of a potential antipsychotic, BMY 14802, on firing of central serotonergic and noradrenergic neurons in rats. Eur J Pharmacol 1990;179:357–366.

32. Campbell BG, Keana JFW, Weber E. Sigma receptor ligand N,N'-di-(ortho-tolyl)guanidine inhibits release of acetylcholine in the guinea pig ileum. Eur J Pharmacol 1991;205:219–223.

33. Junien J-L, Roman FJ, Brunelle G, Pascaud X. JO1784, a novel sigma ligand, potentiates [^{3}H]acetylcholine release from rat hippocampus slices. Eur J Pharmacol 1991;200:343–345

34. Monnet FP, Debonnel G, Junien JL, De Montigny C. N-Methyl-D-aspartate-induced neuronal activation is selectively modulated by σ receptors. Eur J Pharmacol 1990;179:441–445.

35. Monnet FP, Debonnel G, De Montigny C. In vivo electrophysiological evidence for a selective modulation of N-methyl-D-aspartate-induced neuronal activation in rat CA3 dorsal hippocampus by sigma ligands. J Pharmac Exp Ther 1992;261:123–130.

36. Monnet FP, Blier P, Debonnel G, De Montigny C. Modulation by sigma ligands of N-methyl-D-aspartate-induced [^{3}H]noradrenaline release in the rat hippocampus: G-protein dependency. Naunyn Schmiedebergs Arch. Pharmacol 1992;346:32–39.

37. Monnet FP, Debonnel G, Fournier A, De Montigny C. Neuropeptide Y potentiates the N-methyl-D-aspartate response in the rat CA$_3$ dorsal hippocampus. II. Involvement of a subtype of sigma receptor. J Pharmac Exp Ther 1992;263:1219–1225

38. Monnet FP, Debonnel G, Bergeron R, Gronier B, De Montigny C. The effects of sigma ligands and of neuropeptide Y on N-methyl-D-aspartate-induced neuronal activation of CA3 dorsal hippocampus neurones are differentially affected by pertussin toxin. Br J Pharmacol 1994;112:709–715.

39. Monnet FP, Mahé V, Robel P, Baulieu E-E. Neurosteroids, via σ receptors, modulate the [^{3}H]norepinephrine release evoked by N-methyl-D-aspartate in the rat hippocampus. Proc Natl Acad Sci USA 1995;92:3774–3778.

40. Matsuno K., Matsunaga K. and Mita S. Increase of extracellular acetylcholine level in rat frontal cortex induced by (+)N-allylnormetazocine as measured by brain microdialysis. Brain Res 1992;575:315–319.

41. Matsuno K, Matsunaga K, Senda T, Mita S. Increase in extracellular acetylcholine level by sigma ligands in rat frontal cortex. J Pharmac Exp Ther 1993;265:851–859.

42. Patrick SL, Walker JM, Perkel JM, Lockwood M, Patrick RL. Increases in rat striatal extracellular dopamine and vacuous chewing produced by two sigma ligands. Eur J Pharmacol 1993;231:243–249.

43. Kobayashi T, Matsuno K, Nakata K, Mita S. Enhancement of acetylcholine release by SA4503, a novel σ$_1$ receptor agonist, in the rat brain. J Pharmac Exp Ther1996;279:106–113.

44. Quirion R, Bowen WD, Itzhak Y, Junien JL, Musacchio JM, Rothman RB, Su T-P, Tam SW, Taylor DP. A proposal for the classification of sigma binding sites. Trends Pharmac Sci 1992;13:85–86.

45. Keana JFW, McBurney RN, Scherz MW, Fischer JB, Hamilton PN, Smith SM, Server AC, Finkeiner S, Stevens CF, Jahr C, Weber E. Synthesis and characterization of a series of diarylguanidines that are noncompetitive N-methyl-D-aspartate receptor antagonists with neuroprotective properties. Proc Natl Acad Sci USA 1989;86:5631–5635.

46. Perregaard J, Moltzen EK, Meier E, Sanchez C, Hyttel J. 4-phenylpiperidines and -spiropiperidines with sub-nanomolar affinity for sigma binding sites and with potent anxiolytic activity. Soc Neurosci Abst 1993;19:1868.

47. Walker JM, Bowen WD, Patrick SL, Williams WE, Mascarella SW Bai X, Carroll FI. A comparison of (-)-deoxybenzomorphans devoid of opiate activity with their dextrorotatory phenolic counterparts suggests role of σ$_2$ receptors in motor function. Eur J Pharmacol 1993;231:61–68.

48. Chavkin C. The sigma enigma: biochemical and functional correlates emerge for the haloperidol-sensitive sigma binding site. Trends Neurosci 1990;11:213–215.

49. Kavanaugh MP, Tester BC, Scherz MW, Keana J.FW, Weber E. Identification of the binding subunit of the sigma-type opiate receptor by photoaffinity labeling with 1-(4-azido–2-methyl[6–^{3}H]phenyl)–3-(2-methyl[4,6–^{3}H]phenyl)guanidine. Proc Natl Acad Sci USA 1988;85:2844–2848.

50. Hellewell SB, Bowen WD. A sigma-like binding site in rat pheochromocytoma (PC12) cells: decreased affinity for (+)-benzomorphans and lower molecular weight suggest a different sigma receptor form from that guinea pig brain. Brain Res 1990;527:244–253.

51. Kahoun JR, Ruoho AE. (^{125}I)Iodoazidococaine, a photoaffinity label for the haloperidol-sensitive sigma receptor. Proc Natl Acad Sci USA 1992;89:1393–1397.

52. Schuster DI, Ehrlich GK, Murphy RB. Purification and partial amino acid sequence of a 28 kDa cyclophilin-like component of the rat liver sigma receptor. Life Sci 1994,55:151–156.

53. Hanner M, Moebius FF, Flandorfer A, Knaus HG, Striessnig J, Kemper E, Glossmann H. Purification, molecular cloning, and expression of the mammalian sigma$_1$-binding site. Proc Natl Acad Sci USA 1996;93:8072–8077.

54. Hanner M, Moebius FF, Weber F, Grabner M, Striessnig J, Glossmann H. Phenylalkylamine Ca^{2+} antagonist binding protein. Molecular cloning, tissue distribution, and heterogenous expression. J Biol Chem 1995;270:7551–7557.

55. Silve S, Dupuy PH, Labit-Lebouteiller C, Kaghad M, Chalon P, Rahier A, Taton M., Lupker J, Shire D, Loison G. Emopamil-binding protein, a mammalian protein that binds a series of structurally diverse neuroprotective agents, exhibits Δ8–Δ7 sterol isomerase activity in yeast. J Biol Chem 1996;271:22434–22440.

56. Moebius FF, Striessnig J, Glossmann H. The mysteries of sigma-receptors: new family members reveal a role in cholesterol synthesis. Trends Pharmacol Sci 1997;18:67–70.

58. Glämsta EL, Marklund A, Hellman U, Wernstedt C, Terenius L, Nyberg F. Isolation and characterization of a hemoglobin derived opioid peptide from the human pituitary gland. Reg Peptides 1991;34:169–179.

57. Su T-P, Weissman AD, Yeh SY. Endogenous ligands for sigma opioid receptors in the brain ("sigmaphin"): evidence from binding assays. Life Sci 1986;38:2199–2210.

59. Contreras PC, DiMaggio DA, O'Donohue TL. An endogenous ligand for the sigma opioid binding site. Synapse 1987;1:57–61.

60. Zhang AZ, Mitchell KN, Cook L, Tam SW. Human endogenous brain ligands for sigma and phencyclidine recepotrs. In: Domino EF, Kamenka, JM, eds. Sigma and Phencyclidine-like Compounds as Molecular Probes in Biology. NPP Books, Ann Arbor, MI, 1988, pp. 335–343.

61. Roman FJ, Martin B, Junien J-L. In vivo interaction of neuropeptide Y and peptide YY with sigma receptor sites in the mouse brain. Eur J Pharmacol 1993;242:305–307.

62. Quirion R, Mount H, Chaudieu I, Dumont Y, Boksa P. Neuropeptide Y, polypeptide YY, phencyclidine and sigma related agents: any relationships? In: Kameyama T, Nabeshima T, Domino EF, eds. NMDA Receptor Related Agents: Biochemistry, Pharmacology and Behavior. NPP Books, Ann Arbor, MI, 1991, pp. 203–210.

63. Tam SW, Mitchell KN. Neuropeptide Y and peptide YY do not bind to brain sigma and phencyclidine binding sites. Eur J Pharmacol 1991;193:121–122.

64. DeHaven-Hudkins DL, Fleissner LC, Ford-Rice FY. Characterization of the binding of [^{3}H]-(+)-pentazocine to sigma recognition sites in guinea pig brain. Eur J Pharmacol 1992;227:371–378.

65. Monnet FP, Fournier A, Debonnel G, De Montigny C. Neuropeptide Y potentiates selectively the N-methyl-D-aspartate response in the rat CA3 dorsal hippocampus. I. Involvement of an atypical neuropeptide Y receptor. J Pharmac Exp Ther 1992;263:1212–1218.

66. Bouchard P, Dumont Y, Fournier A, St.-Pierre S, Quirion R. Evidence for in vivo interactions between neuropeptide Y-related peptides and σ receptors in the mouse hippocampal formation. J Neurosci 1993;13:3926–3931.

67. Bouchard P, Roman F, Junien J-L, Quirion R. Autoradiographic evidence for the modulation of in vivo sigma receptor labeling by neuropeptide Y and calcitonin gene-related peptide in the mouse brain. J Pharmacol Exp Ther 1996;276:223–230.

68. Su TP, London ED, Jaffe JH. Steroid binding at σ receptors suggest a link between endocrine, nervous, and immune systems. Science 1988;240:219–221.

69. McCann DJ, Su TP. Solubilization and characterization of haloperidol-sensitive (+)-[^{3}H]-SKF–10,047 binding sites (sigma sites) from rat liver membranes. J Pharmac Exp Ther 1991;257:547.

70. Klein M, Musacchio JM. Effects of cytochrome P-450 ligands on the binding of [^{3}H] dextrometorphan and sigma ligands to guinea-pig brain. In: Itzhak Y, ed. Sigma Receptors. Academic, San Diego, CA, 1994, pp. 243–262.

71. Cagnotto A, Bastone A, Mennini T. [^{3}H](+)-pentazocine binding to rat brain σ$_1$ receptors. Eur J Pharmacol 1994;266:131–138.

72. McCann DJ, Weissman AD, Su T-P. Sigma–1 and Sigma–2 sites in rat brain: comparison of regional, ontogenic, and subcellular patterns. Synapse 1994;17:182–186.

73. Yamada M, Nishigami T, Nakasho K, Nishimoto Y, Miyaji H. Relationship between sigma-like site and progesterone-binding site of adult male rat liver microsomes Hepatology 1994;20: 1271–1280.

74. Ramamoorthy JD, Ramamoorthy S, Mahesh VB, Leibach FH, Ganapathy V. Cocaine-sensitive σ-receptor and its interaction with steroid hormones in the human placental syncytiotrophoblast and in choriocarcinoma cells. Endocrinology 1995;136:924–932.

75. Muldoon T.G. Role of receptors in the mechanism of steroid hormone action in the brain. In: Motta M, ed. The endocrine functions of the brain. Raven, New York, NY, 1980, pp. 51–93.

76. Yamamoto KR. Steroid receptor regulated transcription of specific genes and gene networks. Ann RevGenet 1985;19:209–252.

77. Schumacher M. Rapid membrane effects of steroid hormones: an emerging concept in neuroendocrinology. Trends Neurosci 1990;13:359–362.

78. Baulieu EE. Neurosteroids: a new function in the brain. Biol Cell 1991;71:3–10.

79. Paul SM, Purdy RH. Neuroactive steroids. FASEB 1992;J6:2311–2322.

80. Robel P, Baulieu EE. Neurosteroids: biosynthesis and function. Trends Endocrinol Metab 1994;5:1–8.

81. Wehling M. Nongenomic actions of steroid hormones. Trends Endocrinol Metab 1994;5:347–353.

82. Gee KW, McCauley L, Lan NC. A putative receptor for neurosteroids on the $GABA_A$ receptor complex: the pharmacological properties and therapeutic potential of epalons. Critical Rev. Neurobiology 1995;9:207–227.

83. Lambert JJ, Belelli D, Hill-Venning C, Peters JA. Neurosteroids and $GABA_A$ receptor function. Trends Pharmacol Sci 1995;16:295–303.

84. Irwin R.P, Lin SZ, Rogawski MA, Purdy RH Paul SM.(1994) Steroid potentiation and inhibition of N-Methyl-D-Aspartate receptor-mediated intracellular Ca^{++} responses: structure-activity studies. J Pharmac Exp Ther 271:677–682.

85. Park-Chung M, Wu FS, Farb DH. (1994) 3α-hydroxy–5β-pregnan–20-one sulfate: a negative modulator of the NMDA-induced current in cultured neurons. Mol Pharmacol 46:146–150.

86. Ffrench-Mullen JMH, Spence KT. 1991 Neurosteroids block Ca^{2+} channel current in freshly isolated hippocampal CA1 neurons. Eur JPharmacol 202:269–272.

87. Spence KT, Plata-Salaman CR, Ffrench-Mullen JMH. (1991) The neurosteroids pregnenolone and pregnenolone-sulfate but not progesterone, block Ca^{2+} currents in acutely isolated hippocampal CA1 neurons. Life Sci 49:PL235–PL239.

88. Wu F-S, Gibbs TT, Farb DH. Pregnenolone sulfate: a positive allosteric modulator at the N-methyl-D-aspartate receptor. Mol Pharmacol 1991,40:333–336.

89. Irwin RP, Maragakis NJ, Rogawski MA, Purdy RH, Farb DH, Paul SM. Pregnenolone sulfate augments NMDA receptor mediated increases in intracellular Ca^{2+} in cultured rat hippocampal neurons. Neurosci Lett 1992;141:30–34.

90. Bowlby Pregnenolone sulfate potentiation of N-Methyl-D-aspartate receptor channels in hippocampal neurons. Mol Pharmacol 1993;43:813–819.

91. Meyer JH, Gruol DL. Dehydroepiandrosterone sulfate alters synaptic potentials in area CA1 of the hippocampal slice. Brain Res 1994;633: 253–261.

92. Fahey JM, Lindquist DG, Pritchard GA, Miller L.G. Pregnenolone sulfate potentiation of NMDA-mediated increases in intracellular calcium in cultured chick cortical neurons. Brain Res 1995;669:183–188.

93. Bonnet KA, Brown RP. Cognitive effects of DHEA replacement therapy. In: Kalimi M, Regelson W, ed. The Biologic Role of DHEA. Walter de Gruyter, Berlin, 1990, pp. 65–79.

94. Wolkowitz OM, Reus VI, Manfredi F, Roberts E. Reply to F. Leblhuber: Antiglucocorticoid effects of DHEA-S in Alzheimer disease (letter). Am J Psychiatry 1992;149:1126.

95. Friess E, Trachsel L, Guldner J, Schier T, Steiger A, Holsboer F. DHEA administration increases rapid eye movement sleep and EEG power in the sigma frequency range. Am J Physiology 1995;268:E107–E113.

96. Roberts E, Bologa L, Flood JF, Smith GE. Effects of dehydroepiandrosterone and its sulfate on brain tissue in culture and on memory in mice. Brain Res 1987;406:357–362.

97. Flood JF, Roberts E. Dehydroepiandrosterone sulfate improves memory in aging mice. Brain Res 1988;448:178–181.

98. Flood JF, Smith GE, Roberts E. Dehydroepiandrosterone and its sulfate enhance memory retention in mice. Brain Res 1988;447:269–278.

99. Flood JF, Morley JE, Roberts E. Memory-enhancing effects in male mice of pregnenolone and steroids metabolically derived from it. Proc Natl Acad Sci USA 1992;89:1567–1571.

100. Flood JF, Morley JE, Roberts E. Pregnenolone sulfate enhances post-training memory processes when injected in very low doses into limbic system structures: The amygdala is by far the most sensitive. Proc Natl Acad Sci USA 1995;92:10806–10810.

101. Roof RL, Havens MD. Testosterone improves maze performance and induces development of a male hippocampus in females. Brain Res 1992;572:310–313.

102. Isaacson RL, Yoder PE, Varner JA. The effects of pregnenolone on acquisition and retention of a food search task. Behav Neural Biol 1994;61:170–176.

103. Isaacson RL, Varner JA, Baars JM, de Wield D. The effects of pregnenolone sulfate and ethylestrenol on retention of a passive avoidance task. Brain Res 1995;689:79–84.

104. Mathis C, Paul SM, Crawley JN. The neurosteroid pregnenolone sulfate blocks NMDA antagonist-induced deficits in a passive avoidance memory task. Psychopharmacology 1994;116:201–206.

105. Cheney DL, Uzunov D, Guidotti A. Pregnenolone sulfate antagonizes dizocilpine amnesia: role for allopregnanolone. Neuroreport 1995;6:1697–1700.

106. Frye CA, Sturgis JD. Neurosteroids affect spacial reference working and long term memory of female rats. Neurobiol Learn Memory 1995;64:83–96.

107. Vallee M, Mayo W, Darnaudéry M, Corpechot C, Young J, Koehl, LeMoal M, Baulieu EE. Cognitive performance in aged rats is linked with the concentration of pregnenolone sulfate in the hippocampus. In: Function and Dysfunction in the Nervous System, Symposium on Quantitative Biology. LXI Cold Spring Harbor, Cold Spring Harbor Laboratory Press, Cold Spring Harbor, NY, 1995.

108. Debonnel G, Bergeron R, de Montigny C. Potentiation by dehydroepiandrosterone of the neuronal response to N-methyl-D-aspartate in the CA_3 region of the rat dorsal hippocampus: an effect mediated via sigma receptors. J Endocrinology 1996;71:977–987.

109. Debonnel G, Bergeron R, Monnet FP, de Montigny C. Differential effects of sigma ligands on the NMDA response in the CA_1 and CA_3 regions of dorsal hippocampus : effect of mossy fiber lesioning. Neuroscience 1997, in press.

110. Bergeron R, de Montigny C, Debonnel G. Potentiation of neuronal NMDA response by dehydro-epiandrosterone and its suppression by progesterone: an effect mediated via sigma receptors. J Neurosci 1996;16:1193–1202.

111. Corpéchot C, Robel P, Axelson M, Sjövall J, Baulieu EE. Characterization and measurement of dehydroepiandrosterone sulfate in rat brain. Proc Natl Acad Sci USA 1981;78:4704–4707.

112. Akwa Y, Young J, Kabbadj K, Sancho MJ, Zucman D, Vourc'h C, Jung-Testas I, Hu ZY, Le Goascogne C, Jo DH, Corpéchot C, Simon P, Baulieu EE, Robel P. Neurosteroids: biosynthesis, metabolism and function of pregnenolone and dehydroepiandrosterone in the brain. J Steroid Bio Chem Molec Biol 1991;40:71–81.

113. Lanthier A, Patwardhan VV. Sex steroids and 5-en–3β-hydroxysteroids in specific regions of the human brain and cranial nerves. J Steroid BioChem 1986;25:445–449.

114. Lacroix C, Fiet J, Benais JP, Gueux B, Bonete R, Villette JM, Gourmel B, Dreux C. Simultaneous radioimmunoassay of progesterone, and rost–4-enedione, pregnenolone, dehydroepiandrosterone and 17-hydroxyprogesterone in specific regions of human brain. J Steroid Biochem 1987;28:317–325.

115. Baulieu EE. Dehydroepiandrosterone (DHEA): a fountain of youth? J Clin Endocrinol Metab 1996;81:3147–3151.

116. Rajkowski K, Robel P, Baulieu EE. Hydroxysteroid sulfotransferase activity in the rat brain and liver as a function of age and sex. Steroids 1997, in press.

117. Baulieu E-E, Robel P. Dehydroepiandrosterone and dehydroepiandrosterone sulfate as neuroactive neurosteroids. J Endocrinol 1996;150:S221-S239.

118. Heap RB, Deanesly R. Progesterone in systemic blood and placentae of intact and ovariectomized pregnant guinea-pigs. J Endocrinol 1966;34:417–423.

119. Challis JRG, Heap RB, Illingworth D. Concentrations of estrogen and progesterone in the plasma of non-pregnant, pregnant and lactating guinea-pigs. J Endocrinol 1971;51:333–345.

120. Smith MS, Freeman ME, Neill JD. The control of progesterone secretion during the estrous cycle and early pseudopregnancy in the rat: prolactin, gonadotropin and steroid levels associated with rescue of the corpus luteum of pseudopregnancy. Endocrinology 1975;96:219–226.

121. Schwarz S, Pohl P, Zhou GZ. Steroid binding at σ-"opioid" receptors. Science 1989;246:1635–1637.

122. Weindenfeld J, Siegel RA, Chomers I. In vitro conversion of pregnenolone to progesterone by discrete areas of the male rat. J Steroid Bio Chem 1980;13:961–963.

123. Robel P, Bourreau E, Corpéchot C, Dang DC, Halberg F, Clarke C, Haug M, Schlegel ML, Synguelakis M, Vourcíh C, Baulieu E-E. Neurosteroids: 3β-hydroxy-Δ5-derivatives in rat and monkey brain. J Steroid Bio Chem 1987;27:649–655.

124. Robel P, Akwa Y, Corpéchot C, Hu ZY, Jung-Testas I, Kabbadj K, Le Goascogne C, Morfin R, Vourcíh C, Young J, Baulieu E-E. Neurosteroids: biosynthesis and function of pregnenolone and dehydroepiandrosterone in the brain. In: Motta M, ed. Brain Endocrinology. Raven, New York, NY, 1991, pp. 105–131.

125. Yamaji T, Ibayashi H. Plasma dehydroepiandrosterone sulfate in normal and pathological conditions. J Clin Endocrinol,1969;29:273–278.

126. De Peretti E, Forest MG. Pattern of plasma dehydroepiandrosterone sulfate levels in humans from birth to adulthood: evidence for testicular production. J Clin Endocrinol Metab 1978;47:572–577.

127. Corpéchot C, Synguelakis M, Talha S, Axelson M, Sjövall J, Vihko R, Baulieu E-E, Robel P. Pregnenolone and its sulfate ester in the rat brain. Brain Res 1983;270:119–125.

128. Robel P, Corpéchot C, Synguelakis M, Groyer A, Clarke C, Schlegel ML, Brazeau P, and Baulieu E-E. Pregnenolone, dehydroepiandrosterone, and their sulfate esters in rat brain. In: Celotti GF, et al., ed. Metabolism of Hormonal Steroids in the Neuroendocrine Structures. Raven, New York, NY, 1984, pp. 185–194.

129. Lanthier A, Patwardhan VV. Effect of heterosexual olfactory and visual stimulation on 5-en–3β-hydroxysteroids and progesterone in the male rat brain. J Steroid BioChem 1987;28:697–701.

130. Orentreich N, Brind JL, Vogelman JH, Andres R, Baldwin H. Long-term longitudinal measurements of plasma dehydroepiandrosterone sulfate in normal men. J Clin Endocrinol Metab 1992;75:1002–1004.

131. Baulieu EE, Robel P. Neurosteroids: a new brain function? J Steroid Bio Chem Mol Biol 1990;37:395–403.

132. Riva MA, Creese I. Effect of chronic administration of dopamine receptor antagonists on D_1 and D_2 dopamine receptors and σ/haloperidol binding sites in rat brain. Mol Neuro Pharmacol 1990;1:17–22.

133. Jansen KLR, Elliot M, Leslie RA. Sigma receptors in rat brain and testes show similar reductions in response to chronic haloperidol. Eur J Pharmacol 1992;214:281–283.

134. Maayani S, Weinstein H. "Specific binding" of ^{3}H-phencyclidine: artifacts of the rapid filtration method. Life Sci 1980;26:2011–2022.

135. Snyder SH. Phencyclidine. Nature 1980;285:355–356.

12

Steroid Modulation of the Nicotinic Acetylcholine Receptor

Bruno Buisson, MD, and Daniel Bertrand, MD

CONTENTS

INTRODUCTION
LIGAND-GATED CHANNELS
STEROID INHIBITION OF THE NEURONAL nAChRs
ACTIVE STEROIDS
STEROID MODE OF ACTION
ALLOSTERIC MODULATION OF LIGAND-GATED CHANNELS
CONCLUSIONS
REFERENCES

INTRODUCTION

Steroid hormones can be divided into five classes: progestins, estrogens, androgens, glucocorticosteroids, and mineralocorticosteroids. The principal site of synthesis are the corpus luteum and the placenta for the progestatifs, the ovary or testes for the estrogens or androgens, and the adrenal glands for the glucocorticosteroids and mineralocorticosteroids. Until rather recently, it was thought that steroid hormones were synthesized exclusively in peripheral tissues, as previously mentioned. Some evidence has, however, demonstrated that steroids are also synthesized in the nervous system *(1–3)*. An important part of the interest in these neurosteroids comes from the fact that their synthesis is independent of the endocrine glands, suggesting that they may represent key modulators of neuronal activities.

Although direct correlations between steroid concentrations and psychological status are not readily established, it is generally accepted that modifications can occur in response to hormonal levels. The mood alterations that take place in women during the ovarian cycle or at menopause can lead to the simple hypothesis that some brain functions may be modulated by sex hormones. Moreover, clinical profiles such as premenstrual syndrome or postpartum depression reinforce the notion that abrupt changes in the levels of sex hormones can be linked with psychological disorders *(4)*. The first experimental evidence of the action of steroid hormones on brain activity was provided in the late 1950s

From: *Contemporary Endocrinology: Neurosteroids: A New Regulatory Function in the Nervous System* Edited by: E.-E. Baulieu, P. Robel, and M. Schumacher
© Humana Press Inc., Totowa, NJ

by the work of Kawakami and Sawyer *(5)*, who observed that thresholds for electroencephalogram (EEG) arousal and for the induction of "paradoxical sleep" in rabbits were influenced by estrogens. Electrophysiological experiments providing an initial demonstration of the action of steroids on neuronal activities were carried out by Lincoln and Cross *(6,7)*. Using electrodes implanted into rat brains, they observed a modification of neuronal activity in the hypothalamus, septum and preoptic area following estrogen administration *(6,7)*. Such observations were later confirmed by other investigators *(8,9)*. More recently, extracellular and/or intracellular recordings from hippocampus slices have demonstrated a direct effect of estrogens, androgens, and corticosteroids on synaptic transmission *(10–12)*. In parallel, numerous histological studies reported that steroids are able to promote and/or modulate dendritic length *(13)*, as well as dendritic spine density *(14–16)*. A decisive step for elucidating the molecular effect of steroids in the brain was achieved by Majewska *(17)*, Harrison *(18)*, and colleagues who showed that steroids modulate the $GABA_A$ receptor ($GABA_A$R) located in the outer membranes of some nerve cells and induce a potentiation of the GABA-evoked currents. Following these crucial observations, numerous studies have dissected the multiple interactions of steroids with the ionotropic $GABA_A$R, which belong to the superfamily of ligand-gated channels *(19–21)*.

LIGAND-GATED CHANNELS

Ligand-gated channels (LGCs) are integral membrane proteins specialized in the transduction of neurotransmitter flux into electrical signal. Upon agonist binding, LGCs undergo fast conformational transitions which, as demonstrated by patch-clamp recordings, must be in the sub-millisecond time scale *(22)*. When observed at the whole cell level, LGCs response times are slowed down to a few milliseconds owing to neurotransmitter diffusion, integration of the activity occurring over thousands of receptors, and the cell time constant. Typical postsynaptic currents can be as large as a several hundred picoamperes and firing of the action potential by the postsynaptic cell depends on summation of many excitatory and/or inhibitory presynaptic signals. It is worth recalling that a neuron can receive as many as 50,000 synaptic endings. The amplitude as well as the timing of each synaptic event can thus become critical. Potentiation or inhibition of a family of LGCs by a diffusible messenger can profoundly modify the activity of neurons and as a result the information processing of the neuronal networks in which they participate.

Following the initial work carried out on the acetylcholine receptor *(23–25)*, a large number of LGCs have been identified as transmembrane proteins resulting from the assembly of different subunits. In each family, various isoforms (or subtypes) of the receptors have been identified and it has been shown that the different subunits can assemble and form a wide diversity of hetero-oligomers. These receptors display distinct pharmacological profiles with a high specificity for agonists, antagonists, and kinetic responses *(26,27)*. Some of the subunit DNA sequences have been cloned. The currently accepted tertiary structure of a LGC subunit *(24,25,28,29)* assumes that a large hydrophilic segment faces the synaptic cleft and comprises the neurotransmitter binding site. Two to four hydrophobic segments, depending on the receptor type, have been identified as transmembrane-spanning domains. One of them appears to line the ionic pore. Some of the intracellular loops can display sites of regulation by phosphorylation/dephospho-

Side View   Top View

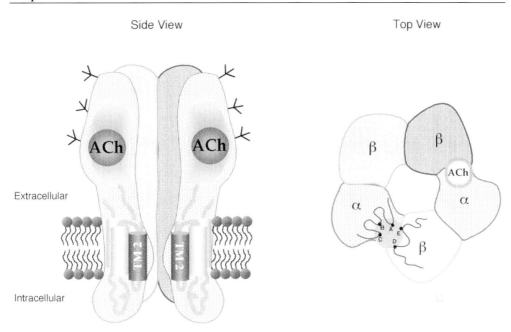

Fig. 1. Schematic representation of the structure of the nAChR. The left panel represents the transmembrane organization of the protein. The ligand-binding site (here ACh) and protein segments spanning the membrane are represented by filled structures. The second transmembrane segments (TM2), which border the aqueous ionic pore, are symbolized by the dark cylinders. The right panel represents the pentameric disposition of a nAChR with two α and three β subunits. Main and complementary parts, or residues, of the ACh-binding site are symbolized **(A–E)**.

rylation mechanisms *(30–33)*. Many features of the tertiary and quaternary structures of the *Torpedo* nicotinic acetylcholine receptor (nAChR) were studied by electron microscopy at 9 Å resolution (34,35), and similar features are thought to be present in neuronal nAChRs and other LGCs such as $GABA_A$ *(36)*, glycine *(37,38)* or serotonin $5HT_3$ receptors *(39)*. The four transmembrane segment scheme illustrated in Fig. 1 represents the currently accepted tertiary structure of the nAChRs and other members of this ionotropic receptors family.

The nAChR is currently the best characterized LGC. Up to the present time, 11 genes coding for putative subunits of the neuronal nAChR have been identified in vertebrates *(24,25,40–44)*, whereas fewer closely related genes have been identified in invertebrates *(25,45,46)*. Sequence analysis of the proteins suggest that all of these subunits derive from a common ancestor molecule by gene duplication and progressive spontaneous mutagenesis *(25,47)*.

Compelling biochemical and electrophysiological evidences suggest that neuronal nAChRs result, as for the muscle receptor, from the assembly of five subunits, which are arranged with an axial pseudosymetry *(29,34,48,49)*. Although single subunit genes (α7–α9) yield functional receptors when expressed in *Xenopus* oocytes or cell lines *(50–55)*, all of the other subunits must co-assemble and produce functional nAChRs only when expressed under adequate combinations of at least two subunits, one α and one β *(25,56)*. It is worth noting that the homomeric forms of nAChRs ($\alpha7$–$\alpha9$) are highly sensitive to the snake toxin α-bungarotoxin (α-Bgt) as is the muscle receptor.

Recent experiments combining molecular biology with both biochemistry and electrophysiology have brought new insights into the acetylcholine (ACh) binding domain. One conclusion of these experiments is that the ACh-binding site lies at the interface between two adjacent subunits (25,57–60). The main component is formed by the α subunit while the complementary component being contributed by the adjacent subunit, which is either a non-α or another segment of an α subunit, as in the case of the homomeric nAChRs.

STEROID INHIBITION OF THE NEURONAL nACHRs

As previously described, it has been firmly established that the activity of the inhibitory GABA$_A$R is modulated by steroids, which exert a fast potentiation of this family of receptors. Comparable studies of native or reconstituted neuronal nAChRs have shown that steroids also modulate the activity of this member of the LGC superfamily. Electrophysiological recordings have illustrated that steroid action leads to a fast and reversible inhibition of the ACh-evoked currents (61–64). Because these studies were carried out on preparations that are known to express different nicotinic subtypes, it can be concluded that steroid inhibition of nAChRs is likely to be an ubiquitous mechanism for this family of LGCs.

Although diverse protocols can be employed to reveal such modulation, one of the most direct experimental paradigms consists of exposing the nAChRs to a steady concentration of ACh and, when the current is stabilized, adding onto it a short pulse of steroid (Fig. 2A). This method offers the advantage of allowing the determination of both the time course of inhibition and recovery, as well as the sensitivity of the receptor for a defined steroid. Studies of chick neuronal nAChRs reconstituted with the major brain subunits $\alpha4\beta2$ have demonstrated that these receptors are inhibited by low concentrations of progesterone (PROG) and display an IC$_{50}$ of about 6 μM with an empirical Hill coefficient close to unity (64). The low empirical Hill coefficient was reported for all tested compounds and can be interpreted by the absence of cooperativity in the process of steroid inhibition. In addition, these experiments illustrate that the time course of inhibition is fast and reaches a steady state within a few seconds. Full recovery of this inhibition is observed within the same time frame (63,64).

The recent isolation and cloning of the human genes encoding for neuronal nAChRs, which correspond to the $\alpha4$, $\beta2$, and $\alpha7$ subunits, opens new possibilities for investigating the role of steroids on these receptors (29,65,66). Moreover, it was also shown that these subunits can be successfully reconstituted in *Xenopus* oocytes or transfected into cell lines (29,55,67). New experiments were thus designed to address the mode of action of steroids on these receptors. PROG effects on human $\alpha4\beta2$ nAChR were first investigated using the coapplication protocols (Fig. 2A) and it was found that, as for the chick receptor, steroid exposure induces a fast and reversible inhibition of the ACh-evoked current. Plots of the current inhibition as a function of the logarithm of the PROG concentration reveal that the current is reduced by half for a concentration of PROG of about 4.75 ± 2.3 μM ($n = 4$, [ACh] test pulse = 0.3 μM). As expected from previous studies (64), increasing the agonist concentration by 10-fold induces no significant shift of the apparent inhibition.

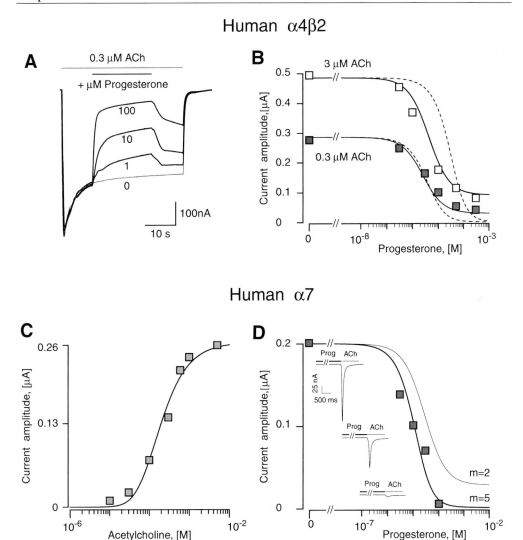

Fig. 2. Human neuronal nAChRs are inhibited by progesterone in the μM range. (**A**) Typical protocol of steroid application on human α4β2 nAChR reconstituted in *Xenopus* oocytes. Exposure of the receptor to a low ACh concentration elicits a steady current. Coapplications of progesterone at three different concentrations induce a fast reduction of the ACh-evoked current. Timing of the applications are symbolized by the bars. The cell was held throughout the experiment at –100 mV. (**B**) Dose-response inhibition of the human α4β2 nAChR for two ACh concentrations. Currents measured as in (A) are plotted as a function of the progesterone concentration. Continuous thick lines are best fits obtained for an allosteric model with respective values $L = 32$, $K_a = 0.041 \; 10^{-6} \, M$, $K_b = 0.394 \; 10^{-6} \, M$, $n = 2$ and $K_a' = 3.9 \; 10^{-6} \, M$, $K_b' = 0.35 \; 10^{-6} \, M$, $m = 2$ (Eq. 1 in Fig. 5). Thin dashed lines correspond to prediction made for a competitive inhibitor *(81)*. (**C**) ACh dose-response of the human α7 nAChR expressed in a *Xenopus* oocytes. (**D**) Progesterone dose-response inhibition curve determined using prepulses. The experimental paradigm is illustrated by the traces presented in the inset. Peak inward currents are plotted as a function of the logarithm of the progesterone concentration. The thick continuous curve is the best fit obtained for an negative allosteric inhibitor using five equivalent binding sites *(81)*. The dashed line was obtained using the same equation and same parameters $L = 10^{6}$, $K_a = 3 \; 10^{-6} \, M$, $K_b = 28.3 \; 10^{-6} \, M$, $n = 5$ and $K_a' = 2.7 \; 10^{-6} \, M$, $K_b' = 0.024 \; 10^{-6} \, M$, $m = 5$ (Eq. 1 in Fig. 5) but with only two binding sites ($m = 2$). All data were recorded at –100 mV in Ba^{2+}-containing medium to minimize contamination by calcium-activated chloride currents *(95)*.

Given the very fast desensitization of receptor reconstituted with the α7 subunit *(29,51,55)*, the experimental protocol employed for the α4β2 nAChR cannot be adapted to determine a possible effect of the steroids on the α7 homomeric nAChR. The experimental design that was retained to explore steroid, effects on this class of receptor is to apply, for a brief time, a prepulse of steroid, which is then followed by a test pulse of ACh. Experiments carried out under these conditions reveal that PROG also inhibits the ACh-evoked current of the human α7 receptor with a half-inhibition concentration at about 12 μ*M*. As distinct from the α4β2 nAchR, the α7 nAChR exhibits a steeper PROG dose-response inhibition curve and ACh-evoked currents are more strongly suppressed by 100 μ*M* progesterone. These receptor subtypes differences cannot be attributed to the specific experimental protocols used.

ACTIVE STEROIDS

Determination of the inhibition dose-response profile of the chick α4β2 nAChR reconstituted in *Xenopus* oocytes yielded a distinct sensitivity profile as a function of the steroid tested. PROG is the most powerful steroid. Half-inhibition concentrations were, respectively, 6 μ*M* for PROG, 46 μ*M* for testosterone (T) and 62 μ*M* for the synthetic steroid dexamethasone. Exposure to cholesterol, pregnenolone (PREG), or allo-pregnanolone (3α-hydroxy-5α-pregnan-20-one) induced no significant reduction of the ACh-evoked currents *(68)*. Comparison of steroids effective on nAChR and GABA$_A$R reveals a clear difference in the pharmacological profile of these two families of receptors. For example neuronal nAChRs are insensitive to pregnenolone sulfate (PREGS), whereas this compound is a potent modulator of the GABA$_A$Rs *(69,70)*.

In addition, it was shown that PROG coupled to bovine serum albumin (BSA) in position 3 (P-3-BSA) or position 11 (P-11-BSA) was as efficient as unmodified PROG. Thus, addition of a molecule as large as BSA in positions 3 or 11 of the molecule had no detectable influence on its biophysiological action, which suggests that PROG is interacting in the extracellular domain of the receptor.

Results obtained with ion flux assays on cell lines expressing nAChRs show pharmacological profiles comparable to those obtained by electrophysiological measurements *(71)*. Namely, rubidium efflux assays of TE671/RD cells, which express muscle nAChR, or SH-SY5Y cells, which are known to express ganglionic nAChR are inhibited by low concentrations of steroids. These cells display an IC$_{50}$ of 6.1 and 11 μ*M*, respectively for PROG. In agreement with results obtained for the chick α4β2, higher values of IC$_{50}$ were found for dexamethasone or T (45 and 100 μ*M*) on cells expressing α3β4. Incubation with P-3-BSA induced a slightly larger inhibition of the ^{86}Rb$^+$ efflux than PROG itself *(71)*. Corticosterone induced a small but significant reduction of cation flux with an IC$_{50}$ in the 100 μ*M* range (71).

It is interesting to note that all data available so far suggest that steroids predominant in females are more active than those found in males and, in turn, might lead to more profound modulation of the neuronal nAChRs under physiological conditions. These fundamental observations, however, still await clinical confirmation.

STEROID MODE OF ACTION

Inhibition by steroids of neuronal nAChRs can occur through several mechanisms illustrated in Fig. 3, which we shall review briefly. Namely, inhibition can be produced either by:

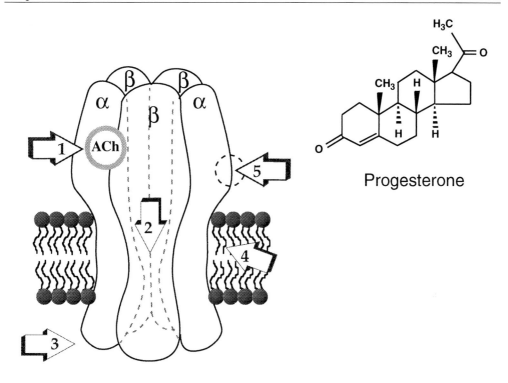

Progesterone

Fig. 3. Possible sites of steroid action. Each arrow symbolizes a possible site where steroids could act on the nAChR and correspond respectively to: 1. ACh-binding site with competitive inhibition, 2. the ionic pore with open channel blockade, 3. phosphorylation sites on the cytoplasmic loops, 4. lipid protein interaction, and 5. putative allosteric sites.

1. A competitive interaction with the natural ligand;
2. A block of the ionic pore (also referred to as open channel blocker: OCB);
3. activation of intracellular second messengers and protein phosphorylation/ dephosphorylation;
4. A partition of the steroid in the membrane lipid environment; and
5. Specific binding of the steroid on the LGC and induction of an allosteric interaction.

Studies designed to elucidate the steroid mode of action clearly demonstrate that active compounds such as PROG do not act as competitive inhibitors *(63,64)*, nor as open channel blockers. In support of this conclusion, it was recently observed on cell lines expressing muscle or neuronal nAChRs that steroid incubation does not alter agonist or toxin binding *(71)*. Furthermore, it was also found that increasing the agonist concentration failed to relieve PROG inhibition, which is another indication that steroids do not act by competition with the natural ligand *(71)*.

Absence of channel blockade was illustrated by the voltage-independence of the inhibition and by determination of the single-channel events in small patches of membrane *(63,64)*. Single-channel measurements can readily be obtained using the method of patch-clamp *(22)*, and excision with a pipet of a small membrane area allows observation of opening and closing of one or a few nAChRs contained in this membrane patch. Typical recordings of single-channel activity, such as those illustrated in Fig. 4, made on membrane patches excised from dissociated quail ciliary ganglion neurons, permitted

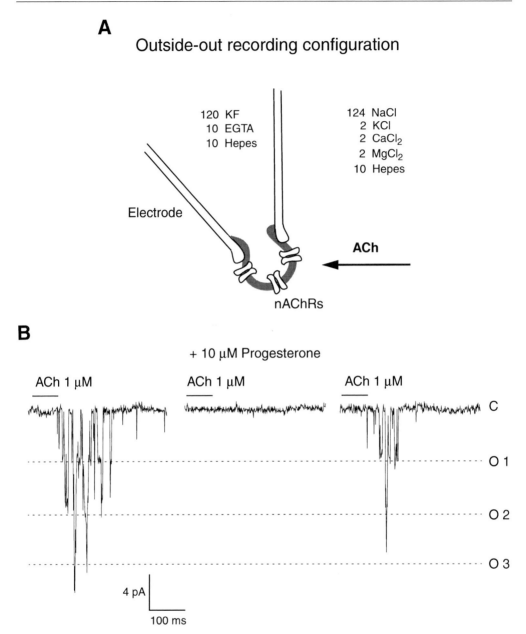

Fig. 4. Progesterone inhibition of single-channels in an outside-out patch. (**A**) Schematic diagram of the experimental procedure used to examine ACh-evoked single channel activity. The media compositions are indicated in mM. (**B**) Application of brief ACh pulses (1 μ*M*) evokes single-channel activity in a membrane patch excised from a ciliary ganglion neuron. Left trace was obtained in control condition, middle trace during progesterone perfusion (10 μ*M*, 55 s), and right trace during recovery (after 45 s of wash). "Open" or "closed" state of the nAChR are indicated by the label on the right. O_1, O_2, and O_3 correspond to the current amplitude relative to the opening of 1, 2, or 3 channels, respectively.

measurements of the amplitude of discrete events activated by short pulses of ACh. Upon exposure to steroids, single-channel activity was profoundly decreased and a progressive recovery was readily observed when returning to the control conditions. Traces illustrated in Fig. 4 show that single-channel amplitudes remained unchanged by these experimental conditions, whereas the mean open-time of nAChRs is decreased.

Two important conclusions were made from these experiments: 1. steroid inhibition cannot be attributed to a reduction of the single channel conductance, and 2. steroid inhibition can take place even in the absence of the cytoplasmic machinery.

Steroids are lipophilic compounds that are known to diffuse through the cellular membrane and induce their action on gene expression by binding to receptors which are then translocated into the nucleus. Thus, addition of steroids in the extracellular medium in the low micromolar concentration range is expected to induce a partition of these molecules within the receptor-lipid environment in the cytoplasmic membrane. In addition, it has been a well-documented that cholesterol plays an important role in the stabilization of integral proteins such as LGCs and that a single muscular receptor can interact with as many as 5–10 cholesterol molecules *(72)*. Thus, it could be expected that steroids act by perturbing the receptor environment. In favor if this hypothesis are recent studies using fluorescent probes and single-channel measurements, revealing that properties of both muscular and neuronal nAChRs depend on their lipid environment *(73)*. Two factors demonstrate, however, that PROG inhibition of the neuronal nAChRs is not mediated by a membrane alteration. First, the inhibition is steroid-specific and addition of cholesterol, even at high doses, does not mimic the PROG inhibition *(63,64)*. Second, PROG coupled with BSA (which is water-soluble and cannot diffuse into the membrane) induces similar or larger effects than free PROG *(64,71)*. Thus, although membrane partitioning of the steroids should occur, it seems unlikely that these modifications could significantly alter the receptor properties, and it was previously concluded that steroids should act as negative allosteric modulators *(63,64)*. A similar conclusion was more recently reached from biochemical and ion-flux assay experiments *(71)*.

ALLOSTERIC MODULATION OF LIGAND-GATED CHANNELS

The first allosteric models, originally proposed to describe enzymatic reactions *(74,75)*, were quickly recognized for their relevance and possible applications to other heteromeric proteins, such as LGCs *(76)*. An important extension to ligand-gated receptors with the introduction of the concept of desensitization was deduced from a series of experiments designed to resolve the receptor kinetics *(77–79)*. It was concluded from these studies that a four-state model was sufficient to describe most of the features of the muscular nAChR (Fig. 5A) *(80)*. The main relevance of such models concerns their capacity to predict the effects induced by different compounds. Any drug that stabilizes the active state (A) will promote a physiological response, whereas compounds that stabilize the (R) or (D) state will reduce the response amplitude that can be evoked by agonist. Another distinction that can be derived from this model is the difference between competitive inhibitors and negative allosteric effectors. Predictions made for competitive inhibitors are that for high concentrations of the inhibitor, the current is reduced to zero and that increase of the agonist concentration removes the inhibition *(81)*. Furthermore, the partial inhibition is consistent with an allosteric mechanism but not with a competitive mechanism or with an open-channel blockade. Negative allosteric effectors do not necessarily abolish the agonist-evoked current, but the inhibition might level off even for very high concentrations of the effector.

Examination of the human $\alpha4\beta2$ PROG dose-response curve reveals that a strong reduction of the ACh-evoked current is observed for low concentrations of PROG, but that even at its highest concentration, this steroid fails to abolish the response to agonists (Fig. 2B). Best fits obtained either with a negative allosteric effector (thick lines) or a competitive inhibitor (dashed lines) clearly illustrate the differences in prediction between these two modes of action. In addition, the effects of a competitive inhibitor should be reduced when the agonist concentration is increased. Comparison of the inhibition obtained at two ACh concentrations differing by 10-fold further illustrates that PROG does not act as a competitive inhibitor of the human neuronal nAChR but rather as a negative allosteric effector at both concentrations. The best fits were obtained with the allosteric model using two sites for the effector.

When comparable experiments are performed with the homomeric human $\alpha7$ receptor, a distinct pattern of inhibition is observed (Fig. 2D). In contrast to the inhibition observed for $\alpha4\beta2$, the $\alpha7$ nAChR is almost fully inhibited by $100 \mu M$ progesterone. The $\alpha7$ dose-response inhibition is also characterized by a steeper slope of the curve (larger apparent Hill coefficient). Fits of this inhibition curve using the allosteric coefficient obtained from the $\alpha7$ dose-response curve (Fig. 2C) reveal that data are adequately described using a value of five for the number of putative effector binding sites (thick line). The power of five, which corresponds to the number of negative effector sites, is necessary for the description of both the curve steepness and the amount of inhibition observed for high PROG concentrations. Results of computations corresponding to identical coefficients but using only a power of two are significantly different from the observed inhibition (thin line in Fig. 2D). Previous analysis of the properties of the $\alpha7$ nAChR have revealed that this homomeric receptor must result from the assembly of five subunits *(48,49,53)*. Thus, it is tempting to conclude that each of the $\alpha7$ nAChR subunits possibly displays one binding site for PROG, which, as for the ACh-binding site, might lay at the interface between the α and its adjacent subunit.

Using the same allosteric model, predictions can also be made for positive allosteric effectors that promote the stabilization of the active (open) state. Interestingly, neuronal nAChRs are modulated by the extracellular calcium and, from the analysis of the dose-response curves recorded at different calcium concentrations, it can be shown that this divalent cation exerts a positive allosteric modulation of the neuronal nAChRs. Namely, addition of calcium in the extracellular medium induces a shift to the left of the dose-response curve, which is accompanied by an increase of the Hill coefficient together with an augmentation of the current evoked at saturating ACh concentrations *(82–86)*. These three observations are in perfect agreement with the predictions made on the basis of allosteric modeling as shown quantitatively by Edelstein et al. *(87)*.

Simulations computed using the allosteric model are presented in Fig. 5. The effects of a fixed concentration of positive or negative allosteric effector on the agonist-dose response profiles are illustrated in Fig. 5B. Figure 5C illustrates the dose-response profiles of a positive or negative allosteric effector at a fixed concentration of agonist. Simulations obtained with either two or five binding sites for the effectors show the difference in the steepness of the dose-response profiles and the lack of complete inhibition ($m = 2$).

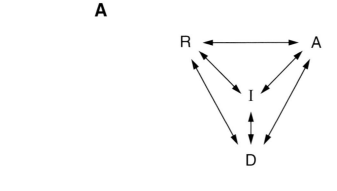

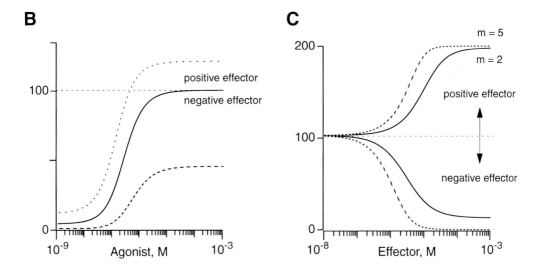

Fig. 5. Allosteric model and theoretical prediction. (**A**) Schematic diagram illustrating the four-state allosteric model developed for the neuromuscular junction *(79)* with: R, resting state, A, active state, I, inactive state and D, desensitized state. The only open state is A. (**B**) Simulation of the agonist dose-response curve. The fraction of the receptor in the open state was computed using Eq. 1 (*see* below) *(75)*. Dashed lines represent the effects induced by the presence of a fixed concentration of positive or negative allosteric effector. (**C**) Simulation of the dose-response curve of an allosteric effector. Values were computed using Eq. 1, but with a fixed concentration of agonist and several effector concentrations. Simulation of the effects of a positive or negative effector are represented. Continuous lines illustrate the results obtained assuming two binding sites for the effector, and dashed lines are the results predicted for five sites.

$$\bar{A} = \cfrac{1}{1 + L \cdot \left(\cfrac{1 + [ACh]/K_b}{1 + [ACh]/K_a}\right)^n \cdot \left(\cfrac{1 + [P]/K_b'}{1 + [P]/K_a'}\right)^m} \tag{1}$$

where: $\bar{A}$, the fraction of receptors in the open state; L = the equilibrium constant in absence of an agonist; K_a, K_b, K_a', and K_b' = the respective microscopic dissociation constants for the agonist and allosteric effector, and [ACh] = the agonist concentration and [P] = the effector concentration. Constants n and m correspond to the number of allosteric sites for the ligand and the effector, respectively.

CONCLUSIONS

Ligand-gated channels represent highly specialized transducer molecules allowing transmission of electrical activities across neuronal membranes. These integral membrane proteins are encoded by a wide family of genes and they share important homologies both in terms of their structural organization as well as their physiological and/or pharmacological properties. LGCs are present in the postsynaptic membrane of cells that receive 1. only one kind of input (single synaptic contact) or 2. several different inputs (multisynaptic connections). A typical example of a single synaptic contact is illustrated by the neuromuscular junction (NMJ). Because it is determinant for the organism that this type of synapse provides a constant transmission, NMJ nAChRs are weakly sensitive to common modulation mechanisms such as phosphorylation *(88,89)*. Critical conditions, such as those encountered in diseases, however, can reveal an increased sensitivity of these receptors to extracellular signals. A clear example is given by the autoimmune disease myasthenia gravis, where antibodies drastically interfere with the functioning of muscle nAChRs *(90)*.

In contrast, signal processing in the brain strongly depends on a multisynaptic organization and on electrical or biochemical interactions between neurons and receptors. Up to now, the most thoroughly studied mechanisms are long-term potentiation (LTP) and long-term depression (LTD), that were proposed to play important roles in the molecular memorization of synaptic events in the hippocampus and other brain areas *(91–93)*. LTP or LTD can be induced at a group of identical glutamatergic synapses. Very schematically, both processes involve activation of the NMDA receptor, calcium entry, and phosphorylation mechanisms; however, LTP is induced by a high-frequency protocol of stimulation whereas LTD is produced by a low-frequency protocol *(92)*. This mechanism illustrates the very high plasticity of brain synapses, even at the level of a single type of neurotransmitter (glutamate). Thus, for synaptic transmission in the brain a "modulable transmission" is at least as important as a "fixed wiring." It is well known that compounds applied systemically can influence animal behavior, and, for instance, relieve stress or anxiety, as shown by the effects of benzodiazepines. Studies of their mode of action have revealed that low doses of those compounds can potentiate the $GABA_A$Rs. Similarly, it was observed that steroids at physiological concentrations (nM to mM range) can also potentiate the $GABA_A$Rs *(18,19)*.

Studies of the steroid effects on neuronal nAChRs carried out in several laboratories with different preparations have revealed, however, that members of this family of LGCs are inhibited by PROG rather than being potentiated as in the case of the $GABA_A$Rs *(61–64,71)*. Furthermore, as previously illustrated, inhibition of the ACh-evoked current induced by a low concentration of progesterone is also observed in two human neuronal nAChRs.

Investigations of the mechanisms of steroid inhibition have shown that neuronal nAChRs have a specific steroid pharmacological profile that differs from that of the $GABA_A$Rs *(64,71)*. Moreover, it was demonstrated that inhibition induced by progesterone does not arise from an open-channel block effect, nor by a mechanism of competitive inhibition or involving second messenger. Conclusions obtained from several studies suggest that steroids rather act as negative allosteric effectors. In agreement with this hypothesis, dose-response inhibition profiles obtained on human neuronal nAChRs can be interpreted with the allosteric scheme.

Although at first surprising, the opposite mode of action of steroids on the $GABA_A$ and neuronal nAChRs represent an interesting mechanism. The presence of a given concentration of an active steroid in the vicinity of synaptic boutons comprising both neuronal nAChRs and $GABA_A R$ would result in an overall reduction of the postsynaptic cell excitation. Given the opposite mode of action of these two receptors, which are, respectively, excitatory and inhibitory, a reduction of the neuronal nAChRs activity would be reinforced by the potentiation of $GABA_A$ receptors. A recent work indicates that nAChRs containing the $\alpha7$ subunits are able to enhance AMPA-mediated synaptic transmission *(56)*. Thus, we propose that steroids could also depress fast glutamatergic transmissions by inhibiting the potentiating effect of presynaptic nAChRs ($\alpha7$-like nAChRs). As a result, weakening of glutamatergic synapses could lead to a morphological rearrangement of the dendritic tree. Such an hypothesis is reinforced by two previous observations. Firstly, $\alpha7$ like nAChRs have been implicated in the modulation of neurite growth *(94)*. Secondly, the long-term effect of PROG in the CA1 region of the hippocampus include a sharp decrease of the dendritic spine density *(15)*. Thus, depending of their cellular localization, nAChRs receptors should have different actions that can be modulated by the presence of neurosteroids.

ACKNOWLEDGMENTS

We are indebted to Prof. J.-P. Changeux and Prof. S. J. Edelstein and Dr. C. Briggs for critical reading and helpful discussion in the elaboration of this manuscript. We also would like to thank specially S. Bertrand for the experiments she performed with the human nAChRs reconstituted in *Xenopus* oocytes and for her constant help in the preparation of this manuscript. Human $\alpha4$ and $\beta2$ cDNAs were kindly provided by L. Monteggia and J. Sullivan from ABBOTT Laboratories, and human $\alpha7$ cDNA was kindly provided by Prof. J. Lindstrom. This work was supported by the Swiss National Foundation and the OFES to D. B.

REFERENCES

1. Baulieu, EE , Robel P. Neurosteroids: a new brain function? J Steroid Biochem Mol Biol 1990;37:395–403.
2. Schumacher M , Baulieu, EE. Neurosteroids: synthesis and functions in the central and peripheral nervous systems. Ciba Found Symp 1995;191:90–106.
3. Baulieu EE, Robel P. Non-genomic mechanisms of action of steroid hormones. Ciba Found Symp 1995;191:24–37.
4. Bancroft J. The premenstrual syndrome-a reappraisal of the concept and the evidence. Psychol Med 1993;24:1–47.
5. Kawakami M, Sawyer CH. Induction of behavioral and electroencephalographic changes in the rabbit by hormones administration or brain stimulation. Endocrinology 1959;65:631–643.
6. Lincoln DW. Unity activity in the hypothalamus septum and preoptic area of the rat: characteristics of spontaneous activity and the effect of oestrogen. J Endocrinol 1967;37:177–189.
7. Lincoln DW, Cross BA. Effect of oestrogen on the responsiveness of neurons in the hypothalamus septum and preoptic area of rats with light-induced persistent oestrus. J Endocrinol 1967;37:191–203.
8. Yagi K. Changes in firing rate of single preoptic and hypothalamic units following an intravenous administration of estrogen in the castrated female rat. Brain Res 1973;53:343–352.
9. Dufy B, Partouche C, Poulain D, Dufy-Barbe L, Vincent JD. Effects of estrogens on the electrical activity of identified and unidentified hypothalamic units. Neuroendocrinology 1976;22:38–47.
10. Teyler TJ, Vardaris RM, Lewis D, Rawitch AB. Gonadal steroids: effects on excitability of hippocampal pyramidal cells. Science 1980;209:1017–1019.

11. Kerr DS, Campbell LW, Hao SY, Landfield PW. Corticosteroid modulation of hippocampal potentials: increased effect with aging Science 1989;245:1505–1509.
12. Wong M, Moss RL. Long-term and short-term electrophysiological effects of estrogen on the synaptic properties of hippocampal CA1 neurons. J Neurosci 1992;12:3217–3225.
13. Kurz EM, Sengelaub DR, Arnold AP. Androgens regulate the dendritic length of mammalian motoneurons in adulthood. Science 1986;232:395–398.
14. Woolley CS, McEwen BS. Estradiol mediates fluctuation in hippocampal synapse density during the estrous cycle in the adult rat. J Neurosci 1992;12:2549–5425.
15. Wolley CS, McEwen BS. Roles of estradiol and progesterone in regulation of hippocampal dendritic spine density during estrous cycle in the rat. J Comp Neurol 1993;336:293–306.
16. Wolley CS, McEwen BS. Estradiol regulates hippocampal dendritic spine density via an N-Methyl-D-Aspartate receptor-dependent mechanism. J Neurosci 1994;14:7680–7687.
17. Majewska MD, Harrison NL, Schwartz RD, Barker JL, Paul SM. Steroid hormone metabolites are barbiturate-like modulators of GABA receptor. Science 1986;232:1004–1007.
18. Barker JL, Harrison NL, Lange GD, Owen DG. Potentiation of γ-amino-butiric-acid-activated chloride conductance by a steroid anaesthetic in cultured rat spinal neurones. J Physiol 1987;386:485–501.
19. Puia G, Santi MR, Vicini S, Pritchett DB, Purdy RH, Paul SM, Seeburg PH, Costa E. Neurosteroids act on recombinant human $GABA_A$ receptors. Neuron 1990; 4:759–765.
20. Majewska MD. Neurosteroids: endogenous bimodal modulators of the $GABA_A$ receptor Mechanism of action and physiological significance. Prog Neurobiol 1992;38:379–395.
21. Lambert JJ, Belelli D, Hill-Vennig C, Callachan H, Peters JA. Neurosteroid modulation of native and recombinant $GABA_A$ receptors. Cell Mol Neurobiol 1996;16:155–174.
22. Hammill OP, Marty A, Neher E, Sakmann B, Sigworth FJ. Improved patch clamp techniques for high resolution current recording from cells and cell-free patches. Pflügers Archives Eur J Physiol 1981;391:85–100.
23. Devillers-Thiéry A, Galzi JL, Eiselé JL, Bertrand S, Bertrand D, Changeux JP. Functional architecture of the nicotinic acetylcholine receptor: a prototype of ligand-gated ion channels. J Membrane Biol 1993;136:97–112.
24. Galzi JL, Changeux JP. Neuronal nicotinic receptors: molecular organization and regulations. Neuropharmacology 1995;34:563–582.
25. Bertrand D, Changeux JP. Nicotinic receptor: an allosteric protein specialized for intercellular communication. Semin Neurosci 1995;7:75–90.
26. Cockcroft VB, Osguthorpe DJ, Barnard EA, Friday AE, Lunt GG. Ligand-gated ion channels: homology and diversity. Mol Neurobiol 1992;4:129–169.
27. Sargent PB. The diversity of neuronal nicotinic acetylcholine receptors. Annu Rev Neurosci 1993;16:403–443.
28. Role LW. Diversity in primary structure and function of neuronal nicotinic acetylcholine receptor channels. Curr Opin Neurobiol 1992;2:254–262.
29. Lindström J. Neuronal nicotinic acetylcholine receptors. In: Narahashi T, ed. Ion Channels. Plenum, New York, NY, 1996, pp. 377–450.
30. Vijayaraghavan S, Schmid HA, Halvorsen SW, Berg DK. Cyclic AMP-dependent phosphorylation of a neuronal acetylcholine receptor alpha-type subunit. J Neurosci 1990;10:3255–3262.
31. Krishek BJ, Xie X, Blackstone C, Huganir RL, Moss SJ, Smart TG. Regulation of $GABA_A$ receptor function by protein kinase C phosphorylation. Neuron 1994;12:1081–1095.
32. McBain CJ, Mayer ML. N-Methyl-D-Aspartic acid receptor structure and function. Physiol Rev 1994;74:723–760.
33. Wyllie DJA, Nicoll RA. A role for protein kinases and phosphatases in the Ca^{2+}-induced enhancement of hippocampal AMPA receptor-mediated synaptic responses. Neuron 1994;13:635–643.
34. Unwin N. The nicotinic acetylcholine receptor at 9Å resolution. J Mol Biol 1993;229:1101–1124.
35. Unwin N. Acetylcholine receptor channel imaged in the open state. Nature 1995;373:37–43.
36. Pritchett DB, Seeburg PH. Gamma-aminobutyric acid type A receptor point mutation increases the affinity of compounds for the benzodiazepine site. Proc Natl Acad Sci USA 1991;88:1421–1425.
37. Betz H. Biology and structure of the mammalian glycine receptor. Trends Neurosci 1987;10:113–117.
38. Betz H. Structure and function of inhibitory glycine receptors. Quarterly Biophysics 1992;25:381–394.
39. Maricq AV, Peterson AS, Brake AJ, Myers RM, Julius D. Primary structure and functional expression of the $5HT_3$ receptor a serotonin-gated channel. Science 1991;254:432–437.

40. Numa S, Noda M, Takahashi H, Tanabe T, Toyosato M, Furutani Y, Kikyotani S. Molecular structure of the nicotinic acetylcholine receptor. Cold Spring Harb Symp Quant Biol 1983;48:57–69.

41. Ballivet M, Nef P, Stalder R, Fulpius B. Genomic sequences encoding the alpha-subunit of acetylcholine receptor are conserved in evolution. Cold Spring Harb Symp Quant Biol 1983;48:83–87.

42. Noda M, Takahashi H, Tanabe T, Toyosato M, Furutani Y, Hirose T, Asai M, Inayama S, Miyata T, Numa S. Primary structure of alpha-subunit precursor of *Torpedo californica* acetylcholine receptor deduced from cDNA sequence. Nature 1982;299:793–797.

43. Devillers-Thiéry A, Giraudat J, Bentaboulet M, Changeux JP. Complete mRNA coding sequence of the acetylcholine binding alpha subunit of *Torpedo marmorata* acetylcholine receptor: a model for the transmembrane organization of the polypeptide chain. Proc Natl Acad Sci USA 1983;80:2067–2071.

44. Barnard EA, Beeson D, Bilbe G, Brown DA, Constanti A, Conti-Tronconi BM, Dolly JO, Dunn SMJ, Mehraban F, Richards BM, Smart TG. Acetylcholine and GABA receptors :subunits of central and peripheral receptors and their encoding nucleic acids. Cold Spring Harb Symp Quant Biol 1983;48:109–124.

45. Sawruk E, Schloss P, Betz H, Schmitt B. Heterogeneity of Drosophila nicotinic acetylcholine receptors: SAD a novel developmentally regulated alpha-subunit. EMBO J 1990;9:2671–2677.

46. Ballivet M, Alliod C, Bertrand S, Bertrand D. Nicotinic acetylcholine receptors in the nematode Caenorhabditis elegans. J Mol Biol 1996;258:261–269.

47. Le-Novère N, Changeux JP. Molecular evolution of the nicotinic acetylcholine receptor: an example of multigene family in excitable cells. J Mol Evol 1995;40:155–172.

48. Cooper E, Couturier S, Ballivet M. Pentameric structure and subunit stoichiometry of a neuronal nicotinic acetylcholine receptor. Nature 1991;350:235–238.

49. Palma E, Bertrand S, Binzoni T, Bertrand D. Neuronal nicotinic α7 receptor expressed in *Xenopus* oocytes presents five putative binding sites for methyllycaconitine. J Physiol (London) 1996;491:151–161.

50. Couturier S, Bertrand D, Matter JM, Hernandez MC, Bertrand S, Millar N, Valera S, Barkas T, Ballivet M. A neuronal nicotinic acetylcholine receptor subunit (alpha 7) is developmentally regulated and forms a homo-oligomeric channel blocked by alpha-BTX. Neuron 1990;5:847–856.

51. Bertrand D, Bertrand S, Ballivet M. Pharmacological properties of the homomeric alpha 7 receptor. Neurosci Lett 1992;146:87–90.

52. Elgoyhen AB, Johnson DS, Boulter J, Vetter DE, Heinemann S. α9:an acetylcholine receptor with novel pharmacological properties expressed in rat cochlear hair cells. Cell 1994;79:705–715.

53. Peng X, Katz M, Gerzanich V, Anand R, Lindstrom J. Human α7 acetylcholine receptor: cloning of the α7 subunit from the SH-SY5Y cell line and determination of pharmacological properties of native receptors and functional α7 homomers expressed in *Xenopus* oocytes. Mol Pharmacol 1994;45:546–554.

54. Séguéla P, Wadiche J, Dineley-Miller K, Dani JA, Patrick JW. Molecular cloning functional properties and distribution of rat brain alpha7:a nicotinic cation channel highly permeable to calcium. J Neurosci 1993;13:596–604.

55. Gopalakrishnan M, Buisson B, Touma E, Giordano T, Campbell JE, Hu IC, Donnelyroberts D, Arneric SP, Bertrand D, Sullivan JP. Stable expression and pharmacological properties of the human (7 nicotinic acetylcholine receptor. Eur J Pharmacol Mol Pharmacol 1995;290:237–246.

56. McGehee DS, Role LW. Physiological diversity of nicotinic acetylcholine receptors expressed by vertebrate neurons. Ann Rev Physiol 1995;57:521–546.

57. Hussy N, Ballivet M, Bertrand D. Agonist and antagonist effects of nicotine on chick neuronal nicotinic receptors are defined by alpha and beta subunits. J Neurophysiol 1994;72:1317–1326.

58. Corringer PJ, Galzi JL, Eisele JL, Bertrand S, Changeux JP, Bertrand D. Identification of a new component of the agonist binding site of the nicotinic alpha 7 homooligomeric receptor. J Biol Chem 1995;270:11749–11752.

59. Martin M, Czajkowski C, Karlin A. The contributions of aspartyl residues in the acetylcholine receptor gamma and delta subunits to the binding of agonists and competitive antagonists J Biol Chem 1996;271:13497–13503.

60. Harvey SC, Luetje CW. Determinants of competitive antagonist sensitivity on neuronal nicotinic receptor beta subunits. J Neurosci 1996;16:3798–3806.

61. Inoue M, Kuriyama H. Glutocorticoids inhibit acetylcholine-induced current in chromaffine cells. Am J Physiol 1989;257:C906-C912.

62. Wu FS, Gibbs TT, Farb DH. Inverse modulation of gaba-aminobutyric acid- and glycine induced currents by progesterone Mol Pharmacol 1990;37:597–602.

63. Bertrand D, Valera S, Bertrand S, Ballivet M, Rungger D. Steroids inhibit nicotinic acetylcholine receptors. Neuroreport 1991;2:277–280.

64. Valera S, Ballivet M, Bertrand D. Progesterone modulates a neuronal nicotinic acetylcholine receptor. Proc Natl Acad Sci USA 1992, 89:9949–9953.

65. Doucette-Stamm L, Monteggia LM, Donelly-Roberts D, Wang MT, Lee J, Tian J, Giordano T. Cloning and sequence of the human α7 nicotinic acetylcholine receptor. Drug Dev Res 1993;30:252–256.

66. Monteggia LM, Gopalakrishnan M, Touma E, Idler KB, Nash N, Arneric SP, Sullivan JP, Giordano T. Cloning and transient expression of genes encoding the human alpha 4 and beta 2 neuronal nicotinic acetylcholine receptor (nAChR) subunits. Gene 1995;155:189–193.

67. Buisson B, Gopalakrishnan M, Arneric SP, Sullivan JP, Bertrand D. Human α4β2 neuronal nicotinic acetylcholine receptor in HEK 293 cells: a patch-clamp study. J Neurosci 1996;16:7880–7891.

68. Valera S. Modulation fonctionnelle des récepteurs nicotiniques par certaines hormones steroides. 1993, PhD Thesis, Geneva.

69. Majewska MD, Mienville JM, Vicini S. Neurosteroid pregnenolone sulfate antagonizes electrophysi-ological responses to GABA in neurons. Neurosci Lett 1988;90:279–284.

70. Mienville J-M, Vicini S. Pregnenolone sulfate antagonizes $GABA_A$ receptor-mediated current via a reduction of channel opening frequency. Brain Res 1989;489:190–194.

71. Ke L, Lukas RJ. Effects of steroid exposure on ligand binding and functional activities of diverse nicotinic acetylcholine receptor subtypes. J Neurochem 1996;67:1100–1112.

72. Jones OT, MacNamee MG. Annular and nonannular binding sites for cholesterol associated with the nicotinic acetylcholine receptor. Biochem 1988;27:2364–2374.

73. Zannello LP, Aztiria E, Antollini S, Barrantes FJ. Nicotinic acetylcholine receptor channels are influ-enced by the physical state of their membrane environment. Biophys J 1996;5:2155–2165.

74. Monod J, Wyman J, Changeux JP. On the nature of allosteric transitions: a plausible model. J Mol Biol 1965;12:88–118.

75. Rubin MM, Changeux JP. On the nature of allosteric transitions; implications of non exclusive ligand binding. J Mol Biol 1966;21:265–274.

76. Changeux JP, Thiéry JP, Tung Y, Kittel C. On the cooperativity of biological membranes. Proc Nat Acad Sci USA 1967; 57:335–341.

77. Grünhagen HH, Changeux JP. Transitions structurales du récepteur cholinergique de Torpille dans son état membranaire mises en évidence à l'aide d'un anesthésique local fluorescent: la quinacrine. CR Acad Sci (Paris) 1975;281D: 1047–1050.

78. Heidmann T, Changeux JP. Structural and functional properties of the acetylcholine receptor protein in its purified and membrane-bound states. Ann Rev Biochem 1978;47:371–357.

79. Heidmann T, Changeux JP. Stabilization of the high affinity state of the membrane-bound acetylcholine receptor from *Torpedo marmorata* by non-competitive blockers. FEBS Lett 1981;131:239–244.

80. Changeux JP. Functional architecture and dynamics of the nicotinic acetylcholine receptor: an allosteric ligand-gated ion channel. In: Changeux JP, Llinàs RR, Purves D, Bloom FE, eds. Fidia Research Foundation Neuroscience Award Lectures. Raven, New York, NY, 1990, pp. 21–168.

81. Karlin A. On the application of "a plausible model" of allosteric proteins to the receptor for acetylcho-line. J Theor Biol 1967;16:306–320.

82. Mulle C, Léna C, Changeux JP. Potentiation of nicotinic receptor response by external calcium in rat central neurons. Neuron 1992;8:937–945.

83. Léna C, Changeux JP. Allosteric modulations of the nicotinic acetylcholine receptor. Trends Neurosci 1993; 16:181–186.

84. Vernino S, Amador M, Luetje CW, Patrick J, Dani JA. Calcium modulation and high calcium perme-ability of neuronal nicotinic acetylcholine receptor. Neuron 1992;8:127–134.

85. Eiselé JL, Bertrand S, Galzi JL, Devillers-Thiéry A, Changeux JP, Bertrand D. Chimaeric nicotinic-serotoninergic receptor combines dictinct ligand binding and channel specificities. Nature 1993; 366:479–483.

86. Galzi JL, Bertrand S, Corringer JP, Changeux JP, Bertrand D. Identification of calcium binding sites which regulate potentiation of a neuronal nicotinic acetylcholine receptor. EMBO J 1996;15:5824–5832.

87. Edelstein SJ, Schaad O, Henry E, Bertrand D, Changeux JP. A kinetic mechanism for nicotinic acetyl-choline receptors based on multiple allosteric transitions. Biol Cybern 75;75:361–379.

88. Mulle C, Benoit P, Pinset C, Roa M, Changeux JP. Calcitonin gene-related peptide enhances the rate of desensitization of the nicotinic acetylcholine receptor in cultured mouse muscle cells. Proc Natl Acad Sci USA 1988;85:5728–5732.
89. Huganir RL, Delcour AH, Greengard P, Hess GP. Phosphorylation of the nicotinic acetylcholine receptor regulates its rate of desensitization. Nature 1986;321:744–776.
90. Tindall RS, Phillips JT, Rollins JA, Wells L, Hall K. A clinical therapeutic trial of cyclosporine in myasthenia gravis. Ann NY Acad Sci 1993;681:539–551.
91. Bliss TVP, Collingridge GL. A synaptic model of memory: long-term potentiation in the hippocampus. Nature 1993;361:31–39.
92. Malenka RC. Synaptic plasticity in the hippocampus: LTP and LTD. Neuron 1994;78:535–538.
93. Collingridge GL, Bliss TVP. Memories of NMDA receptors and LTP. Trends Neurosci 1995;18:54–56.
94. Pugh PC, Berg DK. Neuronal acetylcholine receptors that bind alpha-bungarotoxin mediate neurite retraction in a calcium-dependent manner. J Neurosci 1994;14:889–896.
95. Galzi JL, Devillers TA, Hussy N, Bertrand S, Changeux JP, Bertrand D. Mutations in the channel domain of a neuronal nicotinic receptor convert ion selectivity from cationic to anionic. Nature 1992;359:500–505.

13 Neuroactive Steroid Modulation of Neuronal Voltage-Gated Calcium Channels

Jarlath M. H. ffrench-Mullen, MD

CONTENTS

INTRODUCTION
STEROID INHIBITION OF VOLTAGE-DEPENDENT CA^{2+} CHANNELS
THE ROLE OF GUANINE NUCLEOTIDE PROTEINS
STEROID MODULATION OF NONVOLTAGE-GATED CA^{2+} INFLUX
CONCLUSIONS
REFERENCES

INTRODUCTION

The Ca^{2+} influx through voltage-gated Ca^{2+} channels (VGCCs) plays a vital role in the control of neuronal neurotransmitter release and membrane excitability. The modulation of Ca^{2+} channels controls the extent of Ca^{2+} entry and provides a way of regulating neuronal function. Multiple classes of VGCCs exist in both peripheral and central mammalian neurons, based on biophysical and pharmacological identification. Electrophysiological studies have described a low voltage-activated T-type current and several pharmacologically defined high voltage-activated currents on neuronal cell bodies such as the L, N, P, Q, and R-type Ca^{2+} channels *(1–3)*. L-type channels are sensitive to the dihydropyridines (e.g., nifedipine), N channels to ω-conotoxin-GVIA, P channels to ω-agatoxin-IVA, Q-type to ω-conotoxin-MVIIC, and an R-type insensitive to all these antagonists *(1–3)*.

The presence and action of both endogenous and synthetic steroids in the mammalian central nervous system (CNS) are well-documented. These neuroactive steroids, including those synthesized in brain (neurosteroids and their sulfate derivatives), have a rapid and direct excitatory or inhibitory action on neuronal membranes that is independent of nuclear transcription *(4)*. Considerable data has emerged demonstrating that some neuroactive steroids can potentiate or inhibit $GABA_A$-activated Cl^- current (GABA), enhance NMDA receptor-mediated excitatory amino acid responses, inhibit glycine-activated Cl^- channels, and inhibit voltage-dependent Ca^{2+} channels *(5–9)*.

From: *Contemporary Endocrinology: Neurosteroids: A New Regulatory Function in the Nervous System* Edited by: E.-E. Baulieu, P. Robel, and M. Schumacher
© Humana Press Inc., Totowa, NJ

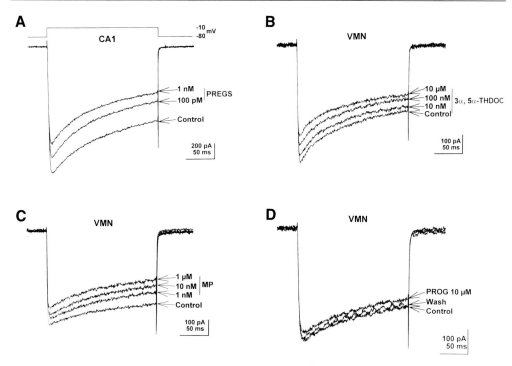

Fig. 1. Neuroactive steroid inhibition of whole-cell Ca^{2+} channel current in freshly isolated guinea-pig hippocampal CA1 neurons and rat hypothalamic ventromedial nucleus (VMN) neurons. **(A)** The neurosteroid pregnenolone sulfate (PREGS) inhibition of the Ca^{2+} channel current, which was fully reversible with wash (not shown) in a CA1 neuron. **(B)** The neurosteroid tetrahydrodeoxycorticosterone ($3\alpha,5\alpha$-THDOC) inhibition of the Ca^{2+} channel current in a VMN neuron. **(C)** The neuroactive steroid medroxyprogesterone acetate (MP; a progesterone derivative) inhibition of the Ca^{2+} channel current in a VMN neuron. **(D)** The steroid progesterone (PROG) had a minimal effect (8% inhibition peak current), which was reversible with wash. All neurons were freshly isolated as previously described; Ca^{2+} channel currents were evoked by 200 ms steps from a holding potential of –80 mV to a test potential of –10 mV with the individual (leak subtracted) currents recorded at –10 mV illustrated, as previously described *(11)*.

STEROID INHIBITION
OF VOLTAGE-DEPENDENT CA²⁺ CHANNELS

The inhibition of VGCCs by endogenous brain steroids was first reported in freshly isolated guinea pig hippocampal CA1 neurons using the whole-cell patch clamp recording technique *(7)*. The 3α-hydroxy ring A-reduced metabolites of progesterone (PROG) and deoxycorticosterone (DOC), namely pregnanolone (3α-hydroxy-5β-pregnan-20-one) and tetrahydrodeoxycorticosterone ($3\alpha,5\alpha$-THDOC; $3\alpha,20$-dihydroxy-5α-pregnan-20-one) and dehydroepiandrosterone sulfate (DHEAS; 3β-hydroxy-androst-5-en-17-one sulfate) were found to inhibit a fraction of the total Ca^{2+} channel current over the concentration range of 10 nM to 100 μM *(7)*. Both pregnanolone (Fig. 1) and $3\alpha,5\alpha$-THDOC had been previously shown to potentiate, and DHEAS to antagonize, the GABA current, respectively *(8)*. Although pregnanolone inhibited only a fraction of the Ca^{2+} channel current (60% at 100 μM) with an IC_{50} of 298

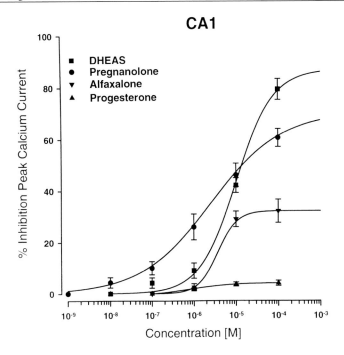

Fig. 2. Concentration-effect curves of certain neuroactive steroid-induced inhibition of the peak whole-cell Ca^{2+} channel current. Ca^{2+} channel currents were evoked in hippocampal CA1 neurons as described in Fig. 1. Each data point represents the mean ± S.E.M. 4–5 neurons for each compound; percent inhibition was calculated as previously described *(11)*. Concentration-effect data were fitted with a nonlinear least-squares program according to the logistical equation $B = 100/1 + (IC_{50}/[DRUG])^{nH}$, where [DRUG] is the drug concentration, IC_{50} is the concentration resulting in 50% inhibition, and nH is an empirical parameter that describes the steepness of the curve and has the same meaning as the Hill coefficient. The IC_{50} were 2.7, 10, and 3 for dihydroepiandosterone sulfate (DHEAS), pregnanolone, and alfaxolone, respectively; $nH = 0.6$, 0.95 and 1.5 for DHEAS, pregnanolone, and alfaxalone.

nM, DHEAS essentially inhibited 80% of the inward current at 100 µM (Fig. 2), which was irreversible; higher concentrations of DHEAS resulted in loss of recording, hence cell death (not shown).

The classical neurosteroids, pregnenolone (PREG) and its sulfate derivative, pregnenolone sulfate (PREGS), which are synthesized and found in intact brain and glial cultures *(9,10)*, appear to have a multitude of actions on various membrane channels *(6)*, including the inhibition of voltage-gated Ca^{2+} channels *(11)*. Both PREG and PREGS inhibited a fraction of the total inward Ca^{2+} current with a maximal inhibition of 64 ± 3% and 57 ± 4%, respectively, at 100 µM and IC_{50} values of 11 and 130 nM, respectively (11). Interestingly, in rat hypothalamic ventromedial nucleus (VMN) neurons, PREGS essentially had no inhibitory effect with a maximal inhibition of 6.5 ± 3% and 7 ± 2% at 1 and 10 µM, respectively (Fig. 3). In contrast to PREGS, 3α,5α-THDOC inhibited the Ca^{2+} current with an $IC_{50} = 673$ nM and an $nH = 0.4$ ($n = 6$) (Fig. 3). The potency of inhibition in rat (VMN) was less than that in guinea-pig CA1 neurons.

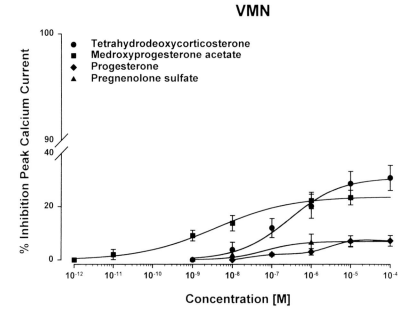

Fig. 3. Concentration-effect curves of certain neuroactive steroids in freshly isolated adult rat hypothalamic ventromedial nulceus (VMN) neurons. Each data point represents the mean± S.E.M. of 5–6 neurons for each compound; *see* Fig. 2 for details. Tetrahydrodeoxycorticosterone and medroxyprogesterone acetate had an IC_{50} = 673 and 4 nM, respectively, and an nH = 0.7 and 0.5, respectively. Progesterone and pregnenolone sulfate had a maximal inhibition of $7\pm2\%$ and 6.9 $\pm\ 2\%$, respectively.

Subsequently, other neuroactive steroids were reported to also inhibit voltage-gated Ca^{2+} channels, such as the glucocorticosteroids cortisol and corticosterone in freshly isolated hippocampal CA1 neurons *(12)*, megestrol acetate in VMN neurons *(13)*, estradiol, estriol and 4-hydroxyestradiol in freshly isolated and cultured neostriatal neurons *(14)*. The steroid anesthetic alfaxolone, which potently (30 nM) potentiates the GABA current *(15)*, at higher concentrations inhibited a fraction of the total Ca^{2+} channel current in hippocampal CA1 neurons (Fig. 2). All of these neuroactive steroids had a rapid and direct action and appeared to exert their inhibitory effect via an extracellular membrane receptor *(11–14)*.

However, PROG, which is also derived from PREG in the brain, had no effect on the Ca^{2+} channel current in either guinea-pig hippocampal CA1 neurons (Figs. 1 and 2) *(11)* or rat VMN neurons (Fig. 3) *(13)*. Other studies have shown that PROG enhances the $GABA_A$-induced responses in Purkinjie and spinal chord neurons *(16,17)*. Megestrol acetate, a synthetic orally active progesterone derivative, is utilized clinically for the treatment of metastatic breast cancer and endometrial cancer *(18)* and also to induce appetite stimulation and weight gain in cancer/AIDS patients with anorexia/cachexia *(19)*. Although its mechanism of action is unknown, megestrol acetate was found to inhibit potently (IC_{50} = 2 nM and an nH = 0.5) a fraction ($24 \pm 3\%$) of the total VGCCs in freshly isolated adult rat VMN neurons with a maximal saturating concentration of 1 and 10 μM *(13)*. The megestrol acetate analogue, medroxyprogesterone acetate (MP) also inhibited the VGCCs in VMN neurons (Figs. 1C and 3). MP showed an identical potency of inhibition to megestrol acetate with a maximal inhibition of $23 \pm 3\%$ at 10 μM of the total VGCCs with an IC$_{50}$ = 4 nM and an nH = 0.5 *(13)*. In contrast, medroxyprogesterone weakly inhibited the VGCCs with a 7% inhibition at 10 mM *(13)*. Furthermore, even in the presence of 10 μM PROG, megestrol acetate showed an identical inhibition of the VGCCs to megestrol acetate alone, suggesting a novel membrane receptor *(13)*.

While inhibiting the Ca^{2+} channel current, some neuroactive steroids also modulated certain parameters of Ca^{2+} channel gating. One commonality observed with those neuroactive steroids was a voltage-dependence of Ca^{2+} channel current inhibition. PREGS, 3α,5α-THDOC, megestrol acetate, and cortisol all showed a voltage-dependent inhibition, specific for negative voltages—that is, greater inhibition at more negative test potentials—typically between –60 and 0 mV *(11–13)*. Another common observation to these same neuroactive steroids was that although there was a lack of effect on the voltage-dependence of activation, there was a slowing of the rate of activation *(11–13)*. The rate or time-course of Ca^{2+} channel activation was slowed by PREGS, 3α,5α-THDOC, megestrol acetate, and cortisol; however, deactivation was slowed by PREGS, 3α,5α-THDOC, and megestrol acetate, but not cortisol *(11–13)*.

With regard to which Ca^{2+} channels these neuroactive steroids inhibited, there was indeed a reasonable lack of specificity. PREG, 3α,5α-THDOC and cortisol were nonselective in that they inhibited both the N- and L-type Ca^{2+} channels, although 3α,5α-THDOC appeared to be more selective in inhibiting the N-type Ca^{2+} channels *(11,12)*. In contrast, in VMN neurons, megestrol acetate selectively inhibited a fraction of the resistant or R-type Ca^{2+} channel current *(13)*. Calcium channel selectivity was also demonstrated with estradiol, which specifically inhibited the L-type Ca^{2+} channel in neostriatal neurons *(14)*.

THE ROLE OF GUANINE NUCLEOTIDE PROTEINS

Guanine nucleotide proteins (G-proteins) appear to regulate many cellular processes, ion channels and neurotransmitter release *(20)*. Several neurotransmitters and several presynaptic receptors are known to modulate voltage-dependent Ca^{2+} channels, through surface receptors coupled to the Ca^{2+} channel via a G-protein-dependent mechanism *(20)*. The actions of certain neuroactive steroids on their respective Ca^{2+} channel current appear to involve signal transduction pathway(s). The actions of the neurosteroids PREG, PREGS, and 3α,5α-THDOC and cortisol on VGCCs are modulated via a G-protein, because their inhibitory effects were significantly reduced by pretreatment with intracellular dialysis of the nonhydrolyzable GTP analog guanosine 5'-O-(2-thiodiphosphate) (GDP-β-S), which inhibits G-proteins *(11)*. Further G-protein involvement was verified by pretreatment with pertussis toxin (PTX), which prevents the interaction of the G-proteins G$_{\alpha i}$ and G$_{\alpha o}$ subclasses by catalyzing their ADP ribosylation *(21)*. In neurons isolated from PTX-treated animals, PTX drastically reduced the inhibitory actions of PREG, PREGS, 3α,5α-THDOC, and cortisol, thus demonstrating either a G$_{\alpha i}$ and/or a G$_{\alpha o}$ involvement; however, further experiments are required to determine precisely which subclass (or both) is involved *(11)*. On the other hand, a specific G-protein was found to modulate the megestrol acetate-induced inhibition. Although intracellular dialysis of GDP-β-S significantly reduced the megestrol acetate effect, PTX had no effect on the megestrol acetate-induced inhibition *(13)*. In neurons isolated from cholera toxin-treated animals, the megestrol acetate-induced inhibition was significantly diminished, suggesting a G-protein α_s-subunit involvement (13). Further confirmation of the $G\alpha_s$-subclass involvement was obtained using antisense phosphothio-oligonucleotides (antisense). In neurons isolated from animals pretreated with antisense-$G\alpha_s$ a significant reduction of the megestrol acetate-induced inhibition of the Ca^{2+} channel current was observed (13). Treatment with either sense-$G\alpha_s$ or antisense-$G\alpha_{11}$ had no effect, confirming a $G\alpha_s$-subunit involvement (13).

The G-protein modulation of Ca^{2+} channels may involve a variety of mechanisms, including a direct action (membrane delimited) or via intracellular kinase mediators (protein kinase C [PKC]; protein kinase A [PKA]), and more than one G-protein may be involved (20). The PREG, $3\alpha,5\alpha$-THDOC, and cortisol G-protein-dependent inhibition of the Ca^{2+} channel current appears to be coupled to PKC. Intracellular dialysis of the specific PKC inhibitors bisindolylmalemide (BIS, 1 mM) and the pseudosubstrate inhibitor PKCI 19–36 (1–2 μM) significantly diminished the PREG, $3\alpha,5\alpha$-THDOC, and cortisol inhibition of the Ca^{2+} channel current; there was no effect by the PKA activators (Sp-cAMPS) or inhibitors (20 AA protein; Rp-cAMPS) (11,12). In contrast, the same PKC and PKA inhibitors both significantly diminished the megestrol acetate-induced inhibition of the voltage-gated R-type Ca^{2+} channel current (13). In addition, internal dialysis of both BIS and the 20AA inhibitors through the patch pipet significantly eliminated the megestrol acetate-induced inhibition thus confirming both a PKC and PKA involvement.

STEROID MODULATION OF NONVOLTAGE-GATED CA²⁺ INFLUX

Steroids also modulate the nonvoltage-gated intracellular Ca^{2+} influx $[Ca^{2+}]_i$ into neuronal cells and tissues. In primary cultures of rat fetal hypothalamic neurons, the neurosteroid allopregnanolone (3α-hydroxy-5α-pregnan-20-one) rapidly and dose-dependently increased $[Ca^{2+}]_i$ with an EC_{50} of 10 nM. Estradiol exhibited a similar effect, but PROG had no effect (22). This effect of allopregnanolone was inhibited by biccuculine and picrotoxin, but not by PTX, thus suggesting a lack of G-protein, but a $GABA_A$ receptor involvement (22). In a clonal pituitary cell line (GH3), PREGS (30 μM), but not PREG, DHEAS, PROG, and estradiol, was found to induce a rapid and transient $[Ca^{2+}]_i$ increase within 1 min (23). This increase was abolished in a Ca^{2+}-free medium, in the presence of the nonselective inorganic Ca^{2+} channel blockers La^{3+} and Co^{2+} and by the organic Ca^{2+} channel blockers methoxyverapamil and nicardipine, suggesting that this Ca^{2+} influx was mediated through L-type VGCCs (23). PREGS also potentiates the N-methyl-D-aspartate (NMDA)-induced Ca^{2+} influx and currents in cultured hippocampal and spinal chord neurons (for review, see ref. 6). In granulosa cells from preovulatory follicles, estradiol increases $[Ca^{2+}]_i$ via phosphinositide hydrolysis (24). In GH3 cells, estradiol rapidly (1–2 min) induces Ca^{2+}-dependent action potentials in GH3 cells (25).

CONCLUSIONS

The neuroactive modulation of both voltage-, and nonvoltage-gated Ca^{2+} influx into cells appears to involve an inhibition or potentiation, respectively. This appears to correspond to a rapid and direct (nongenomic) action on a membrane receptor; however, these nongenomic actions could also have long-term effects on neuronal function. A common mechanism of action for neuroactive steroid inhibition of VGCCs is a modulation via G-proteins, and in some instances, also includes the intracellular messengers PKA and PKC. These diverse actions of some neuroactive steroids such as potentiation/inhibition of GABA-induced currents, potentiation of NMDA-induced currents and inhibition of VGCCs, raises the possibility of a variety of functional roles, such as regulation of CNS excitability. Indeed, some neuroactive steroids, such as PREG, PREGS, and cortisol modulate VGCCs at concentrations found in certain physiological and pathophysiological conditions (*see* refs. *5,6,11,12*). Recently, it was shown that there were brain region-specific effects of neuroactive steroids on the affinity and density of the GABA$_A$-binding site (26). A similar situation may exist regarding Ca^{2+} channels. Although estradiol was found to preferentially reduce neostriatal VGCCs in female versus male animals *(14)*, it had no effect on hippocapal CA1 neuronal VGCCs (unpublished results). Similarly, PREGS depressed VGCCs in hippocampal CA1 *(11)*, but not VMN neurons (Fig. 3). In contrast, 3α,5α-THDOC reduced VGCCs in both CA1 and VMN neurons (ref. *1* and Fig. 3, respectively).

It is now well-documented that certain neuroactive steroids, including both neurosteroids and some steroid hormones, reduce neuronal voltage-gated Ca^{2+} channels or enhance [Ca^{2+}]$_i$ in some cell types. However, further studies are required to clarify this modulatory effect in both physiological and/or pathophysiological conditions.

REFERENCES

1. Wheeler DB, Randall AD, Tsien RW. Roles of N-type and Q-type Ca^{2+} channels in supporting hippocampal transmission. Science 1994;264:107–111.
2. Mintz IM, Adams ME, Bean BP. P-type calcium channels in rat central and peripheral neurons. Neuron 1992;9:85–95.
3. Isibashi H, Rhee JS, Akaike N. Regional differences of high voltage-activated Ca^{2+} channels in rat CNS neurones. Neuroreport 1995;6:1621–1624.
4. McEwen BS. Non-genomic and genomic effects of steroids on neural activity. Trends Pharmacol Sci 1991;12:141–147.
5. Mellon SH. Neurosteroids: biochemistry, modes of action, and clinical relevance. J Clin Endocrinol Metab 1994;78:1003–1008.
6. Kulkarni SK, Reddy DS. Neurosteroids: a new class of neuromodulators. Drugs Today 1995;31:433–455.
7. ffrench-Mullen JMH, Spence K. Neurosteroids block Ca^{2+} channel current in freshly isolated hippocampal CA1 neurons. Eur J Pharmacol 1991;202:269–272.
8. Majewska MD, Demigoren S, Spivake CE, London ED. The neurosteroid dehydroepiandrosterone sulfate is an allosteric modulator of the GABA$_A$ receptor. Brain Res 1990;526:143–146.
9. Corpéchot C, Synguelakis M, Talha S, Axelson M, Sjövall J, Vihko R, Baulieu EE, Robel P. Pregnenolone and its sulfate ester in the rat brain. Brain Res 1983;270:119–125.
10. Lanthier A, Patwardham VV. Sex steroids and 5-en–3β-hydroxysteroids in specific brain regions of the human brain and cranial nerves. J Steroid Biochem 1986;25:445–449.
11. ffrench-Mullen JMH, Danks P, Spence K. Neurosteroids modulate calcium currents in hippocampal CA1 neurons via a pertussis toxin-sensitive G-protein-coupled mechanism. J Neurosci 1994;14:1963–1977.
12. ffrench-Mullen JMH. Cortisol inhibition of calcium curents in guinea-pig hippocampal CA1 neurons via a G-protein-coupled activation of protein kinase C. J Neurosci 1995;15:903–911.
13. Costa AMN, Spence KT, Plata-Salamán CR, ffrench-Mullen JMH. Residual Ca^{2+} channel modulation by megestrol acetate via a G-protein α$_S$-subunit in rat hypothalamic neurones. J Physiol 1995;487:291–303.
14. Mermelstein PG, Becker JB, Surmeir DJ. Estradiol reduces calcium currents in rat neostriatal neurons via a membrane receptor. J Neurosci 1996;15:595–604.
15. Lodge D, Anis NA. Effects of ketamine and three other anesthetics on spinal reflexes and inhibitions in the cat. Brit J Anesth 1984;56:1143–1151.

16. Smith SS, Waterhouse BD, Woodward DJ. Locally applied progesterone metabolites alter neuronal responsiveness in the cerebellum. Brain Res Bull 1987;18:739–747.

17. Wu FS, Gibbs TT, Farb DH. Inverse modulation of gamma-aminobutyric acid- and glycine-induced currents by progesterone. Mol Pharmacol 1987;37:597–602.

18. Gregory EJ, Cohen SC, Oines DW, Mims CH. Megestrol acetate therapy for advanced breast cancer. J Clin Oncol 1985;3:155–160.

19. Graham KK, Mikolich DJ, Fisher AE, Posner MR, Dudley MN. Pharmacologic evaluation of megestrol acetate oral suspension in cachetic AIDS patients. J Acquir Immune Defic Synd 1995;7:580–586.

20. Hille B. G-protein coupling mechanisms and nervous system signalling. Neuron 1992;9:187–195.

21. Gilman AG. G proteins: transducers of receptor generated signals. Ann Rev Biochem 1987;56:615–649.

22. Dayanithi G, Tapia-Arancibia L. Rise in intracellular calcium via a nongenomic effect of allo-pregnanolone in fetal rat hypothalamic neurons. J Neurosci 1996;16:130–136.

23. Büküsoglu C, Sarlak F. Pregnenolone sulfate increases intracellular Ca^{2+} levels in a pituitary cell line. Europ J Pharmacol 1996;298:79–85.

24. Morley P, Whitfield BC, Vanderhyden BC, Tsang BK, Schwartz JL. A new nongenomic estrogen action: the rapid release of intracellular calcium. Endocrinology 1992;131:1305–1309.

25. Dufy B, Vincent JD, Fleury PD, Pasquier D, Gourdji D, Tixer-Vidal A. Membrane effects of thyrotropin-releasing hormone and estrogen shown by intracellular recording from pituitary cell lines. Science 1979;204: 509–511.

26. Jussofie A. Brain region-specific effects of neuroactive steroids on the affinity and density of the GABA-binding site. Biol Chem Hoppe Seyler 1993;374:265–270.

14 Gonadal Hormone Regulation of Synaptic Plasticity in the Brain
What Is the Mechanism?

Bruce S. McEwen, MD

CONTENTS

INTRODUCTION
THREE PHASES OF RESEARCH CHARACTERIZE THE INVESTIGATION
    OF HORMONE ACTION IN BRAIN
ACTIONS OF GONADAL HORMONES IN HYPOTHALAMUS
THE HIPPOCAMPUS AS A SEX HORMONE-SENSITIVE LIMBIC BRAIN
    REGION INVOLVED IN COGNITION AND THE COGNITIVE ASPECTS
    OF EMOTION
CELLULAR AND MOLECULAR PROCESSES REGULATED
    BY CIRCULATING HORMONES
A NEW VIEW OF HIPPOCAMPAL INTERNEURONS
ESTROGEN SENSITIVITY OF AFFERENTS TO THE HIPPOCAMPUS
NONGENOMIC ACTIONS OF ESTROGENS AND VARIANTS
    ON THE GENOMIC ACTIONS
APPROACHES TO THE STUDY OF SYNAPTOGENESIS IN THE MATURE
    NERVOUS SYSTEM
MOLECULAR EVENTS ASSOCIATED WITH SYNAPSE FORMATION
CONCLUSIONS
REFERENCES

INTRODUCTION

Throughout the life span, the brain continues to be shaped and modified by the external world acting through the release and actions of circulating hormones and endogenous growth factors and neurotransmitters. Receptors for steroid hormones and thyroid hormone were the first transcription regulators discovered for eukaryotic cells *(1)*. Besides helping to catalyze the discovery of other transcription regulators *(2,3)*, the steroid-thyroid hormone family of receptors has provided an important tool for elucidating the sites and cellular mechanisms by which circulating hormones exert permanent develop-

From: *Contemporary Endocrinology: Neurosteroids: A New Regulatory Function
in the Nervous System* Edited by: E.-E. Baulieu, P. Robel, and M. Schumacher
© Humana Press Inc., Totowa, NJ

mental effects (e.g., sexual differentiation) and reversible and often cyclic effects on the mature brain (4).

Recent research is showing that the brain is more widely responsive to gonadal hormones than previously thought, e.g., not only is the hypothalamus affected by circulating estrogens and androgens, but also structures like the hippocampus undergo sexual differentiation and are hormone-responsive in maturity (5). Moreover, major projecting neurons such as cholinergic, serotonergic, noradrenergic, and dopaminergic systems are responsive to gonadal hormones (5). It is therefore not so surprising that a variety of nervous and mental disorders and recovery of the brain from damage are subject to sex differences and to gonadal hormone regulation (5).

One of the most striking effects of ovarian steroids is the cyclic induction of synapses in the hypothalamus and hippocampus of female rats, and this chapter briefly summarizes information relevant to understanding possible mechanisms, as well as the significance for behavior and also for human brain function.

THREE PHASES OF RESEARCH CHARACTERIZE
THE INVESTIGATION OF HORMONE ACTION IN BRAIN

Studies of the mechanism of hormone action have provided important insights into the control of eukaryotic gene expression, and studies of steroid receptors in brain showed that the brain responds by the same mechanism as the nonneural tissues. There have been three phases of investigation of steroid hormone effects on the brain. First, there has been the characterization and mapping of steroid and thyroid hormone receptors in brain, establishing that the nervous system has receptors for all six classes of steroid hormones (estrogens, androgens, glucocorticoids, mineralocorticoids, progestins, and vitamin D) as well as thyroid hormone and retinoic acid. Each receptor class is expressed in its own unique, developmentally regulated regional pattern in the brain (6); Second, the role of steroid receptors in behavioral and neuroendocrine events, including developmental programming of sex differences, has been elucidated by pharmacological means, using agonists and antagonists applied systemically or locally into brain regions having receptors and known roles in a behavioral or neuroendocrine event (7). Third, specific cellular and molecular processes have been identified in brain regions linked to specific functions. These include hormonal regulation of neuropeptide gene expression (8–15) and aspects of signal transduction (16) and structural plasticity, involving synaptogenesis (17–19), the retraction and expansion of dendrites (20) and neuronal cell death and neurogenesis (21,22). Besides the hypothalamus and bulbocavernosus nucleus of the spinal cord, one of the brain regions that has emerged as having considerable hormone-regulated plasticity is the hippocampus. This brain region has unique features and relevance to human cognitive process and neurological disorders.

ACTIONS OF GONADAL HORMONES IN HYPOTHALAMUS

Ovarian hormone actions on neurons of the ventromedial hypothalamus, which are important for the regulation of sexual behavior in female rats, include regulation of neuropeptide gene expression (23) and second messenger systems (16), and induction of oxytocin receptors, progestin receptors, and the regulation of cyclic synaptogenesis (18,24–26). There are also developmentally programmed sex differences involving both neuronal wiring as well as programming of responses to hormonal activation of gene expression *(25,27)*. All of these actions occur in neurons that express high levels of estrogen and progestin receptors, in contrast to the hippocampus in which estrogen receptors are very scarce and are found in interneurons and in afferents to the hippocampus such as the entorhinal cortex and the midbrain raphe.

THE HIPPOCAMPUS AS A SEX HORMONE-SENSITIVE LIMBIC BRAIN REGION INVOLVED IN COGNITION AND THE COGNITIVE ASPECTS OF EMOTION

The hippocampus is implicated in spatial and explicit memory functions *(28)* and is part of the limbic system and therefore a participant in the affective and vegetative states *(29)*. It is a brain region that provides "context" and cognitive meaning to many appetitive and aversive events *(30,31)*, and it is a major target for circulating adrenal steroids and or for their actions during stress and in the diurnal sleep-waking cycle *(32)*. Sex differences have been described in hippocampal morphology involving the size of the dentate gyrus *(33–35)*, and spatial learning with global spatial cues is faster in males than in females *(7)*. This trait can be reduced in newborn male rats by castration, and it is enhanced in newborn female rats by neonatal treatment with estrogens *(7)*; this may be the pathway for sexual differentiation, because the hippocampus transiently expresses estrogen receptors and aromatizing enzymes during the first 2 wk of neonatal life *(36,37)*. Estrogen receptors are largely absent from the adult hippocampus, except for scattered interneuron-like cells in Ammon's horn *(38,39)* and some unidentified estrophilic cells in the entorhinal cortex. Yet there are some remarkable effects of estrogens on synaptogenesis *(see* below). Androgen receptors are expressed in the hippocampus of the male and female rat *(40)*. The dentate gyrus is larger in males than in females, owing in part to sexual differentiation *(33,41)*, and there is some preliminary evidence for sex differences in neurogenesis and granule cell death in adult voles captured in the wild *(42)*.

Thyroid hormone treatment immediately after birth has specific effects on the basal forebrain, dentate gyrus, and CA3 region of the hippocampus that last into adult life. Transient neonatal hyperthyroidism enhances basal forebrain cholinergic markers and increases the size of the dentate gyrus and branching of dendrites of CA3 pyramidal neurons *(35,43,44)*. There are sex differences, in that the developing male cholinergic system is much more enhanced by the neonatal hyperthyroid state *(43)*. Moreover, the direction of the thyroid hormone effect in the hippocampal formation is very much like that of testosterone (T), namely, to increase the size of the dentate gyrus and increase innervation of the CA3 pyramidal neurons *(33)*.

CELLULAR AND MOLECULAR PROCESSES REGULATED BY CIRCULATING HORMONES

There have been a number of discoveries that have revealed a much greater degree of structural plasticity in the adult brain than previously imagined. After the discovery that estrogens regulate synapse density in the adult rat hypothalamic ventromedial nucleus (VMN) in a sexually-dimorphic fashion, we showed that the ovarian cycle regulates cyclic synaptogenesis on excitatory spine synapses in hippocampal CA1 pyramidal neurons *(45)*. Male rats show much less estrogen-induced synapse formation unless they are treated at birth with an aromatase (P450aro) inhibitor, and this suggests that the developmentally regulated estrogen receptors and aromatase activity in hippocampus are involved in programming the response of the adult hippocampus (36,37). One of the surprises of the synaptogenesis story is that estrogen-induction of synapses is blocked by N-methyl-D-aspartate (NMDA) receptor antagonist treatment, indicating that excitatory amino acids and NMDA receptors are involved in synapse formation. Progesterone (PROG) secreted at the time of ovulation appears to be responsible for down-regulation of estrogen-induced synapses in the CA1 region, and the cellular location of the progestin receptors as well as of the estrogen receptors is a prime question.

The hippocampus also undergoes two other forms of plasticity, in which circulating hormones and excitatory amino acids acting via NMDA receptors are involved. One of these is the ongoing neurogenesis in the adult rat dentate gyrus, which continues for at least 1 yr after birth and can be increased either by adrenalectomy or by treatment with an NMDA receptor antagonist (46). Although the male dentate gyrus is larger than that of the female (33), there is no information at present concerning the role of gonadal hormones in adult life in ongoing neurogenesis, although preliminary data has noted sex differences in neurogenesis in the adult prairie vole (42). Dentate gyrus granule neurons innervate the CA3 region of Ammon's horn, and stress causes apical dendrites of CA3 pyramidal neurons to undergo atrophy by a process that is dependent in part on circulating adrenal steroids and in part on excitatory amino acids acting via NMDA receptors (47). Hibernation also causes dendrites of CA3 pyramidal neurons to undergo an atrophy that is reversed within as little as 1 h of wakening (48,49), but the pharmacology of this process is unknown at present. Stress-induced dendritic atrophy is also reversible (Magarinos and McEwen, unpublished), albeit more slowly than after hibernation, but severe and prolonged social stress (in vervet monkeys) and cold-swim stress (in rats) causes CA3 pyramidal neuron loss in males that is not evident in females (50,51). Thus, there is the possibility that intrinsic sex differences in hippocampal morphology or in response to hormones or excitatory amino acids may have a protective role in the female. Besides the larger dentate gyrus of the male (33), male CA3 neurons have more excrescences for mossy fiber contacts, whereas female CA3 apical dendrites are more extensively branched (35).

A NEW VIEW OF HIPPOCAMPAL INTERNEURONS

One of the unique features of estrogen sensitivity of the hippocampus is that the mature CA1 pyramidal neurons, where synapse formation is taking place, do not appear to have intracellular estrogen receptors. Instead, a subset of interneurons express estrogen receptors and/or show specific responses to estrogen treatment that suggest that they are estrogen sensitive (38,39). Because there are many types of interneurons in hippocampus (52–55), the identity of these neuron types is not clear, but among the likely candidates are inhibitory basket cells, neuropeptide Y (NPY)-somatostatin-containing interneurons, and excitatory mossy cells. Although basket cells and chandelier cells are interneurons with relatively local projections, recent evidence indicates that some types of interneurons have much more extensive ramifications than previously suspected and may function independently from the principal neurons (55–57). So-called nonprincipal neurons, including inhibitory interneurons and excitatory mossy cells, contribute to the commissural associational pathway (58) and have extensive, but anatomically specific, ramifications within large regions of the septo-temporal extent of the hippocampus or through its lamellar structure (55,58–60).

Many types of interneurons make gamma-aminobutyric acid (GABA) as a neurotransmitter, along with neuropeptides such as NPY, somatostatin, and cholecystokinin and calcium-binding proteins such as parvalbumin, calbindin, and calretinin (55,61–66). However, GABA does not always function as an inhibitory neurotransmitter: recent evidence suggests that GABA can cause excitation and that this may be related to shifts in anionic gradients (67,68).

Many GABA interneurons receive major input from the ascending serotonergic system of the midbrain raphe, and this innervation is selective for cell type, being predominantly of the calbindin type in CA1 and CA3 and of the nonparvalbumin basket cell or fusiform cell type in the dentate gyrus (69,70). There appear to be two types of serotonin (5HT) effects on interneurons: hyperpolarization through 5HT1A receptors and excitation via 5HT3 receptors (71–74). The former effect would disinhibit by blocking interneuron excitation, whereas the latter effect would excite the interneurons. However, in CA1 there are additional 5HT effects that must be considered: 1. 5HT reduces both fast and slow inhibitory postsynaptic potentials (IPSP) produced by interneurons and does so via 5HT1A receptors (75); 2. CA1 pyramidal neurons are excited by 5HT via 5HT1C or 5HT4 receptors if 5HT1A receptors are blocked (73,76,77). Because turnover in hippocampus is strongly affected by ovarian steroids (see next section), the link between 5HT and the hippocampus via the interneurons is particularly important.

ESTROGEN SENSITIVITY OF AFFERENTS
TO THE HIPPOCAMPUS

Besides interneurons, several afferents to the hippocampus show estrogen sensitivity and must be considered as potential sources of the ovarian hormone regulation of pyramidal neuron function. The entorhinal cortex is the major afferent to the hippocampus (78) in which estrogen receptor-containing neurons have been detected. Estrogen receptors are found in scattered cells in the entorhinal cortex (38,79), and these cells may be interneurons, although a careful neuroanatomical study needs to be carried out. Entorhinal projections via the perforant pathway reach not only the dentate gyrus but also terminate in the CA3 and CA1 fields of Ammon's horn (78).

Another important afferent system is the midbrain serotonergic system, which is regulated by ovarian steroids by as-yet-undefined mechanisms. Findings from numerous studies indicate a sex difference in the central serotonergic system of the adult rat brain, with females displaying elevated 5HT levels, synthesis, and turnover compared to male rats. Higher concentrations of 5HT and/or of the primary 5HT metabolite, 5-hydroxyindolacetic acid (5-HIAA), have been reported in the female rat whole brain (80), forebrain (81), raphe (82), frontal cortex (83), hypothalamus (82–84), and hippocampus (83,85) compared to values measured in the male rat brain. A considerably higher rate of 5HT synthesis has also been reported in the hippocampus of adult female rats (85). A similar sex difference in rat brain 5HT turnover, an indication of serotonergic activity, has also been reported (81,86). Brain 5HT levels and activity are altered during periods of physiological ovarian hormone fluctuation, including the estrous cycle, in the rodent (87–91). In addition, estrogen and/or PROG treatment of ovariectomized rats has been shown to affect positively the serotonergic system of the female rat brain (92–104).

In addition to reporting significant increases in hippocampal serotonin levels and synthesis rate in females, Haleem and colleagues *(85)* found that female rats are much more responsive to the 5HT1A receptor-mediated inhibition of 5HT synthesis. That is, female rats exhibited a percentage decrease in hippocampal 5HT synthesis twice that seen in males, following the administration of the 5HT1A receptor agonist 8 hydroxy-2-(di-n-propylamino) tetralin *(8*-OH-DPAT). This may be partly explained by the finding that estrogen treatment increases the efficiency of the 5HT1A receptor to inhibit cyclic AMP formation in isolated membrane fractions in the hippocampus *(105)*.

Although this ovarian hormone modulation of the central 5HT system is not surprising, the mechanism(s) by which estrogen and PROG exert these neuromodulatory effects remain(s) unknown. Estrogen concentrating cells, determined by autoradiography, have been previously reported in the raphe nucleus in the male and female lizard, Anolis carolinensis, but it was not determined whether the cells were serotonergic *(106)*. Very recently, Bethea *(107)* has demonstrated the presence of estrogen-inducible progestin receptors on a majority of 5HT neurons in the dorsal and ventral raphe of intact, and ovariectomized, estrogen and PROG treated macaques, utilizing a double immunohistochemical procedure, and PROG treatment to estrogen-primed primates increases prolactin release via a serotonergic mechanism *(108,109)*.

NONGENOMIC ACTIONS OF ESTROGENS AND VARIANTS ON THE GENOMIC ACTIONS

The puzzle that estradiol affects hippocampal pyramidal neurons that do not appear to have intracellular estrogen receptors might be explainable if there were cell-surface estrogen receptors. Rapid estrogen effects on CA1 pyramidal neurons of the hippocampus have been described in electrophysiological studies on slices, and these appear to involve non-NMDA excitatory amino acid receptors *(110,111)*, that are very likely to be α-amino-3-hydroxy-5-methyl-4-isoxasole propionic acid (AMPA) receptors *(112)*. One approach to rule in or out of nongenomic actions of estradiol would be to study mice lacking intracellular estrogen receptors *(113)*; however, these mice do have some estrogen binding, although they lack a number of known genomic estradiol actions in the reproductive tract *(113)*. Another approach to discriminate between classical estrogen receptor and membrane estrogen receptor is to use anti-estrogens that bind to the intracellular estrogen receptor, but that do not block the rapid membrane effects *(114)*.

Anti-estrogens also have another use—namely, to discriminate between the response elements that the estrogen receptor uses to activate transcription. Nonsteroidal anti-estrogens bind to estrogen receptors and activate transcription via AP-1 response elements *(115)*, while blocking transcriptional activation through the classical estrogen response element (ERE) and not producing any agonist effect via this pathway *(116)*.

A final note on the question of genomic estrogen receptor is that some cells may express a low level of estrogen receptors that is undetectable by conventional means. Such a possibility has been investigated using a transgenic animal with an estrogen receptor promoter attached to a reporter gene *(117)*. Although the distribution of the estrogen receptor-directed reporter gene generally agrees with the estrogen receptor itself, an overall low level of expression in brain tissue that did not manifest itself as discrete labeled cells keeps open the possibility that a low level of expression of estrogen receptors may exist in ubiquitous cell types, including glia *(117)*.

APPROACHES TO THE STUDY OF SYNAPTOGENESIS IN THE MATURE NERVOUS SYSTEM

Synaptogenesis in the Adult Nervous System

Whereas synapses are formed and eliminated during development, synaptogenesis is believed to be more limited in the adult nervous system. However, recent evidence has shown a greater degree of synaptic turnover than previously believed. Cyclic synaptic turnover in the hippocampus and hypothalamus during the estrous cycle of a female rat shows a high degree of specificity: e.g., in hypothalamus neurons of the VMN show cyclic synaptogenesis directed by ovarian steroids; in CA1 pyramidal neurons, estrogen-induced synaptogenesis occurs on dendritic spines and not on shafts, and there are no estrogen effects on dendritic length or branching; moreover, as far as we can tell, such synaptic plasticity is extremely specific and does not occur on CA3 pyramidal neurons or dentate gyrus granule neurons. The discreteness and specificity of this synapse formation implies that molecular markers may be very specific or subtle and that the mechanism may involve changes in a limited number of cellular events, including transcription of discrete structural genes and posttranscriptional events such as translation of mRNAs for structural proteins. Moreover, local regulation, as via afferent input or interneurons, may be very important.

Role of the NMDA Receptors

Antagonists of NMDA receptors block estrogen-induced synaptogenesis on dendritic spines in ovariectomized female rats. Because estrogen treatment increases the density of NMDA receptors in the CA1 region of hippocampus, it is possible that activation of NMDA receptors by glutamate leads the way in causing new excitatory synapses to develop. Spines are occupied by asymmetric, excitatory synapses, and they are sites of Ca^{++} ion accumulation and thus ideal sites for NMDA receptors *(118)*. NMDA receptors are expressed in large amounts in CA1 pyramidal neurons and can be imaged by conventional immunocytochemistry as well as by confocal imaging, in which individual dendrites and spines can be studied for co-localization with other markers *(119,120)*. NMDA receptor mRNA can also be measured by *in situ* hybridization, and four different forms show different regional patterns and developmental regulation *(121)*. As previously noted, adult CA1 neurons lack detectable estrogen receptors as shown by autoradiography *(38)*, immunocytochemistry *(39)*, or *in situ* hybridization *(122)*, leading to the conclusion that a trans-synaptic mechanism is involved from afferent projections and interneurons or that estradiol acts via a novel nongenomic mechanism, or that there are low and undetectable levels of genomic estrogen receptors. Although there is no basis at present to infer a nongenomic action of estradiol, the trans-synaptic notion is more credible and attractive, because both entorhinal cortex cells and hippocampal interneurons have estrogen receptors and project to the CA1 neurons and provide an anatomical pathway for the trans-synaptic estrogen induction of synapses. It should also be noted that the serotonergic system may play a role (*see* earlier).

NMDA receptors are implicated in other morphogenetic processes in the adult brain, such as suppressing neurogenesis in the dentate gyrus *(46)*, and they are also involved in the developing nervous system as facilitators of neuronal migration *(123,124)*. However, there is a noteworthy paradox, in that NMDA receptors are implicated during visual system development in the reduction of synaptic contact in the developing retinal axon arbors *(125)* and NMDA receptor blockade results in rapid acquisition of dendritic spines by visual thalamic neurons *(40)*. It appears likely that hippocampus and visual-system neurons respond in opposite ways to NMDA receptors, because a recent report on embryonic hippocampal neurons in culture indicates that NMDA receptor blockade prevents estrogen-induced synaptogenesis induced by albeit, very high (μmol) levels of estradiol *(126)*.

One problem with the dissociated cell-culture system for studies of mechanism, as opposed to an anatomically-organized hippocampus, is that cells in culture are difficult to characterize with respect to their neurochemical specialization and their synaptic connections with each other. Moreover, they are more of a model for developmental events, rather than regions- and cell-specific synaptogenesis in the adult hippocampus. Studies on hippocampal slices prepared from postnatal brains may be an useful way of studying the synaptogenesis phenomenon, because slices of the 14-d-old ferret thalamus have been used to study the opposite effect to that in hippocampus, namely a rapid increases in spine density after NMDA receptor blockade, and viable hippocampal slice preparations from 25-d-old rat brains have been described *(127,128)*. A model of synaptogenesis in the hippocampus is presented in Fig. 1, emphasizing the role of NMDA receptors and the possible role of afferents from the entorhinal cortex and 5HT input, as well as the possible role of the interneurons in which the estrogen receptors have been found.

The Functional Significance of Synaptogenesis in the Hippocampus

The functional significance of synaptogenesis in the hippocampal CA1 region has been shown in electrophysiological studies, indicating that estradiol treatment of ovariectomized rats produces a delayed facilitation of synaptic transmission in CA1 neurons that is NMDA-mediated *(111)* and leads to an enhancement of voltage-gated Ca^{++}-currents *(110,111)*. This approach has now been taken to a new level by Woolley *(128a)*, who has used biocytin injection and immunostaining after recording from CA1 pyramidal neurons in order to visualize estradiol-induction of spines. She found that spine density correlates negatively with input resistance and that input/output curves show an increased slope under conditions where NMDA receptor-mediated currents predominate, whereas there is no increased slope where AMPA receptor currents predominate. Moreover, in intact female rats, there is a peak of long-term potentiation (LTP) sensitivity on the afternoon of proestrus in female rats at exactly the time when excitatory synapse density has reached its peak *(129)*. Proestrus is also the time of the estrous cycle when seizure thresholds in dorsal hippocampus are the lowest *(130)*. Because activation of NMDA receptors in hippocampus is enhanced via AMPA receptors in some cases but not in others *(68)*, it remains to be seen how plastic the AMPA receptor system is to ovarian steroid manipulations or whether the estradiol-induced synapses are so-called "silent" synapses or ones in which AMPA receptors are induced by LTP. Blockade of AMPA receptors with NBQX during estradiol treatment failed to block synaptogenesis *(131)*.

Effects of Estrogens on Learning and Memory

Besides reducing seizure thresholds and enhancing LTP in hippocampus, estradiol treatment is reported to exert effects on hippocampal-dependent learning and memory.

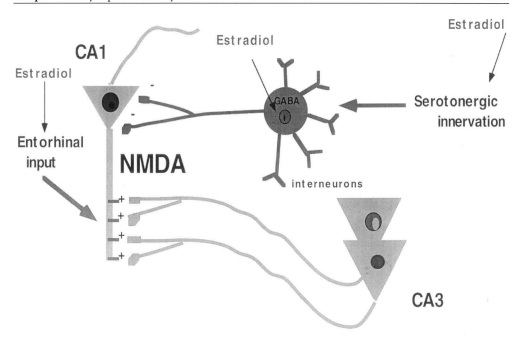

Fig. 1. This model of synaptogenesis in the hippocampus emphasizes the role of NMDA receptors and the possible role of afferents from the entorhinal cortex and serotonin input, as well as the possible role of the interneurons in which the estrogen receptors have been found.

Three types of effects have been reported. First, estradiol treatment of ovariectomized female rats has been reported to improve acquisition on a radial maze task as well as in a reinforced T-maze alternation task *(132,133)*. Second, sustained estradiol treatment is reported to improve performance in a working memory task *(134)* as well as in the radial arm maze *(133,135)*. Third, estradiol treatment is reported to promote a shift in the strategy that female rats use to solve an appetitive two-choice discrimination, with estradiol treatment increasing the probability of using a response as opposed to a spatial strategy *(136)*. Fourth, aging female rats that have low estradiol plasma levels in the estropause are reported to perform significantly worse in a Morris water maze than female rats with high estradiol levels *(137)*. The effects of estrogen replacement in rats are reminiscent of the effects of estradiol treatment in women whose ovarian function has been eliminated by surgical menopause or by GnRH antagonist used to shrink the size of fibroids prior to surgery *(138–140)*. Moreover, these effects are consistent with the findings that estradiol treatment of postmenopausal women appears to have a protective effect on the brain in Alzheimer's disease *(141–145)*. It should also be noted that, in the natural estrous cycle of the female rat, it has been difficult to detect cyclicity of performance in spatial tasks, with either no effect reported *(146)*, or differences reported in motivational or attentional parameters *(147)*, or an impairment reported in performance on proestrus *(148)*. This lack of agreement and paucity of effects may be a reflection of the relative insensitivity of the measures used to detect behaviors that female rats actually use in their natural environments at the time of mating.

MOLECULAR EVENTS ASSOCIATED
WITH SYNAPSE FORMATION

Synapse formation on dendritic spines is a collaborative process involving ingrowth of a presynaptic element on a site where a postsynaptic spine is either present or ready to form *(118)*. There is evidence for a localization of excitatory and inhibitory receptors as clusters opposite to synaptic terminals, and movement of receptors to such clusters is a likely mechanism *(149)*. Division of dendritic spines has been postulated as a mechanism for spine formation, and actin filaments may assist in the division process *(118,150)*. Vacant spines are not seen in vivo, and spine-like processes in cells in culture are much longer than normal spines when they are unoccupied by synapses *(118,126)*. Dendritic spine synapses are overwhelmingly of the Type 1 or asymmetric type and therefore excitatory, although there are occasional synaptic contacts with symmetrical, and therefore inhibitory, synapses on spines with asymmetric synapses, thus providing an excitatory and inhibitory dual control *(118)*.

Presynaptic Markers of Synapses

There are a number of presynaptic molecular markers of synapse formation. GAP43 is a marker of the growth cone and has been shown to increase in the VMN after estrogen treatment *(151)*; however, no studies of this type have been done on the hippocampus. SNAP-25 is a marker of synaptic vesicles *(152,153)*, as are the synaptotagmins *(154–156)*, synaptoporin *(157,158)*, synaptophysin *(159)*, and the synapsins *(160–162)*. Overexpression of synapsins in cultured cells increases synapse formation, suggesting that they may be rate-limiting and that enhanced expression could drive new synapse production *(160,163)*, although synapsins are not essential for synapse formation, because knock-outs lacking two forms of synapsin are viable and form synaptic connections *(161)*.

It is possible to use antibodies to visualize markers of synapses, such as synaptoporin, and of growth cones, such as GAP43, to study reactive synaptogenesis by means of conventional immunocytochemistry and confocal imaging *(164)*. However, to look at the mRNAs for presynaptic proteins, it is necessary to study the cell bodies of afferent projections. Principal afferents to hippocampal CA1 neurons include the Schaffer collateral from CA3 and efferents from the entorhinal cortex *(78)*.

Molecular Events Associated with Dendritic Spine Formation

The estrogen-induced increase in density of dendritic spines on CA1 neurons results in spines that are occupied by synapses; and because estrogen treatment does not reduce the density of shaft synapses, this implies that synapse conversion (shaft to spine) is unlikely and that new spines are formed together with new synapses on the spines. Whether this occurs by a division process or by *de novo* formation, it is likely that new protein components are formed. The postsynaptic machinery for spine formation is believed to center around polyribosomal clusters containing a select population of mRNAs for structural proteins such as MAP-2 *(165)*, ARC *(166)* and BC1 *(167,168)* located in dendrites near the site of dendritic spines. Changes in the expression of these messages or in the translation of proteins in the dendrites might be expected to accompany the formation of new spine synapses. Actin filaments are markers of dendritic spines, and both actin mRNA and MAP-2 mRNA are present in dendrites of hippocampal pyramidal neurons *(165,169,170)*. However, these cytoskeletal markers may be too abundant to be used as a marker of spine formation. Perhaps the most specific markers of dendritic spines thus far described are the a and g1 isoforms of protein phosphatase 1 *(171)*, although an isoform of adenylate cyclase *(172)* and calmodulin-dependent phosphodiesterase also show postsynaptic localization *(173)*.

Involvement of Astroglial Cells

Astrocyte volume in the CA1 region fluctuates in an opposite manner to synapse density, being lowest on proestrus when synapse density is highest *(174)*. On the other hand, in the hilus of the dentate gyrus, the surface area/volume occupied by GFAP-positive processes (an astrocyte marker) is increased on the afternoon and evening of proestrus, more or less in parallel with the increased synapse density *(175)*. There are other instances of increased synaptic density where astrocytic processes increase in parallel *(174,176)*. Do astrocytes contribute to synapse formation? Because astrocytes produce apolipoprotein E (ApoE) *(177,178)*, they are likely to play a role in the formation of membranes via their regulation of cholesterol and fatty acid availability. Indeed, ApoE mRNA levels increase rapidly in response to entorhinal cortex lesions that cause denervation and collateral sprouting within the hippocampus *(177)*. Moreover, ApoE3 stimulates neurite outgrowth in a neuronal cell line *(179)*. ApoE alleles are linked to Alzheimer's disease susceptibility *(180)* and the expression of certain alleles may increase or decrease cytoskeletal protein interactions that lead to formation of neurofibrillary plaques and tangles *(181)*.

Role of Growth Factors

Neurotrophins are expressed in hippocampus, including interneurons *(182)*, and promote cell survival and differentiation *(183)*. At least one neurotrophin, brain-derived neurotrophic factor (BDNF), has been reported to have a putative ERE *(184)*. Neurotrophin expression is regulated in hippocampus by excitatory amino acids released during physiological activity as well as after trauma *(183,185–191)*. Although there have been studies of long-term estrogen regulation of neurotrophin expression in hippocampus and basal forebrain *(192–194)*, no study has thus far considered the rapid estrogen modulation of neurotrophin expression.

CONCLUSIONS

Hormonally-regulated gene expression in the brain is an important mechanism by which the internal environment of the body modifies the structure and function of the brain in response to external demands, and the study of hormone action on brain has provided novel insights for fundamental neuroscience as well as information relevant to reproduction, coping with stressful life experiences, aging, recovery from brain damage, and the pathophysiology of a number of neurological diseases and mental disorders.

From the standpoint of fundamental neuroscience—molecular and cellular neurobiology and endocrinology—hormones have provided many lessons for understanding the mechanism of the regulation of gene expression, and they have provided new insights into the degree and nature of the structural and neurochemical plasticity of the adult as well as developing brain. The hormonally-regulated synaptogenesis and stress-regulated dendritic remodeling in hippocampus—discoveries in our laboratory—are systems in which fundamental mechanisms of cellular plasticity can be studied under physiological conditions.

Hormone actions on the brain have many implications for normal physiology and for disease states. For gonadal hormones, hormonal signaling to the brain is, of course, an essential part of the reproductive process, but there are much broader implications beyond reproduction. Our discovery of estrogen-induced synapse formation in hippocampus and hypothalamus is relevant to postmenopausal changes in brain function, including decline of short-term verbal memory *(195)*, as well as to the occurrence of dementia, which becomes more prevalent in women than in men after the menopause *(141)*. Recent epidemiological studies have suggested a possible protective role for postmenopausal estrogen therapy towards Alzheimer's disease *(142,145)*, whereas estrogen treatment trials have indicated some benefit to demented woman as far as global cognitive function and mood *(196,197)* as well as to normal women *(138–140)* as far as verbal memory. Moreover, estradiol- and PROG-induced regulation of synapse formation and excitability may play a role in catamenial epilepsy, which varies in frequency during the menstrual cycle *(198)*. Sex differences and estradiol effects upon the serotonergic, cholinergic, dopaminergic, and noradrenergic systems all may contribute to many aspects of brain function that are affected by ovarian hormones, including affective state *(199)*, movement disorders *(200)* and cognitive function *(195,201)*. The presence or absence of hormones also contributes to aging of the brain, e.g., loss of hippocampal neurons as a result of elevated glucocorticoid activity *(202,203)*, and consequences of estrogen loss in females, which may include loss of synaptic connections in hippocampus *(204)* or decline in basal forebrain cholinergic function in the absence of circulating estrogens *(205)*.

Sex differences in brain structures and mechanisms are programmed early in life by gonadal hormones and are permanent for the life of the individual. Sex differences occur in other brain regions besides hypothalamus, such as hippocampus, and they appear to be involved in aspects of cognitive function and other processes that go beyond the reproductive process itself. Understanding the cellular and molecular basis of sex differences and of sex differences in the actions of gonadal hormones is vitally important for assessing how pharmaceutical agents differentially affect the brains of males and females *(206)*, as well as in understanding other male–female differences relevant to health and disease, such as the higher incidence of depression in women and of substance abuse in males *(199)*. There are also sex differences in the severity of brain damage resulting from transient ischemia *(207)* and sex differences in the response of the brain to lesions *(208)* and to severe, chronic stress *(50,51)*.

REFERENCES

1. Jensen E, Suzuki T, Kawashima T, Stumpf W, Jungblut W, DeSombre E. A two-step mechanism for the interaction of estradiol with rat uterus. Proc Natl Acad Sci 1968;59:632–638.
2. Yamamoto K. Steroid receptor regulated transcription of specific genes and gene networks. Ann Rev Genet 1985;19:209–252.
3. Miner J N, Diamond MI, Yamamoto KR. Joints in the regulatory lattice: composite regulation by steroid receptor-AP1 complexes. Cell Growth Differ 1991;2:525–530.
4. Becker J, Breedlove SM, Crews D. Behavioral Endocrinology. MIT Press, Cambridge, MA, 1992.
5. McEwen BS, Gould E, Orchinik M, Weiland NG, Woolley CS. Oestrogens and the structural and functional plasticity of neurons: implications for memory, ageing and neurodegenerative processes. In:

Goode J, ed. Ciba Foundation Symposium, vol 191. The Non-Reproductive Actions of Sex Steroids. Wiley, Chichester, UK, 1995, pp. 52–73.

6. McEwen BS, Coirini H, Westlind-Danielsson A, Frankfurt M, Gould E, Schumacher M, Woolley C. Steroid hormones as mediators of neural plasticity. J Steroid Biochem Mol Biol 1991;39:223–232.

7. McEwen BS, Biegon A, Davis P, Krey L, Luine V, McGinnis M, Paden C, Parsons B, Rainbow T. Steroid hormones: humoral signals which alter brain cell properties and functions. Recent Prog Horm Res 1982;38:41–92.

8. Romano GJ, Harlan RE, Shiverst BD, Howells RD, Pfaff DW. Estrogen increases proenkephalin messenger ribonucleic acid levels in the ventromedial hypothalamus of the rat. Mol Endocrinol 1988;2:1320–1328.

9. Simerly RB. Prodynorphin and proenkephalin gene expression in the anteroventral periventricular nucleus of the rat: sexual differentiation and hormonal regulation. Mol Cell Neurosci 1991;2:473–484.

10. Langub MC, Watson RE. Estrogen receptive neurons in the preoptic area of the rat are postsynaptic targets of a sexually dimorphic enkephalinergic fiber plexus. Brain Res 1992;573:61–69.

11. McEwen BS. Cellular biochemistry of hormone action in brain and pituitary. In: Adler N, ed. Primer of Neuroendocrine Function and Behavior. Plenum, New York, NY, 1981, pp. 485–518.

12. Herbison AE. Somatostatin-immunoreactive neurones in the hypothalamic ventromedial nucleus possess oestrogen receptors in the male and female rat. J Neuroendocrinology 1994;6:323–328.

13. Popper P, Priest CA, Micevych PE. Effects of sex steroids on the cholecystokinin circuit modulating reproductive behavior. In: Micevych PE, Hammer RPJ, ed. Neurobiological effects of sex steroid hormones. Cambridge University Press, Cambridge, UK, 1995, pp. 160–183.

14. Akesson TR, Micevych PE. Sex steroid regulation of tachykinin peptides in neuronal circuitry mediating reproductive functions. In: Micevych PE, Hammer RPJ, ed. Neurobiological effects of sex steroid hormones. Cambridge University Press, Cambridge, UK, 1995, pp. 207–233.

15. De Vries GJ. Studying neurotransmitter systems to understand the development and function of sex differences in the brain: the case of vasopressin. In: Micevych PE, Hammer RPJ, ed. Neurobiological Effects of Sex Steroid Hormones. Cambridge University Press, Cambridge, UK, 1995, pp. 254–278.

16. Kow LM, Mobbs CV, Pfaff DW. Roles of second-messenger systems and neuronal activity in the regulation of lordosis by neurotransmitters, neuropeptides and estrogen: a review. Neurosci Biobehav Rev 1994;18:251–268.

17. Carrer H, Aoki A. Ultrastructural changes in the hypothalamic ventromedial nucleus of ovariectomized rats after estrogen treatment. Brain Res 1982;240:221–233.

18. Frankfurt M, Gould E, Wolley C, McEwen BS. Gonadal steroids modify dendritic spine density in ventromedial hypothalamic neurons: a golgi study in the adult rat. Neuroendocrinology 1990;51:530–535.

19. Stephan F. Coupling between feeding-and light-entrainable circadian pacemakers in the rat. Physiol Behav 1986;38:537–544.

20. Forger NG, Breedlove SM. Steroid influences on a mammalian neuromuscular system. Semin Neurosci 1991;3:459–468.

21. Sloviter R, Valiquette G, Abrams G, Ronk E, Sollas A, Paul L, Neubort S. Selective loss of hippocampal granule cells in the mature rat brain after adrenalectomy. Science 1989;243:535–538.

22. Gould E, McEwen BS. Neuronal birth and death. Curr Opin Neurobiol 1993;3:676–682.

23. Harlan RE. Regulation of neuropeptide gene expression by steroid hormones. Mol Neurobiol 1988;2:183–200.

24. McEwen BS, Davis P, Gerlach J, Krey L, MacLusky N, McGinnis M, Parsons B, Rainbow T. Progestin receptors in the brain and pituitary gland. In: Bardin CW, Mauvais-Jarvis P, Milgrom E, eds. Progesterone and Progestin. Raven, New York, NY, 1983, pp. 59–76.

25. McEwen BS, Coirini H, Frankfurt M, Gerlach J, Johnson A, Schumacher M. Neural gonadal steroid receptors and actions: chemical anatomy of the ventromedial hypothalamus in relation to sexual differentiation and sexual behavior. In: Carlstedt-Duke J, Eriksson H, Gustafsson J, eds. The Steroid/Thyroid Hormone Receptor Family and Gene Regulation. Birkhauser, Basel, Switzerland, 1989, pp. 263–270.

26. Schumacher M, Coirini H, Flanagan L, Frankfurt M, Pfaff D, McEwen BS. Ovarian steroid modulation of oxytocin receptor binding in the ventromedial hypothalamus. Ann NY Acad Sci 1992;374–386.

27. McEwen BS, Biegon A, Fischette C, Luine V, Parsons B, Rainbow T. Sex differences in programming of response to estradiol in the brain. In: M Serio, M Motta, M Zanisi, L Martini, eds. Sexual Differentiation. Raven, New York, NY, 1983, pp. 93–98.

28. Eichenbaum H, Otto T. The hippocampus: what does it do? Behav Neural Biol 1992;57:2–36.
29. Gray JA. Precis of the neuropsychology of anxiety: an enquiry into the functions of the septo-hippocamal system. Behav Brain Sci 1982;5:469–534.
30. LeDoux JE. In search of an emotional system in the brain: leaping from fear to emotion and consciousness. In: M Gazzaniga, ed. The Cognitive Neurosciences. MIT Press, Cambridge, MA, 1995, pp. 1049–1061.
31. Phillips RG, LeDoux JE. Differential contribution of amygdala and hippocampus to cued and contextual fear conditioning. Behav Neurosci 1992;106:274–285.
32. McEwen BS, Sakai RR, Spencer RL. Adrenal steroid effects on the brain: versatile hormones with good and bad effects. In: Schulkin J, ed. Hormonally-Induced Changes in Mind and Brain. Academic, San Diego, CA, 1993, pp 157–189.
33. Roof RL. The dentate gyrus is sexually dimorphic in prepubescent rats: testosterone plays a significant role. Brain Res 1993;610:148–151.
34. Juraska J, Fitch J, Washburne J. The dendritic morphology of pyramidal neurons in the rat hippocampal CA3 area II. Effects of gender and the environment. Brain Res 1989;479:115–119.
35. Gould E, Westlind-Danielsson A, Frankfurt M, McEwen BS. Sex differences and thyroid hormone sensitivity of hippocampal pyramidal neurons. J Neurosci 1990;10:996–1003.
36. O'Keefe JA, Handa RJ. Transient elevation of estrogen receptors in the neonatal rat hippocampus. Dev Brain Res 1990;57:119–127.
37. MacLusky N, Clark AS, Naftolin F, Goldman-Rakic PS. Oestrogen formation in the mammalian brain: possible role of aromatase in sexual differentiation of the hippocampus and neocortex. Steroids 1987;50:459–474.
38. Loy R, Gerlach J, McEwen BS. Autoradiographic localization of estradiol-binding neurons in rat hippocampal formation and entorhinal cortex. Dev Brain Res 1988;39:245–251.
39. DonCarlos LL, Monroy E, Morrell JI. Distribution of estrogen receptor-immunoreactive cells in the forebrain of the female guinea pig. J Comp Neurol 1991;305:591–612.
40. Kerr JE, Allore RJ, Beck SG, Handa RJ. Distribution and hormonal regulation of androgen receptor (ar) and ar messenger ribonucleic acid in the rat hippocampus. Endocrinology 1995;136:3213–3221
41. Sherry DF, Jacobs LF, Gaulin SJC. Spatial memory and adaptive specialization of the hippocampus. Trends Neurosci 1992;15:298–303.
42. Galea LAM, McEwen BS. Sex differences in adult neurogenesis in the wild-trapped meadow vole. Abstract Soc Neurosci 1995.
43. Westlind-Danielsson A, Gould E, McEwen BS. Thyroid hormone causes sexually distinct neurochemical and morphological alterations in rat septal-diagonal band neurons. J Neurochem 1991;56:119–128.
44. Gould E, Woolley C, McEwen BS. The hippocampal formation: morphological changes induced by thyroid, gonadal and adrenal hormones Psychoneuroendocrinology 1991;16:67–84.
45. Gould E, Woolley C, Frankfurt M, McEwen BS. Gonadal steroids regulate dendritic spine density in hippocampal pyramidal cells in adulthood. J Neurosci 1990;10:1286–1291.
46. Cameron HA, McEwen BS, Gould E. Regulation of adult neurogenesis by excitatory input and NMDA receptor activation in the dentate gyrus. J Neurosci 1995;15:4687–4692.
47. Magarinos AM, McEwen BS. Stress-induced atrophy of apical dendrites of hippocampal ca3c neurons: involvement of glucocorticoid secretion and excitatory amino acid receptors. Neuroscience 1995;69:89–98.
48. Popov VI, Bocharova LS. Hibernation-induced structural changes in synaptic contacts between mossy fibres and hippocampal pyramidal neurons. Neuroscience 1992;48:53–62.
49. Popov, VI, Bocharova LS, Bragin AG. Repeated changes of dendritic morphology in the hippocampus of ground squirrels in the course of hibernation. Neuroscience 1992;48:45–51.
50. Mizoguchi K, Kunishita T, Chui DH, Tabira T. Stress induces neuronal death in the hippocampus of castrated rats. Neurosci Lett 1992;138:157–160.
51. Uno H, Ross T, Else J, Suleman M, Sapolsky R. Hippocampal damage associated with prolonged and fatal stress in primates J Neurosci 1989;9:1705–1711.
52. Halasy K, Somogyi P. Subdivision in the multiple GABAergic innervation of granule cells in the dentate gyrus of the rat hippocampus. Eur J Neurosci 1993;5:411–429.
53. Amaral DG. A Golgi study of cell types in the hilar region of the hippocampus in the rat. J Comp Neur 1978;182:851.

54. Soriano E, Nitsch R, Frotscher M. Axo-axonic chandelier cells in the rat fascia dentata: Golgi-electron microscopy and immunocytochemical studies. J Comp Neurol 1990;293:1–25.

55. Sik A, Pentonen M, Ylinen A, Buzsaki G. Hippocampal CA1 interneurons: an in vivo intracellular labelling study. J Neuroscience 1995;15:6651–6665.

56. Buckmaster PS, Schwartzkroin PA. Interneurons and inhibition in the dentate gyrus of the rat *in vivo*. J Neurosci 1995;15:774–789.

57. Sik A, Ylinen A, Penttonen M, Buzsaki G. Inhibitory CA1-CA3-Hilar region feedback in the hippocampus. Science 1994;265:1722–1724.

58. Ribak C, Seress L, Peterson GM, Seroogy KB, Fallon JH, Schmued LC. A GABAergic inhibitory component within the hippocampal commissural pathway. J Neurosci 1986;6:3492–3498.

59. Li, X, P Somogyi, J M Tepper, and G Buzsaki 1992 Axonal and dendritic arborization of an intracellularly labeled chandelier cell in the CA1 region of rat hippocampus Exp Brain Res 90:519–525

60. Gulyas A I, Toth K, Danos P, Freund TF. Subpopulations of GABAergic neurons containing parvalbumin, calbindin D28k, and cholecystokinin in the rat hippocampus J Comp Neurol 1991;312:371–378.

61. Nitsch R, Leranth C. Subcortical innervation of hippocampal non-principal cells. Anat Embryol Berlin 1990;181:413–425.

62. Kosaka T, WU JY, Benoit R. GABAergic neurons containing somatostatin-like immunoreactivity in the rat hippocampus and dentate gyrus. Exp Brain Res 1988;71:388–398.

63. Toth K, Freund T. Calbindin D28k containing nonpyramidal cells in the rat hippocampus: their immunocreativity for gaba and projection to the medial septum. Neuroscience 1992;49:793–805.

64. Gulyas AI, Miettinen R, Jacobowitz DM, Freund TF. Calretinin is present in non-pyramidal cells of the rat hippocampus. I. New type of neuron specifically assoicated with the mossy fibre system. Neuroscience 1992;48:1–27.

65. Sloviter RS, Nilaver G. Immunocytochemical localizationof GABA-, cholecystokinin-, vasoactive intestinal polypeptide-, and somatostatin-like immunoreactivity in the area dentata and hippocampus of the rat. J Comp Neurol 1987;256:42–60.

66. Miettinen R, Gulyas AI, Baimbridge KG, Jacobowitz DM, Freund TF. Calretinin is present in non-pyramidal cells of the rat hippocampus- II. Co-existence with other calcium binding proteins and GABA. Neuroscience 1992;48:29–43.

67. Michelson HB, Wong RKS. Excitatory synaptic responses mediated by GABAA receptors in the hippocampus. Science 1995;253:1420–1423.

68. Staley KJ, Soldo BL, Proctor WR. Ionic mechanisms of neuronal excitation by inhibitory GABAA receptors. Science 1995;269:977–985.

69. Halasy K, Miettinen R, Szabat E, Freund TF. GABAergic interneurons are the major postsynaptic targets of median raphe afferents in the rat dentate gyrus. Eur J Neurosci 1992;4:144–153.

70. Freund TF, Gulyas AI, Acsady L, Gorcs T, Toth K. Serotonergic control of the hippocampus via local inhibitory interneurons.Proc Natl Acad Sci USA 1990;87:8501–8505.

71. Ghadimi BM, Jarolimek W, Misgeld U. Effects of serotonin on hilar neurons and granule cell inhibition in the guinea pig hippocampal slice. Brain Res 1994;633:27–32.

72. Ropert N, Guy N. Serotonin facilitates GABAergic transmission in the CA1 region of the rat hippocampus *in vitro*. J Physiol 1994;121–136.

73. Beck SG. 5-Hydroxytryptamine increases excitability of CA1 hippocampal pyramidal cells. Synapse 1992;10:334–340.

74. Zeise ML, Batsche K, Wang RY. The 5-HT3 receptor agonist 2-methyl–5HT reduces postsynaptic potentials in rat CA1 pyramidal neurons of the hippocampus *in vitro*. Brain Res 1994;651:337–341.

75. Schmitz D, Empson RM, Heinemann U. Serotonin reduces inhibition via 5-HT1A receptors in area CA1 of rat hippocampal slices in vitro. J Neurosci 1995;15:7217–7225.

76. Woolley C; McEwen BS. Roles of estradiol and progesterone in regulation of hippocampal dendritic spine density during the estrous cycle in the rat. J Comp Neurol 1993;336:293–306.

77. Andrade R; Chaput Y. 5-Hydroxytryptamine 4-like receptors mediate the slow excitatory response to serotonin in the rat hippocampus. J Pharmacol Exp Ther 1991;257:930–937.

78. Witter MP. Organization of the entorhinal-hippocampal system: a review of current anatomical data. Hippocampus 1993;3:33–44.

79. Sibug RM, Stumpf WE, Shughrue PJ, Hochberg RB, Drews U. Distribution of estrogen target sites in the 2-day-old mouse forebrain and pituitary gland during the 'critical period' of sexual differentiation. Dev Brain Res 1991;61:11–22.

80. Dickinson SL, Curzon G. 5-Hydroxytryptamine mediated behavior in male and female rats. Neurop-harmacology 1986;771–776.

81. Rosencrans JA. Differences in brain area 5-hydroxytryptamine turnover and rearing behavior in rats and mice of both sexes. Eur J Pharmacol 1970;9:379–382.

82. Watts AG, Stanely HF. Indoleamines in the hypothalamus and area of the midbrain raphe nuclei of male and female rats throughout postnatal development. Neuroendocrinology 1984;38:461–466.

83. Kawakami M, Yoshioka E, Konda N, Arita J, Visessuvan S. Data on the sites of stimulatory feeedback action of gonadal steroids indispensable for luteinizing hormone release in the rat. Endocrinology 1978;102:791–798.

84. Carlsson M; Carlsson A. A regional study of sex differences in rat brain serotonin. Prog Neuro-psychopharmacol Biol Psychiat 1988;12:53–61.

85. Halem DJ, Kennett GA, Curzon G. Hippocampal 5-hydroxytryptamine synthesis is greater in female rats than in males and more decreased by the 5-HT_{1A} agonist 8-OH-DPATJ. Neural Transm 1990;79:93–101.

86. Carlsson M, Svensson K, Eriksson E, Carlsson A. Rat brain serotonin: biochemical and functional evidence for a sex difference. J Neural Transm 1985;63:297–313.

87. Biegon A, Bercovitz H, Samuel D. Serotonin receptor concentration during the estrous cycle of the rat. Brain Res 1980;187:221–225.

88. Kueng W, Wirz-Justice A, Menzi R, Chappuis-Arndt E. Regional brain variations of tryptophan, monoamines, monoamine oxidase activity, plasma free and total tryptophan during the estrous cycle of the rat. Neuroendocrinology 1976;21:289–296.

89. Myer DC, Quey WB. Hypothalamic and suprachiasmatic uptake of serotonin in vitro: twenty-four-hour changes in male and proestrus female rats. Endocrinology 1975;98:1160–1165.

90. Uphouse L, Williams J, Eckols K, Sierra V. Variations in binding of (^{3}H)5-HT to cortical membranes during the female rat estrous cycle. Brain Res 1986;381:376–381.

91. Vitali ML, Parisi MN, Chiocchio SR, Tramezzani JH. Median eminence serotonin involved in the proestrus gonadotropin release. Neuroendocrinology 1984;39:136–141.

92. Biegon A, Reches A, Snyder L, McEwen BS. Serotonergic and noradrenergic receptors in the rat brain: modulation by chronic exposure to ovarian hormones. Life Sciences 1983;2015–2021.

93. Chomicka LK. Effect of oestradiol on the responses of regional brain serotonin to stresses in the ovariectomized rat. J Neural Transm 1986;67:267–273.

94. Cone RI, Davis GA, Goy RW. Effects of ovarian steroids on serotonin metabolism within grossly dissected and microdissected brain regions of the ovariectomized rat. Brain Res Bull 1981;7:639–644.

95. Crowley WR, O'Donohue TL, Muth EA, Jacobowitz DM. Effects of ovarian hormones on levels of luteinizing hormone in plasma and on serotonin concentrations in discrete brain nuclei. Brain Res Bull 1979;4:571–574.

96. Di Paolo T, Daigle M, Picard V, Barden N. Effect of acute and chronic 17β-estradiol treatment on serotonin and 5-hydroxy-indole acetic acid content of discrete brain nuclei of overariectomized rats. Exp Brain Res 1983;51:73–76.

97. James MD, Hole DR, Wilson CA. Differential involvement of 5-hydroxytryptamine (5-HT) in specific hypothalamic areas in the mediation of steroid-induced changes in gonadotropin release and sexual behavior in female rats. Neuroendocrinology 1989;49:561–569.

98. Johnson MD, Crowley WR. Acute effects of estradiol on circulating luteinizing hormone and prolactin concentrations and on serotonin turnover in individual brain nuclei. Endocrinology 1983;113:1935–1941.

99. King TS, Steger RW, Morgan WW. Effect of ovarian steroids to stimulate region-specific hypothalamic 5-hydroxytryptamine synthesis in ovariectomized rats. Neuroendocrinology 1986;42:344–350.

100. Ladisich W. Effect of progesterone on regional 5-hydroxytryptamine metabolism in the rat brain. Neuropharmacology 1974;13:877–883.

101. Luine VN, Khylchevcskaya RI, McEwen, BS. Effect of gonadal steroids on activities of monoamine oxidase and choline acetylase in rat brain. Brain Res 1975;86:293–306.

102. Mendelson SD, McKittrick CR, McEwen BS. Autoradiographic analyses of the effects of estradiol benzoate on (^{3}H)-paroxetine binding in the cerebral cortex and dorsal hippocampus of gonadectomized male and female rats. Brain Res 1993;601:299–302.

103. Munaro, NI. The effect of ovarian steroids on hypothalamic 5-hydroxytryptamine neuronal activity. Neuroendocrinology 1978;26:270–276.

104. Walker RF, Wilson CA. Changes in hypothalamic serotonin associated with amplification of LH surges by progesterone in rats. Neuroendocrinology 1983;37:200–205.

105. Clarke WP, Maayani S. Estrogen effects on 5-HT1A receptors in hippocampal membranes from ovariectomized rats: functional and binding studies. Brain Res 1990;518:287–291.

106. Morrell JI, Crews D, Ballin A, Morgentaler A, Pfaff DW. ^{3}H-Estradiol, ^{3}H-testosterone and ^{3}H-dihydrotestosterone localization in the brain of the lizard *Anolis carolinensis*: an autoradiographic study. J Comp Neurol 1979;188:201–244.

107. Bethea CL. Regulation of progestin receptors in raphe neurons of steroid-treated monkeys. Neuroendocrinology 1994;60:50–61.

108. Mistry AM, Voogt JL. Serotonin synthesis inhibition or receptor antagonism reduces pregnancy-induced nocturnal prolactin secretion. Life Sci 1990;47:693–701.

109. Williams RF, Gianfortoni JG, Hodgen GD. Hyperprolactinemia induced by an estrogen-progesterone synergy: quantitative and temporal effects of estrogen priming in monkeys. J Clin Endocrinol Metab 1985;60:126–132.

110. Wong M, Moss RL. Electrophysiological evidence for a rapid membrane action of the gonadal steroid, 17β-estradiol, on CA1 pyramidal neurons of the rat hippocampus. Brain Res 1991;543:148–152.

111. Wong M, Moss RL. Long-term and short-term electrophysiological effects of estrogen on the synaptic properties of hippocampal CA1 neurons. J Neurosci 1992;12:3217–3225.

112. Gu Q, Moss RL. 17β-estradiol potentiates kainate-induced currents via activation of the camp cascade. J Neurosci 1996;16:3620–3629.

113. Korach KS. Insights from the study of animals lacking functional estrogen receptor. Science 1994;266:1524–1527.

114. Mermelstein PG, Becker JB, Surmeier DJ. Estradiol reduces calcium currents in rat neostriatal neurons via a membrane receptor. J Neurosci 1996;16:595–604.

115. Webb P, Lopez GN, Uht RM, Kushner PJ. Tamoxifen activation of the estrogen receptor/ap–1 pathway: potential origin for the cell-specific estrogen-like effects of antiestrogens. Mol Endocrinol 1995;9:443–456.

116. McDonnell DP, Clemm DL, Hermann T, Goldman ME, Pike JW. Analysis of estrogen receptor function *in vitro* reveals three distinct classes of antiestrogens. Mol Endocrinol 1995;9:659–669.

117. Cicatiello L, Cobellis G, Addeo R, Papa M, Altucci L, Sica V, Bresciani F, LeMeur M, Lakshimi-Kumar V, Chambon P, Weisz A. In vivo functional analysis of the mouse estrogen receptor gene promotor: a transgeneic mouse model of study tisse-specific and developmental regulation of estrogen gene transcription. Mol Endocrinol 1995;9:1077–1090.

118. Horner CH. Plasticity of the dendritic spine. Prog Neurobiol 1993;41:281–321.

119. Siegel SJ, Janssen WG, Tullai JW, Rogers SW, Moran T, Heinemann SF, Morrison JH. Distribution of the excitatory amino acid receptor subunits GluR2(4) in monkey hippocampus and colocalization with subunits GluR5–7 and NMDAR1. J Neurosci 1995;15:2707–2719.

120. Siegel SJ, Brose N, Janssen WG, Gasic P, Jahn R, Heineman S, Morrison JH. Regional, cellular, and ultrastructural distribution of N-methyl-D-aspartate receptor subunit 1 in monkey hippocampus. Neurobiology 1994;91:564–568.

121. Monyer H, Burnashev N, Laurie DJ, Sakmann B, Seeburg PH. Developmental and regional expression in the rat brain and functional properties of four NMDA receptors. Neuron 1994;12:529–540.

122. Simerly RB, Chang C, Muramastsu M, Swanson LW. Distribution of androgen and estrogen receptor mrna-containing cells in the rat brain: an *in situ* hybridization study. J Comp Neurol 1990;29:76–95.

123. Komuro H, Rakic P. Selective role of N-type calcium channels in neuronal migration. Science 1995;257:806–809.

124. Komuro H, Rakic P. Modulation of neuronal migration by NMDA receptors. Science 1995;260:95–97.

125. Yen L, Sibley JT, Constantine-Paton M. Analysis of synaptic distribution within single retinal axonal arbors after chronic NMDA treatment. J Neurosci 1995;15:4712–4725.

126. Collin C, Miyaguchi K, Segal M. Dendritic spines in hippocampal neurons: correlating structure and function. Abstract Soc Neurosci 1995;1811.

127. Diekmann S, Nitsch R, Ohm TG. The organotypic entorhinal-hippocampal complex slice culture of adolescent rats. A model to study transcellular changes in a circuit particularly vulnerable in neurodegenerative disorders. J Neural Transm 1994;44:61–71.

128. Yu T, Brown TH. Three-dimensional quantification of mossy-fiber presynaptic boutons in living hippocampal slices using confocal microscopy. Synapse 1994;18:190–197.

128a. Woolley CS, Weiland NG, MCEwen BS, Schwartzkroin PA. Estradiol increases the sensitivity of hippocampal CA1 pyramidal cells to NMDA receptor-mediated synaptic input: correlation with dendritic spine density. J Neurosci 1997;17:1848–1859.

129. Warren SG, Humphreys AG, Juraska JM, Greenough WT. LTP varies across the estrous cycle: enhanced synaptic plasticity in proestrus rats. Brain Res 1995;703:26–30.

130. Terasawa E, Timiras P. Electrical activity during the estrous cycle of the rat: cyclic changes in limbic structures. Endocrinology 1968;83:207–216.

131. Woolley C, McEwen BS. Estradiol regulates hippocampal dendritic spine density via an N-methyl-D-aspartate receptor dependent mechanism. J Neurosci 1994;14:7680–7687.

132. Fader A J, Hendricson AW, Dohanich GP. Effects of estrogen treatment on t-maze alternation in female and male rats. Abstract Soc Neurosci 1996: 1386.

133. Daniel JM, Fader AJ, Spencer A, Wee BEF. Effects of estrogen and environment on radial maze acquisition. Abstract Soc Neurosci 1996;1386.

134. O'Neal MF, Means LW, Poole MC, Hamm RJ. Estrogen affects performance of ovariectomized rats in a two-choice water-escape working memory task. Psychoneuroendocrinology 1996; 21:51–65.

135. Luine VN, Rentas J, Sterbank L, Beck K. Estradiol effects on rat spatial memory. Abstract Soc Neurosci 1996;1387.

136. Korol DL, Couper JM, McIntyre CK, Gold PE. Strategies for learning across the estrous cycle in female rats. Abstract Soc Neurosci 1996;1386.

137. Juraska JM, Warren SG. Spatial memory decline in aged, non-cycling female rats varies with the phase of estropause. Abstract Soc Neurosci 1996;1387.

138. Sherwin BB. Estrogenic effects on memory in women. Ann NY Sci 1994;743:213–231.

139. Robinson D, Friedman L, Marcus R, Tinklenberg J, Yesavage J. Estrogen replacement therapy and memory in older women J Am Geriatr Soc 1994;42:919–922.

140. Sherwin BB, Tulandi T. "Add-Back" estrogen reverses cognitive deficits induced by a gonadot-ropin-releasing hormone agonist in women with leiomyomata uteri. J Clin Endocrinol Metab 1996;81:2545–2549.

141. Birge SJ. The role of estrogen deficiency in the aging central nervous system. In: Lobo RA, ed. Treatment of the Postmenopausal Woman: Basic and Clinical Aspects. Raven, New York, NY, 1994, pp. 153–157.

142. Henderson VW, Paganini-Hill A, Emanuel CK, Dunn ME, Buckwalter JG. Estrogen replacement therapy in older women: comparisons between alzheimer's disease cases and nondemented control subjects. Arch Neurol 1994;51:896–900.

143 Paganini-Hill A, Henderson VW. Estrogen deficiency and risk of alzheimer's disease in women. Am J Epidemil 3;3:3–16.

144. Henderson VW, Watt L, Buckwalter JG. Cognitive skills associated with estrogen replacement in women with alzheimer's disease. Psychoneuroendocrinology 1996;12:421–430.

145. Tang MX, Jacobs D, Stern Y, Marder K, Schofield P, Gurland B, Andrews H, Mayeux R. Effect of oestrogen during menopause on risk and age at onset of Alzheimer's disease. Lancet 1996;348:429–432.

146. Berry B, McMahan R, Gallagher M. The effects of estrogen on performance of a hippocampal-dependent task. Abstract Soc Neurosci 1996;22:1386.

147. Blasberg ME, Stackman RW, Langan CJ, Clark AS. Dynamics of working memory across the estrous cycle. Abstract Soc Neurosci 1996;22:1386.

148. Frye CA. Estrus-associated decrements in a water maze task are limited to acquisition. Physiol Behav 1995;57:5–14.

149. Craig A M, Blackstone CD, Huganir RL, Banker G. Selective clustering of glutamate and γ-amino-butyric acid receptors on opposite terminals releasing the corresponding neurotransmitters. Proc Nat Acad Sci USA 1994;91:12373–12377.

150. Carlin RK, Siekevitz P. Plasticity in the central nervous system: do synapses divide? Proc Nat Acad Sci USA 1983;80:3517–3521.

151. Lustig RH, Hua P, Wilson MC, Frederoff HJ. Ontogeny, sex dimorphism, and neonatal sex hormone determination of synapse-associated messenger RNAs in rat brain. Mol Brain Res 1993;20:101–110.

152. Catsicas S, Larhammar D, Blomqvist A, Paolo Sanna P, Millner RJ, Wilson MC. Expression of a conserved cell-type-specific protein in nerve terminals coincides with synaptogenesis. Neurobiology 1991;88:785–789.

153. Day JR, Min BH, Laping NJ, Martin III G, Osterburg HH, Finch CE. New mRNA probes for hippocampal responses to entorhinal cortex lesions in the adult male rat: a preliminary report. Exp Neurol 1992: 97–99.

154. Vician L, Lim IK, Ferguson G, Tocco G, Baudry M, Herschman HR. Synaptotagmin IV is an immediate early gene induced by depolarization in PC12 cells and in brain. Neurobiology 1995;92:2164–2168.

155. Marqueze B, Boudier JA, Mizuta M, Inagaki N, Seino S, Seagar M. Cellular localization of synaptotagmin i, ii, and iii mrnas in the central nervous system and pituitary and adrenal glands of the rat. J Neurosci 1995;15:4906–4917.

156. Lou X, Bixby JL. Patterns of presynaptic gene expression define two stages of synaptic differentiation. Mol Cell Neurosci 1995;6:252–262.

157. Knaus P, Marqueze-Pouey B, Scherer H, Betz H. Synaptoporin, a novel putative channel protein of synaptic vesicles. Neuron 1990;5:453–462.

158. Marqueze-Pouey B, Wisden W, Malosio Luisa M, Betz H. Differential expression of synaptophysin and synaptoporin mRNAs in the postnatal rat central nervous system. J Neurosci 1991;11:3388–3397.

159. Wiedenmann B, Franke WW. Identification and localization of snyaptophysin, an integral membrane glycoprotein of m_r 38,000 characteristic of presynaptic vesicles. Cell 1985;41:1017–1028.

160. Han H, Nichols RA, Rubin MR, Bahler M, Greengard P. Induction of formation of presynaptic terminals in neuroblastoma cells by synapsin IIb. Nature 1991;349:697–700.

161. Rosahl TW, Spillane D, Missler M, Herz J, Selig DK, Wolff JR, Hammer RE, Malenka RC, Sudhof TC. Essential functions of snyapsins I and II in synaptic vesicle regulation. Nature 1995;375:488–493.

162. Han H, Greengard P. Remodeling of cytoskeletal architecture of nonneuronal cells induced by synapsin. Cell Biol 1994;91:8557–8561.

163. Ferreira A, Han HQ, Greengard P, Kosik KS. Suppression of synapsin II inhibits the formation and maintenance of synapses in hippocampal culture. Proc Nat Acad Sci USA 1995;92:9225–9229.

164. Masliah E, Fagan AM, Terry RD, DeTeresa R, Mallory M, Gage FH. Reactive synaptogenesis assessed by synaptophysin immunoreactivity is associated with GAP–43 in the dentate gyrus of the adult rat. Exp Neurol 1991;113:131–142.

165. Chicurel M, Terrian DM, Potter H. mRNA at the synapse:analysis of a synaptosomal preparation enriched in hippocompal dendritic spines. J Neurosci 1993;13:4054–4061.

166. Lyford GL, Yamagata K, Kaufmann WE, Barnes CA, Sanders LK, Copeland NG, Gilbert DJ, Jenkins NA, Lanahan AA, Worley PF. *Arc*, a Growth factor and activity-regulated gene, encodes a novel cytoskeleton-associated protein that is enriched in neuronal dendrites. Neuron 1995;14:433–445.

167. Tiedge H, Fremeanu RT, Weinstock PH, Arancio OI, Brosius J. Dendritic location of neural BC1 RNA. Proc Nat Acad Sci USA 1991;88:2093–2097.

168. Tiedge H, Zhou A, Thorn NA, Brosius J. Transport of BC1 RNA in hypothalamo-neurohypophyseal axons. J Neurosci 1993;13:4214–4219.

169. Kleiman R, Banker G, Steward O. Subcellular distribution of rRNA and poly(A) RNA in hippocampal neurons in culture. Mol Brain Res 1993;20:305–312.

170. Matus A, Ackermann M, Pehling G, Byers HR, Fujiwara K. High actin concentrations in brain dendritic spines and postsynaptic densities. Proc Natl Acad Sci USA 1982;79:7590–7596.

171. Ouimet CC, Da Curz E Silva EF, Greengard P. The alpha and gamma1 isoforms of protein phosphatase 1 are highly and specifically concentrated in dendritic spines. Proc Nat Acad Sci USA 1995;92:3396–3400.

172. Mons N, Harry A, Dubourg P, Premont RT, Iyengar R, Cooper DMF. Immunohistochemical localization of adenylyl cyclase in rat brain indicates a highly selective concentration at synapses. Proc Nat Acad Sci USA 1995;92:8473–8477.

173. Ludvig N, Burmeister V, Jobe PC, Kincaid RL. Electron microscopic immunocytochemical evidence that the calmodulin-dependent cyclic nucleotide phosphodiesterase is localized predominantly at postsynaptic sites in the rat brain. Neuroscience 1991;44:491–500.

174. Klintsova A, Levy WB, Desmond NL. Astrocytic volume fluctuates in the hippocampal CA1 region across the estrous cycle. Brain Res 1995;690:269–274.

175. Luquin S, Naftolin F, Garcia-Segura LM. Natural fluctuation and gonadal hormone regulation of astrocyte immunoreactivity in dentate gyrus. J Neurobiol 1992;24:913–924.

176. Laping NJ, Teter B, Nichols NR, Rozovsky I, Finch CE. Glial fibrillary acidic protein: regulation by hormones, cytokines, and growth factors. Brain Pathology 1994;1:259–275.

177. Poirier J, Hess M, May PC, Finch CE. Astrocytic apolipopprotein E mRNA and GFAP mRNA in hippocampus after entorhinal cortex lesioning. Mol Brain Res 1991;11:97–106.

178. Poirier J. Apolipoprotein E in animal models of CNS injury and in Alzheimer's disease. Trends Neurosci 1994;17:525–530.

179. Holtzman DM, Pitas RE, Kilbridge J, Nathan B, Mahley RW, Bu G, Schwartz AL. Low density lipoprotein receptor-related protein mediates apolipoprotein E-dependent neurite outgrowth in a central nervous system-derived neuronal cell line. Proc Natl Acad Sci USA 1995;92:9480–9484.

180. Strittmatter WJ, Roses AD. Apolipoprotein E and Alzheimer disease. Neurobiology 1995; 92:4725–4727.

181. Goedert M, Strittmatter WJ, Roses AD. Risky apolipoprotein in brain. Nature 1995;372:45–46.

182. Lauterborn JC, Tran TMD, Isackson PJ, Gall CM. Nerve growth factor mRNA is expressed by GABAergic neurons in rat hippocampus. Neuro Report 1994;5:273–276.

183. Cheng B, Mattson MP. NT–3 and BDNF protect CNS neurons against metabolic/excitotoxic insults. Brain Res 1994;640:56–67.

184. Sohrabji F, Miranda RCG, Toran-Allerand CD. Identification of a putative estrogen response element in the gene encoding brain-derived neurotrophic factor. Proc Nat Acad Sci USA 1995;92:11110–11114.

185. Gall C. Regulation of brain neurotrophin expression by physiological activity Trends Pharmacol Sci 1992;13:401–403.

186. Patterson SL, Grover LM, Schwartzkroin PA, Bothwell M. Neurotrophin expression in rat hippocampal slices: a stimulus paradigm inducing LTP in CA1 evokes increases in BDNF and NT-3 mRNAs. Neuron 1992;9:1081–1088.

187. Lindvall O, Ernfors P, Bengzon J, Kokaia Z, Smith ML, Siesjo BK, Persson H . Differential regulation of mRNAs for nerve growth factor, brain-derived neurotrophic factor, and neurotrophin 3 in the adult rat brain following cerebral ischemia and hypoglycemic coma. Proc Natl Acad Sci USA 1992;89:648–652.

188. Wetmore C, Olson L, Bean AJ. Regulation of brain-derived neurotrophic factor (BDNF) expression and release from hippocampal neurons is mediated by non-NMDA type glutamate receptors. J Neurosci 1994;14:1688–1700.

189. Neeper SA, Gomez-Pinilla F, Choi J, Cotman C. Exercise and brain neurotrophins. Nature 1995;373:109.

190. Kokaia Z, Bengzon J, Metsis M, Kokaia M, Persson H, Lindvall O. Coexpression of neurotrophins and their receptors in neurons of the central nervous system. Proc Natl Acad Science USA 1993;90:6711–6715.

191. Springer JE, Gwag BJ, Sessler FM. Neurotrophic factor mRNA expression in dentate gyrus is increased following in vivo stimulation of the angular bundle. Mol Brain Res 1994;23:135–143.

192. Gibbs RB, Pfaff DW. Effects of estrogen and fimbria/fornix transection on p75NGFr and ChAT expression in the medial septum and diagonal band of broca. Exp Neurol 1992;116:23–29.

193. Gibbs RB, Wu D, Hersh LB, Pfaff DW. Effects of estrogen replacement on the relative levels of choline acetyltransferase, trkA, and nerve growth factor messenger RNAs in the basal forebrain and hippocampal formation of adult rats. Exp Neurol 1994;129:70–80.

194. Singh M, Meyer EM, Simpkins JW. The effect of ovariectomy and estradiol replacement on brain-derived neurotrophic factor messenger ribonucleic acid expression in cortical and hippocampal brain regions of female sprague-dawley rats. Endocrinology 1995;136:2320–2324.

195. Phillips SM, Sherwin BB. Effects of estrogen on memory function in surgically menopausal women. Psychoneuroendocrinology 1992;17:485–495.

196. Fillit H, Weinreb H, Cholst I, Luine V, McEwen BS, Amador R, Zabriskie J. Observations in a preliminary open trial of estradiol therapy for senile dementia–Alzheimer's type. Psychoneuroendocrinology1986;11:337–345.

197. Honjo H, Ogino Y, Naitoh K, Urabe M, Kitawaki J, Yasuda J, Yamamoto T, Ishihara S, Okada H, Yonezawa T, Hayashi K, Nambara T. In vivo effects by estrone sulfate on the central nervous system-senile dementia. J Steroid Biochem Mol Biol 1989;34:521–525.

198. Bonuccelli U, Melis GB, Paoletti AM, Fioretti P, Murri L, Muratoria A. Unbalanced progesterone and estradiol secretion in catamenial epilepsy. Epil Res 1989;3:100–106.
199. Regier DA, Boyd JH, Burke JD, Rae DS, Myers JK, Kramer M, Robbins LN, George LK, Karno M, Locke BZ. One-month prevalence of mental disorders in the US. Arch Gen Psychiat 1988;45:977–986.
200. Bedard P, Langelier P, Villeneuve A. Oestrogens and extrapyramidal system. The Lancet 1977;1367.
201. Kimura D. Sex differences in the brain. Sci Amer 1992;267:119–125.
202. Landfield P. Modulation of brain aging correlates by long-term alterations of adrenal steroids and neurally-active peptides. Prog Brain Res 1987;72:279–300.
203. Sapolsky R. Stress, The Aging Brain and the Mechanisms of Neuron Death. MIT Press, Cambridge, MA, 1992;1–423.
204. Woolley C, McEwen BS. Estradiol mediates fluctuation in hippocampal synapse density during the estrous cycle in the adult rat. J Neurosci 1992;12:2549–2554.
205. Luine VN. Estradiol increases choline acetyltransferase activity in specific basal forebrain nuclei and projection areas of female rats. Exp Neurol 1985;89:484–490.
206. Hamilton JA. Reproductive pharmacology: perspectives on gender as a complex variable in clinical research. Social Pharmacol 1989;3:181–200.
207. Hall ED, Pazara KE, Linseman KL. Sex differences in postischemic neuronal necrosis in gerbils. J Cereb Blood Flow Metab 1991;11:292–298.
208. Morse JK, Dekosky ST, Scheff SW. Neurotrophic effects of steroids on lesion-induced growth in the hippocampus. Exp Neurol 1992;118:47–52.

15 Steroid Effects on Brain Plasticity
Role of Glial Cells and Trophic Factors

Luis Miguel Garcia-Segura, MD
Julie Ann Chowen, MD, *Frederick Naftolin,* MD
and Ignacio Torres-Aleman, MD

CONTENTS

INTRODUCTION
STEROIDS AND GLIA
INTERACTION OF STEROIDS AND GROWTH FACTORS IN THE BRAIN
CONCLUSIONS
REFERENCES

INTRODUCTION

It is well established that circulating steroids produced by the adrenal gland and the gonads affect the development, structure, and function of the central nervous system (CNS). The mechanism of action of hormonal steroids in the brain involves their binding to specific intranuclear receptors that then act as transcription factors for specific genes *(1,2)*. Furthermore, steroid hormones may modulate neuronal excitability by having rapid nongenomic actions *(3)*. Neural activity is also modulated by local steroids that are synthesized de novo in the brain from cholesterol *(4)*. Neurosteroids affect neuronal excitability by modulating calcium channel currents and by acting on GABA and other ionotrophic receptors *(5–10)* (*see* also previous chapters).

To understand the effect of steroids on brain tissue, it is necessary to remember that cellular interactions are fundamental for brain function. Brain activity depends on the coordinated activity of neurons and on the coordinated interaction of neurons with glial cells. Effects of neuroactive steroids on one cell may be transmitted to other cells in the brain, even to those located at a considerable distance. It is now clearly established that in addition to their effects on neurons, circulating steroids *(11,12)* and neurosteroids *(11,13,14)* may affect brain function by acting on glial cells as well. All types of glial cells—microglia, Schwann cells, oligodendroglia, and astroglia—have been shown to be affected by steroids *(11)*. Glial cells in vitro express receptors for gonadal steroids *(15,16)*

From: *Contemporary Endocrinology: Neurosteroids: A New Regulatory Function in the Nervous System* Edited by: E.-E. Baulieu, P. Robel, and M. Schumacher
© Humana Press Inc., Totowa, NJ

and estrogen receptor immunoreactivity has been detected in hypothalamic glia *in situ* *(17)*. Steroid hormones and neurosteroids affect myelination by acting on oligodendrocytes and Schwann cells *(12,18–21)* and modulate the response of nerve tissue to pathological insults by acting on microglia and astroglia *(11,22–24)*. In addition, glial cells participate in the metabolism of hormonal steroids *(25,26)* and in the synthesis of neurosteroids *(27–29)*. Here we focus on a subtype of glial cells, the astroglia, and we examine recent studies that indicate that these cells may mediate steroid effects on neurons through the release of growth factors.

STEROIDS AND GLIA

Effects of Astroglia on Hormonal Steroids and Neurosteroids

Astroglia play a critical role in the CNS by providing metabolites, trophic factors, and neuromodulators to neurons and by regulating extracellular ion concentrations and local cerebral blood flow. Furthermore, recent studies have shown that astroglia have a fundamental role in neural signaling by modulating synaptic transmission and synaptic plasticity. Therefore, astroglia are a crucial element to take into consideration when trying to understand the cellular mechanisms involved in the physiological action of steroids on brain function. It is also important to keep in mind the participation of astroglia in the response to injury, in regard to the therapeutical implications of steroids as promoters of neural regeneration and prevention of neuronal death.

Astroglia in several brain areas are affected by gonadal hormones. For instance, administration of estradiol to adult ovariectomized rats, castration of newborn males and testosterone (T) administration to newborn females result in significant changes in the distribution of the astrocytic marker glial fibrillary acidic protein (GFAP), a specific component of the astroglia cytoskeleton, in the striatum and hippocampus *(11,30)*, whereas castration of adult male rats results in elevated levels of GFAP mRNA in the hippocampus *(31)*. In adult females, the surface density of GFAP-immunoreactive cells in the hilus of the dentate gyrus fluctuates during the estrous cycle following the physiological variations in the circulatory levels of ovarian hormones, decreases after removal of circulating gonadal steroids by ovariectomy, and increases after the pharmacological administration of either 17β-estradiol or progesterone (PROG), but not 17α-estradiol, to ovariectomized animals *(32)*. In contrast to the significant modifications in the surface density of GFAP-immunoreactive cells, the number of GFAP-immunoreactive astrocytes is not affected by experimental manipulations of the levels of gonadal steroids and does not change during the estrous cycle *(32)*. This suggests that differences in the extent of branching and/or immunoreactivity of astrocytic processes are the most likely source for the observed modifications in the surface density of GFAP-immunoreactive cells. This is also supported by studies on explant hippocampal cultures showing that 17β-estradiol and T induce an increase in the growth of GFAP-immunoreactive processes *(14)*. In these cultures, it was also shown that pregnenolone (PREG) and its sulfated derivative induced the growth of GFAP-immunoreactive processes. Thus, the effect of this neurosteroid on hippocampal astroglia was qualitatively similar to that exerted by the gonadal hormones 17β-estradiol and T. In contrast, PREG oleate was without effect on hippocampal astroglia. Dehydroepiandrosterone, in contrast to its effect on primary brain cell cultures where it enhances astroglia differentiation *(33)*, did not affect the extension of GFAP-immunoreactive processes in hippocampal cultures, but induced the forma–

tion of hypertrophied astrocytes, highly immunoreactive for GFAP and with an appearance similar to reactive astroglia *(14)*.

These findings indicate that astroglia are affected not only by peripheral steroid hormones, but also by endogenous steroids. This opens the possibility for interactions among the effects of circulating hormones and endogenous steroids on astroglia. For instance, PROG is among the steroids that induce astroglia plastic changes and this steroid is produced by glial cells from cholesterol *(19,29)* and is also an ovarian hormone that enters the brain from the circulation. PROG and estradiol have complex interactions on astroglia in vivo when both steroids are administered simultaneously to ovariectomized rats. In the hippocampus an initial additive effect during the first 24 h after steroid administration is followed by an antagonistic effect by 48 h *(32)*. In contrast, in the hypothalamus, PROG completely blocks the effect of estradiol on astroglia *(34)*.

The differing effects of PROG on hippocampal and hypothalamic astroglia suggest a heterogeneity in the response of these cells to steroids. This is also supported by the fact that astroglia from the granular layer of the cerebellar cortex of adult female rats fail to respond to natural and experimental changes in gonadal steroids *(32)*. Furthermore, Day et al. *(31)* have detected regional differences in the responses of astroglia to castration and sex hormone replacement in adult male rats. These regional differences in the effects of steroids on astroglia may reflect the existence of astroglia subpopulations with differing degrees of sensitivity to steroids or may be the consequence of neuron to glia interactions (*see* Neuron to Astroglia Signaling Mediated by Adhesion Molecules May Be Implicated in the Effect of Steroids).

Steroids Modulate Astroglia Plasticity after Brain Injury

Gonadal steroids and neurosteroids not only modulate physiological astroglial plasticity, but also affect astroglial responses in pathological conditions *(22,35)*. The effect of steroids on astroglia has been studied in rats after a penetrating injury of the cerebral cortex and hippocampus. Such a lesion results in the proliferation and hypoertrophy of astrocytes in the proximity of the wound. Castration of rats of both sexes increases the proliferation of astrocytes after injury. In contrast, administration of high physiological levels of estradiol or PROG to ovariectomized females, or the administration of T to castrated males, decreases the proliferation and hypertrophy of astrocytes in the injured brain. This effect was observed either after systemic administration of the hormones or after their intracerebroventricular administration. Intracerebroventricular administration of neurosteroids, such as PREG and dehydroepiandrosterone, also decreased astroglial proliferation *(22,22a)*.

The participation of astrocytes in the wounding response is considered to be in part detrimental and in part beneficial for the restoration of functional neuronal circuits after the lesion. Astrocytes located near the site of injury help to restore the structural integrity of the neural parenchyma, are a source of peptides and trophic factors that promote neuronal survival and neuritic growth, and secrete basal lamina components involved in regenerating axonal guidance. On the other hand, the reactive astrocytes form a physical barrier between the wound and the nerve parenchyma that impedes axonal growth. The modulation of reactive gliosis and astrocyte proliferation by gonadal steroids and neurosteroids is of important practical interest because there is limited knowledge regarding substances that reduce astrocyte reaction to injury.

The mechanisms involved in the effect of steroids on astroglia proliferation after brain injury are yet unknown. Recent studies on hippocampal cultured slices *(36)* have revealed that the response of astroglia to neurosteroids and gonadal hormones is affected by the extracellular concentration of K^+. Because extracellular K^+ levels rise in the brain parenchyma after injury, this may be one of the reasons why androgens affect astroglia proliferation after injury, but do not affect astroglia proliferation during normal development of the hypothalamic arcuate nucleus *(37)*.

Astroglia Involvement in Synaptic Plasticity Induced by Sex Steroids and in the Sexual Differentiation of Synaptic Connectivity

As mentioned previously, normal functioning of the brain depends on the existence of a specific pattern of connectivity among neurons. The formation of synaptic connections is affected by gonadal hormones in several brain areas, resulting in specific sex differences in neuronal connectivity that are probably the basis of sex differences in behavior and neuroendocrine function. In addition, synapses are plastic structures that may be modified in the adult brain in response to changing physiological conditions, including modifications in hormone levels (*see* Chapter 13 in this volume).

Cellular mechanisms mediating steroid actions on synapses and glial cells have been extensively studied in the rat arcuate nucleus, a hypothalamic center involved in the feedback regulation of gonadotropins. Perinatal androgens, probably after its conversion to estrogens in the brain *(38)*, induce the sexual differentiation of synaptic connectivity in the arcuate nucleus *(37,39)*. Furthermore, in postpubertal females, there is an estrogen-induced transient disconnection of inhibitory GABAergic inputs to the somas of arcuate neurons during the preovulatory and ovulatory phases of the estrous cycle *(11,40,41)*. This synaptic remodeling is blocked by PROG and begins with the onset of female puberty *(42)*. Astroglia appear to play a significant role in these synaptic changes by stripping off the synaptic terminals from the neuronal surface *(34,42)*. In the afternoon of proestrus, estradiol induces synthesis of GFAP *(34,42,43)* and the growth of glial processes, which ensheathe the neuronal membrane and displace the synaptic terminals. Glial processes retract and synapses reform in the afternoon of estrus *(34,42)*. Similar changes are observed after the administration of estradiol to ovariectomized rats. PROG, in contrast, blocks the effect of estradiol on glial cells and synaptic plasticity *(34,42)*.

Glial cells also may be involved in the organizational effects of sex steroids on brain synaptic connectivity *(37,44)*. Perinatal steroids appear to regulate the number of synaptic inputs to arcuate neurons by affecting the expression of cytoskeletal components of astroglia and the amount of neuronal membrane covered by glial processes and, therefore, the amount of membrane available for the formation of synaptic contacts *(29,44)*.

Neuron to Astroglia Signaling Mediated by Adhesion Molecules May Be Implicated in the Effect of Steroids

The signaling mechanisms involved in the steroid effects on neurons and glia have been investigated in hypothalamic cultures *(42,45)*. Estradiol induces the growth of GFAP immunoreactive astroglial processes in mixed primary cultures of hypothalamic neurons and glial cells. This effect is detected as early as 30 min after the addition of the hormone to the cultures, is dose-dependent, reversible, and specific to hypothalamic cells.

The estradiol-induced growth of astroglial processes in vitro depends on the presence of neurons because it is not observed in pure glial cultures. Moreover, this effect is dependent on preexisting direct membrane-to-membrane contact between living neurons and glia and appears to involve specific hypothalamic neuroglia interactions, because it is not observed in co-cultures of hypothalamic neurons with astroglia from other brain areas *(42,45)*. Furthermore, the expression of a specific form of the neural cell adhesion molecule (N-CAM) on the neuronal membranes is essential for the glial plastic changes induced by estradiol.

N-CAM exists in a variety of isoforms differing in the length of their cytoplasmic domain and/or their carbohydrate content. In embryonic brain, N-CAM is enriched in polysialic acid (PSA). This PSA-N-CAM isoform is gradually replaced in most brain areas during the perinatal and early postnatal periods by less sialylated N-CAM isoforms. However, PSA-N-CAM expression persists in areas of the adult brain that can undergo neuronal-glial changes, such as the hypothalamo-neurohypophysial system, arcuate nucleus, and median eminence.

In hypothalamic monolayer cultures, PSA-N-CAM is expressed on the surface of neurons, whereas astrocytes are not PSA-immunoreactive *(42,45)*. Enzymatic removal of PSA from neuronal surfaces prevents the effect of estradiol on astroglial shape but not the effect of other signals such as fibroblast growth factor, which act directly on astroglia *(42,45)*. This indicates that PSA-N-CAM on the neuronal surface is necessary for the manifestation of the hormonal effect on astroglia and suggests that a neuron to glia signaling pathway, mediated by adhesion molecules, participates in the plastic effects of gonadal hormones. The role of PSA-N-CAM on astroglia shape changes may be related, in part, to a modulation of cell adhesion properties. PSA can exert broad steric effects at the cell-surface and may modulate not only the homophilic binding of N-CAM to other N-CAM molecules, but the interaction of other cell-surface molecules as well. In addition, the role of PSA may be related to the activation of second messenger pathways *(42,45)*.

INTERACTION OF STEROIDS AND GROWTH FACTORS IN THE BRAIN

Steroid Effects May Be in Part Mediated by Trophic Factors

In addition to direct neuron to glia signaling mediated by adhesion molecules, soluble factors may also be involved in the effects of steroids on brain cells. Glial cells may release different growth factors that could alter neuronal function and that may be involved in the regulation of synaptic connectivity. For instance, it has been shown that estrogen receptors co-localize with low-affinity nerve growth factor (NGF) receptors in cholinergic neurons of the basal forebrain of developing rodents *(46)* and that estrogen modulates the expression of transforming growth factor-α (TGFα) in the hypothalamus *(47)* and the levels of NGF receptors in PC12 cells and dorsal root ganglion neurons of adult female rats *(48,49)*. Furthermore, astroglia are a source of trophic factors, such as TGF-α and -β, and insulin-like growth factor I (IGF-I), substances that may mediate some of the neuroendocrine effects of gonadal hormones *(47,50–52)*.

We have recently studied the interaction of gonadal hormones with IGF-I. This factor has paracrine trophic effects on neural cells and also acts as a hormonal signal involved in the regulation of hypothalamic hormone secretion. IGF-I is locally synthesized by glia and neurons of the hypothalamus and other brain areas *(53,54)* and has prominent trophic actions, including stimulation of survival, proliferation and differentiation of specific neural cell populations *(55,56)*. IGF-I may also participate in neuroendocrine events at the level of the hypothalamus because it has been shown to be involved in the feed-beck regulation of growth hormone by affecting the synthesis or the release of growth hormone-releasing hormone and somatostatin by hypothalamic neurons *(57,58)*. IGF-I may also affect the reproductive axis by modulating the secretion of gonadotrophin-releasing hormone by hypothalamic cells and, therefore, the release of gonadotrophins *(50,59)*.

In several tissues, such as rodent uterus and pituitary, and in several cell types, such as human breast cancer cells, estrogen up-regulates IGF-I gene expression *(60–65)* and modulates IGF-I action by affecting the levels of IGF-I receptors *(66)* and IGF binding proteins (IGFBPs) *(67–70)*. Likewise, IGF-I may regulate steroid hormone action by stimulating the synthesis of steroid hormones *(71–73)* and steroid hormone receptors *(74–76)*. In addition, estrogen and anti-estrogens regulate several cellular responses induced by IGF-I *(74,77–79)*. As in other cell types, IGF-I and estrogen may have interactive effects on neurons. The first evidence was provided by Toran-Allerand and coworkers *(80)*, showing that in explant cultures of fetal rodent hypothalamus, estrogen, and insulin have synergistic effects on neurite growth, an effect probably mediated by IGF-I receptors. More recent data from our laboratory indicates that estrogen modulates IGF-I receptors and binding proteins in monolayer hypothalamic cultures *(81)*.

Trophic Effects of Estradiol
on Hypothalamic Neurons are Mediated by IGF-I

We have recently studied whether the effects of estrogen on hypothalamic neuronal survival and neurite growth are mediated by IGF-I *(82)*. Hypothalamic cultures exposed to estradiol or IGF-I showed a significant increase in neuronal survival and in the growth of MAP-2 immunoreactive processes. The simultaneous incubation of cultures with 17β-estradiol and IGF-I also resulted in increased neuronal survival and differentiation. The effect of estradiol and IGF-I acting together was similar to that observed when cultures were treated separately with either factor. Therefore, the effects of 17β-estradiol and IGF-I were not additive, suggesting that both factors may be acting through a common mechanism. We decided to test whether the effect of estradiol was dependent on IGF-I synthesis. Incubation of the cultures with an antisense oligonucleotide to IGF-I resulted in a significant decrease in the stimulatory effects of 17β-estradiol on the number of neurons and the extension of neuronal processes *(82)*. These results indicate that IGF-I synthesis in the cultures is necessary for the manifestation of the sex steroid effect, suggesting that estradiol may induce neuronal survival and differentiation by the activation of IGF-I signaling cascades.

Trophic Effects of IGF-I
on Hypothalamic Neurons are Mediated by Estrogen Receptors

Recent studies indicate that IGF-I *(83–88)* and other trophic factors may activate the estrogen receptor in different cell types. Activation of the estrogen receptor appears to be essential for the mitogenic effect of IGF-I on the prolactin-secreting, pituitary tumor cell line GH3 *(87)* and for the IGF-I induced growth and differentiation of the human neuroblastoma cell line SK-ER3 *(86)*. In uterine cell cultures transfected with a simple estrogen-responsive reporter gene, not only estrogen, but also IGF-I is able to stimulate estrogen receptor-mediated trans-activation and estrogen receptor phosphorylation, suggesting that IGF-I could be acting to stimulate estrogen receptor-mediated transcription in these cells through direct modification of the estrogen receptor protein *(83)*. This activation of the estrogen receptor occurs in the absence of the hormone *(83–88)*, is mediated by the membrane-associated receptor tyrosine kinase-Ras-Raf-mitogen-activated protein kinase cascade *(85,88)*, involves the activation function 2 domain of the estrogen receptor in neuroblastoma cells *(88)*, and the activation function 1 domain in other cell types *(84,85)*.

Based on these studies, we decided to determine if the effect of IGF-I on the survival and differentiation of hypothalamic neurons was dependent on the estrogen receptor *(82)*. Hypothalamic cultures were incubated with IGF-I in the presence of the pure estrogen receptor antagonist ICI 182,780 or an antisense oligodeoxynucleotide to the estrogen receptor. A nonsense sequence was used as a control. Both the antisense oligonucleotide directed against the estrogen receptor and the estrogen receptor antagonist ICI 182,780 blocked the effects of estradiol and IGF-I. These parameters were not significantly affected by the nonsense control sequence *(82)*. This indicates that estrogen receptors are necessary for the action of IGF-I on hypothalamic survival and neuritic growth. A possible explanation of these results is that IGF-I may activate, either directly or indirectly, estrogen receptors in hypothalamic neurons.

IGF-I Receptors are Involved in the Activation of Astroglia by Estradiol

One of the most prominent effects of estrogen on the hypothalamic arcuate nucleus is the increase in GFAP levels that occurs on the afternoon of proestrus *(34,42,43)*. The estrogen-induced increase in GFAP protein and mRNA levels during the afternoon of proestrus is associated with the redistribution of astroglia cytoskeletal components, the growth of astroglial processes, the ensheathing of neuronal somas by glial processes, and the transient disconnection of inhibitory GABAergic synapses from neuronal somas by the interposed glial processes. These changes are also elicited by the administration of estradiol to adult ovariectomized rats *(34,42)*.

We have recently tested whether astroglia activation by estrogen in arcuate nucleus is dependent on IGF-I. Hypothalamic tissue fragments from ovariectomized rats, containing the arcuate nucleus and the median eminence, were incubated in an artificial cerebrospinal fluid for 6 h in the presence or in the absence of estradiol. In contrast to what is observed in vivo, the hormone was unable to induce a significant increase in GFAP immunoreactive levels. However, when insulin was present in the medium, estradiol was able to induce an increase in GFAP immunoreactivity *(88a)*. The effect of estradiol in the presence of insulin was blocked by a specific IGF-I receptor antagonist peptide *(89)*. These findings suggest that the effect of estradiol on arcuate nucleus astroglia depends on the activation of IGF-I receptors. However, insulin at concentrations that act on IGF-I receptors was unable to induce an increase in GFAP immunoreactive levels, suggesting that activation of IGF-I receptors by itself is not enough to activate glial cells. This further supports the existence of coordinated cross-talk between the IGF-I and estradiol signaling pathways in the hypothalamus.

Steroids Modulate IGF-I Levels in Astroglia in the Hypothalamus

Studies in vivo also suggest an interaction of IGF-I with gonadal steroids and an active participation of glial cells in this interaction. Tanycytes, a specific form of astroglia present in the arcuate nucleus and median eminence, are IGF-I immunoreactive (90). IGF-I immunoreactive levels in tanycytes show sex differences in the rat arcuate nucleus, with adult females showing significantly lower IGF-I levels than males of the same age. This sex difference is abolished by early postnatal androgenization of females (90), suggesting that it may be dependent on the burst of androgen production by the testis of developing rats that occurs perinatally. Furthermore, IGF-I levels in tanycytes increase in male and female rats at the time of puberty. Females show an abrupt increase in IGF-I immunoreactive levels in tanycytes between the morning and the afternoon of the first proestrus. Henceforth, IGF-I immunoreactivity fluctuates according to the different stages of the estrus cycle. IGF-I immunoreactive levels are high in the afternoon of proestrus, after the peak of estrogen in plasma, remain increased by the morning of the following day and then decrease to basal conditions by the morning of metestrus (90). In addition, IGF-I levels decrease in tanycytes when gonadal steroid levels are reduced by ovariectomy and increase in a dose-dependent manner when ovariectomized rats are injected with 17β-estradiol (90).

Tanycytes are specialized astroglia cells whose function is still unclear. It has been proposed that these cells may be involved in endocrine regulation (22,47,91). This function may be mediated in part by the transport by tanycytes of substances from the cerebrospinal fluid or from the capillaries of the median eminence to the brain parenchyma. In agreement with this possibility, previous studies have shown that tanycytes are able to take up β-endorphin from the cerebrospinal fluid (92). Furthermore, processes of tanycytes are closely associated with neurosecretory terminals in the median eminence (93,94). Encapsulation of neurosecretory terminals by tanycyte endfeet may regulate neuronal contact with portal capillaries (93,95–97) and may also result in a focal concentration of factors, such as IGF-I that may affect neurohormone release. In addition to IGF-I other factors may be involved in the endocrine effects of tanycytes. Ma et al. (47) have reported a marked increase in TGF-α gene expression in tanycytes during the initiation of puberty in the rat. TGF-α mRNA levels increase gradually after the anestrous phase of puberty, reaching peak values on the afternoon of the first proestrus.

An interesting question in regard to the hormonal-induced changes in IGF-I immunoreactivity in tanycytes is the source of IGF-I. Because tanycytes do not express mRNA for IGF-I (90), the modifications in IGF-I levels may be the result of the hormonal modulation of its uptake from blood or cerebrospinal fluid. To test this possibility, IGF-I was labeled with digoxigenin and injected intravenously or in the lateral cerebral ventricle. In both cases, we found that various subsets of neurons and glial cells throughout the CNS, including tanycytes, specifically accumulate the labeled IGF-I (98). The accumulation of IGF-I was specific because it was substantially decreased by the administration of unlabeled IGF-I or unlabeled insulin, which also acts on IGF-I receptors (90), and was blocked by the specific IGF-I receptor antagonist JB1 (98). The distribution of IGF-I accumulating cells varied depending on the time after the intravenous administration of labeled IGF-I. By 5 min, IGF-I accumulation was observed in the choroid plexus, median eminence, and area postrema, structures with high local levels of IGF-I receptors. By 90 min, IGF-I was accumulated in cells located in different CNS areas, such as the olfactory bulb, cerebral cortex, striatum, islands of Calleja, hippocampal formation, habenula, hypothalamus, midbrain, cerebellum, pons, medulla oblongata, and spinal cord. The time elapsed between the intravenous injection of the peptide and the labeling of many brain areas suggests that the peptide is first taken up by areas devoid of blood brain barrier and then released to the cerebral ventricles. IGF-I may then be accumulated by specialized cells such as ependymal cells and tanycytes.

In 1974, Brawer et al. *(99)* reported ultrastructural modifications in the ventricular surface of tanycytes in the arcuate nucleus of female rats at different stages of the estrous cycle. The number of microvilli increases during proestrus, remains elevated during estrus, and decreases in metestrus. The significance of these changes is still unknown, but may well be related to the uptake of substances from the cerebrospinal fluid. By using colloidal gold ultrastructural immunolocalization techniques, we have recently observed that the IGF-I receptor is enriched in the microvilli of tanycytes (L. M. Garcia-Segura et al., unpublished results). Therefore, changes in the extension of microvilli may be related to changes in the number of IGF-I receptors exposed in the lumen of the third ventricle and this, in turn, may influence the uptake of IGF-I by tanycytes. In order to test whether IGF-I uptake by tanycytes fluctuates during the different stages of the estrous cycle, we injected IGF-I labeled with digoxigenin in the lateral cerebral ventricle of cycling female rats *(98)*. Six animals were injected for each day of the estrous cycle, three of them in the morning and the other three in the afternoon. Animals were killed 1 h after the injection and the number of digoxigenin-labeled tanycytes was counted *(98)*.

The number of tanycytes labeled with digoxigenin showed prominent changes according to the different phases of the estrous cycle. Compared with diestrus and metestrus, the number of labeled tanycytes showed a significant decrease in the afternoon of proestrus. A recover in IGF-I accumulation was observed by the morning of estrus, and this was followed by a significant increase by the afternoon of estrus *(98)*.

The decrease in the number of tanycytes that accumulate digoxigenin-labeled IGF-I in the afternoon of proestrus was unexpected, since at this stage of the estrous cycle there is a significant increase in IGF-I immunoreactivity in these cells *(90)*. Differences in IGF-I accumulation most likely reflect differences in IGF-I transport and release and not only differences in IGF-I uptake. It is therefore possible that the rate of transport and release of IGF-I to cerebral parenchyma is increased in the afternoon of proestrus. Another possible explanation is that exogenous IGF-I had to compete with increased levels of endogenous IGF-I. Further studies are necessary to determine the cause of the differences observed in the number of tanycytes that accumulate IGF-I after its intracerebroventricular injection. Nevertheless, these findings suggest that tanycytes may play a key role in the neural effects of gonadal steroids, by regulating the availability of IGF-I to hypothalamic neurons.

CONCLUSIONS

In summary, the data examined in this chapter indicate that neurosteroids and hormonal steroids affect brain function not only by direct effects on neurons, but also that glial cells may participate in the effects of neuroactive steroids by modulating neuronal responses under physiological and pathological conditions. Gonadal steroids and neurosteroids promote astroglia plasticity in several areas of the CNS, including the hypothalamus, the striatum, and the hippocampus, and modulate astroglia proliferation and the formation of reactive astroglia after brain injury. Under physiological conditions, the effects of steroids on astroglia may be involved in the sexual differentiation of synaptic connectivity and in synaptic plastic events during adult life. Recent evidence indicates that the effects of neuroactive steroids in brain may be in part mediated by growth factors, such as IGF-I. Astroglia also may play a crucial role by regulating the availability of such factors to neurons.

ACKNOWLEDGMENTS

This work was supported by Fundación Ramón Areces, DGICYT, NIH (HD13587), and Fundación Endocrinologia y Nutrición.

REFERENCES

1. Beato M. Gene regulation by steroid hormones. Cell 1989;56:335–344.
2. Evans RM. The steroid and thyroid hormone receptor superfamily. Science 1988;240:889–895.
3. McEwen BS. Non-genomic and genomic effects of steroids on neural activity. Trends Pharmacol Sci 1991;12:141–147.
4. Baulieu EE, Robel P. Neurosteroids: a new brain function? J Steroid Biochem Mol Biol 1990,37:395403.
5. ffrench-Mullen J, Danks P, Spence KT. Neurosteroids modulate calcium currents in hippocampal CA1 neurons via a pertussis toxin-sensitive G-protein-coupled mechanism. J Neurosci 1994;14:1963–1977.
6. Lambert JJ, Peters J, Cottrell A. Actions of synthetic and endogenous steroids on the GABA$_A$ receptor. Trends Pharmacol Sci 1987;8:224–227.
7. Majewska MD. Neurosteroids: endogenous bimodal modulators of the GABA$_A$ receptor. Mechanism of action and physiological significance. Prog Neurobiol 1992;38:379–395.
8. Meyer JH, Gruol DL Dehydroepiandrosterone sulfate alters synaptic potentials in area CA1 of the hippocamapal slice. Brain Res 1994;633:253–261.
9. Puia G, Santi MR, Vicini S, Pritchett DB, Purdy RH, Paul SM, Seeburg PH, Costa E. Neurosteroids act on recombinant GABA$_A$ receptors. Neuron 1990;4:759–765.
10. Wu F, Gibbs TT, Farb DH. Pregnenolone sulfate: a positive allosteric modulator at the N-methyl-D-aspartate receptor. Mol Pharmacol 1991;40:333–336.
11. Garcia-Segura LM, Chowen JA, Naftolin F. Endocrine glia: roles of glial cells in the brain actions of steroid and thyroid hormones and in the regulation of hormone secretion. FrontNeuroendocrinol 1996;17:180–211.
12. Jung-Testas I, Schumacher M, Robel P, Baulieu EE. Actions of steroid hormones and growth factors on glial cells of the central and peripheral nervous system. J Steroid Biochem Mol Biol 1994;48:145–154.
13. Chvatal A, Kettenmann H. Effects of steroids on gamma-aminobutyrate-induced currents in cultured rat astrocytes. Pflugers Arch 1991;419:263–266.
14. Del Cerro S, Garcia-Estrada J, Garcia-Segura LM. Neuroactive steroids regulate astroglia morphology in hippocampal cultures from adult rats. Glia 1995;14:65–71.
15. Jung-Testas I, Renoir JM, Gasc JM, Baulieu EE. Estrogen-inducible progesterone receptor in primary cultures of rat glial cells. Exp Cell Res 1991;193:12–19.
16. Santagati S, Melcangi RC, Celotti F, Martini L, Maggi A. Estrogen receptor is expressed in different types of glial cells in culture. J Neurochem 1994;63:2058–2064.
17. Langub MC, Watson RE. Estrogen receptor-immunoreactive glia, endothelia, and ependyma in guinea pig preoptic area and median eminence: electron microscopy. Endocrinology 1992; 130:364–372.
18. Jung-Testas I, Schumacher M, Bugnard H, Baulieu EE. Stimulation of rat Schwann cell proliferation by estradiol: synergism between the estrogen and cAMP. Dev Brain Res 1993;72:282–290.
19. Koenig HL, Schumacher M, Ferzaz B, Do Thi AN, Ressouches A, Guennoun R, Jung-Testas I, Robel P, Akwa Y, Baulieu EE. Progesterone synthesis and myelin formation by Schwann cells. Science 1995; 268:1500–1503.
20. Kumar S, Cole R, Chiappelli F, de Vellis J. Differential regulation of oligodendrocyte markers by glucocorticoids: post-transcriptional regulation of both proteolipid protein and myelin basic protein and transcriptional regulation of glycerol phosphate dehydrogenase. Proc Natl Acad Sci USA 1989;86:6807–6811.

21. Tsuneishi S, Takada S, Motoike T, Ohashi T, Sano K, Nakarnura H. Effects of dexamethasone on the expression of myelin basic protein, proteolipid protein, and glial fibrillary acidic protein genes in developing rat brain. Dev Brain Res 1991;61:117–123.

22. Garcia-Estrada J, Del Rio JA, Luquin S, Soriano E, Garcia-Segura LM. Gonadal hormones down-regulate reactive gliosis and astrocyte proliferation after a penetrating brain injury. Brain Res 1993;628:271–278.

22a. Garcia-Estrada J, Luquin S, Fernández AM, Garcia-Sequra LM. Dehydroepiandrosterone, pregnenolone and sex steroids down-regulate reactive astroglia in the male rat brain after a penetrating brain injury. Int J Dev Neurosci, 1999;17:145–151.

23. Genter S, Northoff H, Mannel D, Gebicke-Harter PJ. Growth control of cultured microglia. J Neursosci Res 1992;33:218–230.

24. Keifer R, Kreutzberg GW. Effects of dexamethasone on microglial activation in vivo: selective down regulation of major histocompatibility complex class II expression in regenerating facial nucleus. J Neuroinmunol 1991;34:99–108.

25. Melcangi RC, Celotti F, Castano P, Martini L Intracellular signalling systems controling the 5α-reductase in glial cell cultures. Brain Res 1992;585 :411–415.

26. Melcangi RC, Celotti F, Castano P, Martini L Differential localization of the 5α-reductase and the 3α-hydroxysteroid dehydrogenase in neuronal and glial cultures. Endocrinology 1993; 132:1252–1259.

27. Akwa Y, Sananes N, Gouezou M, Robel PI, Baulieu EE, Le Goascogne C. Astrocytes and neurosteroids: Metabolism of pregnenolone and dehydroepiandrosterone. Regulation by cell density. J Cell Biol 1993;121:135–143.

28. Hu ZY, Bourreau E, Jung-Testas I, Robel P, Baulieu EE. Neurosteroids: Oligodendrocyte mitochondria convert cholesterol to pregnenolone. Proc Natl Acad Sci USA 1987;84:8215–8219.

29. Jung-Testas I, Hu ZY, Baulieu EE, Robel P. Neurosteroids: Biosynthesis of pregnenolone and progesterone in primary cultures of rat glial cells. Endocrinology 1989;125 :2083–2091.

30. Garcia-Segura LM, Suarez I, Segovia S, Tranque PA, Cales JM, Aguilera P, Olmos G, Guillamon A. The distribution of glial fibrillary acidic protein in the adult rat brain is influenced by the neonatal levels of sex steroids. Brain Res 1988;456:357–363.

31. Day JR, Laping NJ, Lampert-Etchells M, Brown SA, O'Callaghan JP, McNeill TH, Finch CE. Gonadal steroids regulate the expression of glial fibrillary acidic protein in the adult male rat hippocampus. Neuroscience 1993;55:435–443.

32. Luquin S, Naftolin F, Garcia-Segura LM. Natural fluctuation and gonadal hormone regulation of astrocyte immunoreactivity in dentate gyrus. J Neurobiol 1993;24:913–924.

33. Bologa L, Sharma J, Roberts E. Dehydroepiandrosterone and its sulfated derivative reduce neuronal death and enhance astrocytic differentiation in brain cell cultures. J Neurosci Res 1987;17:225–234.

34. Garcia-Segura LM, Luquin S, Parducz A, Naftolin F. Gonadal hormone regulation of glial fibrillary acidic protein immunoreactivity and glial ultrastructure in the rat neuroendocrine hypothalamus. Glia 1994;10:59–69.

35. Day JR, Laping NJ, McNeil TH, Schreiber SS, Pasinetti G, Finch CE. Castration enhances expression of glial fibrillary acidic protein and sulfated glycoprotein-2 in the intact and lesion-altered hippocampus of the adult male rat. Mol Endocrinol 1990;4: 1995–2002.

36. Del Cerro S, Garcia-Estrada J, Garcia-Segura LM. Neurosteroids modulate the reaction of astroglia to high extracellular potassium levels. Glia 1996;18:293–305.

37. Garcia-Segura LM, Duenas M, Busiguina S, Naftolin F, Chowen JA. Gonadal hormone regulation of neuronal-glial interactions in the developing neuroendocrine hypothalamus. J Steroid Biochem Molec Biol 1995,53 :293–298.

38. Naftolin F, MacLusky NJ. Aromatization hypothesis revisited. In: Serio M, Motta M, Zanisi M, Martini L, eds. Sexual differentiation: Basic and Clinical Aspects, Raven, New York, NY, 1984, pp. 79–82.

39. Matsumoto A. Synaptogenic action of sex steroids in developing and adult neuroendocrine brain. Psychoneuroendocrinology 1991;16: 25–40.

40. Olmos G, Naftolin F, Pérez J, Tranque PA, Garcia-Segura LM. Synaptic remodelling in the rat arcuate nucleus during the estrous cycle. Neuroscience 1989;32:663–667.

41. Párducz A, Pérez J, Garcia-Segura LM. Estradiol induces plasticity of GABAergic synapses in the hypothalamus. Neuroscience 1993;53:395–401.

42. Garcia-Segura LM, Chowen JA, Parducz A, Naftolin F. Gonadal hormones as promoters of structural synaptic plasticity: cellular mechanisms. Prog Neurobiol 1994;44: 279–307.

43. Kohama SG, Goss JR, McNeill TH, Finch CE. Glial fibrillary acidic protein mRNA increases at proestrus in the arcuate nucleus of mice. Neurosci Lett 1995;183:164–166.

44. Chowen JA, Busiguina S, Garcia-Segura LM. Sexual dimorphism and sex steroid modulation of glial fibrillary acidic protein messenger RNA and immunoreactive levels in the rat hypothalamus. Neuroscience 1995,69:519–532.

45. Garcia-Segura LM, Cañas B, Parducz A, Rougon G, Theodosis D, Naftolin F, Torres-Aleman I. Estradiol promotion of changes in the morphology of astroglia growing in culture depends on the expression of polysialic acid on neuronal membranes. Glia 1995;13:209–216.

46. Toran-Allerand CD, Miranda RC, Bentham W, Sohrabji F, Brown EJ, Hochberg RB, MacLusky NJ. Estrogen receptors co-localize with low-affinity NGF receptors in cholinergic neurons of the basal forebrain. Proc Natl Acad Sci USA 1992;89:4668–4672.

47. Ma YJ, Junier MP, Costa ME, Ojeda SR. Transforming growth factor-α gene expression in the hypothalamus is developmentally regulated and linked to sexual maturation. Neuron 1992,9: 657–670.

48. Sohrabji F, Greene LA, Miranda RC, Toran-Allerand D. Reciprocal regulation of estrogen and NGF receptors by their ligands in PC12 cells. J Neurobiol 1994;25:974–988.

49. Sohrabji F, Miranda C, Toran-Allerand CD. Estrogen differentially regulates estrogen and nerve growth factor receptor mRNA in adult sensory neurons. J Neurosci 1994;14:459–471.

50. Hiney JK, Ojeda SR, Les Dees W. Insufin-like growth factor I: a possible metabolic signal involved in the regulation of female puberty. Neuroendocrinology 1991,54:420423.

51. Melcangi RC, Galbiati M, Messi E, Piva F, Martini L, Motta M. Type 1 astrocytes influence luteinizing hormone-releasing hormone release from the hypothalamic cell line GT1-1: is transforming growth factor β the principle involved? Endocrinology 1995 ;136:679–686.

52. Ojeda SR, Urbanski HF, Costa ME, Hill DF, Moholt-Siebertdd M. Involvement of transforming growth factor α in the release of luteinizing-hormone releasing hormone from the developing female rat hypothalamus. Proc Natl Acad Sci USA 1990;87:9698– 9702.

53. Bondy C, Werner H, Roberts CT, LeRoith D. Cellular pattern of type-I insulin-like growth factor receptor gene expression during maturation of the rat brain: comparison with insulin-like growth factors I and II. Neuroscience 1992; 46:909–923.

54. Garcia-Segura LM, Perez J, Pons S, Rejas MT, Torres-Aleman I. Localization of insulin-like growth factor I (IGF-I)-like immunoreactivity in the developing and adult ret brain. Brain Res 1991; 560:167–174.

55. Lenoir D, Honegger P. Insulin-like growth factor I stimulates DNA synthesis in fetal rat brain cell cultures. Dev Brain Res 1983;7:205–213.

56. Torres-Aleman I, Naftolin F, Robbins RJ. Trophic effect of insulin-like growth factor-I on fetal rat hypothalamic cells in culture. Neuroscience 1990; 35:601–608.

57. Berelowitz M, Szabo M, Frohrnan LA, Firestone S, Chu L, Hintz RL. Somatomedin C mediates growth hormone negative feedback by effects on both the hypothalamus and the pituitary. Science 1981; 212:1279–1281.

58. Tannenbaum GS, Guyda HJ, Posner BI. Insulin-like growth factors: A role in growth hormone negative feedback and body weight regulation via brain. Science 1983,220:77–79.

59. Bourguignon JP, Gerard A, Alvarez Gonzalez ML, Franchimont P. Acute suppression of gonadotropin-releasing hormone secretion by insulin-like growth factor I and subproducts: an age-dependent endocrine effect. Neuroendocrinology 1993,58:525–530.

60. Gahary A, Chakrabarti S, Murphy LJ. Localization of the sites of synthesis and action of insulin-like growth factor-1 in the rat uterus. Mol Endocrinol 1990;4:191–195.

61. Kapur S, Tamada H, Dey SK, Andrews GK. Expression of insulin-like growth factor-I (IGF-I) and its receptor in the pert-implantation mouse uterus, and cell-specific regulation of IGF-I gene expression by estradiol and progesterone. Biol Reprod 1992;46: 208–219.

62. Michels KM, Lee WH, Seltzer A, Saavedra JM, Bondy CA. Up-regulation of pituitary [125I] insulin-like growth factor-I (IGF-I) binding and IGF-I gene expression by estrogen. Endocrinology 1993;132: 23–29.

63. Murphy LJ, Murphy LC, Friesen HG. Estrogen induces insulin-like growth factor-I expression in the rat uterus. Mol Endocrinol 1987;1 :445–450.

64. Simmen RCM, Simmen FA, Hofig A, Farmff SJ, Bazer FW. Hormonal regulation of insulin-like growth factor gene expression in pig uterus. Endocrinology 1990; 127:2166–2174.

65. Umayahara Y, Kawamori R, Watada H, Imano E, Iwama N, Morishima T, Yamasaki Y, Kajirnoto Y, Kamada T. Estrogen regulation of the insulin-like growth factor I gene transcription involves an AP-1 enhancer. J Biol Chem 1994; 269: 16433–16442.

66. Wimalasena J, Meehan D, Dostal R, Foster JS, Cameron M, Smith M. Growth factors interact with estradiol and gonadotrophins in the regulation of ovarian cancer cell growth and growth factor receptors. Oncol Res 1993;5:325–337.

67. Krywicki RF, Figueroa JA, Jackson JG, Kozelsky TW, Shimasaki S, Von Hoff DD, Yee D. Regulation of insulin-like growth factor binding proteins in ovarian cancer cells by oestrogen. Eur J Cancer 1993;29A:2015–2019.

68. Molnar P, Murphy LJ. Effects of oestrogen on rat uterine expression of insulin-like growth factor-binding proteins. J Mol Endocrinol 1994;13: 59–67.

69. Owens PC, Gill PG, De Young NJ, Weger MA, Knowels SE, Moyse KJ. Estrogen and progesterone regulate secretion of insulin-like growth factor binding proteins by human breast cancer cells. Biochem Biophys Res Commun 1993;193: 467–473.

70. Yallampalli C, Rajaraman S, Nagarnani M. Insulin-like growth factor binding proteins in the rat uterus and their regulation by oestradiol and growth hormone. J Reprod Fertil 1993;97: 501–505.

71. Constantino CX, Keyes PL, Kostyo JL. Insulin-like growth factor-I stimulates steroidogenesis in rabbit luteal cells. Endocrinology 1991;128: 1702–1708.

72. Erickson GF, Garzo VG, Magoffin DA. Insulin-like growth factor-I (IGF-I) regulates aromatase activity in human granulosa luteal cells. J Clin Endocrinol Metab 1989;69:716–724.

73. Hernandez ER, Resnick CE, Svoboda ME, Van Wyk J, Payne DW, Adashi EY. Somatomedin-C/insulin-like growth factor I as an enhancer of androgen biosynthesis by cultured rat ovarian cells. Endocrinology 1988; 122: 1603–1612.

74. Aronica SM, Katzenellenbogen BS. Progesterone receptor regulation in uterine cells: stimulation by estrogen, cyclic adenosine 3',5'-monophosphate, and insulin-like growth factor I and suppression by antiestrogens and protein kinase inhibitors. Endocrinology 1991 ;128 :2045–2052.

75. Cho H, Aronica SM, Katzenellenbogen BS. Regulation of progesterone receptor gene expression in MCF-7 breast cancer cells: a comparison of the effects of cyclic adenosine 3',5'-monophosphate, estradiol, insulin-like growth factor I, and serum factors. Endocrinology 1994; 134: 658–664.

76. Katzenellenbogen BS, Norman MJ. Multihormonal regulation of the progesterone receptor in MCF-7 human breast cancer cells: interrelationships among insulin/insulin-like growth factor-I, serum, and estrogen. Endocrinology 1990;126: 891–898.

77. Freiss G, Prebois C, Rochefort H, Vignon F. Anti-steroidal and anti-growth factor activities of anti-estrogens. J Steroid Biochem Molec Biol 1990;37: 777–781.

78. Thorsen T, Lahood H, Rasmussen M, Aakvaag A. Estradiol treatment increases the sensitivity of MCF-7 cells for the growth stimulatory effect of IGF-1. J Steroid Biochem Molec Biol 1992; 41:537–540.

79. Wosikowski K, Kung W, Hasmann M, Loser R, Eppenberger U. Inhibition of growth-factor-activated proliferation by anti-estrogens and effects on early gene expression of MCF-7 cells. Int J Cancer 1993;53: 290–297.

80. Toran-Allerand CD, Ellis L, Pfenninger KH. Estrogen and insulin synergism in neurite growth enhancement in vitro: Mediation of steroid effects by interactions with growth factors? Dev Brain Res 1988;41:87–100.

81. Pons S, Torres-Aleman I. Estradiol modulates insulin-like growth factor I receptors and binding proteins in neurons from the hypothalamus. J Neuroendocrinol 1993;55:267–271.

82. Duenas M, Torres-Aleman I, Naftolin F, Garcia-Segura LM. Interaction of insulin-like growth factor-I and estradiol signalling pathways on hypothalamic neuronal differentiation. Neuroscience 1996;74:531–539.

83. Aronica SM, Katzenellenbogen BS. Stimulation of estrogen receptor-mediated transcription and alteration in the phosphorylation state of the rat uterine estrogen receptor by estrogen, cyclic adenosine monophosphate, and insulin-like growth factor-I. Mol Endocrinol 1993;7:743–752.

84. Ignar-Trowbridge DM, Pimentel M, Parker MG, McLachlan JA, Korach KS. Peptide growth factor cross-talk with the estrogen receptor requires the A/B domain and occurs independently of protein kinase C or estradiol. Endocrinology 1996;137:1735–1744.

85. Kato S, Endoh H, Masuhiro Y, Kitamoto T, Uchiyama S, Sasaki H, Masushige S, Gotoh Y, Nishida E, Kawashima H, Metzger D, Chambon P. Activation of the estrogen receptor through phosphorylation by mitogen-activated protein kinase. Science 1995;270:1491–1494.

86. Ma ZQ, Santagati S, Patrone C, Pollio G, Vegeto E, Maggi A. Insulin-like growth factor activates estrogen receptor to control the growth and differentiation of the human neuroblastoma cell line SK-ER3. Mol Endocrinol 1994;8: 910–918.

87. Newton CJ, Buric R, Trapp T, Brockmeier S, Pagotto U, Stalla GK. The unligand estrogen receptor (ER) transduces growth factor signals. J Steroid Biochem Molec Biol 1994;48: 481–486.
88. Patrone C, Ma ZQ, Pollio G, Agrati P, Parker MG, Maggi A. Cross-coupling between insulin and estrogen receptor in human neuroblastoma cells. Molec Endocrinol 1996;10:499–507.
88a. Fernandez-Galaz MC, Morschl E, Chowen JA, Torres-Aleman I, Naftolin F, Garcia-Segura LM. Role of astroglia and insulin-like growth factor-I in gonadal hormone-dependent synaptic plasticity. Brain Res Bull 19997;44:525–531.
89. Pietrzkowski Z, Wernicke D, Porcu P, Jameson BA, Baserga R. Inhibition of cellular proliferation by peptide analogues of insulin-like growth factor I. Cancer Res 1992;52:6447–6451.
90. Duenas M, Luquin S, Chowen JA, Torres-Aleman I, Naftolin F, Garcia-Segura LM. Gonadal hormone regulation of insulin-like growth factor-I-like immunoreactivity in hypothalamic astroglia of developing and adult rats. Neuroendocrinology 1994;59:528–538.
91. McQueen JK. Glial cells and neuroendocrine function. J Endocrinol 1994;143:411–415.
92. Bjelke B, Fuxe K. Intraventricular β-endorphin accumulates in DARPP-32 immunoreactive tanycytes. NeuroReport 1993;5:265–268.
93. Kozolowski GP, Coates PW. Ependymoneuronal specializations between LHRH fibers and cells of the cerebroventricular system. Cell Tiss Res 1985;242:301–311.
94. Oota Y, Kobayashi H, Nishioka RS, Bern HA. Relationship between neurosecretory axon and ependymal terminals on capillary walls in the median eminence of several vertebrates. Neuroendocrinol 1974;16:127–136.
95. King JC, Letourneau RJ. Luteinizing hormone-releasing hormone terminals in the median eminence of rats undergo dramatic changes after gonadectomy, as revealed by electron microscopic image analysis. Endocrinology 1994; 134: 1340–1351.
96. King JC, Rubin BS. Dynamic changes in LHRH neurovascular terminals with various endocrine conditions in adults. Horm Behav 1994; 28:349–356.
97. Meister B, Hökfelt T, Tsuruo Y, Hemmings H, Ouimet C, Greengard P, Goldstein M. DARP-32, a dopamine- and cyclic AMP-regulated phosphoprotein in tanycytes of the mediobasal hypothalamus: distribution and relation to dopamine and luteinizing hormone-releasing hormone neurons and other glial elements. Neuroscience 1988; 27:607–622.
98. Fernandez-Galaz MC, Torres-Aleman I, Garcia-Segura LM. Endocine-dependent accumulation of IGF-I by hypothalamic glia. NeuroReport 1996;8:373–377.
99. Brawer JR, Lin PS, Sonnenschein C. Morphological plasticity in the wall of the third ventricle during the estrous cycle in the rat: a scanning electron microscopic study. AnatRec 1974;179:481–489.

16

Steroid Receptors
in Brain Cell Membranes

Victor D. Ramírez, MD
and Jianbiao Zheng, PhD

CONTENTS

INTRODUCTION
EVIDENCE THAT A mER MEDIATES ESTRADIOL-EVOKED DOPAMINE
    RELEASE FROM FEMALE RAT STRIATAL TISSUE
EVIDENCE THAT THERE ARE SPECIFIC BINDING SITES FOR ESTRADIOL
    IN CS-P₃ MEMBRANE PREPARATIONS
EVIDENCE THAT THE MEMBRANE ESTRADIOL-BINDING SITES IN THE
    CNS ARE PHYSIOLOGICALLY RELEVANT PROTEINS
SUMMARY
REFERENCES

INTRODUCTION

There is abundant but circumstantial evidence indicating that brain cells possess putative membrane steroid receptors (for review, *see* refs. *1* and *2*). It seems appropriate to emphasize once more the several criteria that need to be fulfilled before accepting the concept that steroid hormones bind to specific sites in cellular membranes of the nervous system (CNS), representing protein molecules with the properties of receptors.

The receptors should have high affinity because physiological hormone concentrations are usually in the namolar range, though in different physiological states *(3–5)*, a broad range of fluctuation in blood levels does exist. Alternately, the local effective concentration of the hormones in a particular region of the CNS may not represent accurately the blood concentration *(6–8)*. They should have also high specificity, so that closely related hormones will still preferentially bind to their cognate receptors and remain functionally distinct. There should be a finite number of receptors in any given membrane preparation so they should become saturable with increased doses of the ligand. The kinetics of the receptor–ligand interaction should follow the laws of mass action, with the ligand binding the receptor in a reversible reaction reaching equilibrium rapidly, at which stage the rate of association equals the rate of dissociation. However,

From: *Contemporary Endocrinology: Neurosteroids: A New Regulatory Function
in the Nervous System* Edited by: E.-E. Baulieu, P. Robel, and M. Schumacher
© Humana Press Inc., Totowa, NJ

under certain condition the hormone-receptor (HR) complex may bind to an effector (X) with a K_d that favors the formation of the trimeric complex (HR:X), complicating the kinetics of a bimolecular reaction *(9,10)*. The receptors should have a tissue distribution appropriate to the action of the hormone; that is, it should be present in the target organs of a particular steroid and absent from the tissue unresponsive to the steroid. Within a particular organ, such as the brain, for instance, the receptor may have a selective distribution in the cell membrane of the neurons or glia and/or in specific compartments of such cells, as it is the case for the mitochondria that bind estradiol (E) through oligomycin sensitivity conferring protein (OSCP), a subunit of the ATP synthase *(11,12)*. The receptor should be an integral membrane protein that can be recovered after detergent solubilization and inactivated by proteolytic enzymes. Within limits, the specific binding should increase linearly with the increase in the number of receptors, i.e., concentration of proteins in the membrane preparation. Eventually, and most importantly, the activation of the receptor by the ligand should be coupled to a biological response. Ultimately, the membrane steroid receptors should be cloned and molecularly characterized.

Though there are strong supporting evidence for specific membrane sites for several steroid hormones in the CNS *(1,2,13)*, in this chapter we describe some of the aforementioned criteria above as applied to one of those membrane steroid receptors, the putative membrane estrogen receptor (mER), as an example of these new series of membrane receptors. Thus, in what follows, and using the estradiol-bovine serum albumin conjugate (E-6-BSA) as a probe for the putative mER, we address the following questions:

1. Is the E-6-BSA conjugate biologically active?
2. Does the conjugate specifically bind to subcellular brain preparations?
3. Are these membrane estradiol binding sites novel or physiologically relevant proteins?

EVIDENCE THAT A mER MEDIATES ESTRADIOL-EVOKED DOPAMINE RELEASE FROM FEMALE RAT STRIATAL TISSUE

Rapid effects of estradiol on all three major dopamine (DA) systems—nigrostriatal, mesolimbic, and tuberoinfundibular—have been reported. For example, an early study *(14)* showed that relatively high concentrations of E and a synthetic estrogen, diethylstilbestrol (DES) produced a concentration-dependent (0.1–20 m*M*) release of DA and norepinephrine (NE) from in vitro hypothalamic preparations, whereas its biologically inactive enantiomer, 17α-estradiol, was ineffective. The effect was observed following a delay of approximately 20–40 min for DA, suggesting mediation of a possible membrane mechanism. In the nigrostriatal DA system, in which the corpus striatum (CS) is the site of major dopaminergic innervation, a variety of behavioral and functional indices are dependent on the gonadal status of the animal, particularly upon E levels. For instance, E has been reported to influence rapidly striatal DA release, DA receptor concentration, and behavior mediated by the striatum *(15–17)*. Becker *(18,19)* showed that physiological concentrations (0.22–3.7 n*M*) of E or DES rapidly (within 20 min) potentiated, the amphetamine-stimulated striatal DA release from striatal tissue of ovariectomized (ovx) rats as measured by microdialysis. This rapid E effect was correlated to rapid effects of E on rat rotational behavior. 17α-estradiol (17α-E) had much less effect, indicating a stereospecific effect of E. This rapid effect of E is sexually dimorphic because it was absent in the striatal tissue of intact male rats *(20)*. A subsequent study also revealed that

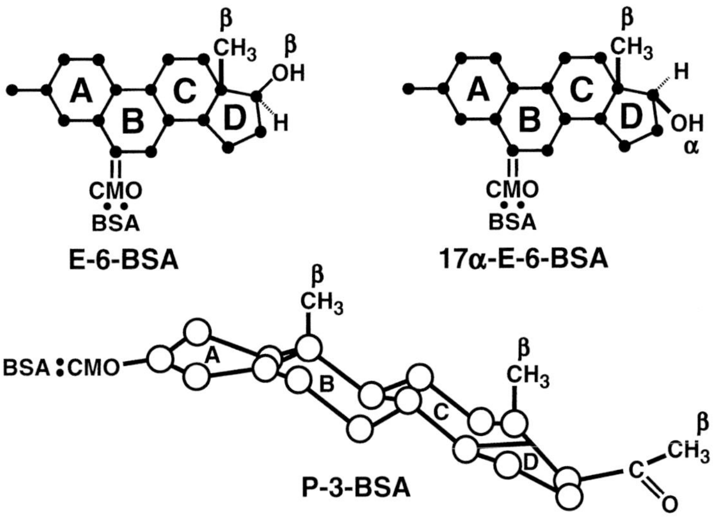

Fig. 1. Structure of novel ligands to study steroid membrane actions. Crystallographically observed structure of the estradiol molecule in a perpendicular view to the phenolic ring; modified from Keasling and Schneler *(33)*. For details *see text.*

E acutely inhibits (within 30 min) the striatal D2-DA receptor binding *(21)*, which might be owing to a rapid conversion of high to low affinity D2-DA receptors, as shown by Levesque and DiPaolo *(22)*. Recently, a rapid stimulation of striatal dopamine synthesis by E but not by 17α-E, was reported in ovx rats in vivo within 15 min of physiological doses of the steroid injected subcutaneously *(23,24)*. In addition, incubation of striatal slices in vitro with 1 nM E (but not 17α-E) evoked a twofold increase in the K_i of one form of the tyrosine hydroxylase (TH) enzyme for DA, suggesting a decrease in TH susceptibility to end-product inhibition, presumably owing to phosphorylation of the enzyme *(23,24)*. However, all these findings were obtained using free E, which can diffuse inside the cells; therefore, the results may not be owing to a membrane-mediated event. In the mesolimbic system, a nongenomic effect of E on DA release from the nucleus accumbens studied by in vivo microdialysis was also observed *(25)*. E hemisuccinate infusion resulted in an initial increase in K+-simulated DA release within 2 min, followed by a later increase at about 1 h after the infusion of the steroid, which, according to the authors, was probably secondary to a genomic stimulation.

Thus, to differentiate between a certain outer-membrane effect of E and one in which the diffusion of this liposoluble steroid can confound those initial membrane events, we decided to study the acute release of DA by estradiol, using the impermeable E-6-BSA conjugate (Fig. 1). To address this issue we utilized an in vitro superfusion system to perifuse CS fragments derived from female rats in specific phases of the estrous cycle, as determined by daily vaginal smears. For technical details, see our previous publications *(26,27)*. Figure 2 shows that E-6-BSA rapidly stimulates (within the first 10 min of infusion at interval #4) basal DA release from CS fragments derived from proestrous rats killed in the morning (9 AM). Noteworthy, the isomer of E-6-BSA, the 17α-E-6-BSA conjugate (Fig. 1), did not stimulate the basal DA release using an identical concentration of 10 nM in parallel experiments. The fact that BSA does not stimulate the release of DA

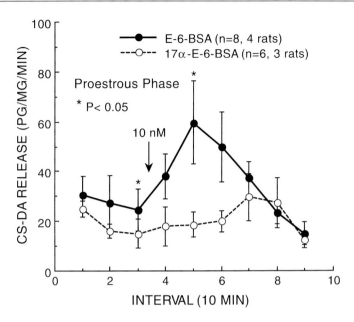

Fig. 2. E-6-BSA stimulates dopamine release from CS fragments from Proestrous rats. Proestrous rats were sacrificed at 900 h and the CS fragments were distributed in four chambers. Two chambers were stimulated with E-6-BSA and two chambers with 17α-E-6-BSA. The experiment was repeated four times; however, in the fourth repetition, two chambers received BSA instead of 17α-E-6-BSA. The data indicate no effect of BSA (31–66; 42–53; 50–18; 25–20; 10–22; 6–24; 14–24, 10–15 pg/mg/min for intervals 1–8 in the two chambers, respectively) and a robust response to E-6-BSA during proestrus. In all figures, values are X ± SE. The stars indicate significant differences between values at intervals 3 and 5. The arrow indicates the time when the infusion of the hormones occurred (starting after interval 3 and ending at interval 4). The same applies to Figs. 3 and 4.

(*see* Fig. 2 legend), together with the lack of effect of 17α-E-6-BSA, indicates that the stimulatory action of the complex is owing to estradiol and not BSA. Interestingly, CS fragments from diestrous and estrous rats are not or less responsive to E-6-BSA, respectively, as shown in Table 1.

In ovx rats (more than 14 d), an optimal effective concentration of the complex (10 nM) evoked a small but not significant increase in DA release (Fig. 3) in spite of a robust response of the preparation to a depolarizing dose of K^+ (30 mM). To test if the reduction of E levels causes the decrease in responsiveness of the CS fragments to the complex, ovx rats were treated with estradiol benzoate for 2 d (0.5 μg on d 1, increased to 1 μg on d 2) and sacrificed on d 3 (at 9 AM). This treatment partially recovers the response of the CS to E-6-BSA (Fig. 4), suggesting a crucial role for E in the function of its own membrane receptor in CS neural membranes; this was probably owing to a genomic activation of the neurons leading to the production of specific transcripts involved in the synthesis of mERs.

The rapid increase in basal DA release by E-6-BSA from striatal fragments derived from proestrous rats is dose-dependent, with a maximal effective concentration of 10 nM, which induces close to a sixfold increase in DA release over control pretreatment values (Fig. 5). The ED$_{50}$ is about 5 nM and a minimal but significant response was observed with

Table 1
Differential Response to E-6-BSA-Evoked DA release
from CS Fragments Superfused In Vitro

Condition	Dose (nM)	Number of Chambers[a]	Percent Response[b]
1. Diestrus	10	4	110 ± 25
2. Proestrus	10	8	562 ± 147^{c}
Proestrus	25	8	333 ± 84^{c}
3. Estrus	10	14	273 ± 69^{c}
4. Constant estrus	5	6	260 ± 55^{c}
Constant estrus	25	6	1022 ± 256^{c}
5. Adult Male	10	4	109 ± 14
Adult Male	25	4	138 ± 19

[a]Each rat generates two CS, one per each chamber.
[b]Maximal response over pretreatment value at interval #3.
[c]$p < 0.05$ at least.

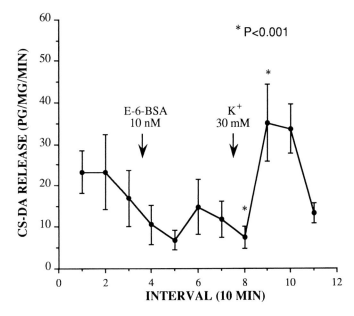

Fig. 3. Rats were ovx and 15–20 d post-ovx received oil and sacrificed on d 3 at 9.00 h. CS fragments were superfused in vitro and at interval 4 stimulated with 10 nM E-6-BSA. To test for viability of the tissue a depolarizing dose of K^+ (30 mM) was applied at interval 8. Note a robust response to K^+ and a nonsignificant response to E-6-BSA, $n = 4$ chambers, two rats. Note a different y scale between Figs. 2 and 3.

1 nM. This membrane-mediated event of E-6-BSA is gender-specific, because similar CS preparations from intact male rats did not respond to a broad range of doses of the conjugate (Fig. 5). A further indication that the hormonal status of the animal appears to be crucial for the expression of this response is the serendipitous finding that CS fragments derived from three rats in constant estrus (with vaginal smear in constant estrus for greater than 12 d) were highly responsive to the infusion of the conjugate, because both

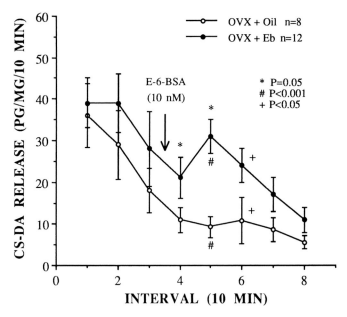

Fig. 4. The effect of ovx and Eb treatment on dopamine release from CS fragments by E-6-BSA. A 2-d treatment with Eb (0.5 μg s.c. on d 1, followed by 1 μg on d 2) led on d 3 to a partial recovery of the response to 10 nM E-6-BSA. Symbols indicate significant differences within (*) and between conditions. (#, +)

a 5 and 25 nM dose were more potent in releasing DA than similar doses in proestrous rats (Table 1).

Hence, it seems that E acts on the extracellular phase of the membranes of the CS neurons to activate a "receptor" that is functionally coupled to DA release only under a certain, critical endogenous hormonal milieu, such as the one present in proestrus, in ovx rats treated with E, or in rats in constant estrus.

EVIDENCE THAT THERE ARE SPECIFIC BINDING SITES FOR ESTRADIOL IN CS-P₃ MEMBRANE PREPARATIONS

The presence of specific membrane E binding sites in the CNS has been documented previously *(1,28)*. However, most authors, including us, have used either a crude synaptosomal preparation *(29)* or purified synaptosomal membranes *(28,30)* from different regions of the brain. The K_d reported are in the low (1–20 nM) and high (>100 nM) nanomolar range, with variation depending on the type of neural tissue. This is an indication of heterogenous sites most likely corresponding to different estrogen-binding proteins. For instance, using a crude synaptosomal preparation (P_2 fraction) we reported *(11,29)* significantly different K_d values of 3 ± 0.7 ($n = 3$), 10 ± 1.5 ($n = 6$) and 34 ± 7 ($n = 6$) nM for the female rat hypothalamus, olfactory bulb, and cerebellum, respectively. These results suggest that different circulating levels of E may activate differentially these putative mERs in these three particular CNS regions and thereby controlling different brain functions.

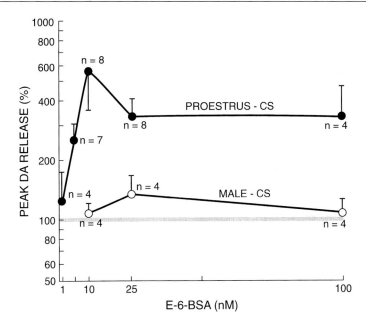

Fig. 5. Dose-response to E-6-BSA. Note that 10 nM elicited a maximal percent dopamine release over dopamine levels at interval 3 (pre-infusion). Peak dopamine release is defined as the difference between values at interval 3 and maximal release after the infusion of the complex. N values represent number of superfusion chambers per dose. In one male rat (4 chambers) the 10 nM dose was ineffective, and in two other rats, neither the 25 (4 chambers) nor the 100 nM doses (4 chambers) were effective.

These neural membrane preparations are by no means "pure" cell membranes and therefore the Kd values and specific binding sites reported are most likely a representation of several estrogen protein binders from different cellular organelles recovered in P_2 fractions. Therefore, it was of interest to repeat those binding studies using a relatively enriched cellular membrane preparation obtained by differential centrifugation according to Darnell et al. *(31)*. Herein, we report data on the so called plasmalemma-microsomal fractions from either the CS or the entire brain (including the CS) of female rats. Plate 1 depicts the ultrastructural features of the three subcellular fractions generated by differential centrifugation as previously mentioned. There are clear-cut electron microscopical differences in these three fractions as expected. First, the so-called P_1 or nuclear fraction generated after 10 min of centrifugation at 600g of a brain homogenate contains a variety of organelles indicating a highly contaminated fraction (*see* **A**). In contrast, the mP_2 fraction (15,000g for 5 min) is enriched in swollen mitochondria showing several degrees of damage, though some large myelin sheaths and synaptic connections are also present (*see* **B**). The plasmalemma- microsomal P_3 fraction (ultracentrifugation of the supernatant of the P_2 fraction for 60–90 min at 125,000g) is enriched in those membrane components with little contamination from mitochondria or other organelles (*see* **C**). Note that at a large magnification, the P_3 fraction shows membranes undergoing endoexocytosis as indicated by the arrowhead in Plate 1, (*see* **D**). The degree of purity of these fractions is also revealed by the amount of protein recovered from the initial brain

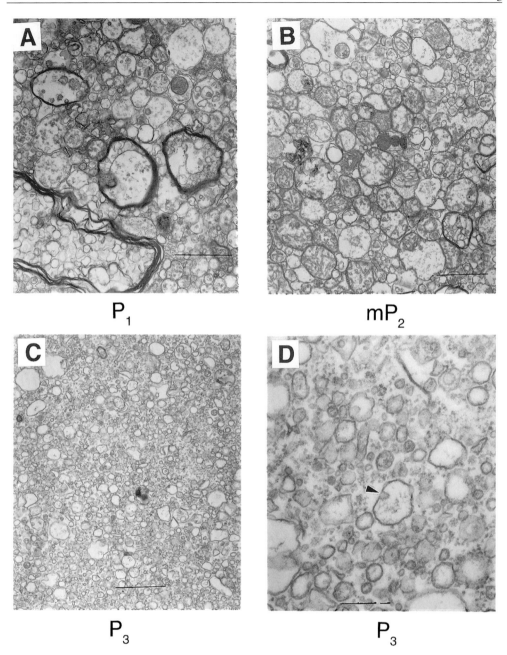

Plate 1. P_1, mP_2, and P_3 fractions from rat brains were prepared according to Darnell et al. *(31)* and pelleted down by ultra centrifugation at 125,000g for 1 h. Then they were fixed in 4% glutaraldehyde, 0.1 M cacodylate buffer, pH 7.2, overnight at 4°C, followed by washing 3 times, 15 min each. The fractions were subsequently postfixed in 1% osmium tetroxide, 0.1 M cacodylate buffer for 50 min followed by addition of KFeCN to a final concentration of 1.5% for 20 min. The materials were rinsed by the same cacodylate buffer, dehydrated in acetone, infiltrated with Polybed 812, and finally in fresh epoxy for polymerization at 60°C for 3 d. Thin sections of these fractions were then examined with a Hitachi H-600 electron microscope at different magnifications. Panels A, B, and C correspond to a typical sample from P_1, mP_2 and P_3, respectively. Panel D is a higher magnification of the P_3 pellet. The scale bar is 1 μm for A, B, and C and 0.2 μm for D.

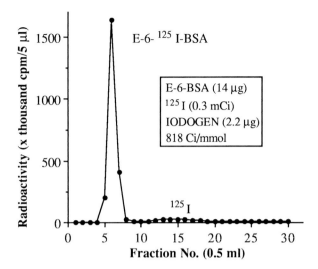

Fig. 6. A typical example of separation of iodinated E-6-BSA (E-^{125}I-BSA) from free ^{125}I by a PD-10 column. Five hundred ml fractions were collected and 5 µL from each fraction were taken and counted in a gamma counter. The first radioactive peak corresponded to bound ^{125}I and the second radioactive peak corresponded to free [125]I.

homogenates. For example, from five rats, the total wet weight of the brain was 7.3 g. In the P_1, mP_2, and P_3 fractions the protein recovered were 3.9, 0.62, and 0.14%, respectively, of the total protein in the homogenate (about 730 mg protein). The X ± SE values for the P_3 fraction in four experiments were 0.19 ± 0.038% corresponding to 3.2 ± 0.85 mg of protein. Thus, the plasmalemma-microsomal fraction contains the least amount of proteins and the largest amount of cell membranes compared to the other two fractions.

Consistent with the ultrastructural differences between the mitochondrial (mP_2) and plasmalemma-microsomal (P_3) enriched fractions, the radioiodinated ligand E-6-^{125}I-BSA (using the iodogen procedure to label the conjugates shown in Fig. 6) differentially binds to these two fractions, as depicted in Fig. 7. Interestingly, the highest affinity ($K_d = 0.14 ± 0.08$ nM, $n = 3$) and the greater number of binding sites ($B_{max} = 31.3 ± 11.8$ pmol/mg protein) correspond to the P_3 fraction with a K_d of at least 10 times lower than the one determined for the mP_2 fraction. This difference indicates that the sought-out mER is probably an estrogen protein binder localized in the cell membrane of neurons or glial cells with high affinity for E, as one would expect because of the low circulatory levels of this hormone in blood *(3)*. Besides the high affinity and abundance of sites, the binding sites are also selective for E, because P-3-BSA, a progesterone–BSA conjugate, shows very little specific binding when low doses of protein of the P_3 fraction are used in the radioreceptor assay (Fig. 8). In addition, unlabeled P-3-BSA is a poor competitor of the ligand binding since the IC_{50} is greater than 1000 nM (Fig. 9).

If one considers what are thought to be classical features of the estradiol structure for binding—that is, "the molecule should be flat with hydrophilic groups (OH groups) at either end of the molecule, that the middle portion of the molecule be hydrophobic and

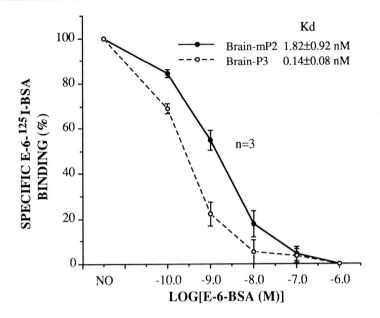

Fig. 7. Homologous competitions curves of E-6-^{125}I-BSA binding to subcellular fractions (mP$_2$ and P$_3$) from the whole female rat brain. The data are analyzed by LIGAND program and the Kds are shown in the figure. The concentrations of specific binding sites for mP$_2$ and P$_3$ are 10.2 ± 4.3 and 31.3 ± 11.8 pmol/mg proteins, respectively. The nonspecific binding was obtained in the presence of 1 μM unlabeled E-6-BSA. Data are expressed as X $\pm$ SD. "No" indicates the absence of competitor.

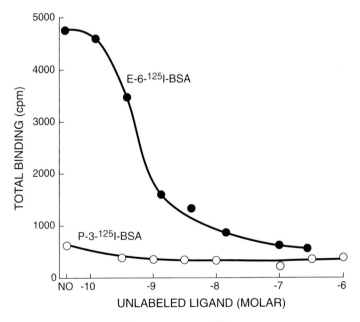

Fig. 8. Differential binding of E-6-^{125}I-BSA and P-3-^{125}I-BSA to CS-P3 fractions (0.5 µg protein). A single experiment in duplicate for each case.

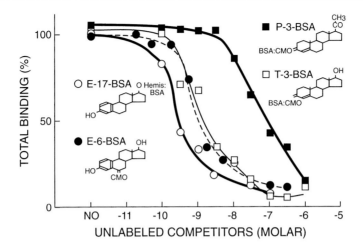

Fig. 9. Competition curve of several steroid-BSA conjugates of ligand binding E-6-[125] I-BSA to CS-P3 fractions (0.5 μg protein). One experiment in duplicate for each case.

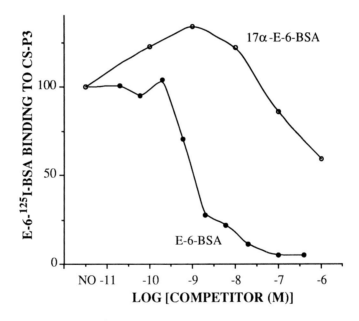

Fig. 10. Specific binding of E-6-^{125}I-BSA *(45,000 cpm/0.5 mL, 0.14 nM)* to CS-P3 (0.5 μg) in duplicates displaced by unlabeled E-6-BSA and 17α-E-6-BSA. The total binding without competitor (about 4000 cpm) is considered as 100%. "NO" indicates the absence of competitor.

that the distance between terminal hydroxyls (1.09 nm) be highly specific" *(32,33)*, it is intriguing that another conjugate testosterone-BSA (T-3-BSA) with the OH (C-3) blocked by the BSA has a comparable high affinity for the E binding sites in these membranes (Fig. 9), indicating that the OH (C-17) is important for the binding. Moreover, if the BSA blocks the OH (C-17) and leaves the OH (C-3) available for binding, higher affinity is observed. In addition, the binding of E-6-BSA is highly sterospecific because its α isomer is a poor competitor (Fig. 10). Therefore, it seems that both hydroxyl groups are required

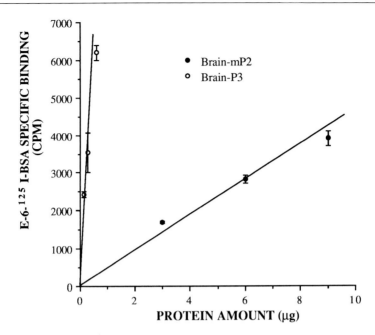

Fig. 11. Specific binding curves for B-mP$_2$ and B-P$_3$ using several doses of proteins. Each point represents three duplicate experiments and the values are expressed as X ± SD.

for binding, and they must be oriented in the β position. It would be of interest to know if E-17-BSA and T-3-BSA are also active in releasing DA from striatal fragments. The specific binding of E-6-^{125}I-BSA represents over 90% of total binding and increases linearly as a function of low doses of protein either in P3 fractions derived from brain or CS tissues (Figs. 11 and 12, respectively). Note that at equivalent concentration of proteins much higher specific binding is detected in the P3 than in the mP2 fractions from brain origin (Fig. 11) This is consistent with the finding that there are greater number of binding sites in the cell membranes than in the mitochondrial fraction, as previously shown.

Further experiments were performed to determine the binding kinetics of E-6-^{125}I-BSA to CS-P3 from female rat brains. Figure 13A shows the association curve of E-6-^{125}I-BSA to CS-P3 membranes over time. The binding was rapid and reached equilibrium by about 20 min at 4°C. This association kinetics is more rapid ($k_1 = 0.33$ nM^{-1} min^{-1}) than that of P$_2$ from brain, which reached equilibrium only after about 30 min (29). Figure 13B shows the dissociation curve of the labeled ligands from their binding sites in CS-P3. This dissociation constant is estimated to have a $k_2 = 0.075$ min^{-1}. The K_d calculated from these data revealed a K_d value of 0.23 nM close to the one obtained by competition binding, demonstrating the validity of the assay.

Though we have reported earlier that free estradiol (but not 17α-E) is a partial competitor (IC$_{50}$ about 1000 n*M*) of the ligand binding to P2 brain fractions (11) and that ^{125}I-BSA does not bind this fraction nor the unlabeled BSA competes, it seems of interest to compare how these estradiol conjugates will behave in a classical uterine cytosolic preparation in which the nuclear estradiol receptor (nER) is labeled with ^{3}H-estradiol. Uterine

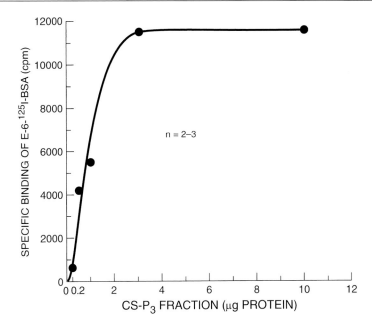

Fig. 12. Similar to Fig. 11, but using CS-P3 fractions.

cytosols (rich in nERs) were prepared from immature female rats in TE buffer (10 mM Tris, 0.2 mM ethylenediaminetetraacetic acid [EDTA], pH 7.5) according to a modified procedure of Bruns et al. *(34)*. Briefly, immature female rats (30 d old) were sacrificed by decapitation and the uteri were removed quickly into cold TE buffer. The uteri were minced and homogenized in the same Teflon glass homogenizer at 1 uterus/mL TE for 2 min. The homogenate was then ultracentrifuged at 125,000g for 60 min; the supernatant (S3) obtained was considered the uterine cytosol. The protein concentration was estimated by the method of Bradford *(35)* using BSA as standard, and stored in aliquots at −70°C. The saturation and competition assay of the binding of [^{3}H]- estradiol (85 Ci-mmol, NEN) to intracellular estradiol receptors (nER) in uterine cytosol of immature rats were performed at 4°C in TE buffer or TE plus 0.08% BSA (TEB). [^{3}H]-estradiol (2 or 10 nM for competition assay and 0.1–10 nM for saturation assay) was incubated for 1.5–3 h with uterine cytosol (80–440 mg proteins) and competing compounds in 500 mL or 250 mL volume. The ethanol used to dissolve the ligand and steroids was in the range of 0.004–0.4%. 200–500-fold E or DES was used to determine the nonspecific binding. The bound [^{3}H]- estradiol was separated from free using the following two methods: 1. Rapid filtration by polyethylenimine (PEI)-treated filters: The rapid filtration using PEI-treated Whatman GF/B glass filters for separation of bound from ligand was based on the method of Bruns et al. *(34)* Briefly, the glass filters were soaked in 0.3% PEI (v/v) for 1–3 h at room temperature and placed on a 1225 sampling manifold. The manifold was then transferred to the cold room (4°C) for about 1 h before use. After the incubation, the reaction solution was poured onto PEI-treated filters in the manifolds under reduced pressure. The tubes and filters were washed with two 5 mL P2-Tris incubation buffer (TE or TEB). The radioactivity retained by the filters was counted using aqueous scintillation

Association

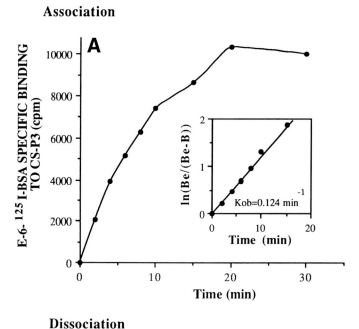

Dissociation

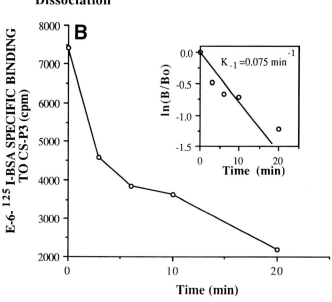

Fig. 13. The kinetics of E-6-^{125}I-BSA binding (0.15 nM) to CS-P3 fraction from adult female rats at 4°C. **(A)** The association curve for the binding of E-6-BSA to CS-P3 (0.5 μg protein). The nonspecific binding was measured in the presence of 1 μM unlabeled E-6-BSA. The specific binding was determined by subtracting the nonspecific binding from the total binding (in the absence of unlabeled E-6-BSA). Note that the specific binding reached equilibrium at about 20 min. The K_{ob} is estimated as 0.124 min⁻¹. **(B)** The dissociation curve for the binding of E-6-^{125}I-BSA to CS-P3 (0.3 μg protein). After preincubation for 10 min, E-6-BSA (final concentration of 1 μM) was added and the tubes were incubated for the time indicated. A rate of dissociation is estimated as 0.075 min⁻¹. For the calculations we have considered the number of moles of estradiol (~30 moles of estradiol)/mole of 6-keto estradiol 6-(0-carboxymethyl) oxime BSA, which gives a total MW of about 76,770. The same is true for the other figures.

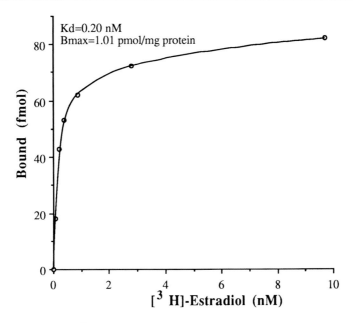

Fig. 14. Saturation curve of [³H]-estradiol *(2 nM)* binding to nuclear ER in the uterine cytosol (S3, 80 μg in a total volume of 500 μL TEB buffer) from immature female rats using a rapid filtration assay with PEI-treated GF/B glass filters. The nonspecific binding was determined in the presence of 300-fold excess of unlabeled 17β-estradiol. The ethanol used to dissolve labeled and unlabeled ligands were in the concentrations of 0.004–0.4% and had no effect on the binding. Inset: Scatchard plot.

cocktail, Bio-Safe II after overnight incubation. 2. Gel filtration: Sephadex G-25 fine beads were equilibrated with TE buffer at room temperature for at least 3 h and then packed in a glass Pasteur pipet with a bed volume of about 1.8 mL. The packed columns were then transferred to the cold room (4°C) and equilibrated with cold TE or TEB. 125 μL reaction solution was removed and loaded to the column without disturbing the gel bed. Two-min fractions were collected with volume of about 250 μL and counted by addition 3–5 mL Bio-Safe II scintillation cocktail. The bound [³H]-estradiol appears in the void volume as the first radioactive peak. The dissociation constant (K_d) and binding sites concentration (B_{max}) for homologous assays as well as saturation assays were determined with the nonlinear curve fitting LIGAND program *(36)*. K_i for different competitors was calculated according to Cheng and Prusoff *(37)*.

Because in all our previous studies 0.08 % BSA (12 μ*M*) is included in the binding buffer to decrease unspecific absorption of the conjugates and BSA itself is an estradiol binding protein with low affinity (K_d in the range of 10–100 μ*M*), the saturation study for [³H]-estradiol was prepared in TE, plus 0.08% BSA as shown in Fig. 14. A K_d and B_{max} (0.2 n*M*, 1.01 picomoles/mg protein) similar to values determined by other authors *(38,39)* was determined with TEB buffer indicating that BSA does not interfere in the assay under these conditions. Using 2 n*M* [³H]-estradiol, the relative affinity of several steroid-BSA conjugates for the nER in TEB buffer in uterine cytosol was then determined (Fig. 15). The K_d of Fig. 14 was used to calculate the K_i according to Chen and Prusoff *(37)*. The K_i of 0.16 n*M* for E is similar to the K_d value obtained by the saturation assay as previously

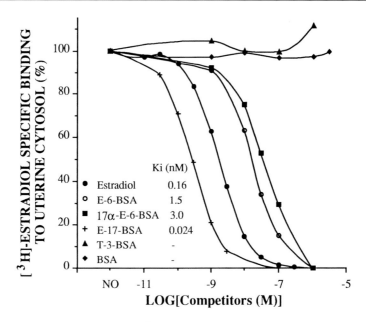

Fig. 15. Competition curves of specific [^{3}H]-estradiol (2 nM) binding to uterine cytosol (80 µg in 500 µL total volume) using various unlabeled competitors in duplicates as determined by a rapid filtration assay with PEI-treated GF/B glass filters. The Kd obtained from the saturation study in TEB of Fig. 14 was used to calculate the Ki values for the different competitors. "NO" indicates the absence of competitors.

shown (Fig. 14). In this classical assay, the 17β-E-6-BSA and its α isomer are good competitors with K_i of 1.5 nM and 3 nM, respectively. Interestingly, E-17-BSA has a very high affinity for the nER (K_i of 0.024 nM, which is sevenfold lower than that of E, the natural ligand though the molecular weight (MW) of the conjugate is calculated considering about 30 moles of E/mole of BSA; Fig. 13). Consistent with the binding properties of the nER preparation, T-3-BSA did not compete, whereas the conjugate is a very good competitor in the mER assay, as shown earlier. As expected, BSA had no effect in this assay nor in the mER assay. In addition, the effect of E-17-BSA was tested in the gel-filtration method using Sephadex G-25 fine in TE buffer (Fig. 16). When [^{3}H]-estradiol and the nER mixture was applied to the column a distinct peak appeared in fractions 3–6, which is significantly reduced by 10 nM E-17-BSA reaching a level close to the small blank peak (buffer + E-17-BSA) most likely owing to the presence of 0.08% BSA in the binding buffer. Therefore, the data obtained in these two classical methods to measure estradiol binding activity to the nER shows that the E-6-BSA or E-17-BSA behaves as good or a better competitor as free estradiol, respectively, indicating that BSA does not interfere in the binding and allowing the OH groups of the estradiol molecule to interact with the receptor.

Overall, these data reinforce the concept that the rapid actions of E are mediated by specific E binding sites in nerve cell membranes from several CNS regions, suggesting the existence of putative receptors for this steroid with different functions. The concept of an heterogeneous group of estradiol protein binders in the CNS is further supported by

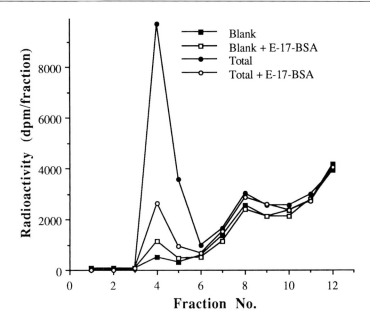

Fig. 16. The binding of [³H]-estradiol *(10 nM)* to uterine cytosol was determined by a gel filtration assay. Half (125 μL) of the total 250 μL reaction solution containing 80 μg uterine cytosol was applied to a Sephadex G-25 fine column. The [³H]-estradiol bound proteins appeared in the first peak from fraction number 3–6. The assay was done in TEB buffer. 10 nM E-17-BSA was used to displace the binding. Note that both BSA and E-17-BSA bound a very small fraction of [³H]-estradiol and appeared from fraction number 3–6. The total binding obtained was 12859 dpm and it was displaced to 2154 dpm in the presence of 10 nM E-17-BSA.

the clear-cut differences between the binding properties of the mitochondrial fractions and the cell membrane preparations of the rat brain. As we will discuss later, these binding characteristics correspond to different proteins. It is also apparent that the binding properties of the unpurified nER and those of the so-called mER are quite different inviting to speculate that the steroid molecule recognizes a different binding pocket in these two receptors. A final answer to this challenging problem will require the cloning of the mER.

EVIDENCE THAT THE MEMBRANE ESTRADIOL-BINDING SITES IN THE CNS ARE PHYSIOLOGICALLY RELEVANT PROTEINS

Progress in this phase of our research has been mainly achieved by the use of an affinity chromatography column constructed with the conjugate E-6-BSA attached to an agarose matrix as reported earlier *(11,40)*. Using this procedure, which leads to at least 1000-fold purification in a single passage of a detergent-solubilized P2 fraction from the rat brain or cerebellum, we were able to identify two proteins in the retained fraction: 1. corresponding to OSCP, a 23 kDa subunit of the ATP synthase complex of mitochondrial origin, and 2. a protein of 18 kDa, also a subunit of this same multimeric enzyme. The OSCP in the eluted fraction retained the capacity to bind E-6-^{125}I-BSA with nanomolar affinity and it appears to be the only subunit of the ATP synthase to be recognized by the

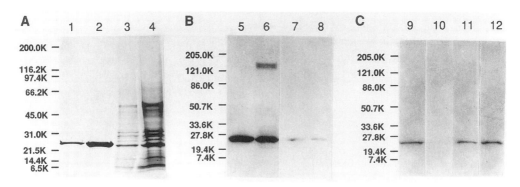

Fig. 17. (A) SDS-PAGE of recombinant bovine OSCP (rbOSCP, lanes 1 and 2, 1 µg and 5 µg, respectively) and E-6-BSA affinity column-retained proteins from digitonin-solubilized B-P2 (lanes 3 and 4, 2 µg and 10 µg, respectively). **(B)** RbOSCP *(5* µg, lanes 5 and 7) and purified B-P2 (10 µg, lanes 6 and 8) were separated in SDS-PAGE and transferred to a nitrocellulose membrane. The binding proteins were detected by incubating the membrane with E-6-^{125}I-BSA $(1 \times 10^6$ cpm/mL, 1.6 n*M*) in the absence (lanes 5 and 6) and presences (lanes 7 and 8) of 1 µ*M* unlabeled E-6-BSA. Curiously, in lane 6 not only the OSCP band was specifically identified, the ligand also labeled a 130 kDa protein. This may represent contamination from plasma membrane. **(C)** Ligand blotting of rbOSCP (1 µg in each lane) using E-6-^{125}I-BSA $(1 \times 10^6$ cpm/mL, 1.6 n*M*) in the absence of competitors (lane 9), and in the presence of 0.5 µ*M* E-6-BSA (lane 10), 0.5 µ*M* 17α-E-6-BSA *(11)*, and 12 µ*M* BSA (lane 12). The broad range Mr markers used in (A) are from high to low molecular weight: myosin, β-galactosidase, phosphorylase B, BSA, ovalbumin, bovine carbonic anhydrase, soybean trypsin inhibitor, lysozyme, and aprotinin. In (B) and (C) and in Figs. 18 and 19, similar but prestained broad range markers were used.

ligand *(1,11,12)*. A further confirmation that the 23 kDa protein is OSCP and that this subunit has high affinity for E comes from recent experiments using a recombinant OSCP of bovine origin (rbOSCP) (kindly provided to us by Dr. Y. Hatefi et al., Scripps Research Institute, La Jolla, CA). This protein in sodium dodecyl sulfate-polyacrimide gel electrophoresis (SDS-PAGE) migrates as a single band in the same position as the 23 kDa protein of the purified brain-P2 (B-P2) fraction as shown in Fig. 17A. Importantly, the E-6-^{125}I-BSA binds specifically to both the rbOSCP as well as the affinity purified 23 kDa protein from B-P$_2$, because both proteins are displaced by 1 µ*M* unlabeled ligand (Fig. 17B). It is noteworthy that in the purified fraction of the B-P$_2$, a strong band in the 130 kDa range is also labeled by the ligand, probably an estradiol protein binder from the cell membranes contaminating the B-P$_2$ fraction. The binding is quite selective and stereospecific because BSA does not compete and the 17α-isomer of E-6-BSA is a poor competitor (Fig. 17C).

The presence of E binding sites in mitochondria has been implicated in early experiments that showed that about 10–20% of total estradiol binding sites in immature female rats were detected in a mitochondrial fraction *(41,42)*. Relevant to this finding is the fact that micromolar concentrations of DES, a synthetic estradiol with similar structure as E, also interacted with F0F1ATP-synthase/ATPase in the rat liver to modulate proton transport *(43,44)*. The OSCP subunit is usually considered an essential contributor to the stalk that links the F0 sector to F1 sector, as well as a transducer that transforms the proton gradient across F0 to ATP synthesis on F1. It is conceivable that OSCP is responsible for

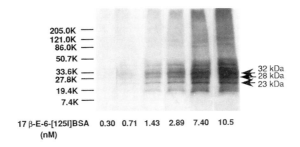

Fig. 18. Dose-dependent E-6-^{125}I-BSA binding to CB-P2 in nanomolar. CB-P2 proteins were separated by SDS-PAGE and electroblotted to a nitrocellulose membrane using Towbin buffer containing 0.005% SDS. The different lanes of the blotted nitrocellulose membrane were incubated for 45 min at 4°C with 0.30–10.5 n*M* (3.0–74 × 105 cpm/mL) E-6-^{125}I-BSA. The blots were exposed to Kodak SB film for 2 h and then developed for 1 min. The prestained protein standards are shown on the left of the figure.

these early observations on E-mitochondria interactions. OSCP could be also involved in some of the rapid or nongenomic effects of E previously mentioned *(1,45)* by regulating ATP synthesis and concentration, since ATP not only serves as the master energy donor *(46–48)*, but is also an important neurotransmitter that can be released by neurons to regulate varieties of brain functions *(49)*. Previous studies have established that E did decrease the ATP concentration of uterus in ovariectomized or immature female rats *(50)*, though this decrease was believed to be mainly owing to E-induced, nuclear estradiol receptor-mediated RNA synthesis *(50)*. However, the involvement of E via mitochondria in decreasing or increasing ATP levels cannot be excluded. Furthermore, this mechanism could participate in the nuclear estradiol receptor-mediated genomic action because several recent studies have emphasized the importance of ATP in the molecular events associated with interaction among steroid hormone, heat shock proteins, and nuclear receptors *(51,52)*.

It remains to be shown that rbOSCP binds [^{3}H]-estradiol. Though rbOSCP binds [^{3}H]-estradiol (about 4% of total), the binding conditions need to be optimized since this protein behaves differently than the classical estradiol receptor from the uterine cytosolic preparation using size exclusion chromatography or filtration assays (unpublished data).

Our results and the aforementioned data suggest a new mechanism by which E can affect the function of diverse cells through binding to F0F1 ATP synthase/ATPase, a key enzyme of the cell energy machinery, as discussed earlier *(11)*. However, this mechanism cannot explain the direct effects of E at the plasma membrane demonstrated previously (for review, *see* refs. *1* and *13*).

So, in our research for the putative mER we ended up isolating an estradiol protein binder that belongs to the multimeric ATP synthase enzyme of mitochondrial origin. This unexpected result was most likely owing to the high level of damaged mitochondrial organelles present in the brain or cerebellum P$_2$ fractions as shown above in the E.M. images of these preparations. In addition, a Western blotting assay of CB-P$_2$ fractions revealed that in addition to the 23 kDa protein, other proteins of different sizes were also identified by this procedure as depicted in Fig. 18. These unidentified proteins may correspond to the mER or mERs. Therefore, recently we have focused our studies to

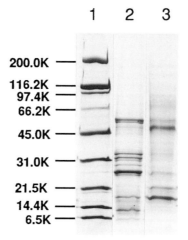

Fig. 19. The SDS-PAGE analysis of affinity column-purified mP$_2$ and P$_3$. Digitonin-solubilized B-mP2 or B-P3 fractions were applied to the E-6-BSA affinity column and the retained proteins by the affinity column were separated by SDS-PAGE. Lane 1, broad range protein markers (Bio-Rad). Lane 2, retained proteins from solubilized B-mP$_2$ (5 μg). Lane 3, retained proteins from solubilized B-P3 (5 μg). *See text* for details.

isolate these estradiol binding proteins from the plasmalemma-microsomal enriched P$_3$ fraction. To this end, a similar E-6-BSA affinity chromatography column was loaded with a detergent-solubilized P$_3$ fraction and the retained proteins were isolated by SDS-PAGE under reducing conditions. Figure 19 compares the size and mobility of these affinity purified protein in mP$_2$ and P$_3$ fractions from the female rat brain. Note that in the mP$_2$ fraction we have a similar pattern of retained proteins in the columns as shown previously, with the 23 kDa protein as a major band. In contrast, the affinity purified P$_3$ fraction contained two different major proteins, one corresponding to a MW of about 48 kDa and the other smaller, an 18 kDa protein. These proteins may correspond to similar estradiol binding proteins detected by Western blot in Fig. 18 from a CB-P$_2$ crude fraction. Current efforts are aiming to microsequencing these protein.

OVERVIEW

In closing, we would like to borrow the "unfolding of a continuing concept" formulated by C. Szego *(41)* many years ago and in a timely recent review *(53)*, to summarize what we have discussed in this chapter. According to the unfolding of the continuous process, E initially faces the extracellular compartment of the cell membrane as depicted in Fig. 20. For a more detailed discussion, the readers are referred to a recent review of us *(1)*. At least, we can distinguish three major initial events corresponding to three distinct pathways: first, the classical diffusion pathway by which E will diffuse inside the cell to bind the nER in an inactive state. The binding dissociates heat shock proteins and E-receptor dimers find its way to the ERE in the DNA to activate gene transcription *(54)*. This intracellular E could also diffuse inside the membrane of the mitochondria to encounter the OSCP subunit of the ATP synthase *(47)* and thereby

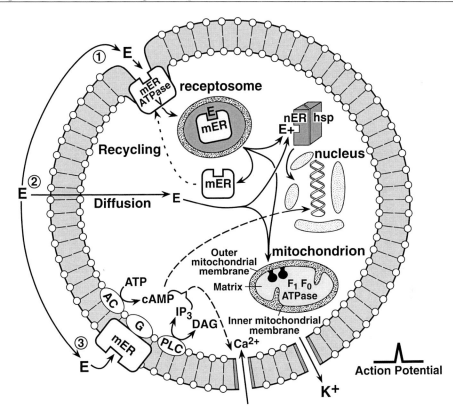

Fig. 20. A model of the "unfolding of a continuum concept" taken and modified from Szego *(41)* of estradiol action at the cellular level. For details, *see text.*

regulate cell energy by altering ATP production *(43,44)*; the second pathway involves an active endocytotic process, which has been initially reported for the uterus *(55)* but also recently detected in the hypothalamus and other brain cells *(56–58)*. In this process, E is internalized by a translocation mechanism most likely involving an E receptor molecule with the formation of a receptosome that after enzymatic digestion by lysosomes *(41)* releases its receptor (which might be recycled) and the free E is then available for intracellular actions, including enzymatic degradation. Recently, we have presented evidence indicating that this process may be present in the liver of ovx adult rats, because in vivo administration of E-6-^{125}I-BSA led to translocation of the ligand from the plasmalemma to the mitochondrial compartment within 5 min postinjection *(59)*; the third pathway probably involves a receptor coupled to a G protein, which either activates an adenylate cyclase system with cAMP production *(60–62)* or a PLC system with secondary production of IP3 and DAG *(63,64)*, two important intracellular messengers controlling intracellular distribution of calcium. Our data on E-6-BSA-evoked DA release from the CS most likely involves either of these two intracellular events.

In summary, in the search for a mER we have rediscovered the concept that E may bind to several unique proteins, either enzymes or typically known or novel receptors, in the regulation of specific cellular functions.

ACKNOWLEDGMENTS

This work was in part funded by a NIH grant #RO1-MH55986-01A1 to Victor D. Ramírez. We wish to thank Lori Heil and Missy Vandersall for editorial and administrative assistance.

REFERENCES

1. Ramírez VD, Zheng J. Membrane sex-steroid receptors in the brain. Frontiers Neuroendocrinol 1996;17:402–439.
2. Orchinik M, McEwen BS. Rapid actions in the brain: A critique of genomic and nongenomic mechanism. In: Wehling, M, ed. Genomic and Non-Genomic Effects of Aldosterone. CRC, London, 1995, pp. 77–108.
3. Smith MS, Freeman ME, Neil JD. The control of progesterone secretion during the estrous cycle and early pseudopregnancy in the rat: prolactin, gonadotropin and steroid levels associated with rescue of the corpus luteum of pseudopregnancy. Endocrinology 1975;96:219–226.
4. Cook B, Beastall GH. Measurement of steroid hormone concentrations in blood, urine and tissues. In: Green B, Leake RE, eds. Steroid Hormones: A Practical Approach. IRL, Oxford, 1987, pp. 1–65.
5. Lufkin EG, Ory SJ. Postmenopausal estrogen therapy. Trends Endocrinol Metabol 1995;6:50–54.
6. Majewska MD, Harrison NL, Schwartz RD, Barker JL, Paul SM. Steroid hormone metabolites are barbiturate-like modulators of the GABA receptor. Science 1986;232:1004–1007.
7. Morissette M, Garcia-Segura LM, Belanger A, and Di Paolo T. Changes of rat striatal neuronal membrane morphology and steroid content during the estrous cycle. Neuroscience 1992;49:893–902.
8. Robel P, Baulieu EE. Neurosteroids: biosynthesis and function. Trends Endocrinol Metabol 1994;5:1–8.
9. DeLean A, Stadel JM, Lefkowitz RJ. A ternary complex model explains the agonist-specific binding properties of the adenylate cylase-coupled β-adrenergic receptor. J Biol Chem 1980;255:7108–7117.
10. Sibley DR, DeLean A, Creese I. Anterior pituitary dopamine receptors: demonstration of interconvertible high and low affinity states of the D–2 dopamine receptor. J Biol Chem 1982;257:6351–6361.
11. Ramírez VD, Zheng J, Khawar MS. Membrane receptors for estrogen, progesterone and testosterone in the rat brain: fantasy or reality? Cell Mol Neurobiol 1996;16:175–197.
12. Zheng J, Ramírez VD. Purification and identification of an estrogen binding protein from rat brain: oligomycin sensitivity-conferring protein (OSCP), a subunit of mitochondrial F_0F_1-ATP synthase/ATPase. J Steroid Biochem Mol Biol, 1999;68:65–75.
13. McEwen BS. Steroid hormone actions on the brain: When is the genome involved? Horm Behav 1994;28:396–405.
14. Paul SM, Axelrod J, Saavedra JM, Skolnick P. Estrogen-induced efflux of endogenous catecholamines from the hypothalamus *in vitro*. Brain Res 1979;178:499–505.
15. Di Paolo T. Modulation of brain dopamine transmission by sex steroids. Rev Neurosci 1994;5:27–42.
16. Di Paolo T, Rouillard C, Bedard P. 17β-estradiol at a physiological dose acutely increases dopamine turnover in rat brain. Eur J Pharmacol 1985;117:197–203.
17. Hruska RE, Silbergeld EK. Estrogen treatment enhances dopamine receptor sensitivity in the rat striatum. Eur J Pharmacol 1980;61:397–400.
18. Becker JB. Estrogen rapidly potentiates amphetamine-induced striatal dopamine release and rotational behavior during microdialysis. Neurosci Lett 1990;118:169–171.
19. Becker JB, Cha J. Estrous cycle-dependent variation in amphetamine-induced behaviors and striatal dopamine release assessed with microdialysis. Behav Brain Res 1989;35:117–125.
20. Becker JB. Direct effect of 17β-estradiol on striatum: Sex differences in dopamine release. Synapse 1990;5:157–164.
21. Bazzett TJ, Becker JB. Sex differences in the rapid and acute effects of estrogen on striatal D–2 dopamine receptor binding. Brain Res 1994;637:163–172.
22. Levesque D, Di Paolo T. Rapid conversion of high into low striatal D2-dopamine receptor agonist binding states after an acute physiological dose of 17B-estradiol. Neurosci Lett 1988;88:113–118.
23. Pasqualini C, Oliver V, Guibert B, Frain O, Leviel V. Acute stimulatory effect of estradiol on striatal dopamine synthesis. Cell Mol Neurobiol 1996;16:411–415.

24. Pasqualini C, Oliver V, Guibert B, Frain O, Leviel V. Rapid stimulation of striatal dopamine synthesis by estradiol. J. Neurochem. 1995;65:1651–1657.
25. Thompson TL, Moss RL. Estrogen regulation of dopamine release in the nucleus accumbens: genomic- and nongenomic-mediated effects. J Neurochem 1994;62:1750–1756.
26. Dluzen DE, Ramírez VD. Bimodal effect of progesterone on *in vivo* dopamine function of the rat corpus striatum. Neuroendocrinology 1984;39: 149.
27. Dluzen DE, Ramírez VD. Modulatory effects of progesterone upon dopamine release from the corpus striatum of ovariectomized estrogen-treated rats are stereospecific. Brain Res 1991;538:176–179.
28. Towle AC, Sze PY. Steroid binding to synaptic plasma membrane: differential binding of glucocorticoids and gonadal steroids. J Steroid Biochem 1993;18:135–143.
29. Zheng J, Ali A, Ramírez VD. The use of steroids conjugated to bovine serum albumin (BSA) as tools to demonstrate the existence of specific steroid neuronal membrane binding sites. J Psychiatry Neurosci 1995;21:187–197.
30. Horvat A, Nikezic G, Martinovic JV. Estradiol binding to synaptosomal plasma membranes of rat brain regions. Experientia 1995;51:11–15.
31. Darnell J, Lodish H, Baltimore D. Molecular Cell Biology. Freeman, New York, NY, 1990.
32. Duax WH, Griffin JF, Rohrer DC, Weeks CM. Steroid agonists and antagonists: molecular conformation, receptor binding and activity. In: Agarwal MK, ed. Hormone Antagonists. Walter de Gruyter, New York, NY, 1982, pp. 3–24.
33. Keasling HH, Schueler FW. The relationship between estrogenic action and chemical constitution in a group of azomethine derivatives. J Am Pharm Assoc 1950;39:87–90.
34. Bruns RF, Lawson-Wendling K, Pugsley TA. A rapid filtration assay for soluble receptors using polyethylenimine-treated filters. Anal Biochem 1983;132:74–81.
35. Bradford MM. A rapid and sensitive method for the quantitation of microgram quantities of protein utilizing the principle of protein-dye binding. Anal Biochem 1976;72:248.
36. Munson PJ, Rodbard D. LIGAND: a versatile computerized approach for characterization of ligand-binding systems. Anal Biochem 1980;107:220–239.
37. Cheng YC, Prusoff WH. Relationship between the inhibition constant (ki) and the concentration of inhibitor which causes 50 percent inhibition (IC_{50}) of an enzymatic reaction. Biochem Pharmacol 1973;22:3099–3108.
38. Sutherland RL, Watts CKW, Murphy LC. Binding properties and ligand specificity of an intracellular binding site with specificity for synthetic oestrogen antagonists of the triphenylethylene series. In: Agarwal MK, ed. Hormone Antagonists. Walter de Gruyter, New York, NY, 1982, pp. 147–161.
39. Clark JH, Shailaja KM. Actions of ovarian steroid hormones. In: Knobil E, Neil J, eds. The Physiology of Reproduction, 2nd ed. Raven, New York, NY, 1994, pp. 1011–1059.
40. Tischkau SA, Ramírez VD. A specific membrane binding protein for progesterone in rat brain: sex differences and induction by estrogen. Proc Natl Acad Sci USA 1993;90:1285–1289.
41. Szego CM, Pietras RJ. Lysosomal functions in cellular activation: Propagation of the actions of hormones and other effectors. Int Rev Cytology 1984;88:1–302. 42.
42. Noteboom WD, Gorski J. Stereospecific binding of estrogens in the rat uterus. Arch Biochem Biophys 1965;111:559–568.
43. McEnery MW, Pedersen PL. Diethylstilbestrol: a novel F_0-directed probe of the mitochondrial proton ATPase. J Biol Chem 1986;261: 1745–1752.
44. McEnery MW, Hullihen J, Pedersen PL. F_0 "proton channel" of rat liver mitochondria: rapid purification of a functional complex and a study of its interaction with the unique probe diethylstilbestrol. J Biol Chem 1989;264:12029–12036.
45. McEwen BS. Non-genomic and genomic effects of steroids on neural activity. Trends Pharmacol Sci 1991;12:141–147.
46. Abrahams JP, Leslie AGW, Lutter R, Walker JE. Structure at 2.8Å resolution of F_1-ATPase from bovine heart mitochondria. Nature 1994;370:21–628.
47. Pedersen PL, Amzel LM. ATP synthases: structure, reaction center, mechanism, and regulation of one of nature's most unique machines. J Biol Chem 1993;268:9937–9940.
48. Walker JE, Collinson I. The role of the stalk in the coupling mechanism of F1Fo-ATPases. FEBS Lett 1994;346:39–43.
49. Zimmerman H. Signalling via ATP in the nervous system. Trends Neurosci. 1994;102:1151–1157.
50. Aaronson SA, Natori Y, Tarver H. Effect of estrogen on uterine ATP levels. Proc Soc Exp Biol Med 1965;120:9–10.

51. Bodwell JE, Hu CM, Hu JM, Orti E, Munck A. Glucocorticoid receptors: ATP-dependent cycling and hormone-dependent hyperphosphorylation. J Steroid Biochem Molec Biol 1993;47:31–38.

52. Smith DF, Stensgard BA, Welch WJ, Toft DO. Assembly of progesterone receptor with heat shock proteins and receptor activation are ATP mediated events. J Biol Chem 1992;267:1350–1356.

53. Szego CM. Cytostructural correlates of hormone action: new common ground in receptor-mediated signal propagation for steroid and peptide agonists. Endocrine 1994;2:1079–1093.

54. O'Malley BW, Tsai SY, Bagchi M,Weigel NL, Schrader WT, Tsai MJ. Molecular mechanism of action of a steroid hormone-receptor. Recent Prog Horm Res 1991;47:1–24.

55. Rambo CO, Szego CM. Estrogen action at endometrial membranes: alterations in luminal surface detectable within seconds. J Cell Biol 1983;97:679–685.

56. Garcia-Segura LM,Olmos G, Tranque P, Naftolin F. Rapid effects of gonadal steroids upon hypothalamic neuronal membrane ultrastructure. J Steroid Biochem 1987;27:615–623.

57. Garcia-Segura LM, Olmos G, Robbins RJ, Hernandez P, Meyer JH, Naftolin F. Estradiol induces rapid remodeling of plasma membranes in developing rat cerebrocortical neurons in culture. Brain Res 1989;498:339–343.

58. Garcia-Segura LM, Chowen JA, Parducz A, Naftolin F. Gonadal hormones as promoters of structural synpatic plasticity: cellular mechanisms. Prog Neurobiol 1994;44:279–307.

59. Moats RK, Ramírez VD. Evidence for a membrane-mediated uptake mechanism for estrogen in the liver of the female rat. Society Study Reproduc 1996, Abs # 278.

60. Aronica SM, Kraus WL, Katzenellenbogen BS. Estrogen action via the cAMP signalling pathway-stimulation of adenylate cyclase and cAMP-regulated gene transcription. Proc Natl Acad Sci USA 1994;91:8517–8521.

61. Zhou Y, Watters JJ, Dorsa DM. Estrogen rapidly induces the phosphorylation of the cAMP response element binding protein in rat brain. Endocrinology 1996;137:2163–2166.

62. Szego CM, Davis JS. Adenosine 3',5'-monophosphate in rat uterus: acute elevation by estrogen. Proc. Natl. Acad. Sci. 1967;58:1711–1718.

63. Lieberherr M, Grosse B. Androgens increase intracellular calcium concentration and inositol 1,4,5-trisphosphate and diacylglycerol formation via a pertussis toxin-sensitive G-protein. J Biol Chem 1994;269:7217–7223.

64. Lieberherr M, Grosse B, Kachkache M, Balsan S. Cell signalling and estrogens in female rat osteoblasts: a possible involvement of unconventional non-nuclear receptors. J Bone Mineral Res 1993;8:1365–1376.

17

Novel Mechanisms of Estrogen Action in the Developing Brain

Role of Steroid/Neurotrophin Interactions

C. Dominique Toran-Allerand, MD

Contents

INTRODUCTION
ESTROGEN
THE ESTROGEN RECEPTORS
THE NEUROTROPHINS
THE NEUROTROPHIN RECEPTORS
NEUROTROPHIN SIGNAL TRANSDUCTION CASCADES
INTERACTIONS OF ESTROGEN AND THE NEUROTROPHINS
CONSEQUENCES OF TYROSINE PHOSPHORYLATION
    OF THE ESTROGEN RECEPTOR
CROSS-COUPLING OF ESTROGEN AND NEUROTROPHIN
    SIGNALING PATHWAYS
MULTIMERIC COMPLEXING OF ESTROGEN RECEPTORS
    WITH SIGNALING PROTEINS
CONCLUSION
REFERENCES

INTRODUCTION

Sex-specific and temporally restricted, differential exposure of the developing male and female central nervous system (CNS) to gonadal steroid hormones such as the estrogens and the androgens has been implicated in the organization of neural circuits controlling a broad spectrum of sexually differentiated neuroendocrine, behavioral, and cognitive functions in the mammalian adult *(1–4)*. Paradoxically, many actions of testosterone in the developing brain depend on its initial intraneuronal conversion, through aromatization, to estradiol. Metabolic conversion results in the subsequent binding of estradiol to high-affinity intranuclear estrogen receptors (ERs) *(3)*, that are located within neurons of brain regions such as the hypothalamus, preoptic area, cerebral cortex, hippocampus and amygdala. These are all regions that are rich in aromatase activity, particularly during

From: *Contemporary Endocrinology: Neurosteroids: A New Regulatory Function in the Nervous System* Edited by: E.-E. Baulieu, P. Robel, and M. Schumacher
© Humana Press Inc., Totowa, NJ

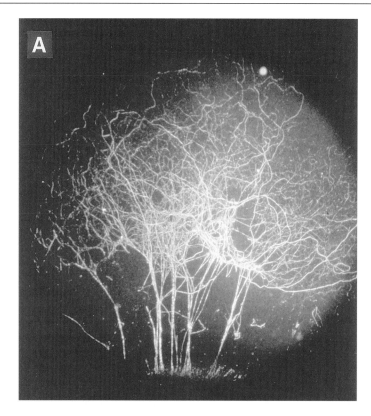

Fig. 1. (A) Neurite-promoting effects of estradiol in hypothalamic explant cultures, 19 d in vitro. Photomicrographs of right and left homologous coronal halves of a Holmes' silver-impregnated pair of explants from the preoptic area. Darkfield microscopy, ×125. Control exposed only to estrogens endogenous to the 25% horse serum component of the nutrient medium. The silver-impregnated neurofibrils (bundles of neuron-specific, neurofilament proteins) course outward from the margin of the explant.

development *(5)*. Increasing evidence, however, suggests that this widely held view of estrogen action in the developing brain is too restrictive and should be expanded beyond the strict confines of sexual differentiation. Thus estrogens, and estradiol in particular, have important consequences for neuronal development, survival, regeneration, plasticity, and even aging of the mammalian CNS.

ESTROGEN

Among its various neural actions, estradiol exhibits growth- or neurite-promoting properties for neurons of the developing brain. Toran-Allerand *(1–4)* first demonstrated that estrogen elicits the selective enhancement of axon and dendrite (neurite) growth and differentiation in developing estrogen target regions of the hypothalamus, preoptic area, and cerebral cortex *(1,2,6–8)* (Fig. 1). This neurite-promoting property of estradiol is expressed only during development and never in the adult brain that is normally exposed to estrogen. However, following damage in the adult to estrogen target brain regions, as

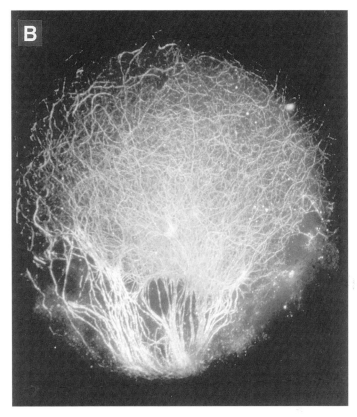

Fig. 1. (B) Exogenous estradiol (50 ng/mL) added to the culture medium. There is a significant enhancement of neurite growth from the same region of the homologous explant half, with extensive arborization of neurites in the outgrowth. (Adapted with permission from ref. 2.)

a result of loss of trophic support, whether through axotomy, deafferentation, or steroid deprivation, responsiveness to estrogen returns and estrogen can again be shown to influence the regrowth and differentiation of neurite-derived structures such as axons, dendrites and their spines, and synapses *(9,10)*. In this respect, therefore, estrogen should be added to the growing list of important growth- or neurite-promoting molecules such as growth factors, including the members of the neurotrophin family of peptides (e.g., nerve growth factor [NGF], brain-derived neurotrophic factor [BDNF], neurotrophin-3 [NT-3], neurotrophin-4/5 [NT-4/5], and neurotrophin-6 [NT-6]*)*.

Overlapping regions of the male and female forebrain that subserve cognitive functions, such as the basal forebrain, cerebral cortex, and hippocampus, are not only targets of estrogen and the neurotrophins, but sites of estrogen and neurotrophin synthesis as well. Such an association directs attention to the possible importance of steroid/neurotrophin interactions for their neurons. In neurons of the developing and adult forebrain, for example, ERs are widely co-expressed with the neurotrophins and their cognate receptors *(11–13)*. This association has led us to question whether the neurotrophic aspects of estrogen's actions in the developing CNS may be mediated, at least in part, by interactions of estrogen with the neurotrophin ligands or their receptors *(14,15)*.

THE ESTROGEN RECEPTORS

There are two rat ER genes, coding respectively for the "classical" receptor ER-α (66/67 kDa) and for the ER-β (54 kDa), which differ significantly with respect to their C-terminal (ligand binding) domain (58% homology) and N-terminal (transactivation) domain (no homology) *(16,17)*, as well as in their binding affinities, ligand specificities and tissue distribution *(18)*. The recent discovery of the ER-β gene complicates matters considerably, because very little is known about its regulation or function, particularly in the developing and adult mammalian nervous system, and its recent identification raises the possibility of additional, as yet unidentified, ER gene(s) as well. Thus, it is not at all clear whether our understanding of any aspects concerning the role and function of the neural "estrogen receptor" applies to ER-α, to ER-β, or to both. The presence of ER-β and its regional distribution have been described incompletely in the adult rat brain *(19)*, whereas the ontogeny and mechanisms of regulation of ER-β during neural development have yet to be addressed. These issues are particularly relevant with respect to the identity of the receptor phenotype of the "estrogen receptor" of the cerebral cortex. The cortical ER is developmentally regulated and its highest levels of expression (comparable to levels of adult preoptic area) are expressed only transiently during a very restricted period of postnatal cortical differentiation *(1,20,21)*. In the discussion that follows, reference will be made only to the ER without attempting to distinguish ER-α from ER-β, which are both likely to be present. However, whatever information has been derived from our own *in situ* hybridization studies of the ontogeny of ER mRNA expression in the developing cerebral cortex *(22)*, and of the regulation of ER mRNA expression in PC12 cells *(23)* and adult sensory ganglia *(24)*, refers to ER-α, at least, because the oligonucleotide probe used in these studies (nucleotides 1923–1970; ligand-binding domain of the rat uterine ER *[25]*) shares no homology with ER-β (M. Singh and D. Toran-Allerand, unpublished observations).

The nonactivated (unliganded) ER has a molecular architecture homologous to the androgen, glucocorticoid, and progesterone receptors, even though phylogenetically the ER genes form a distinct subgroup within the gene superfamily of nuclear hormone receptors. This family also includes thyroid hormone, retinoic acid, aldosterone, vitamin D receptors, and the "orphan" receptors whose ligands and/or target genes are unknown *(26–28)*. Estrogen receptor/ligand interactions trigger a cascade of events including hormone binding, dissociation from heat shock proteins (hsp90 in particular), homodimer formation, and phosphorylation, resulting in the association of the hormone-activated receptor with specific regulatory DNA sequences, or estrogen-responsive elements (EREs), in target genes *(26,27,29)*. Ligand-independent activation of steroid receptors has also been described *(30–33)*.

The classical ER is a phosphoprotein that exhibits basal levels of phosphorylation. The ER becomes rapidly hyperphosphorylated (2–7-fold) within 2 min upon binding of estrogen. Maximum levels of phosphorylation are reached at 30–40 min *(29,34–39)*. There appears to be controversy in the literature whether phosphorylation of the ligand-activated ER occurs exclusively on tyrosine, on serine, or on both tyrosine and serine residues *(29,34–39)*. Most studies agree that both estrogen-dependent and estrogen-independent tyrosine phosphorylation of the ER occurs only on tyrosine residue 537 *(40–42)*, a step required for ligand binding to the receptor, homodimerization and binding to EREs in DNA *(43,44)*. Serine, on the other hand, is reportedly phosphorylated at residue 167 in an estrogen-dependent manner *(39,40,45)*, whereas serine 118 appears to be critical in non-neural tumor cells for full steroid-independent activation of the ER activation function 1 (AF-1) by growth factors such as insulin-like growth factor-1 (IGF-1) and epidermal growth factor (EGF) *(46)*, and is the site of growth factor-induced phosphorylation by mitogen-activated protein (MAP) kinases (extracellular-regulated kinases, ERKs) directly *(31,47)*.

We have recently shown for the first time in brain tissue (cerebral cortical explants), that estrogen hyperphosphorylate the ER on both tyrosine and serine residues *(48,49)*. This response occurs within 5 min, becomes maximal at 30 min, and persists for at least 4 h. These findings are very important because they document that tyrosine phosphorylation of the ER does occur in wild-type (normal) ERs of the postnatal-d 2 rat brain (cerebral cortex) developing under quasi-normal conditions and is not just a property of tumor cell lines that may overexpress the ER or that have been transfected with mutant or truncated receptors. Whether the increase in estrogen binding also results from an increase in ER protein content is currently under study. However, whether or not the receptor molecules are actually increased in number, translational and posttranslational effects on their own can modify estrogen binding so that the resulting effect of estradiol on neurons would be augmented.

Of the members of the steroid receptor family, it is noteworthy that only the ER becomes phosphorylated on both tyrosine and serine *(29,39)*. The other steroid receptors are phosphorylated almost exclusively on serine, occasionally on threonine as well *(29)*. Ligand-induced phosphorylation on tyrosine residues places the ER in a steroid class by itself and puts it in the same category as growth factor receptor tyrosine kinases. Although the ligand-activated ER was initially thought not to exhibit intrinsic kinase activity *(34)*, the analogy with growth factor receptor tyrosine kinases becomes even stronger with the recent surprising finding that the plasma membrane-associated nonactivated (unliganded) goat uterine ER is a receptor tyrosine kinase and does, in fact, apparently exhibit intrinsic tyrosine kinase activity and tyrosine autophosphorylation *(50,51)*. It is tempting to speculate that the ability of estrogen to elicit tyrosine phosphorylation of its own receptor, which appears to be unique to estrogen and the ER, may relate to the growth- or neurite-promoting actions of estrogen, a property that also appears to be unique among the steroid hormones.

Until several years ago, the dogma of estrogen action was that estrogen regulation of gene expression is mediated through the classical intranuclear receptor to stimulate transcriptional activity directly via EREs *(26,27)*. The classical ER is said to shuttle constantly between the nucleus and cytoplasm, although under steady-state conditions it is predominantly intranuclear in both the presence and absence of its ligand *(52–55)*. However, increasing evidence suggests that there may be multiple types of ERs, including, in particular, estrogen-binding proteins, associated with the cell surface membrane and organelles *(56–62)*, which can mediate extracellular signals in both a steroid-dependent and steroid-independent manner by means of growth factor signaling pathways *(32,33)*. For example, in breast cancer and other non-neural cell lines, estrogen has been shown to elicit very rapid and transient responses, (ranging from seconds to min) similar to those evoked by mitogenic peptide growth factors such EGF and IGF-1 *(63–65)*. This time course is inconsistent with transcriptional modulation but is consistent with the sharing of estrogen and growth factor (IGF-1 and EGF) signaling pathways for cell proliferation and ER phosphorylation *(31,47,66–70)*. Migliaccio et al. *(63)*, moreover, have shown that, in MCF-7 cells, estradiol elicits maximal phosphorylation of *src* within 10 s, an effect which apparently required only 10–20% ER occupancy *(65)*. This level of occupancy has been reported to correspond to the percentage of ER estimated to be associated with the plasma membrane *(59)*. Findings such as these have led to the hypothesis that rapid signaling of this type may be mediated by a membrane-associated ER.

Some studies *(60)* suggest that there is a strong immunoreactive similarity between the classical ER and a membrane-associated subpopulation that appears to mediate rapid estrogen responses. Other studies *(51)*, however, report that the nonactivated (unliganded) goat uterine ER is a unique membrane-associated receptor whose primary structure is distinctly different from the "classical" ER, even though all ER antibodies apparently do cross-react with it. This finding may explain the reported apparent immunological similarities with the classical ER *(60)*.

In contrast, little is known about the nature of the ER in the postmitotic CNS, where estrogen elicits differentiative rather than proliferative effects, or about estrogen signaling pathways in the brain. Thus, as will be considered later, although the ER is generally considered a classical, ligand-induced transcriptional enhancer, the ER may, in fact, also act as a tyrosine kinase, even as a receptor tyrosine kinase with intrinsic kinase activity, in much the same manner as the receptors for peptide growth factors such as the neurotrophins.

THE NEUROTROPHINS

Expression of the neurotrophins and their cognate receptors is widespread throughout the developing and adult CNS, including forebrain regions such as the basal forebrain, cerebral cortex, and hippocampus. The neurotrophins NGF, BDNF, NT-3, NT-4/5, and NT-6 are structurally and functionally related proteins with important growth and trophic actions on the development and maintenance of the CNS and peripheral nervous system (reviewed in ref. *71*). Despite their strong homology, each neurotrophin exhibits restricted spatial and temporal patterns of expression, different, often sequential, functions; and different stages of central and peripheral target responsiveness. Although NGF, BDNF, and NT-3 mRNAs, for example, are expressed in distinct neuronal subpopulations of the developing and adult brain, neurotrophin functions in the CNS are far from being fully understood, particularly during development. We have recently documented extensive co-localization of ERs with the neurotrophins and their receptors in regions of the developing forebrain and diencephalon, including, in particular, the basal forebrain, cerebral cortex, hippocampus, hypothalamus, and preoptic area *(11–13)*.

THE NEUROTROPHIN RECEPTORS

The biological activities of the neurotrophin family of growth factors are mediated by two structurally distinct classes of cell membrane receptors, which are preferentially expressed in neural tissues *(72–74)*; one class consists of members of the *trk* family of ligand-specific, transmembrane receptor protein tyrosine kinases, each of which mediates neurotrophin signaling to the nucleus and cytoskeleton through increased tyrosine autophosphorylation of its cognate receptor. NGF binds to *trkA*, BDNF and NT-4/5 to *trkB*, and NT-3 primarily to *trkC*. Although dogma currently holds that normal *trkA* mRNA and protein expression in vivo are restricted to subsets of spinal and cranial sensory neurons and to neurons of the basal forebrain *(75-78)*, we have also found *trkA* mRNA and protein expression throughout the developing forebrain, particularly in the basal forebrain, cerebral cortex, and hippocampus *(12,13,79)*.

The second receptor, p75, a 75-kDa transmembrane protein, appears to have a modulatory role on *trk* activity and function *(74,80)*. Like the *trk* receptors, p75 has been found to be co-expressed with ERs *(11,13)*. P75 is related to the tumor necrosis factor-1 (TNF-1)/Fas/CD40 receptor family and, when overexpressed or stimulated in the absence of *trk*, has been recently implicated in the regulation of neuronal apoptotic death *(74,80)* and the activation of NFkB *(81)* and in the production of the ICE-like protease ceramide *(82)*.

NEUROTROPHIN SIGNAL TRANSDUCTION CASCADES

Signals from polypeptide growth and trophic factors such as the neurotrophins are propagated to the nucleus by an essentially linear flow of sequential protein phosphorylation and dephosphorylation events. These second messenger enzyme cascades, which involve both tyrosine and serine/threonine kinases and phosphatases, serve to funnel, amplify, and propagate signals generated at the cell surface into complex biological responses, including the regulation of target transcription factors such as CREB and *Elk* and the induction of immediate early genes such as c-*fos* and c-*jun (83–87)*. Virtually all that is known about neurotrophin signaling in neural tissue is derived from studies of nerve growth factor (NGF), the prototypical neurotrophin, in PC12 cells, a cell line derived from a rat pheochromocytoma and prototypical NGF target *(88)*. As illustrated in Fig. 2, NGF treatment of PC12 cells elicits dimerization of *trkA* and activates its catalytic *src*-homology1 (SH*1*) domain, resulting in autophosphorylation of *trkA* on tyrosine residues *(89–92)*. Tyrosine autophosphorylation regulates interactions of the activated *trkA* with multiple intracellular proteins with *src*-homology2 (SH2) domains that either function as enzymes (kinases), such as phospholipase C-γ1 (PLC-γ1) and c-*src*, or as docking proteins, such as Shc and Grb2. Shc and Grb2 with the glutamyl transpeptidase/gel diffusion precipitin (GTP/GDP) exchange protein SOS connect activated *trkA* to the authentic signaling enzyme p21^{Ras}. *Ras*, a small guanine nucleotide-binding protein, then activates members of the MAP kinase cascade by sequential phosphorylation on tyrosine or serine/threonine residues. The MAP kinase cascade is triggered by *Ras* activation of the cell-type specific *Raf* family *(93, 94)* (b-*Raf* in PC12 cells; c-*Raf* in sympathetic neurons; b- and/or c-*Raf* in the CNS?); followed by activation of MAP Kinase kinase, or MEK [MAP kinase/extracellular-regulated kinase (ERK) Kinase kinase], then MAP Kinase (MAPK), or ERK, which phosphorylates other kinases such as p90^{Rsk} or transcription factors *(95)*. Phosphorylated ERK (ERK2 in particular) and *Rsk* both translocate to the nucleus and are the means by which growth factor signaling regulates transcription. The MAP kinase cascade and *suc*-associated neurotrophic factor-induced tyrosine-phosphorylated target (SNT) *(96)*, a parallel, growth factor- and differentiation-specific pathway, form two major growth factor signaling pathways whose prolonged activation is necessary but not sufficient for PC12 neuronal differentiation *(84,86,97–99)*. Neurotrophin signaling pathways in the CNS, on the other hand, are very ill-defined.

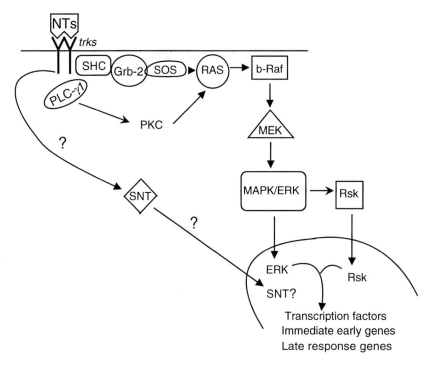

Fig. 2. Some *trkA* signaling cascades activated by NGF. In PC12 cells, treatment with NGF, the prototypical neurotrophin, elicits dimerization of *trkA* and activates its catalytic *src*-homology1 (SH1) domain, resulting in autophosphorylation of *trkA* on tyrosine residues. Autophosphorylation regulates interactions of the activated *trkA* with multiple intracellular proteins with SH2 domains that either function as enzymes (kinases), such as PLC-γ1 and c-*src*, or as docking proteins, such as Shc and Grb2. Shc and Grb2 with the GTP/GDP exchange protein SOS connect activated *trkA* to the authentic signaling enzyme p21^{Ras}. *Ras* then activates members of the MAP kinase cascade, b-*Raf*, MEK, and ERK (MAPK) by sequential phosphorylation on tyrosine, serine/threonine residues. ERK then phosphorylates other kinases such as *Rsk*, and the phosphorylated ERKs and *Rsk* both translocate to the nucleus to regulate immediate early and late response genes and transcription factors. The MAP kinase cascade and SNT, a parallel, growth factor- and differentiation-specific pathway, form two major growth factor signaling pathways whose prolonged activation is necessary but not sufficient for PC12 neuronal differentiation.

INTERACTIONS OF ESTROGEN AND THE NEUROTROPHINS

The cascade of molecular events in the brain that follows estrogen activation of the neural ER are largely unknown, as are the signaling pathways mediating the differentiative actions of estrogen and the neurotrophins in the CNS. A critical and as yet unanswered question is whether the developmental actions of estrogen in the brain, such as enhancement of neurite growth and differentiation, are mediated directly or as a consequence of a large cascade of intracellular events initiated by interactions of estrogen with endogenous growth factors such as the neurotrophins and their receptors *(1,100)*. The findings of estrogen and neurotrophin receptor co-expression in the developing forebrain *(11,13)* and of putative EREs in the genes for NGF *(13)*, BDNF *(101)*, NT-3 (M. Singh and D. Toran-Allerand, unpublished observations), p75 *(11)*, and *trkA (24)* suggest that estrogen

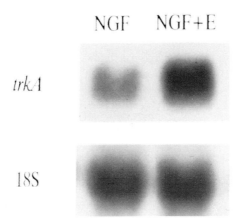

Fig. 3. Estrogen up-regulation of *trkA* mRNA in PC12 cells. Northern blot analysis of PC12 mRNA probed for *trkA*. Top: Total RNA (20 mg) was size-fractionated on a 1.2% agarose gel and transferred to nylon. Blots were hybridized to a random-primed (^{32}P) cDNA probe of approximately 0.5 kb (gift of Dr. Luis F. Parada) for 48 h, washed at high stringency (0.2 × SSC, 50°C, 2 h) and apposed to film (Kodak X-RP). PC12 cells were exposed to either NGF (100 ng/mL) alone for 18 d or to NGF alone for 10 days, followed by NGF plus estrogen (10^{-9} *M*) concurrently for an additional 8 days. Bottom: Same blot probed for β-actin mRNA, using a 40 base oligonucleotide (Dupont), 3'-labeled with ^{32}P, using terminal deoxynucleotidyl transferase. Densitometric measurements, normalized to β-actin, suggest that, in the presence of NGF, estrogen appears to increase *trkA* mRNA expression significantly. (Adapted with permission from ref. *14*).

may regulate neurite growth and differentiation by interactions with neurotrophins through autocrine or local paracrine mechanisms.

Estrogen and the neurotrophins may influence each other's actions to regulate receptor and/or ligand availability by actions at the transcriptional, translational, and posttranslational levels. In this regard, differential and reciprocal regulation of estrogen and NGF receptor mRNAs (both p75 and *trkA*) by their ligands has been shown in both adult sensory neurons *(24)* and PC12 cells *(23)*. In both PC12 cells (Fig. 3) and following estrogen treatment of the ovariectomized adult female rat, p75 mRNA was transiently down-regulated; whereas *trkA* mRNA expression was significantly up-regulated and sustained. NGF was also found to up-regulate estrogen binding in both PC12 cells *(23)* and cerebral cortical explants *(80)* (Fig. 4). Unlike the pattern seen in PC12 cells, however, there was no apparent associated change in cortical ER mRNA expression.

Interactions of estrogen and the neurotrophins may also be involved in the as yet unknown mechanisms that underlie differential regulation by estrogen of its own receptor in the brain. The direction of the responses of the neural ER to estrogen appears to be developmental-stage dependent. Thus, although estrogen classically down-regulates its receptor in the adult brain *(102,103)*, a considerable degree of ER mRNA expression is seen in the developing postnatal brain until around postnatal d 28 *(22)*, despite postnatal levels of estrogen normally sufficient for receptor down-regulation in the adult. One way of interpreting such regulatory patterns would be to consider that they may result, during the postnatal period, from either estrogen up-regulation of its receptor or from the inability of estrogen to regulate its own receptor (nonregulation) *(14)*. One might further speculate that developmental stage-dependent differences in the direction of estrogen

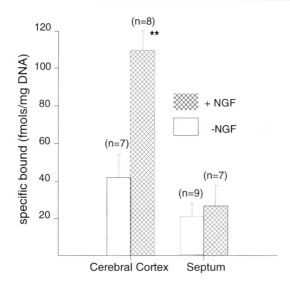

Fig. 4. NGF regulates estrogen binding by the unliganded estrogen receptor. Specific, nuclear [³H]moxestrol binding (normalized to DNA content) was observed in both postnatal d 2 (P2) cortical and basal forebrain cultured explant slices, maintained for 8 d in vitro in the absence of estradiol. The addition of human recombinant NGF led to a significant increase (**) in nuclear estrogen binding sites in cortical but not basal forebrain explants. NGF regulation of estrogen binding under estrogen-deficient conditions appears to be region-specific in the explants. This apparent specificity, however, may reflect differences in the ontogeny of estrogen binding in these regions. Cortical receptors develop significantly earlier than those of the basal forebrain. Maximal receptor levels are reached ~P8-10 in the cortex; ~puberty in the basal forebrain (D. Toran-Allerand, unpublished observations). *n* = sample size in each group. (Adapted with permission from ref. 79.)

regulation of its own receptor may perhaps be a consequence of interactions with other transcription-regulating molecules, including the neurotrophins. To explain this discrepancy in the responses of the ER during development and in the adult, I have proposed that the neurotrophins may serve as regulatory switches whereby their modulatory role on ER expression may influence the direction of estrogen regulation of its own receptor (Fig. 5) *(14,15)*. For example, during CNS development, the ability of the neurotrophins to increase ER protein levels and binding significantly may be sufficient alone (or even in synergy with estrogen) to influence or even override the intrinsic suppressive action of estrogen on its own receptor. Maturation of the CNS is associated with significant alterations in the spatial, temporal, and functional expression of the neurotrophins and their receptors *(104,105)*, as well as in their physiological role(s) *(106)*. Such changes may serve to "free" the ER from the regulatory influences of the neurotrophins, resulting in the emergence of the intrinsic (adult) pattern of estrogen-induced receptor down-regulation and loss of estrogen's neurite-promoting effects. However, in the adult, following injury to estrogen target regions or in the presence of estrogen deficiency (e.g., ovariectomy, menopause), there may be a "switch" in the direction of estrogen regulation of its receptor back to the developmental pattern that is manifested by a re-expression of the growth-promoting properties of estrogen which is never seen in the normal adult. Because various forms of trauma and injury to the brain (perhaps including steroid deficiency) also

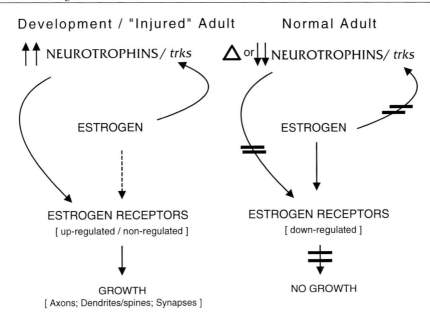

Fig. 5. Neurotrophins as regulatory switches. During development, the ability of neurotrophins to increase estrogen binding significantly may be sufficient alone or in synergy with estrogen to influence or override the intrinsic suppressive action of estrogen on its own receptor and enhance the growth and differentiation of neurite-derived structures. In contrast, maturation of the CNS is accompanied by alterations in the spatial, temporal, and functional expression of the neurotrophins and their receptors, as well as by age-related changes in their physiological roles. Such changes may "free" the ER from the regulatory or modifying influences of the neurotrophins, resulting in the emergence of the intrinsic (adult) pattern of receptor down-regulation and a loss of estrogen's neurite-promoting effects. However, enhanced neurotrophin sensitivity in the injured or steroid-deficient adult brain may result in a return ("switch") of neurotrophin modulation of the ER back to the developmental pattern that is manifested by a re-expression of the growth-promoting properties of estrogen on axons, dendrites and synapses. (Adapted with permission from ref. *15*.)

elicit up-regulation of neurotrophin ligand and receptor expression *(107–109)*, the enhanced sensitivity to neurotrophins of the injured or estrogen-deficient adult brain may result in a return of neurotrophin modulation of the ER and estrogen enhancement of neurite growth and differentiation.

CONSEQUENCES OF TYROSINE PHOSPHORYLATION OF THE ESTROGEN RECEPTOR

We have recently shown in explants of the cerebral cortex that the cortical ER becomes phosphorylated on tyrosine. Phosphorylation of the ER synthesized in vitro on tyrosine specifically has been shown to result in an acquisition of or increase in estrogen binding sites *(38,110)*. One predicted consequence of this event in the brain would be to increase the number of activated neuronal estrogen binding sites. One possible mechanism, therefore, for the observed NGF-induced increases in estrogen binding in explants of the cerebral cortex *(79)* and PC12 cells *(23)* may be tyrosine phosphorylation of the cortical ER. That the ER of the cerebral cortex does become phosphorylated on tyrosine residues by the neurotrophins NGF, BDNF, NT-3, and NT4/5, as well as by its own ligand estrogen, has been documented recently by immunoprecipitation with antibodies to the ER, followed by Western immunoblotting using anti-phosphotyrosine antibodies (4G10) *(48,49)*. Because mutation of tyrosine 537 to phenylalanine reportedly eliminated immunodetection of tyrosine phosphorylation of the extra-neural ER *(44)*, our very ability to detect immunologically tyrosine phosphorylation of the cortical ER *(48,49)* suggests that tyrosine 537 is the residue that also becomes phosphorylated by both estrogen and the neurotrophins in the brain.

NGF up-regulation of cortical estrogen binding, without influencing mRNA levels, could be explained by a reapportioning of the ER to the activated (hyperphosphorylated) form. The resultant increased affinity for DNA, which is a consequence of ER tyrosine phosphorylation, is a posttranslational event that does not require a change in steady-state mRNA *(38,39,110)*. Whether the increase in estrogen binding also results from an increase in ER protein content is not yet known. However, whether or not the receptor protein molecules are also actually increased in number, translational and posttranslational effects on their own can modify estrogen binding so that neurotrophin regulation of the ability of cells to bind estrogen would serve to regulate neuronal responsiveness to this steroid hormone.

Neurotrophin-induced acquisition of estrogen binding may have developmental significance for the development of both estrogen and neurotrophin receptors and suggests a reciprocal role for their ligands in this process. For example, in the rodent the temporal expression of the neurotrophins and their receptors in the developing cerebral cortex is present earlier than that of the cortical ER *(104*; D. Toran-Allerand, unpublished observations). Neurotrophin-induced increases in the acquisition of estrogen binding by target neurons would thus initiate or enhance their responsiveness to estrogen. In a reciprocal manner, enhanced neuronal responsiveness to estrogen would have consequences for estrogen up-regulation of neurotrophin ligand and receptor expression. Increased neurotrophin levels, in turn, would further influence the levels of estrogen binding by its receptor, and so forth. Thus, reciprocal regulation of the estrogen and neurotrophin receptors by their ligands at transcriptional, translational, and even posttranslational levels suggest the potential for reciprocal regulatory loops that may influence the ontogeny of both receptor systems.

CROSS-COUPLING OF ESTROGEN
AND NEUROTROPHIN SIGNALING PATHWAYS

An additional way by which estrogen may interact with the neurotrophins is through reciprocal regulation at the level of signal transduction. Convergence or cross-coupling of estrogen and neurotrophin signaling pathways (receptor cross-talk) may lead to nuclear end- points that regulate the same broad array of growth-associated and cytoskeletal genes related to neuronal differentiation and neurite growth. Cross-coupling of ERs with growth-factor signaling pathways has been shown in non-neural estrogen target tissues and does not involve binding to DNA (reviewed in refs. *67* and *111*).

The potential for cross-coupling of the estrogen and neurotrophin signaling pathways in the developing brain is suggested by our recent studies, which provide the first example in nervous tissue that estrogen elicits rapid and prolonged tyrosine phosphorylation of both ERK1 and ERK2 (p44 and p42 MAP kinase isoforms, respectively) *(48,49)*. Activation of the ERKs in PC12 cells by EGF and IGF-1, for example, is very transient, a pattern that is associated with cell proliferation *(87)*. Prolonged activation of ERK1 and ERK2, as elicited by NGF in PC12 cells, on the other hand, has been found to lead to neuronal differentiation *(84,86,95,97–99)*. The prolonged time-course of ERK activation, which follows estrogen exposure, is consistent with its observed differentiative actions with respect to neurite growth and differentiation *(1,6–8)* (Fig. 1). Estrogen-induced tyrosine phosphorylation of ERK in the cerebral cortex occurred within 5 min, became maximal at 30 min, and persisted for at least 4 h. Thirty minute pulses of the neurotrophins NGF-, BDNF-, NT-3-, and NT-4/5-induced tyrosine phosphory-lation of ERK1 and ERK2 in the cortical explants to levels that were qualitatively and quantitatively similar to those following comparable exposure to estrogen. There were no additive effects, suggesting that the cells responding to each ligand were the same and not additional ER-containing subsets. Because ERK2 (and possibly ERK1) translocate to the cell nucleus *(97–99)*, convergence or cross-coupling of the estro-gen and neurotrophin receptor systems provides novel and unconventional signaling pathways to the nucleus to mediate estrogen and neurotrophin actions in the devel-oping brain. Confirmation of estradiol-induced activation of the phosphorylated ERK, a process that is required for nuclear translocation, was established with the in-gel kinase assay, utilizing myelin basic protein (MBP) as the substrate for ERK activity *(49)*. The E-induced, tyrosine phosphorylated ERKs were much more active in their ability (ERK2 > ERK1) to phosphorylate MBP as a substrate than the untreated controls.

The ability of estradiol to tyrosine phosphorylate and activate a component of the MAP kinase cascade (ERK) represents a novel finding in the CNS. This observation supports the idea of alternative pathways for estrogen action in the brain, which could explain both the rapid effects of estrogen and the regulation of non-ERE-containing genes. Protein tyrosine phosphorylation represents a nongenomic way by which estrogen may elicit direct effects in its target neurons. Ligand-activation of tyrosine kinases is a property shared by several membrane growth factor receptors. In some instances, the stimulated kinase is intrinsic to the receptor molecule, e.g., the *trk (90)* and EGF receptors *(64)*. In other cases, ligand-activated tyrosine kinases such as *src* have been described that are not intrinsic to membrane receptors, but appear functionally associated with the ER *(40,63,65)*. Membrane estrogen-binding sites could interact rapidly with the steroid and, in neurons where estrogen and neurotrophin receptors co-localize, perhaps activate con-tiguous tyrosine kinases.

MULTIMERIC COMPLEXING OF ERS WITH SIGNALING PROTEINS

Critical and as yet unanswered questions concern the identity of the pathways that may mediate estrogen-induced activation of the ERKs in the brain and by which neurotrophins elicit tyrosine phosphorylation of the unliganded neural ER. The MAP kinase cascade is an important pathway for NGF-induced differentiation in PC12 cells. Although it is presumed that neurotrophin signaling pathways in the brain are likely to be similar to those of PC12 cells, the actual cascades used have never really been characterized in the CNS. In PC12 cells, signal transduction through the MAP kinase cascade is dependent on activation of *Ras*, which binds directly to the *Raf* family of protein kinases to mediate their translocation to the membrane, essential for *Raf* activation. The *Raf* kinases (b-*Raf* in PC12 cells; c-*Raf* (*Raf*-1) in sympathetic neurons; ?? b- and/or c-*Raf* in the CNS) initiate the MAP kinase (MAPK) cascade by phosphorylating MEK (MAPK kinase) which in turn phosphorylates and activates MAPK or ERK. The b-*Raf* is the only one of the *Raf* family members to become phosphorylated in response to NGF exposure of PC12 cells *(112)*. In PC12 cells, b-*Raf* has been found to be present as a component of a putative high molecular weight (>300 kDa) complex, consisting of at least b-*Raf* and heat shock protein (hsp) 90, whose assembly is constitutive and independent of NGF activation *(113)*. Hsp90 is highly abundant in unstressed eukaryotic cells and represents 1–2% of the cytosolic protein *(114)*.

We have recently found evidence that this putative complex is present in the CNS (cerebral cortex) as well *(49,116)*. Because the unliganded ER is believed to be kept inactive in the cytosol and from forming homodimers by becoming complexed with the hsp90-based chaperone system *(28,114)*, we started investigating whether the putative b-*Raf*/hsp90 complex may also include the unliganded ER. Like the ER, hsp90 becomes tyrosine-phosphorylated by estrogen. In addition, because hsp90 has also been reported to form stable complexes with pp60^{src} *(28,114)* as well as the ER, we hypothesized that *src*, a nonreceptor protein tyrosine kinase, would also be a good candidate, because estrogen has been reported to elicit tyrosine phosphorylation of *src* within 10 s *(63)*. In fact, Migliaccio et al. *(65)* have suggested that estrogen-induced tyrosine phosphorylation of the ER is a consequence of the very rapid phosphorylation of *src*. We further questioned whether, in the CNS, other protein kinases downstream of *Raf* in the MAP kinase cascade, e.g., MEK and ERK, might also be associated with both hsp90 and the ER in a multimeric complex or even in more than one complex, depending on the ER type.

Preliminary immunoprecipitation experiments in explants of the cerebral cortex and a PC12 cell variant, PC12-E2 *(116)*, which expresses high levels of ERs (M. Singh and D. Toran-Allerand, unpublished observations) show evidence by Western analysis of co-immunoprecipitation of b-*Raf*, *src*, and hsp90 with the ER and of MEK with *src* *(49,115)*. Surprisingly, co-precipitation of hsp90 with ERK and of the ER with ERK has also been documented in the cortical explants *(117)*. The sum of these findings implies that these signaling proteins may also be components of the putative complex or complexes. One might speculate, as illustrated in Fig. 6, that, following neuronal exposure to E, dissociation and conformational changes within the complex(es), resulting from tyrosine phosphorylation of the ER, hsp90, and *src*, may lead to direct phosphorylation and activation of MEK and thence ERK. Alternatively, estrogen exposure could even lead to phosphorylation and activation of ERK directly via a putative ERK/ER/hsp90 complex.

Conversely, because activation of *trkA* following NGF exposure also elicits tyrosine phosphorylation and activation of MEK via *Ras/Raf* activation, this hypothesis also suggests a reciprocal signaling pathway by which the unliganded ER, bound by hsp90 to the rest of the putative multimeric complex(es), could become tyrosine phosphorylated by the neurotrophins. Thus, regardless of the ligand, dissociation of the ER from these putative complexes, consequent to tyrosine phosphorylation within the complex, would be not only ER activation but activation of ERK as well, followed by nuclear translocation of both the ER and ERK, and gene regulation.

Despite the issues of ER subtypes and affinities raised earlier, that the ER may be complexed directly with MEK, the kinase immediately upstream of ERK, or complexed

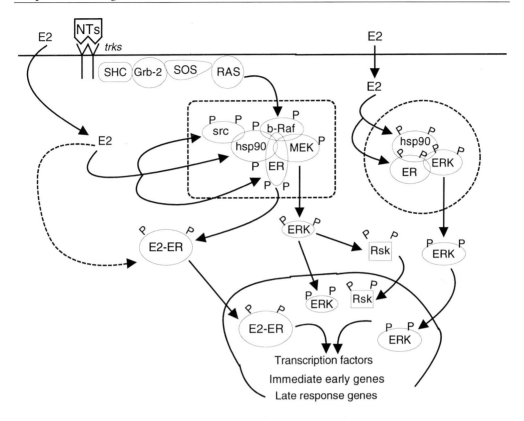

Fig. 6. Sites of potential cross-coupling of the estrogen and neurotrophin receptor systems. Estrogen and the neurotrophin-induced activation of the putative multimeric b-*Raf* complex by tyrosine phosphorylation, which would be accompanied by changes in the configuration of its hsp90/*src*/ ER components, may phosphorylate MEK and lead to rapid activation of MAPK/ERK. Alternatively, estrogen-induced activation of the putative ER/hsp90/ERK complex may phosphorylate ERK directly. These changes would be followed in both instances by nuclear translocation of both ERK and the now-activated ER, resulting in activation of immediate and late response genes and transcription. On the other hand, activation of the *trk* receptors and of the downstream putative b-*Raf* complex by NGF and the other neurotrophins could lead, conversely, to tyrosine phosphorylation of the unliganded ER.

directly with ERK itself has strong implications for estrogen activation of ERK. Direct activation of these putative complexes by both estrogen and the neurotrophins would also have significant implications for the rapidity and specificity of their activation of immediate-early genes and nuclear transcription factors. Segnitz and Gehring *(28)* have suggested that the nonactivated ER of human MCF-7 mammary carcinoma cells has a heterotetrameric structure consisting of one receptor polypeptide, two hsp90 molecules, and one p59 subunit, for which the molecular mass adds up to approximately 300 kDa. No other proteins, including the heat-shock protein hsp70 and the 40-kDa cyclophilin, were reportedly detected as components of this highly purified cross-linked ER complex. Whether our two putative multimeric complexes are related to this ER complex or whether our complexes are characteristic of developing neural tissue in particular or of the wild-type ER is currently unknown.

Such an hypothesis is in no way meant to imply that estrogen activation of other substrates such as adenylate cyclase- *(36,118)* or Ca^{2+}-dependent channels *(119)* or of other pathways *(120)*, which also lead to phosphorylation of the ERKs via PKA/PKC *(121)* or via *Ras (120)*, for example, may not also be occurring concurrently in the brain. It is also highly probable that there are influences from concurrent interactions of estrogen with other growth factors in the postnatal brain whose receptors, as tyrosine kinases, may also activate many of the same differentiative signaling cascades, utilized by the neurotrophins (e.g., the *Ras/Raf*-Map kinase cascade or SNT). On the other hand, other routes, involving the *trk*, PLC-γ1/PKCa cascade, for example, which also phosphorylate and activate p21^{Ras} *(36,118,120,121)* and thence the entire MAP kinase cascade may be important in recruiting and prolonging the initial rapid responses through the variety of pathways with which PKC interacts. And, because ER-containing cortical neurons also co-express the neurotrophin ligand mRNAs *(13)*, it is entirely possible that the patterns of signaling we have observed may also reflect estrogen regulation of neurotrophin synthesis and release rather than direct activation of signaling intermediates. Such a mechanism may well explain estrogen regulation of genes such as NGF *(122)*, BDNF *(123)* and the cholinergic enzymes, for example *(124,125)*. However, our preliminary results document that, among its postulated CNS actions, estrogen does activate signaling proteins rapidly and directly, supporting the hypothesis of cross-coupling of the estrogen and neurotrophin signaling systems.

Because it has been suggested that complete activation of the ER requires both the intracytoplasmic and intranuclear action of at least six protein kinases *(38)*, kinases such as ERK and *Rsk*, which translocate to the nucleus, may also act as signaling intermediates to phosphorylate the ER. Through nuclear translocation of ERK and *Rsk*, convergence or cross-coupling of the estrogen and neurotrophin signaling pathways to the nucleus, via the putative multimeric complexes and/or via individual components of the MAP kinase cascade, would provide alternative, novel, and unconventional routes to the nucleus to mediate estrogen and neurotrophin actions in the developing brain. Although the ligand-activated ER undoubtedly acts as a transcription factor, cross-coupling of estrogen and neurotrophin signalling pathways could explain how estrogen and the neurotrophins could each regulate the same broad array of ERE- and non-ERE-containing genes, involved in neuronal differentiation and neurite growth. For example, the neurite- and growth-related genes, β-tubulin MAP-2, *tau* microtubule-associated protein, and GAP-43 are regulated not only by estrogen *(126–129)* but by the neurotrophins as well *(85,130–134)*.

Whether the actions of NGF and the other neurotrophins in neural tissues are mediated only by *trk* receptors or also involve the ER as well is currently unknown. Evidence supporting each possibility has been reported in non-neural tumor cell lines. Cross-coupling of the ER with growth factor signaling pathways appears to be a general property of the ER. Estrogen-dependent and estrogen-independent interactions of the ER with neurotransmitters (e.g., dopamine) *(32,33,135)* and growth factor signaling pathways (e.g., EGF, IGF-I, insulin) *(31,46,47,70,136,137)* have been shown to activate the ER via the cell surface and to be implicated in the mediation of an increasing number of estrogen-induced/estrogen-like differentiative processes. For example, EGF reportedly interacts in the adult mouse uterus with both estrogen and EGF receptors independently of estrogen to elicit responses attributed to estrogen actions *(44,46,69,71,137,138)*. Interdependency of estrogen and growth factor (EGF, IGF-1) signaling pathways through the intermediary of MAP kinase has recently been implicated in the mediation of cell proliferation in non-neural estrogen targets, such as the uterus and tumor cell lines *(138)*. IGF-1 and EGF caused phosphorylation of the unliganded ER on serine[118], an action attributed to direct activation by MAP kinase (ERK) *(31,46,47)*. On the other hand, Migliaccio et al. *(65)* have suggested that estradiol-induced phosphorylation of EGF and IGF-1 signaling pathways in MCF-7 cells requires ligand occupation of the classical ER, because the pure anti-estrogen ICI 182 780 inhibited estrogen activation (phosphorylation) of each component of the MAP kinase cascade. Moreover, very preliminary findings suggest that in the absence of estrogen the anti-estrogen ICI 164 384 blocked NGF phosphorylation of the ERKs completely (M. Singh and D. Toran-Allerand, unpublished observations), suggesting that in the brain both estrogen and neurotrophin receptors may be required for estrogen and neurotrophin activation of the ERKs and perhaps the upstream signaling proteins as well.

That estrogen and the neurotrophins each cause tyrosine phosphorylation and activation of the ER and the ERKs suggests multiple potential routes by which different signal transduction pathways may converge and influence one another. Cross-coupling of the estrogen and neurotrophin receptor systems may have great importance for the regulatory mechanisms underlying autocrine and paracrine responses in both the developing and adult brain. Convergence of the estrogen and neurotrophin signaling pathways may have relevance not only for the ontogeny of both the estrogen and neurotrophin receptor systems, but for neurodegenerative disorders and brain injury and the potential for regeneration and repair as well. Regenerative responses, which follow injury, also represent stages when functional neuronal contacts, ensuring target-derived (trans-synaptic) neurotrophin availability, have yet to be made. Thus, the ER may use multiple, possibly redundant, signaling pathways in mediating estrogen and neurotrophin responses, as has been shown for NGF and *trkA* in PC12 cells *(139,140)*.

CONCLUSION

Mediation of estrogen actions by interactions with locally synthesized growth factors and their receptors, such as the neurotrophins in the brain, may represent a universal mechanism by which the effects of steroid hormones, such as estrogen, whose actions are widespread and varied, may exert local control and exhibit specificities at both tissue and developmental-stage levels. Cross-coupling of the ER and neurotrophin regulatory pathways may be relevant to understanding the mechanisms underlying not only the developmental actions of estrogen in the brain but also estrogen actions on neuronal survival, regeneration, repair and aging in brain regions that underlie learning, memory, and other cognitive functions. Estrogen and the neurotrophins may stimulate the synthesis of proteins required for neuronal differentiation, survival, and maintenance of function. In humans of both sexes, moreover, the natural decline in gonadal steroid levels, particularly in women, may contribute to the loss of neuronal systems vital to cognitive functions, whether this occurs to the extreme extent observed in Alzheimer's disease or follows the less traumatic path associated with the postmenopausal state and normal aging. Estrogen and neurotrophin interactions, latent since development, may be recruited, following loss of trophic support whether from injury or steroid deprivation, as occurs following the menopause, gonadectomy (especially ovariectomy), and anti-estrogen (tamoxifen) treatment for breast cancer, for example. Through their reciprocal interactions at transcriptional, translational, and posttranslational levels, estrogen and the neurotrophins may have not only important and intertwined roles during brain development, but may also decrease the vulnerability of their target neurons to the consequences of neuro-degenerative disease processes such as Alzheimer's disease.

ACKNOWLEDGMENTS

Many thanks are owed to Drs. Rajesh Miranda, Farida Sohrabji, Meharvan Singh, and Gyorgy Sétáló, Jr. (Past and present Postdoctoral Fellows, Department of Anatomy and Cell Biology, Columbia University) for much of the work described in this chapter; to Dr. Wayne D. L. Bentham, for expert technical assistance throughout his many years as a student in my laboratory; to Mr. Matthew M. Warren and Ms. Cynthia Leung for valuable technical support, and to Dr. Lloyd A. Greene (Columbia University) for many helpful discussions. This work has been supported in part by grants from NIH, NIMH, and NSF, and an ADAMHA Research Scientist Award to DT-A.

REFERENCES

1. Toran-Allerand CD. On the genesis of sexual differentiation of the central nervous system: morpho-genetic consequences of steroidal exposure and possible role of α-fetoprotein. Prog Brain Res 1984;61:63–98.
2. Toran-Allerand CD, Gerlach J, McEwen B. Autoradiographic localization of ^{3}H-estradiol related to steroid responsiveness in cultures of the newborn mouse hypothalamus and preoptic area. Brain Res 1980;184:517–522.
3. Kawata M. Roles of steroid hormones and their receptors in structural organization in the nervous system. Neurosci Res 1995;24:1–46.
4. MacLusky NJ, Naftolin F. Sexual differentiation of the central nervous system. Science 1981; 211:1294–1303.
5. MacLusky NJ, Walters MJ, Clark AS, Toran-Allerand CD. Aromatase in the cerebral cortex, hippocampus and mid-brain: ontogeny and developmental implications. Mol Cell Neurosci 1994;5:691–698.
6. Toran-Allerand CD. Sex steroids and the development of the newborn mouse hypothalamus and preoptic area *in vitro*: implications for sexual differentiation. Brain Res 106;1976:407–412.
7. Toran-Allerand CD. Sex steroids and the development of the newborn mouse hypothalamus and preoptic area *in vitro*: II. Morphological correlates and hormonal specificity. Brain Res 1980;189:413–427.
8. Toran-Allerand CD, Hashimoto K, Greenough WT, Saltarelli M. Sex steroids and the development of the newborn mouse hypothalamus and preoptic area *in vitro*: III. Effects of estrogen on dendritic differentiation. Dev Brain Res 1983;7:97–101.
9. Matsumoto A, Arai Y. Neuronal plasticity in the deafferented hypothalamic arcuate nucleus of adult female rats and its enhancement by treatment with estrogen. J Comp Neurol 1981;197:197–206.
10. Gould E, Woolley CS, Frankfurt M, McEwen, BS. Gonadal steroids regulate dendritic spine density in hippocampal pyramidal cells in adulthood. J Neurosci 1990;10:1286–1291.
11. Toran-Allerand CD, Miranda RC, Bentham W, Sohrabji F, Brown TJ, Hochberg RB, MacLusky NJ. Estrogen receptors co-localize with low-affinity nerve growth factor receptors in cholinergic neurons of the basal forebrain. Proc Natl Acad Sci USA 1992;89:4668–4972.
12. Miranda RC, Sohrabji F, Toran-Allerand CD. Neuronal co-localization of the mRNAs for the neurotrophins and their receptors in the developing CNS suggests the potential for autocrine interactions. Proc Natl Acad Sci USA 1993;90:6439–6443.
13. Miranda RC, Sohrabji F, Toran-Allerand CD. Estrogen target neurons co-localize the mRNAs for the neurotrophins and their receptors during development: a basis for the interactions of estrogen and the neurotrophins. Mol Cell Neurosci 1993;4:510–525.
14. Toran-Allerand CD. Mechanisms of estrogen action during neural development: Mediation by inter-actions with the neurotrophins and their receptors ? J Steroid Biochem Mol Biol 1995;56:169–178.

15. Toran-Allerand CD. The estrogen/neurotrophin connection during neural development: is co-localization of estrogen receptors with the neurotrophins and their receptors biologically relevant? Dev Neurosci 1996;18:36–48.

16. Kuiper GGJM, Enmark E, Pelto-Huikko M, Nilsson S, Gustafsson J-A. Cloning of a novel estrogen receptor expressed in rat prostate and ovary. Proc Natl Acad Sci USA 1996;93:5925–5930.

17. Mosselman S, Polman J, Dijkema R. estrogen receptor beta: identification and characterization of a novel human estrogen receptor. FEBS Lett 1996;392:49–53.

18. Kuiper GG, Carlsson B, Grandien K, Enmark E, Haggblad J, Nilsson S, Gustafsson JA. Comparison of the ligand binding specificity and transcript tissue distribution of estrogen receptors alpha and beta. Endocrinology 1997;138:863–870.

19. Shughrue PJ, Komm B, Merchenthaler I. The distribution of estrogen receptor-beta mRNA in the rat hypothalamus. Steroids 1996;61:678–681.

20. Gerlach J, McEwen B, Toran-Allerand CD, Friedman W. Perinatal development of estrogen receptors in mouse brain assessed by radioautography, nuclear isolation and receptor assay. Brain Res 1983;11:7–18.

21. Shughrue PJ, Stumpf WE, MacLusky NJ, Zielinski JE, Hochberg RB. Developmental changes of estrogen receptors in mouse cerebral cortex between birth and post-weaning: studied by autoradiography with 11β-methoxy-16α-^{125}I iodoestradiol. Endocrinology 1990;126:1112–1124.

22. Miranda RC, Toran-Allerand CD. Developmental expression and regulation of estrogen receptor mRNA in the rat cerebral cortex: a non-isotopic in situ hybridization histochemistry study. Cereb Cortex 1992;2:1–15.

23. Sohrabji F, Greene LA, Miranda RC, Toran-Allerand CD. Reciprocal regulation of estrogen and nerve growth factor receptors by their ligands in PC12 cells. J Neurobiol 1994;22:974–988.

24. Sohrabji F, Miranda RC, Toran-Allerand CD Ovarian hormones differentially regulate estrogen and nerve growth factor mRNAs in adult sensory neurons. J Neurosci 1994;14:459–471.

25. Koike S, Sakai M, Muramatsu M. Molecular cloning and characterization of rat estrogen receptor cDNA. Nucleic Acids Res 1987;15:2499–2513.

26. Evans RM. The steroid and thyroid hormone receptor superfamily. Science 1988;240:889–896.

27. Landers JP, Spelsberg TC. New concepts in steroid hormone action: transcription factors, proto-oncogenes and the cascade model for steroid regulation of gene expression. Crit Rev Eukaryotic Gene Expression 1992;2:19–63.

28. Segnitz B, Gehring U. Subunit structure of the nonactivated human estrogen receptor. Proc Natl Acad Sci USA 1995;92:2179–2183.

29. Orti E, Bodwell JE, Munck A. Phosphorylation of steroid hormone receptors. Endocrine Rev 1992;13:105–127.

30. Newton CJ, Buric R, Trapp T, Brockmeir S, Pagotto U, Stalla G. The unliganded estrogen receptor (ER) transduces growth factor signals. J Biol Chem 1994;48:481–486.

31. Kato S, Endoh H, Masuhiro Y, Kitamoto T, Uchiyama S, Sasaki H, Masushige S, Gotoh Y, Nishida E, Kawashima H, Metzger D, Chambon P. Activation of the estrogen receptor through phosphorylation by mitogen-activated protein kinase. Science 1995;270:1491–1494.

32. Power RF, Mani SK, Codina J, Conneely OM, O'Malley BW. Dopaminergic and ligand-independent activation of steroid receptors. Science 1991;254:1636–1639.

33. O'Malley BW, Schrader WT, Mani S, Smith C, Weigel NL, Conneely OM, Clark JH. An alternative ligand-independent pathway for activation of steroid receptors. Rec Prog Horm Res 1995;50:333–347.

34. Auricchio F. Phosphorylation of steroid receptors. J Steroid Biochem 1989;32:613–622.

35. Auricchio F, Migliaccio A, Castoria G, Di Domenico M, Pagano M. Phosphorylation of uterus estradiol receptor on tyrosine. Prog Clin Biol Res 1990;322:133–155.

36. Aronica SM, Katzenellenbogen BS. Stimulation of estrogen receptor-mediated transcription and alteration in the phosphorylation state of the rat uterine estrogen receptor by estrogen, cyclic adenosine monophosphate and insulin-like growth factor-I. Mol Endocrinol 1993;7:743–752.

37. LeGoff P, Montano MM, Schodin DJ, Katzenellenbogen BS. Phosphorylation of the human estrogen receptor. J Biol Chem 1994;269:4458–4466.

38. Arnold SF, Obourn JD, Yudt MR, Carter TH, Notides AC. In vivo and in vitro phosphorylation of the human estrogen receptor. J Steroid Biochem Molec Biol 1995;52:159–171.

39. Kuiper GGJM, Brinkmann AO. Steroid hormone receptor phosphorylation: is there a physiological role? Mol Cell Endol 1994;100:103–107.

40. Arnold SF, Obourne JD, Jaffe H, Notides AC. Phosphorylation of the human estrogen receptor on tyrosine 537 in vivo and by *src* family tyrosine kinases *in vitro*. Mol Endocrinol 1995;9:24–33.

41. Arnold SF, Vorojeikina DP, Notides AC. Phosphorylation of tyrosine 537 on the human estrogen receptor is required for binding to an estrogen response element. J Biol Chem 1996;270:30205–30212.

42. Weis KE, Ekena K, Thomas JA, Lazennec G, Kateznellenbogen BS. Constitutively active human estrogen receptors containing amino acid substitutions for tyrosine 537 in the receptor protein. Mol Endocrinol 1996;10:1388–1398.

43. Arnold SF, Notides AC. An antiestrogen: a phosphotyrosyl peptide that blocks dimerization of the human estrogen receptor. Proc Natl Acad Sci U S A 1995;92:7475–7479.

44. Arnold SF, Melamed M, Vorojeikina DP, Notides AC, Sasson S. Estradiol-binding mechanism and binding capacity of the human estrogen receptor is regulated by tyrosine phosphorylation. Mol Endocrinol 1997;11:48–53.

45. Arnold SF, Obourn JD, Jaffe H, Notides AC. Serine 167 is the major estradiol-induced phosphorylation site on the human estrogen receptor. Mol Endocrinol 1994;8:1208–1214.

46. Arnold SF, Obourne, Jaffe H, Notides AC. Phosphorylation of the human estrogen receptor by mitogen-activated protein kinase and casein kinase II: consequences on DNA binding. J Steroid Biochem Mol Biol 1995;55:163–172.

47. Bunone G, Briand P-A, Miksicek RJ, Picard D. Activation of the unliganded estrogen receptor by EGF involves the MAP kinase pathway and direct phosphorylation. EMBO J 1996;15:2174–2183.

48. Toran-Allerand CD, Mauri E, Leung C, Warren M, Singh M. Activation of MAP kinases (ERKs) by estradiol in cerebral cortical explants: Cross-coupling of the estrogen and neurotrophin signalling pathways. Soc Neurosci Abstr 1996;22:555.

49. Singh M, Sétáló Jr G, Guan X-P, Warren M, Toran-Allerand CD. Estrogen activation of MAP Kinase (ERK) in cerebral cortical explants: cross-coupling of estrogen and neurotrophin signaling pathways. J Neurosci 1999;19:1179–1188.

50. Anuradha P, Khan SM, Karthikeyan N, Thampan RV. The nonactivated estrogen receptor (naER) of the goat uterus is a tyrosine kinase. Arch Biochem Biophys 1994;309:195–204.

51. Karthikeyan N, Thampan RV. Plasma membrane is the primary site of localization of the nonactivated estrogen receptor in the goat uterus: hormone binding causes receptor internalization. Arch Biochem Biophys 1996;325:47–57.

52. Dauvois S, White R, Parker MG. The antiestrogen ICI 182780 disrupts estrogen receptor nucleocytoplasmic shuttling. J Cell Sci 1993;106:1377–1388.

53. King WJ, Greene GL. Monoclonal antibodies localize estrogen receptor in the nuclei of target cells. Nature 1984;307:745–747.

54. Welshons WV, Lieberman ME, Gorski J. Nuclear localization of unoccupied estrogen receptors. Nature 1984;307:747–749.

55. Blaustein JD. Cytoplasmic estrogen receptors in rat brain. immunocytochemical evidence using three antibodies with distinct epitopes. Endocrinology 1992;131:1336–1342.

56. Pietras RJ, Szego CM. Specific binding sites for oestrogen at the outer surfaces of isolated endometrial cells. Nature 1977;265:69–72.

57. Zheng J, Ramirez VD. Purification and identification of estrogen-binding proteins from neuronal membranes of female rat brain. Soc Neurosci Abstr 1994;20:95.

58. Muldoon TG, Watson GH, Evans Jr AG, Steinsapir J. Microsomal receptor for steroid hormones: functional implications for nuclear activity. J Steroid Biochem 1988;30:23–31.

59. Watson CS, Pappas TC, Gametchy B. The other estrogen receptor in the plasma membrane: implications for the actions of environmental estrogens. Env Health Perspect 1995;103(Suppl 7):41–50.

60. Pappas TC, Gametchu B, Watson CS. Membrane estrogen receptors identified by multiple antibody labeling and impeded-ligand binding. FASEB J 1995;9:404–410.

61. Berthois Y, Pourreau-Schneider, Gandilhon P, Mittre H, Tubiana N, Martin PM. Estrogen membrane binding sites on human breast cancer cell lines: use of a fluorescent estradiol conjugate to demonstrate plasma membrane binding systems. J Steroid Biochem 1986;25:963–972.

62. Pappas TC, Gametchu B, Watson CS. Membrane estrogen receptor-enriched GH3/B6 cells have an enhanced non-genomic response to estrogen. Endocrine 1995;3:743–749.

63. Migliaccio A, Pagano M, Auricchio F. Immediate and transient stimulation of protein tyrosine phosphorylation by estradiol in MCF-7 cells. Oncogene 1993;8:2183–2191.

64. Reddy KB, Mangold GL, Tandon AK, Yoneda T, Mundy GR, Zilberstein A, Osborne K. Inhibition of breast cancer cell growth *in vitro* by a tyrosine kinase inhibitor. Cancer Res 1992;52:3636–3641.

65. Migliaccio A, Di Domenico M, Castoria G, de Falco A, Bontempo P, Nola E, Auricchio F. Tyrosine kinase/p21^{ras}/MAP kinase pathway activation by estrogen-receptor complex in MCF-7 cells. EMBO J 1996;15:1292–1300.

66. Katzenellenbogen BS. Estrogen receptors: bioactivities and interactions with cell signaling pathways. Biol Reprod 1996;54:287–293.

67. Schule R, and Evans RM. Cross-coupling of signal transduction pathways. Trends Genet 1991;7:377–381.

68. Ignar-Trowbridge DM, Nelson KG, Biwell MC, Curtis SW, Washburn TF, McLachlan JA, Korach KS. Coupling of dual signaling pathways: epidermal growth factor actions involves the estrogen receptor. Proc Natl Acad Sci USA 1992;89:4658–4662.

69. Patrone C, Ma ZQ, Pollio G, Agrati P, Parker MG, Maggi A. Cross-coupling between insulin and estrogen receptor in human neuroblastoma cells. Mol Endocrinol 1996;10:499–507.

70. Ignar-Trowbridge DM, Pimentel M, Teng CT, Korach KS, McLachlan JA. Cross talk between peptide growth factor and estrogen receptor signaling systems. Env Health Perspect 1995;103(Suppl 7):35–38.

71. Barde Y-A. Trophic factors and neuronal survival. Neuron 1989;2:1525–1534.

72. Chao MV. Neurotrophin receptors: a window into neuronal differentiation. Neuron 1992;9:583–593.

73. Raffioni S, Bradshaw RA, Buxer SE. The receptors for nerve growth factor and other neurotrophins. Annu Rev Biochem 1993;62:823–850.

74. Chao MV, Hempstead BL. p75 and *Trk*: a two receptor system. Trends Neurosci 1995;18:321–326.

75. Martin-Zanca D, Barbacid M, Parada LF. Expression of the *trk* proto-oncogene is restricted to sensory cranial and spinal ganglia of neural crest origin in mouse development. Genes Dev 1990;4:683–694.

76. Vasquez ME, Ebendal T. Messenger RNAs for *trk* and the low-affinity NGF receptor in rat basal forebrain. NeuroReport 1991;2:593–596.

77. Holtzman DM, Li Y, Parada LF, Kinsman S, Chen C-K, Valetta J, Zhou J, Long JB, Mobley WC. p140trk mRNA marks NGF-responsive forebrain neurons: evidence that *trk* gene expression is induced by NGF. Neuron 1992;9:465–478.

78. Koh JY, Gwag BJ, Lobner D, Choi DW. Potentiated necrosis of cultured cortical neurons by neurotrophins. Science 1995;268:573–575.

79. Miranda RC, Sohrabji F, Singh M, Toran-Allerand CD. Nerve growth factor (NGF) regulation of estrogen receptors in the developing nervous system. J Neurobiol 1996;31:77–87.

80. Bothwell M. p75NTR: a receptor after all. Science 1996;272:506–507.

81. Carter BD, Kaltschmidt C, Kaltschmidt B, Offenhauser N, Bohm-Matthaei R, Baeuerle PA, Barde YA. Selective activation of NF-kappa B by nerve growth factor through the neurotrophin receptor p75. Science 1996;272:542–545.

82. Rao P, Hsu KC, Chao MV. Upregulation of NF-kappa B-dependent gene expression mediated by the p75 tumor necrosis factor receptor. J Interferon Cytokine Res 1996;15:71–177.

83. Schlessinger J, Ullrich A. Growth factor signaling by receptor tyrosine kinases. Neuron 1992;9:383–391.

84. Hill CS, Treisman R. Transcriptional regulation by extracellular signals: mechanisms and specificity. Cell 1995;80 199–211.

85. Hershman HR. Primary response genes induced by growth factors and tumor promoters. Annu Rev Biochem 1991;60:281–319.

86. Egan SE, Weinberg RA. The pathway to signal achievement. Nature 1993;365:781–783.

87. Szeberenyi J, Erhardt P. Cellular components of nerve growth factor signaling. Biochem Biophy Acta 1994;1222:187–202.

88. Greene LA, Tischler AS. PC12 pheochromocytoma cultures in neurobiological research. Adv Cell Neurobiol 1982;3:373–414.

89. Kaplan DR, Hempstead BL, Martin-Zanca D, Chao MV, Parada LF. The *trk* proto-oncogene product: signal transducing receptor for nerve growth factor. Science 1991;252:554–557.

90. Kaplan DR, Martin-Zanca D, Parada LP. Tyrosine phosphorylation and tyrosine kinase activity of the *trk* proto-oncogene product induced by NGF. Nature 1991;350:158–160.

91. Chao MV. Growth factor signaling: where is the specificity? Cell 1992;68:995–997.

92. Greene LA, Kaplan DR. Early events in neurotrophin signalling via *Trk* and p75 receptors. Curr Opin Neurobiol 1995;5:579–587.

93. Borasio GD, Markus A, Wittinghofer A, Barde YA, Heumann R. Involvement of Ras p21 in neurotrophin-induced response of sensory, but not sympathetic neurons. J Cell Biol 1993; 121:665–672.

94. Chao TS, Foster DA, Rapp UR, Rosner MR. Differential *Raf* requirement for activation of mitogen-activated protein kinase by growth factors, phorbol esters, and calcium. J Biol Chem 1994;269:7337–7341.

95. Blenis J. Signal transduction via the MAP kinases: Proceed at your own RSK. Proc Natl Acad Sci USA 1993;90:5889–5892.

96. Rabin SJ, Clehon V, Kaplan DR. SNT, a differentiation-specific target of neurotrophic factor-induced tyrosine kinase activity in neurons and PC12 cells. Mol Cell Biol 1993;13:2203–2213.

97. Marshall CJ. Specificity of receptor tyrosine kinase signalling: transient versus sustained extracellular signal-regulated kinase activation. Cell 1995;80:179–185.

98. Traverse S, Gomez N, Paterson H, Marshall C, Cohen P. Sustained activation of the mitogen-activated protein (MAP) kinase cascade may be required for differentiation of PC12 cells. Comparison of the effects of nerve growth factor and epidermal growth factor. Biochem J 1992;288:351–355.

99. Pang L, Sawada T, Decker SJ, Saltiel AR. Inhibition of MAP kinase kinase blocks the differentiation of PC12 cells induced by nerve growth factor. J Biol Chem 1995;270:13585–13588.

100. Toran-Allerand CD, Pfenninger K, Ellis L. Estrogen and insulin synergism in neurite growth enhancement *in vitro*: mediation of steroid effects by interactions with growth factors? Dev Brain Res 1988;41:87–100.

101. Sohrabji F, Miranda RC, Toran-Allerand CD. Identification of a potential estrogen response element in the gene encoding brain-derived neurotrophic factor. Proc Natl Acad Sci USA 1995;92:11110–11114.

102. Shughrue PJ, Refsdal CD, Dorsa DM. estrogen receptor messenger ribonucleic acid in female rat brain during the estrus cycle: a comparison with ovariectomized females and intact males. Endocrinology 1992; 131:381–388.

103. Shupnik MA, Gordon MS, Chin WW. Tissue specific regulation of rat estrogen receptor mRNAs. Mol Endocrinol 1991;3:660–665.

104. Knusel B, Rabin SJ, Hefti F, Kaplan DR. Regulated neurotrophin receptor responsiveness during neuronal migration and early differentiation. J Neurosci 1994;14:1542–1554.

105. Segal RA, Takahashi H, McKay RDG. Changes in neurotrophin responsiveness during the development of cerebellar granule cells. Neuron 1992;9:1041–1052.

106. Lewin GR, Mendell LM. Nerve growth factor and nociception. Trends Neurosci 1993;16:353–359.

107. Higgins GA, Koh S, Chen KS, Gage FH. NGF induction of NGF receptor gene expression and cholinergic neuronal hypertrophy within the basal forebrain of the adult rat. Neuron 1989;3:247–256.

108. Gage FH, Batchelor P, Chen KS, Chin D, Higgins GA, Koh S, Deputy S, Rosenberg MB, Fisher W, Björklund A. NGF receptor re-expression and NGF-mediated cholinergic neuronal hypertrophy in the damaged adult neostriatum. Neuron 1989;2:177–184.

109. Merlio JP, Ernfors P. Kokaia Z, Middlemas DS, Bengzon J, Kokaia M, Smith ML, Siesjo BK, Hunter T, Lindvall O. Increased production of the TrkB protein tyrosine kinase receptor after brain insults. Neuron 1993;10:151–164.

110. Migliaccio A, Di Domenico M, Green S, de Falco A, Kajtaniak E, Blasi F, Chambon P, Auricchio F. Phosphorylation on tyrosine of *in vitro* synthesized human estrogen receptor activates its hormone binding. Mol Endocrinol 1989;3:1061–1069.

111. Brann DW, Hendry LB, Mahesh VB. Emerging diversities in the mechanism of action of steroid hormones. J Steroid Biochem Mol Biol 1995;52:113–133.

112. Jaiswal RK, Moodie SA, Wolfman A, Landreth GE. The mitogen activated protein kinase cascade is activated by B-*Raf* in response to nerve growth factor through interaction with p21[Ras]. Mol Cell Biol 1994;14:6944–6953.

113. Jaiswal RK, Weissinger E, Kolch W, Landreth G. Nerve growth factor-mediated activation of the mitogen-activated protein (MAP) kinase cascade involves a signaling complex containing B-*Raf* and hsp90. J Biol Chem 1996;271:23626–23629.

114. Pratt WB. The role of the hsp90-based chaperone system in signal transduction by nuclear receptors and receptors signaling via MAP kinase. Annu Rev Pharmacol Toxicol 1997;37:297–326.

115. Singh M, Warren MF, Sétáló Jr G, Toran-Allerand CD. The estrogen receptor exists in a multimeric complex consisting of at least B-*raf*, MEK and hsp90 in explants of the cerebral cortex. Soc Neurosci Abstr 1997;23:1709.

116. Wu YY, Bradshaw RA. PC12-E2 cells: a stable variant with altered responses to growth factor stimulation. J Cell Physiol 1995;164:522–532.

117. Sétáló Jr G, Singh M, Warren MF, Toran-Allerand CD. Direct association of heat shock protein hsp90 and the extracellular signal regulated kinases, ERK1/2. A possible link between estrogen and neurotrophin signaling. Soc Neurosci Abstr 1997;23:1709.

118. Aronica SM, Kraus WI, Katzenellenbogen BS. Estrogen action via the cAMP signaling pathway: Stimulation of adenylate cyclase and c-AMP-regulated gene transcription. Proc Natl Acad Sci USA 1994;91:8517–8521.

119. Morley P, Whitfield JF, Vanderhyden BC, Tsang BK, Schwartz J. A new, nongenomic estrogen action: the rapid release of intracellular calcium. Endocrinology 1992;131:1305–1312.

120. Finkbeiner S, Greenberg ME. Ca^{2+}-dependent routes to Ras: mechanisms for neuronal survival, differentiation, and plasticity? Neuron 1996;16:233–236.

121. Frodin M, Peraldi P, Van Obberghen E. Cyclic AMP activates the mitogen-activated protein kinase cascade in PC12 cells. J Biol Chem 1994;269:6207–6214.

122. Singh M, Meyer EM, Huang FS, Millard WJ, Simpkins JW. Ovariectomy reduces ChAT activity and NGF mRNA levels in the frontal cortex and hippocampus of the female Sprague Dawley rat. Soc Neurosci Abstr 1993;19:1254.

123. Singh M, Meyer EM, Simpkins JW. The effect of ovariectomy and estradiol replacement on brain-derived neurotrophic factor messenger ribonucleic acid expression in cortical and hippocampal brain regions of female Sprague-Dawley rats. Endocrinology 1995;136:2320–2324.

124. Singh M, Meyer EM, Millard WJ, Simpkins JW. Ovarian steroid deprivation results in a reversible learning impairment and compromised cholinergic function in female Sprague Dawley rats. Brain Res 1994;644:305–312.

125. Luine VN. Estradiol increases choline acetyltransferase activity in specific basal forebrain nuclei and projection areas of female rats. Exp Neurol 1985;89:484–490.

126. Lustig RH, Sudol M, Pfaff DW, Federoff HJ. Estrogen regulation of sex dimorphism in growth-associated protein 43 Kda (GAP-43) mRNA in the rat. Mol Brain Res 1991;11:125–132.

127. Stanley HF, Borthwick NM, Fink G. Brain protein changes during development and sexual differentiation in the rat. Brain Res 1986;370:215–222.

128. Ferreira A, Caceres A. Estrogen-enhanced neurite growth: evidence for a selective induction of tau and stable microtubules. J Neurosci 1991;11:293–400.

129. Weisz A, Cicatiello L, Persico E, Scalona M, Bresciani F. Estrogen stimulates transcription of the c-jun protooncogene. Mol Endocrinol 1990;4:1041–1050.

130. Sheng M, Greenberg ME. The regulation and function of Fos and other immediate early genes in the nervous system. Neuron 1990;4:477–485.

131. Wu BY, Fodor EJ, Edwards RH, Rutter WJ. Nerve growth factor induces the proto-oncogene c-jun in PC12 cells. J Biol Chem 1989;264:9000–9003.

132. Drubin DG, Feinstein SC, Shooter EM, Kirschner MW. Nerve growth factor-induced neurite outgrowth in PC12 cells involves the coordinate induction of microtubule assembly and alpha assembly promoting factors. J Cell Biol 1985;101:1799–1807.

133. Federoff HJ, Grabczyk E, Fishman MC. Dual regulation of GAP-43 gene expression by NGF and glucocorticoids. J Biol Chem 1988;263:19290–19295.

134. Hanemaaijer R, Ginzburg I. Involvement of mature tau isoforms in the stabilization of neurites in PC12 cells. J Neurosci Res 1991;30:163–171.

135. Mani SK, Allen JM, Clark JH, Blaustein JD, O'Malley BW. Convergent pathways for steroid hormone- and neurotransmitter-induced rat sexual behavior. Science 1994;265:1246–1249.

136. Ignar-Trowbridge DM, Nelson KG, Biwell MC, Curtis SW, Washburn TF, McLachlan JA, Korach KS. Coupling of dual signaling pathways: epidermal growth factor actions involves the estrogen receptor. Proc Natl Acad Sci USA 1992;89:4658–4662.

137. Nelson KG, Takahashi T, Bossert NL, Walmer DK, McLachlan JA. Epidermal growth factor replaces estrogen in the stimulation of female genital tract growth and differentiation. Proc Natl Acad Sci USA 1991;88:21–25.

138. Cho H, Katzenellenbogen BS. Synergistic activation of estrogen receptor-mediated transcription by estradiol and protein kinase activators. Mol Endocrinol 1993;7:441–452.

139. Batistatou A, Volonte C, Greene LA. Nerve growth factor employs multiple pathways to induce primary response genes in PC12 cells. Mol Biol Cell 1992;3:363–371.

140. Stephens RM, Loeb DM, Copeland TD. Pawson T, Greene LA, Kaplan DR. *Trk* receptors use redundant signal transduction pathways involving SHC and PLC-γl to mediate NGF responses. Neuron 1994;12:691–705.

18 Neurosteroids
Behavioral Studies

Willy Mayo, MD, Monique Vallée, MD,
Muriel Darnaudéry, MD, and Michel Le Moal, MD

CONTENTS

INTRODUCTION
NEUROSTEROIDS AND AFFECTIVE RESPONSES: ANXIETY, STRESS,
    AND AGGRESSION
NEUROSTEROIDS AND COGNITION: LEARNING AND MEMORY
REFERENCES

INTRODUCTION

The reports of higher concentrations of certain steroids in the brain than in blood and of their accumulation in brain independently of adrenal and gonadal sources led to the discovery of steroid biosynthetic pathways in the central nervous system (CNS). As a result, the term "neurosteroids" was proposed, referring to steroids synthesized in the brain, either de novo from cholesterol or by in situ metabolism of blood-borne precursors *(1)*. In this chapter, we summarize the behavioral effects—on affective and cognitive functions—of systemic or intra-cerebral administration of these neurosteroids. In addition to these pharmacological studies, we focus on recent physiological data indicating a possible role of certain neurosteroids in age-related memory deficits. Neurosteroids and affective responses: anxiety, stress, and aggression

Rationale

Neurosteroids have been shown in vitro to modulate the gamma amino butyric/benzodiazepine (GABA/BZD) receptor-chloride ionophore complex *(2)*. Some of these steroids, particularly the ring-A-reduced metabolite of progesterone (PROG), 3α-hydroxy-5α-pregnan-20-one (allopregnanolone) increase the binding of [³H] muscimol to the GABA recognition site *(3,4)* and stimulate [³H] flunitrazepam binding to the allosteric-linked benzodiazepine receptor *(5)*. Allopregnanolone stimulates GABA-mediated Cl⁻ uptake in cortical synaptosomes *(5–7)* and potentiates GABA-activated Cl⁻ currents in hippocampal neurons in primary culture *(3,5)* and potentiates GABA-acti-

From: *Contemporary Endocrinology: Neurosteroids: A New Regulatory Function
in the Nervous System* Edited by: E.-E. Baulieu, P. Robel, and M. Schumacher
© Humana Press Inc., Totowa, NJ

vated Cl⁻ currents in hippocampal neurons in primary culture *(3,5)* and in human cell lines transfected with $GABA_A$ receptor subunits *(8)*. A second class of neurosteroids represented by pregnenolone (PREG) and dehydroepiandrosterone (DHEA) and their sulfate esters have been shown to behave as negative modulators of the $GABA_A$ receptor *(9,10)* with possible anxiogenic properties. The GABAergic properties of neurosteroids are similar to those of anxiolytic or anxiogenic compounds acting at the $GABA_A$ receptor like BZD or β-carbolines. Thus a possible role of neurosteroids in the neurophysiological regulation of adaptive responses can be hypothesized. Consequently numerous studies have focused on the role of neurosteroids mainly on affective responses.

Behavioral studies of the anxiolytic/anxiogenic properties of neurosteroids have used a large panel of classical "anxiety" *(11)* including stress paradigms.

Anxiety-like Measurement Paradigms

Several different behavioral paradigms have been proposed to reflect pharmacologically sensitive anxiety levels in animals. These include a variety of tests related to spontaneous behavior: exploratory behavior (elevated plus-maze, light-dark transition chamber, mirror chamber test) or spontaneous avoidance (burying test). Other procedures employ punishment responses as operant conflict tests.

ELEVATED PLUS MAZE

This task widely cited in the literature and used for the evaluation of anxiety-like behavior *(12,13)* is based on the natural agoraphobic behavior of rodents.

Apparatus and response measurements. The apparatus consists of two open arms and two enclosed arms with an open roof, arranged such that the two open arms are opposite one to the other. The maze is elevated above the floor (≥50 cm). Anxiolytic effects of treatments are noted as an increase in the number of entries into the open arms and/or an increase in the time spent in these open arms as compared to control animals. Conversely anxiogenic compounds decrease these parameters.

Neurosteroid Administration. In this task, allopregnanolone administered intraperitoneally (ip) (1–20 mg/kg) in male mice elicited clear anxiolytic effects, i.e., an increase in the number of open-arm entries and of the time spent in these arms *(14)*. When injected icv (1.25–10 μg) in adult female rats, the same anxiolytic properties were observed *(15)*. The highest dose (10 μg) resulted in sedation as measured by decreased locomotor activity. In another study, 5 or 10 μg of allopregnanolone administered icv in male Wistar rats were able to counteract the anxiogenic action of corticotropin releasing hormone (CRH) with an increase in the time spent in open arms *(16)*.

PROG administered subcutaneously (sc) 4 h prior to the task (1–4 mg/animal, i.e., approximately 4–16 mg/kg) in ovariectomized female rats also had anxiolytic properties *(17)*. Following an immobilization stress (2 h), PROG (acute administration of 10 mg/kg sc or 9 d pretreatment with 1 mg/kg) increased the proportion of entries and the time spent in open arms *(18)*. In contrast low doses (1 and 5 mg/kg had no effect. The anxiolytic effect of PROG (1 mg/kg × 9 d) was abolished by pretreatment with bicuculline (1 mg/kg ip), a specific $GABA_A$ antagonist or with picrotoxin (1 mg/kg ip) a $GABA_A$ receptor-gated Cl⁻ channel antagonist indicating an involvement of $GABA_A$ receptors in the anxiolytic properties of PROG. This effect of picrotoxin administration (0.75 mg/kg ip) on the anxiolytic activity of PROG has also been reported in ovariectomized rats

(1 mg sc 4 h prior to the task) by Bitran et al. *(19)*. Reddy and Kulkarni *(18)* also reported that in their protocol a pretreatment with flumazenil (2 mg/kg ip) an antagonist of the BZD recognition site of the $GABA_A$ receptor failed to antagonize the anxiolytic effects of PROG, indicating that PROG or its metabolites modulate the $GABA_A$ receptor by acting on sites distinct from the BZDs. The anxiolytic effect of PROG besides a specific action on central GABAergic transmission demonstrated by its potentiating effect on the electrophysiological responses to GABA in vitro *(20)* and in vivo *(21)*, can also result from a central bioconversion into allopregnanolone. Indeed, the anxiolytic effects of PROG have been correlated with an increase in cortical allopregnanolone levels associated with an increase in cortical $GABA_A$ receptor function (decrease of EC_{50} and increase of E_{max}) *(17)*. This can be blocked by pretreatment with 4-MA, a 5α-reductase inhibitor, i.e., a molecule inhibiting the conversion of PROG into allopregnanolone *(19)*.

Neurosteroids with negative modulatory action at the $GABA_A$ receptor were also investigated in this task. Melchior and Ritzmann *(22)* have shown in mice that low doses of PREG (10 ng/kg ip) caused an anxiogenic response, i.e., a decreased number of entries into the open arms. Pregnenolone sulfate (PREGS) produced a biphasic response: 1 and 10 µg/kg caused an anxiogenic response whereas 100 ng/kg produced anxiolytic one. Moreover PREG and its sulfate (1 µg/kg) were able to block the anxiolytic effect of ethanol (1.5 g/kg). The biphasic action of PREGS on anxiety could be related to the mixed agonist/antagonist action of this compound at the $GABA_A$ receptor complex *(23)*. DHEA and its sulfate (DHEAS) when administered intraperitoneally, showed anxiolytic activity, however, DHEAS (1 mg/kg), as well as PREG and its sulfate, blocked the anxiolytic effect of ethanol *(24)*. These results are somewhat surprising in light of the known antagonist activity of DHEA and its sulfate at the $GABA_A$ receptor *(9,25,26)*. However the peripheral route of administration can partly explain these results. Indeed, DHEA attenuates the stress-induced increase in plasma corticosterone levels *(27)* and animals with naturally low corticosterone response to stress exhibit low anxiety in the plus maze *(28)*. Moreover DHEA when administered peripherally decreases brain levels of PREGS *(29)* leading thus to an anxiolytic effect.

LIGHT-DARK TRANSITION CHAMBER

This task was originally proposed by Crawley and Goodwin *(30)* for the study of the anxiolytic properties of BZD.

Apparatus and Response Measurements. The animals are allowed to run free in a two-chambered arena where one area is illuminated and the other is darkened. The number of transitions between the light and the dark chamber is interpreted as an anxiolytic effect of the substance studied.

Neurosteroid Administration. Allopregnanolone, when administered to male mice (10–40 mg/kg ip), increased the number of transitions between the light and the dark chamber *(31)*, the activity in light box and the time spent in the light box *(14)*. Interestingly $3\beta,5\alpha$-THPROG, the stereoisomer of allopregnanolone (20 mg/kg ip), was devoid of effect in this task, demonstrating the stereospecific requirements for the functional activation induced by allopregnanolone.

MIRROR-CHAMBER TEST

This task, originally proposed by Toubas et al. *(32)* measures approach-conflict behavior.

Apparatus and Response Measurements. The chamber of mirrors consists of a mirrored cube open on one side, which is placed into a square box. The mirrored cube is made of 5 pieces of mirrored glass. Three parameters can be recorded in this task:

1. latency to enter the chamber,
2. number of entries, and
3. total time spent in the chamber during the test.

This task is based on the fact that a wide spectrum of vertebrate species show approach and withdrawal responses on the placement of mirrors into their environment *(33)*.

Neurosteroid Administration. In this test the effect of various doses of allo-pregnanolone, PROG, PREGS, and DHEAS were evaluated in male mice *(34)*. Allopregnanolone (0.5 and 1 mg/kg ip) produced a dose-dependent decrease in the latency to enter, and increased the number of entries as well as the time spent in the mirrored chamber as compared to controls. This effect was prevented by picrotoxin, indicating that the anxiolytic effect of allopregnanolone is mediated via potentiation of $GABA_A$ receptors. This is in line with the results of Bitran et al. *(15)* in the plus maze *(see* earlier). By contrast, flumazenil had no effect on the anxiolytic properties of allopregnanolone, indicating an action at the $GABA_A$ receptor at a site distinct from the BZD binding site, perhaps on a specific site as suggested by Gee et al. *(35)*. PROG (1, 5, and 10 mg/kg sc) elicited a dose-dependent anxiolytic effect, possibly resulting from an indirect action on $GABA_A$ receptor function mediated by its reduced metabolite allopregnanolone. DHEAS (1 and 2 mg/kg ip) increased the latency to enter the chamber and reduced the number of entries and the total time spent in the mirrored chamber indicating a clear anxiogenic action of this neurosteroid. These results are in agreement with those of Melchior and Ritzmann *(24)* showing that the same doses of DHEAS blocked the anxiolytic effects of ethanol. The anxiogenic responses observed with DHEAS could be partly attributed to its positive allosteric modulation of the N-methy-D-aspartate (NMDA) receptor complex at the sigma site *(36)*. Indeed Reddy and Kulkarni *(34)* have shown that dizocilpine (a noncompetitive NMDA receptor antagonist) when injected ip (0.5 mg/kg), elicited an anxiolytic effect in the mirrored chamber test that was blocked by pretreatment with DHEAS (2 mg/kg). This indicates that in addition to the antagonist action on $GABA_A$ receptors, a positive modulation of NMDA receptors could explain in part the anxiogenic properties of DHEAS.

Curiously in this task, PREGS (0.5 and 2 mg/kg ip) produced anxiolytic effects, i.e., a decrease in the latency to enter and an increase of the number of entries and of the time spent in the mirrored chamber was observed as compared to controls. Low doses of PREGS (100 ng/kg ip) have previously been shown to have an anxiolytic action in the plus maze *(22)*. By contrast an anxiogenic effect was observed at 1 and 10 µg/kg. More-over a dose of 1 µg/kg blocked the anxiolytic action of ethanol (1.5 g/kg). This effect can be partly explained by the biphasic modulation of the $GABA_A$ receptor by PREGS *(23)*. In the study of Reddy and Kulkarni *(34)*, high doses were used (i.e., 2 mg/kg) albeit these doses are low compared with those used in the memory studies *(see* below). Interestingly 4'-chlordiazepam (4'CD) a specific ligand for the mitochondrial diazepam binding inhibitor (DBI) receptor (MDR) exhibited anxiolytic properties in the mirrored chamber that were attributed by the authors to its agonistic effect on MDR-mediated neurosteroidogenesis and a resulting action on $GABA_A$ receptors via increased mito-chondrial synthesis of PREG and resulting release of allopregnanolone.

Burying Behavior

Apparatus and Response Measurements. Rodents display a natural defense reaction to a strange and/or a dangerous object by burying it with bedding material from the floor of the cage *(37)*. Anxiolytic drugs inhibit this behavior. Although it is possible to use objects that provoke burying spontaneously *(38)*, the classical procedure employs an object on which a first contact induces a mild electric shock (usually 0.3 mA). Two parameters can be recorded in this task: (1) the burying behavior latency, i.e., the time elapsed between the first shock and the burying behavior display and (2) the duration of the burying behavior, i.e., the time that the rat spends burying the object.

Neurosteroid Administration. PROG administered to female Wistar rats at a dose of 4 mg/kg ip increases the burying behavior latency *(39)*. However neither lower doses, nor allopregnanolone, $3\beta,5\alpha$-THPROG, 5α-dihydroprogesterone (5α-DHPROG), or PREGS had an effect on this parameter. A decrease in the duration of burying behavior was obtained in a dose-dependent manner with PROG and allopregnanolone (with a minimal dose of 1 mg/rat and 0.125 mg/rat respectively). $3\beta,5\alpha$-THPROG, 5α-DHPROG, and PREGS had no effect. The anxiolytic effect of PROG (1 mg/rat sc) was also observed in ovariectomized females *(19)*. Interestingly this effect was prevented by pretreatment with 4-MA, indicating that the anxiolytic property is mediated by the action of the reduced metabolite, i.e., allopregnanolone.

In summary, experiments using the burying behavior paradigm confirm the anxiolytic action of PROG and allopregnanolone. However allopregnanolone seems to be the substance effectively responsible for the effect in view of the fact that blockade of the bioconversion of PROG to allopregnanolone abolished the anxiolytic effect of PROG on the duration of burying behavior. Moreover the minimally active dose on burying behavior was 10-fold lower for allopregnanolone than for PROG.

Operant Conflict Tests

Apparatus and Response Measurements. These procedures involve punishment in the form of an electric shock. For example in the Geller-Seifter procedure *(40)*, periods of responding for pellets or an appetitive liquid (e.g., sweetened condensed milk) on a variable interval schedule were interrupted by periods where the reward could be obtained more frequently but was accompanied by a low intensity electric shock. An anxiolytic drug should enhance responding only in the conflict periods and have no effect on normal responding *(11)*. In another paradigm called the Vogel test or licking suppression test *(41)*, a water-deprived animal has free access to a drinking tube but every tenth lick is punished (0.1 mA).

Neurosteroid Administration. With this procedure, allopregnanolone (7.5 mg/kg, subcutaneous) induced anti-anxiety activity in male Sprague-Dawley rats, revealed by a significant increase in punished behavior *(14)*. Recently Brot et al. *(42)* found that allopregnanolone injected 30 min prior to the conflict test in female ovariectomized rats (8 mg/kg sc) exhibited anxiolytic-like effects. These effects were reversed by the prior injection of RO15-4513 (a benzodiazepine receptor, partial inverse agonist), indicating that stimulation of the chloride channel in $GABA_A$ receptors is an important component mediating the effects of allopregnanolone. Similar anxiolytic-like effects were obtained using a Vogel paradigm. Allopregnanolone (20 mg/kg ip) produced a significant increase in punished responding (235%) comparable to that obtained with chlordiazepoxide (197%)(10 mg/kg ip) *(31)*.

Neurosteroids in Anxiety Paradigms: A Synthesis

These studies clearly demonstrate the anxiolytic properties of allopregnanolone irrespective of the route of administration (ip, sc or icv) or the task used (plus-maze, light-dark chamber, mirror chamber, burying, or operant conflict test). The anxiolytic action of PROG (ip or sc) is also consistent, but could result from its bioconversion into allopregnanolone *(17,19)*. These compounds probably modulate anxiety through positive modulation of the $GABA_A$ receptors in specific brain regions. The prefrontal cortex and particularly the mesocortical dopaminergic system could be a plausible candidate. Indeed stress-induced activation of the prefrontal cortical dopaminergic innervation is antagonized by icv administration of the "neuroactive steroid" tetrahydro-corticosterone ($3\alpha,5\alpha$-THDOC), the major metabolite of deoxycorticosterone (DOC) *(43)*. For the neurosteroids with a negative modulatory action at the $GABA_A$ receptor, the results are less clear. DHEAS and PREGS exhibit either anxiolytic or anxiogenic actions depending on the dose used. The mixed agonist/antagonist action of PREGS at the $GABA_A$ receptor complex *(23)* could partly explain its biphasic modulation of anxiety.

Effects of Stress or Anxiety on Neurosteroid Expression

Various procedures can be used to induce acute stress or anxiety. Among these, swim stress and CO_2 inhalation have been used to study the relationships between stress or anxiety and the cerebral concentrations of some neurosteroids.

Swim-Stress Paradigm

Apparatus and Response Measurements. The swim stress paradigm consists of placing animals in a container filled with water (ambient or cold temperature) for 5 or 10 min.

Neurosteroid Concentrations. Using this procedure, Purdy et al. *(44)* showed that an acute stress induces in male Sprague-Dawley rats a rapid (<5 min) increase (twofold) in allopregnanolone in the cerebral cortex (5 ng/g), the hypothalamus (4 ng/g) and in plasma (3ng/mL) as compared to controls. This stress also induces a 20-fold increase in cerebral $3\alpha,5\alpha$-THDOC. However $3\alpha,5\alpha$-THDOC should be considered as a neuroactive steroid, and not as a neurosteroid *stricto sensu*, although produced in brain from DOC, because THDOC becomes undetectable in the brain following an adrenalectomy (ADX) whereas allopregnanolone is still present. The hypothesis of a biosynthesis of allopregnanolone from PROG formed in situ (brain) was supported in this study by the fact that in intact animals the levels of PROG and allopregnanolone in the cerebral cortex are equal. Conversely, stressed ADX animals exhibit allopregnanolone levels that greatly exceed those of PROG, reinforcing the hypothesis of an *in situ* (brain) biosynthesis of allopregnanolone from PROG. Consistent with the anxiolytic effect of allopregnanolone, the stress-induced cerebral increase of this substance may represent an adaptive response of the organism to stress. In accordance with this hypothesis, Guo et al. *(45)* demonstrated (using the same procedure but with cold water, i.e., 4°C) that icv administration of an anti-allopregnanolone serum (10 μL) potentiated the stress-induced corticosterone release. This effect was observed in prepubertal, adult fertile rats, as well as castrated male rats compared to control or anti-serum treated rats, and in prepubertal and fertile female rats throughout the estrous cycle, but not in aged male or female animals (16 mo). An enhanced adrenocortical response to stress was previously observed following icv or ip administration of $GABA_A$ antagonists such as picrotoxin or bicuculline *(46)*. An inhibitory role of allopregnanolone on the stress-related response of corticosterone may thus be explained by the GABA-mimetic effects of this neurosteroid. Studies by Guo et al. *(45)* also suggest that the effect of allopregnanolone is probably independent of changes in gonadal steroid plasma levels indicated by the lack of difference in stress-related corticosterone secretion following immunoneutralization of allopregnanolone between adult castrated and fertile male rats and confirmed by the same lack of difference in female rats undergoing different phases of the estrous cycle.

INHALATION OF CO_2

Apparatus and Response Measurements. This procedure induces anxiety and panic attacks in humans *(47)*. Animals are briefly exposed to a mixture of O_2 and CO_2 in an hermetically closed box for 1 min.

Neurosteroid Concentrations. This stress induces an increase in the content of PREG and PROG in the cerebral cortex and the hippocampus *(48)*. Although an increase in DOC was also reported, no changes in DHEA concentrations were observed. However, these increases could result not only from an enhancement of brain steroidogenesis but also from an increased adrenal steroid output (particularly for DOC). Further studies using ADX animals would thus be of interest in addressing these question.

NEUROSTEROID EXPRESSION INDUCED BY STRESS OR ANXIETY: A SYNTHESIS

Taken together, these works demonstrate that a stressful event induces an increase in cerebral allopregnanolone, which could attenuate the corticosterone stress-related response via the modulation of $GABA_A$ receptors. However, the stress/anxiety-induced PREG and PROG increases in the brain (i.e., formed *in situ*) need to be confirmed.

Aggressive Behavior

Adult female mice display an aggressive behavior towards lactating intruders. This behavior does not depend on ovarian hormones because it persists after ovariectomy *(49)*. This aggressive behavior is reduced in intact males but is amplified by castration *(49)*. DHEA injected chronically (sc, 80 µg/d/2 wk) significantly reduced the aggressive response of castrated males. This effect does not result from a transformation of DHEA into sex hormones (i.e., testosterone (T) or estradiol). Indeed the synthetic steroid CH_3-DHEA (3β-methyl-Δ5-androstene-17-one)—which is devoid of hormonal action—had an inhibitory effect on the attack similar to that of DHEA *(50)*. Interestingly, both molecules significantly decrease PREGS concentrations in the brain of treated, castrated mice *(29)*. A possible explanation for the anti-aggressive effect of DHEA could be an increased GABAergic tone secondary to the decrease of PREGS. Indeed, high levels of GABA have been described in the hypothalamus, olfactory bulbs, and amygdala of some particularly aggressive strains of mice *(51)*. However, the mechanism by which DHEA decreases brain levels of PREGS remains unknown.

Age-Related Effects of Neurosteroids on Stress and Anxiety

Previously described studies have been performed on adult rodents. In order to determine whether the anxiolytic effect of allopregnanolone could be demonstrated in infant animals, Zimmerberg et al. *(52)* investigated the consequence of icv injections of different doses of allopregnanolone (1.25–5 µg) on ultrasonic vocalization production induced after maternal separation. These vocalizations classically occur following maternal deprivation *(53)* and anxiolytic compounds, such as BZD, reduce it *(54,55)*. Allopregnanolone caused a dose-dependent decrease in these ultrasonic vocalizations in 1-wk-old Wistar rats. These results suggest that the $GABA_A$ receptor site for this neurosteroid is behaviorally active in neonates as well as in adult rats.

Concerning aging studies, the work of Guo et al. *(45)* (*see* earlier) has shown that anti-allopregnanolone treatment had no effect on corticosterone levels after stress in aged males or females rats, although the mechanisms underlying this phenomenon remain unclear. In fact, to date, the only report of an altered mechanism of steroidogenesis in aged animals (reproductive senescence) comes from a study of Hodges and Karavolas *(56)*, which showed that 5α-reductase (5α-R; the enzyme that converts PROG into 5α-DHPROG) and 3α hydroxysteroid oxydoreductase (3α-HOR; the enzyme that converts 5α-DH PROG into allopregnanolone) are altered in the pituitary of anestrus females compared to constant estrus ones.

Concluding remarks in summary, studies using anxiety-like measurements have shown that

1. Peripheral/central allopregnanolone administration induces anxiolytic behavior or reverses the anxiogenic effects of CRH.
2. The anxiolytic effects of exogenous PROG are owing at least in part to its bioconversion into cerebral allopregnanolone.
3. Results obtained with PREGS and DHEA and its sulfate remain difficult to interpret in light of their biphasic modulation of the $GABA_A$ receptor.

Collectively, these results demonstrate that neurosteroids with a $GABA_A$-agonist profile exhibit clear anxiolytic properties. Conversely neurosteroids with an antagonist-like action at the $GABA_A$ receptor seem to act as anxiogenic compounds although some of them display biphasic effects i.e., anxiogenic/anxiolytic depending of the dose used.

In addition to animal studies, a few studies has been performed in humans. Following a single oral dose of micronized PROG (1.2 mg) in female subjects (18–25 ye), the peak plasma level of PROG was correlated with plasmatic levels of allopregnanolone and pregnanolone (3α-hydroxy-5β-pregnan-20-one) *(57)*. The levels of allopregnanolone were significantly correlated with measures of fatigue and confusion. Although these and pregnanolone levels correlated with reduced tension-anxiety, changes in these parameters were no greater than those observed with placebo. However the normal subjects used in this study had very low anxiety scores and had no mood distress at baseline. Studies in anxious patients may better demonstrate the anxiolytic effects of these molecules, as suggested by the authors.

NEUROSTEROIDS AND COGNITION: LEARNING AND MEMORY

The consequences of neurosteroid administration on learning and memory processes are not easy to summarize. In fact a great number of paradigms involving different memories (spatial/nonspatial, working/reference, and so on) have been used and different steps of the information processing (acquisition, consolidation, retention) have been studied. However, owing to the previously demonstrated effect of neurosteroids on the emotional status of the animals, we decided to use a classification based on the nature of the task in terms of avoidance vs approach.

Avoidance-Based Paradigms

In these paradigms, animals learn a behavior in order to avoid some noxious stimulus. However in these tasks, emotional factors may play a critical role *(58)*, making it impossible to interpret solely the "memory" component of the animal's performance.

PASSIVE AVOIDANCE

In passive avoidance paradigms, the animals remember that a certain response terminated in an unpleasant event and will therefore hesitate to repeat it in the future. An increase in response latency reflects the strength of the memory trace for the aversive event (*see* ref. *59* for review).

Apparatus and Response Measurements. In some procedures called "step-through passive avoidance," a lighted compartment (naturally aversive) is coupled directly or through a runway to a dark opaque compartment (naturally secure). Following habituation trials, the animals are placed in the lighted compartment. They naturally quickly run to the dark compartment, where this time, they are confined and receive an electric shock that is applied through the floor (usually 0.3–0.4 mA, for a 2 s duration). The animal is then returned to its home cage. This trial is called the acquisition trial and following a variable time interval (hours, days, or even weeks) the animal is again placed in the lighted compartment and the latency to enter the dark compartment is measured. The longer is this latency, the better is the "memory" performance. Pharmacological treatments can be administered before the acquisition trial or after it (retention). Another procedure is called "step-down passive avoidance." In this procedure, there are no compartments or runways, only an insulated platform located in the center of an open field with a grid floor. The animal is placed onto the platform and when he steps down an electric shock is applied through the grid floor of the open-field. Following a variable time interval, the animal is again placed onto the platform and the latency to "step-down" is recorded.

Neurosteroid Administration *Before the Acquisition Trial.* In these experiments, the use of pre-training injection procedures limits the interpretation in terms of direct interactions with learning and memory process.

PREGS when injected alone (0.3–700 ng icv) had no effect on the acquisition or the retention (24 h later) performance in male Sprague-Dawley rats *(60)*. However using the same procedure, PREGS (175 or 351 ng icv) reversed the deficit induced by prior administration of the competitive NMDA receptor antagonist CPP 3-([±]-2-carboxypiperazin-4-yl)-propyl-1-phosphonic acid (CPP) *(60)*. The same effect was reported by Cheney et al. *(61)* in CPP (2.5 mg/kg) or dizocilpine (MK801, a noncompetitive NMDA receptor antagonist, 0.15 mg/kg)-treated adrenalectomized/castrated male rats following iv injections of PREGS (0.5–20 mg/kg) 30 min prior to the acquisition trial, and by Romeo et al. *(62)* in dizocilpine-treated intact male rats following an ip injection of PREGS (20 mg/kg). These results may be explained by the ability of PREGS to potentiate the activation of the NMDA subtype of excitatory amino-acid receptors as demonstrated in cultured rat hippocampal neurons *(63,64)*.

DHEAS (10 or 20 mg/kg sc) was also shown to attenuate dizocilpine-induced impairments in this task *(65)*; this effect was antagonized by the co-administration of the σ antagonist BMY-14802 (5 mg/kg ip) or by a sub-chronic treatment with haloperidol (4 mg/kg/day sc for 7 d) suggesting an interaction between DHEAS and σ_1 receptors.

Allopregnanolone (15 μmol iv) had the same effect as PREGS or DHEAS in dizocilpine-induced deficits *(62)*. For these authors, this quite surprising cognitive-enhancing effect of a neurosteroid acting as a positive modulator at the $GABA_A$ receptor suggests that either another receptor mediates the allopregnanolone effect or perhaps the involvement of different $GABA_A$ receptor subtypes.

After the Acquisition Trial. These experiments focus mainly on the consolidation/retrieval action of neurosteroids. When injected subcutaneously to male Wistar rats immediately following the avoidance trial, PREGS (1, 10, and 100 ng) facilitates the retention of a passive avoidance 24 h later. With a delay of 48 h only the dose of 100 ng was effective *(66)*. When PREGS was injected 1 h prior the retention trial (i.e., 23 h or 47 h after the acquisition) no clear effect was observed.

ACTIVE AVOIDANCE

In active avoidance paradigms, the animals are required to make some measurable response in order to avoid a noxious stimulus (generally an electric footshock).

Apparatus and Response Measurements. The more simple paradigms require an animal to run from one compartment of an apparatus to another (one-way step through) or to jump onto a pole to avoid a footshock. Rats and mice can acquire the appropriate responses within a limited number of trials. In the two-way shuttle avoidance paradigm, the animal has to shuttle from one compartment of an avoidance chamber to another. On each trial, the direction of the response is reversed. In T-maze or Y-maze active avoidance paradigms, boxes are placed at the end of each alley (one start box and two goal boxes). The animal is placed in the start box and must learn to walk quickly through the maze in order to reach one of the goal boxes designated as correct; otherwise, an electric shock is applied through the floor of the maze. The animal is shocked until it reaches the correct box. In these tasks, it is possible to measure a temporal component (i.e., the latency to leave the start alley) and a discrimination component (i.e., to choose the correct goal box). Facilitating or deleterious effects of various drugs on the retention of these active avoidance paradigms can be evaluated by modulating the strength of the acquisition in control animals (for example, a low shock intensity during acquisition trials led to a poor performance in retention. Conversely, higher electrical shocks during acquisition trials induce an optimal retention performance).

Neurosteroid Administration. The effects of neurosteroids in these tasks were evaluated by retention performance (i.e., administration made at the end of acquisition trials). DHEAS enhances retention 1 wk after training in a T-maze active avoidance paradigm when injected subcutaneously in mice *(67)*. This effect seems to follow an inverted U-shaped curve, i.e., intermediate doses having a significant effect on retention (525–700 μg/mouse), whereas lower (175 and 350 μg/mouse) or higher doses (875 and 1400 μg/mouse) had no significant effect. Similar dose-effects were reported following icv (108–271 ng active, 55 and 324 ng inactive) or intra-hippocampal administration (0.4 ng active, 0.04 and 4 ng inactive) and also following an oral administration during 1 wk (0.7 and 1.4 mg/mouse active, 0.36 and 2–3 mg/mouse inactive) *(67,68)*. Subcutaneous DHEAS (20 mg/kg) can also reverse spontaneous retention deficits in old mice (18 or 24 mo-old) *(69)*. Experimentally-induced amnesia in these tasks is sensitive to treatment with DHEAS. Retention deficits induced by scopolamine, dimethyl sulfoxide (DMSO), or anisomycin (inhibitor of protein synthesis) are abolished by DHEAS (icv 162 ng) *(67)*. DHEA and PREG (icv 350 pmol/mouse) reverse DMSO-induced amnesia in the

T-maze active avoidance paradigm *(70)*. PREGS was shown to be very potent in these paradigms. When administered icv in mice, a dose of 1.47 pg is already active on memory performance *(70)*. Local administration in various limbic structures (amygdala, hippocampus, mammillary bodies and septum) confirms the potency of this neurosteroid. Amygdala infusions reveal that 15 molecules of PREGS (2.4×10^{-23} mol, i.e., 10–20 g) are able to significantly enhance the retention of mice as compared to control animals *(68)*. Effects seen in amygdala are 10^4 times more potent than those in the hippocampus or 10^5 times more potent than those in the septum or the mammillary bodies. In all these limbic structures, the effects of PREGS exhibit an inverted U-shaped dose response curve. If these U-shaped response curves are typical of memory-enhancing compounds, the range of effective doses of PREGS (4–6 orders of magnitude) extends the usual range (2–5). These results show that PREGS is by far the most potent memory enhancer in this task yet reported. For the authors, some effects of this compound could imply the existence of an as yet unidentified receptor that has a high affinity for PREGS. An action on NMDA receptors can also be envisaged in light of the work of Mathis et al. *(71)*, which showed that in a Y-maze active avoidance paradigm icv infusions of PREGS (4.2–42 ng) blocked the retention deficits induced by the competitive NMDA receptor antagonist D-AP5 (D-2-amino-5-phosphonovalerate).

WATER MAZE

The learning of this task originally proposed by Morris *(72)*, involves the storage and the retrieval of spatial information and the planning of navigational strategies.

Apparatus and Response Measurements. In this task, animals are trained to escape from the water of a swimming pool by swimming to a hidden platform. The location of this hidden platform needs the use of distal extra-maze cues. Normal animals learn the location of the platform rapidly (usually a dozen trials spaced over several days). At the end of the learning phase, the strength of the memory for the location of the platform can be assessed by removing the platform and measuring the time to find (or the distance traveled to) the previous location of the platform.

Neurosteroid Administration. When administered subcutaneously to female ovariectomized rats, DHEAS or PREGS (3.2 or 6.4 mg/kg) have no effect on the latency to find the platform but reduce the distance to find this platform compared to control animals *(73)*. When administered icv (1–2 μg), they reduce both the latency and the distance to escape onto the platform during the first trials of the task. Allopregnanolone (sc 3.2 or 6.4 mg/kg) in the same experiment reduced the latency to find the platform but was devoid of effect when administered icv These results are difficult to interpret in terms of memory owing to the protocol used, i.e., icv administrations made before the first trial of a 1-d water-maze procedure. Nevertheless an indirect enhancing effect of some neurosteroids in this task can be derived from the work of Romeo et al. *(62)*, which showed that administration of FGIN 1–27—a ligand at the mitochondrial diazepam-binding inhibitor receptor complex (MDRC) that stimulates neurosteroidogenesis—reverses the memory deficit induced by dizocilpine in this task.

NEUROSTEROIDS AND AVOIDANCE-BASED PARADIGMS: A SYNTHESIS

As previously mentioned, emotional factors can play a critical role in these tasks and the results obtained are difficult to interpret solely in terms of memory performance. However, when administered during the consolidation/retention phase, PREGS and

DHEAS facilitate the retention of the task. The facilitating effects of PREGS were obtained with extremely low dose, but in this case the mechanisms underlying this effect remains largely unknown.

Approach-Based Paradigms

In these tasks, animals usually learn a response in order to get some appetitive reinforcement. However some paradigms can imply spontaneous approach behaviors.

SPONTANEOUS EXPLORATION OF NOVELTY

Apparatus and Response Measurements. Rodents have a natural drive to explore novel environments. This behavior implies that the animal must memorize a previously explored environment in order to discriminate it from a novel one. A classical paradigm for studying this behavior is the spontaneous alternation task in a Y-maze or a T-maze. The animal freely explores the maze during a period of time (usually 10 min) and the percentage of alternation (an entry into all three arms on consecutive occasions) is recorded. The alternation score reflects attentional and short-term memory abilities. Another procedure recently proposed by Dellu et al. *(74)* requires the animal to explore 2 of the 3 arms of a Y-maze during a period of time (usually 10 min) which corresponds to the acquisition phase. Following a variable time interval (usually several hours), the animal is then replaced in the maze but this time he can explore all the three arms. Increased exploration of the "novel" arm reflects memorization of the previously explored places.

Neurosteroid Administration. In the Dellu's task (two-trial recognition task) an infusion of PREGS (5 ng) into the nucleus basalis magnocellularis (NBM) of male rats immediately following the acquisition trial enhances recognition performance as compared to control *(75)*. When administered before the acquisition trial, PREGS had no effect. These results suggest an action of PREGS mainly on consolidation/retrieval processes and not on acquisition. DHEAS (sc 10–20 mg/kg) attenuates the dizocilpine-induced impairment in a Y-maze alternation task *(65)*. Conversely, allopregnanolone infused into the NBM (0.2 or 2 ng) disrupts performance in the two-trial recognition task. These results suggest a memory-enhancing action of neurosteroids acting as negative allosteric modulators at the $GABA_A$ receptor and, conversely, a deleterious action of positive modulators (i.e., allopregnanolone). The effect at the NBM level also suggests possible modulation of cholinergic systems by neurosteroids. Indeed the NBM is the major source of the cortical cholinergic innervation.

SPATIAL FOOD/WATER-SEARCH TASKS

Apparatus and Response Measurements. In these tasks, animals are required to find food reinforcement using spatial cues. The classical paradigm is the radial-maze task *(76)*. This maze consists of an octagonal central area from which eight arms radiate outwards. A food cup is located at the end of each arm. Food-deprived rats must learn to avoid choosing arms they have already visited during the test session. Another paradigm of spatial food search uses a hole-board *(77)*, where the animal must find food reinforcement placed in one hole. These paradigms require the use of spatial extra maze cues by the animal. Some procedures using delayed nonmatching to sample (DNMTS) involving spatial discriminations are also used *(78)*; for example, a Y-maze in which the animal must choose the opposite arm from that which it forced down in a previous run.

Neurosteroid Administration. In a hole board task, PREGS when administered (100 µg ip) 8 d before exposure to the test and during the 5 d of acquisition, failed to modify significantly acquisition performance as compared to control animals *(79)*. A subsequent 10-d treatment of these animals with subcutaneous PREG pellets (100 µg daily) until the retention phase, also failed to modify retention performance. Similar results were obtained in a second set of experiments in which the animals were implanted with PREG pellets during 21 d. However, when treated, animals of the two experiments were pooled and compared to controls for retention performance, a significant treatment-effect was noticed in the middle trials of the retention phase (trials 4–6). However, in view of the statistical analysis of these results (pooling of experimental groups) and the experimental design (PREGS and PREG administration), caution should be used when interpreting the results.

In the radial-maze paradigm, no direct investigations were done, however, Romeo et al. *(62)* have shown that the deficit induced in this task by dizocilpine (i.e., an increase in the number of errors made in the fifth to eighth visits) was abolished by pretreatment with FGIN 1-27 indicating a positive effect of an enhanced steroidogenesis on this pharmacologically induced spatial memory deficit.

Using a DNMTS procedure in a Y maze, Frye and Sturgis *(73)* showed in ovariectomized rats that DHEAS (6.4 mg/kg ip) enhanced the percentage of correct choices made on d 5 of the task, but when injected on d 3 (3.2 mg/kg), the latency to the goal box was increased. This apparent discrepancy could be explained by an anxiogenic effect of DHEAS on the third day and a promnesic effect on the fifth day. However, the use of different doses of DHEAS in the same animal complicates the interpretation of the data. Using a similar paradigm in a T maze, Melchior and Ritzman *(80)* have shown that subcutaneous injections in mice of neurosteroids with a GABA antagonist profile (DHEA, DHEAS, PREG, PREGS), enhance performance in the task with an inverted U-shaped dose-response curve. Moreover, each neurosteroid at a dose of 0.05 mg/kg blocked the amnesic effect of ethanol (0.5 g/kg). Conversely, neurosteroids with a GABA agonist profile, i.e., pregnanolone or epipregnanolone (3β,5β-THPROG) disrupted the memory performance in this DNTMS task. Epipregnanolone had no effect on ethanol-induced amnesia. Surprisingly pregnanolone, which disrupted memory by itself, was also effective, in a wide range of doses, in blocking the amnesic action of ethanol. The authors explain this paradoxical effect by the fact that low levels of ethanol could counteract the GABA agonist properties of pregnanolone, as has been previously demonstrated for allopregnanolone *(81)*.

NONSPATIAL FOOD/WATER REINFORCED TASKS

Apparatus and Response Measurements. In these tasks the animal must discriminate between two (or more) differentiated compartments of an apparatus in order to find reinforcement. Two kinds of procedures are currently used in these tasks : the "forced choice," in which the two compartments are shown together and the animal must select one of them, and the "go/no go" procedure, in which the different compartments are shown one at a time and the subject decides whether or not to make a response. Another classical nonspatial food-reinforced task involves operant behavior in Skinner boxes. In the simplest procedures the animal must press a lever in order to receive a food pellet. The number of reinforced responses increases with time, reaching a plateau that reflects acquisition of the task. A retention test is administered following a variable delay (24 h or more) and the number of reinforced responses during the beginning of the retention test is compared to the number of reinforced responses obtained during the last phase of the acquisition.

Neurosteroid Administration. In a go/no go paradigm, Meziane et al. *(82)* showed that PREGS administered icv (0.2 µg) to male mice after the first learning session enhanced the subsequent learning performance during the second and third learning sessions. Administration of 0.04 µg or 0.4 µg had no effect on learning performance reflecting an inverted U-shaped response curve. However all these doses are effective in blocking the amnesic action of scopolamine (3 mg/kg sc) in this task. In the lever-press task, PREGS administered to male mice (41.8 ng icv) immediately after the acquisition session had no effect on retention performance measured 24 h later *(71)*. However, the same injection can block the D-AP5-induced deficit in the retention phase. This positive result can be explained by the fact that PREGS blocks the effect of D-AP5 through its positive modulatory action on NMDA receptors.

NEUROSTEROIDS AND APPROACH-BASED PARADIGMS: A SYNTHESIS

The use of these paradigms demonstrate the memory-enhancing properties of PREGS and DHEAS. Conversely THPROG, pregnanolone, and epipregnanolone disrupted the memory performance, suggesting that the positive/negative effects of neurosteroids on memory processes could involve their positive/negative modulation of $GABA_A$ receptors. However, a modulation of NMDA receptors could also participate in the effects observed, particularly for PREGS.

PHYSIOLOGICAL DATA

Despite the great number of pharmacological studies indicating a promnesic action of some neurosteroids, and particularly of those having a GABA antagonist profile, little if nothing is known about the link between the cerebral concentrations of these steroids and memory performances. In order to define this relationship, we have first evaluated the learning/memory performances of a group of old male rats (24 mo) in the water-maze task and in the Y-maze spontaneous recognition task. Classical variability in the performances of old rats was noticed. Performances in the two tasks were correlated, i.e., animals that explored preferentially the novel arm in the Y-maze covered a shorter distance to escape onto the platform in the water maze (Spearman's $\rho = -0.67, p < 0.001$). We then measured the concentrations of PREGS in various brain areas. A significant correlation was found between the performance of the animals in the water maze and the concentrations of PREGS in the hippocampus ($r = -0.53, p < 0.003$) (Fig. 1).

This relationship seems to be specific to the hippocampus. Indeed no correlation was found in the amygdala, prefrontal cortex, parietal cortex, or striatum *(83)*.

In order to determine the causative role of hippocampal PREGS in memory performance, PREGS (5ng/0.5 µL) was infused directly into the dorsal hippocampus of old cognitively impaired rats immediately after the acquisition trial in the two-trial recognition task (Y maze). Animals treated with PREGS performed better than the vehicle injected group ($t = 3.1, df = 10, p < 0.01$) (Fig. 2).

These results suggest that neurosteroids could be studied in the context of prevention and/or treatment of age-related memory disorders.

Conclusions

All these experiments clearly demonstrate that neurosteroids—particularly those having a GABA antagonist profile—have memory-enhancing properties. Among these,

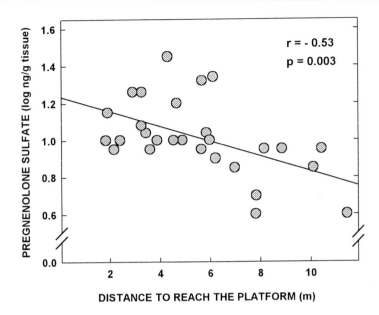

Fig 1. Learning performance of aged rats in the water-maze: correlation with PREGS levels in the hippocampus. PREGS concentrations were expressed in log (ng/g). Performance was expressed as the mean distance to reach the hidden platform during the last 3 d of the test. Low PREG S levels were linked with longer distances, i.e., worse performances ($y = [-7.01 \pm 2.18] x + 12.61$).

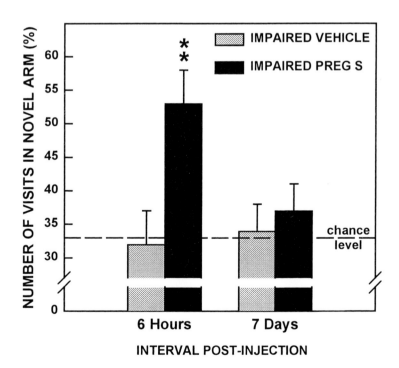

Fig. 2. Effects of bilateral injection of PREG S into the hippocampus on the performance of impaired aged rats in the Y-maze. The subgroup treated with PREGS ($n = 7$) performed significantly above chance level 6 h post-injection ($t = 4.1$, $df = 5$, **$p < 0.01$), and returned to chance level 7 d later ($t = 1.1$, $df = 5$, ns).

PREGS is probably the most potent. The mechanisms underlying these properties are presently unknown, but it could be hypothesized that the neuromodulatory pathways of PREGS may reinforce neurotransmitter systems that decline with age. Central cholinergic transmission represents a plausible candidate for these steroid effects. Indeed cholinergic systems in the basal forebrain, thought to be involved in the regulation of memory processes, are altered in normal aging, and degenerative changes in cholinergic nuclei correlate with memory impairments in old rats *(84)*. Previous results of Mayo *(75)* and Meziane *(82)* are in agreement with this hypothesis. Moreover, it has recently been demonstrated that icv infusions of PREGS stimulated, in a dose-dependent manner the release of acetylcholine in the cortex and the hippocampus *(85)*. The effects of neurosteroid administration on cholinergic transmission in old, cognitively impaired rats are currently under investigation, and could provide new insights into therapeutic strategies against age-related degenerative diseases, including senile dementia of the Alzheimer's type.

REFERENCES

1. Baulieu EE, Robel P. Neurosteroids: a new brain function? J Steroid Biochem Mol Biol 1990;37:395–403.
2. Gee KW. Steroid modulation of the GABA/benzodiazepine receptor- linked chloride ionophore. Mol Neurobiol 1988;2:291–317.
3. Harrison NL, Majewska MD, Harrington JW, Barker JL. Structure-activity relationships for steroid interaction with the gamma-aminobutyric acid A receptor complex. J Pharmacol Exp Ther 1987; 241:346–353.
4. Lopez-Colomè AM, McCarthy M, Beyer C. Enhancement of [^{3}H]muscimol binding to brain synaptic membranes by progesterone and related pregnanes. Eur J Pharmacol 1990;176:297–303.
5. Majewska MD, Harrison NL, Schwartz RD, Barker JL, Paul SM. Steroid hormone metabolites are barbiturate-like modulators of the GABA receptor. Science 1986;232:1004–1007.
6. Morrow AL, Pace JR, Purdy RH, Paul SM. Characterization of steroid interactions with gamma-aminobutyric acid receptor-gated chloride ion channels: evidence for multiple steroid recognition sites. Mol Pharmacol 1990;37:263–270.
7. Purdy RH, Morrow AL, Blinn JR, Paul SM. Synthesis, metabolism, and pharmacological activity of 3 alpha- hydroxy steroids which potentiate GABA-receptor-mediated chloride ion uptake in rat cerebral cortical synaptoneurosomes. J Med Chem 1990;33:1572–1581.
8. Puia G, Santi MR, Vicini S, Pritchett DB, Purdy RH, Paul SM, Seeburg PH, Costa E. Neurosteroids act on recombinant human GABA$_A$ receptors. Neuron 1990;4:759–765.
9. Carette B, Poulain P. Excitatory effect of dehydroepiandrosterone, its sulphate ester and pregnenolone sulphate, applied by iontophoresis and pressure, on single neurones in the septo-preoptic area of the guinea pig. Neurosci Lett 1984;45:205–210.
10. Majewska MD, Schwartz RD. Pregnenolone-sulfate: an endogenous antagonist of the gamma-aminobutyric acid receptor complex in brain? Brain Res 1987;404:355–360.
11. Andrews JS, Broekkamp CLE. Procedures to identify anxiolytic or anxiogenic agents. In: Sahgal A, ed. Behavioral Neuroscience: A Practical Approach. Oxford University Press, New York, NY, 1993, pp. 37–54.
12. Pellow S, Chopin P, File SE, Briley M. Validation of open:closed arm entries in an elevated plus-maze as a measure of anxiety in the rat. J Neurosci Methods 1985;14:149–167.
13. Pellow S, File SE. Anxiolytic and anxiogenic drug effects on exploratory activity in an elevated plus-maze: a novel test of anxiety in the rat. Pharmacol Biochem Behav 1986;24:525–529.
14. Wieland S, Belluzzi JD, Stein L, Lan NC. Comparative behavioral characterization of the neuroactive steroids 3 alpha-OH,5 alpha-pregnan–20-one and 3 alpha- OH,5 beta- pregnan–20-one in rodents. Psychopharmacology (Berlin) 1995;118:65–71.
15. Bitran D, Hilvers RJ, Kellogg CK. Anxiolytic effects of 3 alpha-hydroxy–5 alpha[beta]-pregnan-20-one: endogenous metabolites of progesterone that are active at the GABA$_A$ receptor. Brain Res 1991;561:157–161.

16. Patchev VK, Shoaib M, Holsboer F, Almeida OF. The neurosteroid tetrahydroprogesterone counteracts corticotropin- releasing hormone-induced anxiety and alters the release and gene expression of corticotropin-releasing hormone in the rat hypothalamus. Neuroscience 1994;62:265–271.

17. Bitran D, Purdy RH, Kellogg CK. Anxiolytic effect of progesterone is associated with increases in cortical allopregnanolone and GABA$_A$ receptor function. Pharmacol Biochem Behav 1993;45:423–428.

18. Reddy DS, Kulkarni SK. Role of GABA-A and mitochondrial diazepam binding inhibitor receptors in the anti-stress activity of neurosteroids in mice. Psychopharmacology (Berlin) 1996;128:280–292.

19. Bitran D, Shiekh M, McLeod M. Anxiolytic effect of progesterone is mediated by the neurosteroid allopregnanolone at brain GABA$_A$ receptors. J Neuroendocrinol 1995;7:171–177.

20. Wu FS, Gibbs TT, Farb DH. Inverse modulation of gamma-aminobutyric acid- and glycine- induced currents by progesterone. Mol Pharmacol 1990;37:597–602.

21. Smith SS, Waterhouse BD, Chapin JK, Woodward DJ. Progesterone alters GABA and glutamate responsiveness: a possible mechanism for its anxiolytic action. Brain Res 1987;400:353–359.

22. Melchior CL, Ritzmann RF. Pregnenolone and pregnenolone sulfate, alone and with ethanol, in mice on the plus-maze. Pharmacol Biochem Behav 1994;48:893–897.

23. Majewska MD. Neurosteroids: endogenous bimodal modulators of the GABA$_A$ receptor. Mechanism of action and physiological significance. Prog Neurobiol 1992;38:379–395.

24. Melchior CL, Ritzmann RF. Dehydroepiandrosterone is an anxiolytic in mice on the plus maze. Pharmacol Biochem Behav 1994;47:437–441.

25. Demirgören S, Majewska MD, Spivak CE, London ED. Receptor binding and electrophysiological effects of dehydroepiandrosterone sulfate, an antagonist of the GABA$_A$ receptor. Neuroscience 1991;45:127–135.

26. Majewska MD, Demirgören S, Spivak CE, London ED. The neurosteroid dehydroepiandrosterone sulfate is an allosteric antagonist of the GABA$_A$ receptor. Brain Res 1990;526:143–146.

27. Ben-Nathan D, Lustig S, Kobiler D, Danenberg HD, Lupu E, Feuerstein G. Dehydroepiandrosterone protects mice inoculated with West Nile virus and exposed to cold stress. J Med Virol 1992;38:159–166.

28. Vallée M, Mayo W, Dellu F, Le Moal M, Simon H, Maccari S. Prenatal stress induces high anxiety and postnatal handling induces low anxiety in adult offspring: correlation with stress-induced corticosterone secretion. J Neurosci 1997;17:2626–2636.

29. Young J, Corpéchot C, Haug M, Gobaille S, Baulieu EE, Robel P. Suppressive effects of dehydroepiandrosterone and 3 beta-methyl-androst–5-en–17-one on attack towards lactating female intruders by castrated male mice. II. Brain neurosteroids. Biochem Biophys Res Commun 1991;174:892–897.

30. Crawley J, Goodwin FK. Preliminary report of a simple animal behavior model for the anxiolytic effects of benzodiazepines. Pharmacol Biochem Behav 1980;13:167–170.

31. Wieland S, Lan NC, Mirasedeghi S, Gee KW. Anxiolytic activity of the progesterone metabolite 5 alpha-pregnan–3 alpha-ol–20-one. Brain Res 1991;565:263–268.

32. Toubas PL, Abla KA, Cao W, Logan LG, Seale TW. Latency to enter a mirrored chamber: a novel behavioral assay for anxiolytic agents. Pharmacol Biochem Behav 1990;35:121–126.

33. Gallup GG Jr. Mirror-image stimulation. Psychol Bull 1968;70:782–793.

34. Reddy DS, Kulkarni SK. Differential anxiolytic effects of neurosteroids in the mirrored chamber behavior test in mice. Brain Res 1997;752:61–71.

35. Gee KW, McCauley LD, Lan NC. A putative receptor for neurosteroids on the GABA$_A$ receptor complex: the pharmacological properties and therapeutic potential of epalons. Crit Rev Neurobiol 1995;9:207–227.

36. Monnet FP, Mahé V, Robel P, Baulieu EE. Neurosteroids, via sigma receptors, modulate the [^{3}H]norepinephrine release evoked by N-methyl-D-aspartate in the rat hippocampus. Proc Natl Acad Sci USA 1995;92:3774–3778.

37. Treit D, Pinel JP, Fibiger HC. Conditioned defensive burying: a new paradigm for the study of anxiolytic agents. Pharmacol Biochem Behav 1981;15:619–626.

38. Broekkamp CL, Rijk HW, Joly-Gelouin D, Lloyd KL. Major tranquillizers can be distinguished from minor tranquillizers on the basis of effects on marble burying and swim- induced grooming in mice. Eur J Pharmacol 1986;126:223–229.

39. Picazo O, Fernandez-Guasti A. Anti-anxiety effects of progesterone and some of its reduced metabolites: an evaluation using the burying behavior test. Brain Res 1995;680:135–141.

40. Geller I, Seifter J. The effects of meprobamate, barbiturates, d-amphetamine and promazine on experimentally induced conflict in the rat. Psychopharmacologia 1960;1:482–492.

41. Vogel JR, Beer B, Clody DE. A simple and reliable conflict procedure for testing anti-anxiety agents. Psychopharmacologia 1971;21:1–7.

42. Brot MD, Akwa Y, Purdy RH, Koob GF, Britton KT. The anxiolytic-like effects of the neurosteroid allopregnanolone: interactions with $GABA_A$ receptors. Eur J Pharmacol 1997;325:1–7.

43. Grobin AC, Roth RH, Deutch AY. Regulation of the prefrontal cortical dopamine system by the neuroactive steroid 3α,21-dihydroxy–5α-pregnane–20-one. Brain Res 1992;578:351–356.

44. Purdy RH, Morrow AL, Moore PH, Jr., Paul SM. Stress-induced elevations of gamma-aminobutyric acid type A receptor-active steroids in the rat brain. Proc Natl Acad Sci USA 1991;88:4553–4557.

45. Guo AL, Petraglia F, Criscuolo M, Ficarra G, Nappi RE, Palumbo MA, Trentini GP, Purdy RH, Genazzani AR. Evidence for a role of neurosteroids in modulation of diurnal changes and acute stress-induced corticosterone secretion in rats. Gynecol.Endocrinol. 1995;9:1–7.

46. Makara GB, Stark E. Effects of gamma-aminobutyric acid (GABA) and GABA antagonist drugs on ACTH release. Neuroendocrinology. 1974;16:178–190.

47. Woods SW, Charney DS, Loke J, Goodman WK, Redmond DE, Jr., Heninger GR. Carbon dioxide sensitivity in panic anxiety. Ventilatory and anxiogenic response to carbon dioxide in healthy subjects and patients with panic anxiety before and after alprazolam treatment. Arch Gen Psychiatry 1986;43:900–909.

48. Barbaccia ML, Roscetti G, Trabucchi M, Cuccheddu T, Concas A, Biggio G. Neurosteroids in the brain of handling-habituated and naive rats: effect of CO_2 inhalation. Eur J Pharmacol 1994;261:317–320.

49. Haug M, Spetz JF, Ouss-Schlegel ML, Benton D, Brain PF. Effects of gender, gonadectomy and social status on attack directed towards female intruders by resident mice. Physiol Behav 1986;37:533–537.

50. Haug M, Ouss-Schlegel ML, Spetz JF, Brain PF, Simon V, Baulieu EE, Robel P. Suppressive effects of dehydroepiandrosterone and 3-beta-methylandrost–5-en–17-one on attack towards lactating female intruders by castrated male mice. Physiol Behav 1989;46:955–959.

51. Haug M, Simler S, Ciesielski L, Mandel P, Moutier R. Influence of castration and brain GABA levels in three strains of mice on aggression towards lactating intruders. Physiol Behav 1984;32:767–770.

52. Zimmerberg B, Brunelli SA, Hofer MA. Reduction of rat pup ultrasonic vocalizations by the neuroactive steroid allopregnanolone. Pharmacol Biochem Behav 1994;47:735–738.

53. Hofer MA, Shair H. Ultrasonic vocalization during social interaction and isolation in 2-week-old rats. Dev Psychobiol 1978;11:495–504.

54. Gardner CR. Distress vocalization in rat pups. A simple screening method for anxiolytic drugs. J Pharmacol Methods 1985;14:181–187.

55. Insel TR, Hill JL, Mayor RB. Rat pup ultrasonic isolation calls: possible mediation by the benzodiazepine receptor complex. Pharmacol Biochem Behav 1986;24:1263–1267.

56. Hodges DR, Karavolas HJ. Pituitary progestin-metabolizing enzyme activities in the aged female rat. J Steroid Biochem Mol Biol 1992;41:79–84.

57. Freeman EW, Purdy RH, Coutifaris C, Rickels K, Paul SM. Anxiolytic metabolites of progesterone: correlation with mood and performance measures following oral progesterone administration to healthy female volunteers. Neuroendocrinology 1993;58:478–484.

58. Heise GA. Learning and memory facilitators: experimental definition and current status. Trends Pharmacol Sci 1981;2:158–160.

59. Sahgal A. Passive avoidance procedures. In: Sahgal A, ed. Behavioural Neuroscience: A Practical Approach. Oxford University Press, New York, NY, 1993, pp. 49–56.

60. Mathis C, Paul SM, Crawley JN. The neurosteroid pregnenolone sulfate blocks NMDA antagonist- induced deficits in a passive avoidance memory task. Psychopharmacology (Berlin) 1994;116:201–206.

61. Cheney DL, Uzunov D, Guidotti A. Pregnenolone sulfate antagonizes dizocilpine amnesia: role for allopregnanolone. Neuroreport. 1995;6:1697–1700.

62. Romeo E, Cheney DL, Zivkovic I, Costa E, Guidotti A. Mitochondrial diazepam-binding inhibitor receptor complex agonists antagonize dizocilpine amnesia: putative role for allopregnanolone. J Pharmacol Exp Ther 1994;270:89–96.

63. Irwin RP, Maragakis NJ, Rogawski MA, Purdy RH, Farb DH, Paul SM. Pregnenolone sulfate augments NMDA receptor mediated increases in intracellular Ca^{2+} in cultured rat hippocampal neurons. Neurosci Lett 1992;141:30–34.

64. Bowlby MR. Pregnenolone sulfate potentiation of N-methyl-D-aspartate receptor channels in hippoc-ampal neurons. Mol Pharmacol 1993;43:813–819.

65. Maurice T, Junien JL, Privat A. Dehydroepiandrosterone sulfate attenuates dizocilpine-induced learn-ing impairment in mice via sigma 1-receptors. Behav Brain Res 1997;83:159–164.

66. Isaacson RL, Varner JA, Baars JM, De Wied D. The effects of pregnenolone sulfate and ethylestrenol on retention of a passive avoidance task. Brain Res 1995;689:79–84.

67. Flood JF, Smith GE, Roberts E. Dehydroepiandrosterone and its sulfate enhance memory retention in mice. Brain Res 1988;447:269–278.

68. Flood JF, Morley JE, Roberts E. Pregnenolone sulfate enhances post-training memory processes when injected in very low doses into limbic system structures: the amygdala is by far the most sensitive. Proc Natl Acad Sci USA 1995;92:10806–10810.

69. Flood JF, Roberts E. Dehydroepiandrosterone sulfate improves memory in aging mice. Brain Res 1988;448:178–181.

70. Flood JF, Morley JE, Roberts E. Memory-enhancing effects in male mice of pregnenolone and steroids metabolically derived from it. Proc Natl Acad Sci USA 1992;89:1567–1571.

71. Mathis C, Vogel E, Cagniard B, Criscuolo F, Ungerer A. The neurosteroid pregnenolone sulfate blocks deficits induced by a competitive NMDA antagonist in active avoidance and lever-press learning tasks in mice. Neuropharmacology 1996;35:1057–1064.

72. Morris R. Developments of a water-maze procedure for studying spatial learning in the rat. J Neurosci Methods 1984;11:47–60.

73. Frye CA, Sturgis JD. Neurosteroids affect spatial/reference, working, and long-term memory of female rats. Neurobiol Learn Mem 1995;64:83–96.

74. Dellu F, Mayo W, Cherkaoui J, Le Moal M, Simon H. A two-trial memory task with automated record-ing: study in young and aged rats. Brain Res 1992;588:132–139.

75. Mayo W, Dellu F, Robel P, Cherkaoui J, Le Moal M, Baulieu EE, Simon H. Infusion of neurosteroids into the nucleus basalis magnocellularis affects cognitive processes in the rat. Brain Res 1993;607:324–328.

76. Olton DS, Samuelson RJ. Remembrance of place passed: spatial memory in rats. J Exp Psychol 1976;2:97–116.

77. Kesner RP, Farnsworth G, DiMattia BV. Double dissociation of egocentric and allocentric space follow-ing medial prefrontal and parietal cortex lesions in the rat. Behav Neurosci 1989;103:956–961.

78. Kelsey JE, Vargas H. Medial septal lesions disrupt spatial, but not nonspatial, working memory in rats. Behav Neurosci 1993;107:565–574.

79. Isaacson RL, Yoder PE, Varner J. The effects of pregnenolone on acquisition and retention of a food search task. Behav Neural Biol 1994;61:170–176.

80. Melchior CL, Ritzmann RF. Neurosteroids block the memory-impairing effects of ethanol in mice. Pharmacol Biochem Behav 1996;53:51–56.

81. Majewska MD. Interaction of ethanol with the $GABA_A$ receptor in the rat brain: possible involvement of endogenous steroids. Alcohol 1988;5:269–273.

82. Meziane H, Mathis C, Paul SM, Ungerer A. The neurosteroid pregnenolone sulfate reduces learning deficits induced by scopolamine and has promnestic effects in mice performing an appetitive learning task. Psychopharmacology (Berlin) 1996;126:323–330.

83. Vallée M, Mayo W, Darnaudery M, Corpechot C, Young J, Koehl M, Le Moal, Baulieu EE, Robel P, Simon H. Neurosteroids: deficient cognitive performance in aged rats depends on low pregnenolone sulfate levels in the hippocampus. Proc Natl Acad Sci USA 1997;94:14865–14870.

84. Rapp PR, Amaral DG. Individual differences in the cognitive and neurobiological consequences of normal aging. Trends Neurosci 1992;15:340–345.

85. Darnaudery, M., Koehl, M., Le Moal, M., Mayo, W. The neurosteroid pregnenolone sulfate increases cortical acetylcholine release. J Neurochem 1998;71:2018–2022.

19 Remarkable Memory-Enhancing Effects of Pregnenolone Sulfate with Pheromone-Like Sensitivity
An Amplificatory Hypothesis

Eugene Roberts, MD

CONTENTS

INTRODUCTION
THE REMARKABLE ME EFFECTS OF PREGS
CAN THE MEMORIAL PATH OF PREGS IN THE NEUROLABYRINTH
   BE TRACED?
HYPOTHESIS: AN AMPLIFICATORY MECHANISM WITH PHEROMONE-
   LIKE SENSITIVITY PROPOSED FOR THE ME EFFECT OF PREGS
CONCLUSIONS
REFERENCES

INTRODUCTION

When it is desired to improve nervous system function, such as enhancing suboptimal learning or accelerating repair of damage as a result of disease, injury, or aging, it is necessary to facilitate adaptive coupling among relevant functional processes by relieving rate-limiting constrictions in mutually shaping interactions among intracellular, intercellular, and extracellular components of the system *(1)*. My colleagues and I have performed many experiments over the years that have shown that some of the steroids found normally in blood have facilitatory effects on aspects of nervous function (e.g., *2–5*). Virtually all aspects of relevant published work have been thoroughly reviewed *(6,7)*. Herein I confine my comments only to the remarkable enhancement by pregnenolone sulfate (PREGS) of memory for footshock active avoidance training (FAAT) in weakly trained mice *(8)*.

Dehydroepiandrosterone (DHEA), dehydroepiandrosterone sulfate (DHEAS), pregnenolone (PREG), PREGS, androstenedione, testosterone, dihydrotestosterone, and aldosterone-produced memory enhancement (ME), whereas estrone, estradiol, progesterone, and 16 β-bromoepiandrosterone did not do so when injected intra-

From: *Contemporary Endocrinology: Neurosteroids: A New Regulatory Function in the Nervous System* Edited by: E.-E. Baulieu, P. Robel, and M. Schumacher
© Humana Press Inc., Totowa, NJ

cerebroventricularly after training. Dose-response curves with PREG, PREGS, and DHEA, showed PREGS to be most potent, with significant ME occurring at 3.5×10^{-15} moles/mouse (5).

Test substances were administered after training so that they could not affect acquisition. Retention was tested 1 wk later so that retention of test performance would not be directly affected by their administration. Lack of differences in escape latencies between vehicle controls and mice receiving test substance indicated that ME in mice receiving the steroids was not attributable to proactive motor facilitatory effects of the steroids. Because the substances tested could not directly affect performance during either training or testing, the changes in retention test performance are interpreted as being the result of changes in memory processing occurring shortly after training.

Substances administered intracerebroventricularly penetrate to several brain regions. Prior to attempting to define mechanisms of action of PREGS, it was necessary to determine whether or not regional differences exist in sensitivity to its action so as to help identify the neural circuitry most importantly involved. Memory-active substances (enhancing or inhibitory) generally have produced differing effects when injected into structures of the forebrain limbic system, e.g., mammillary bodies, septum, amygdala, and hippocampus (see 9,10). The latter regions, which are implicated variously in learning as exemplified by retention of FAAT, differ in structure and in distribution of neurotransmitter and neuromodulator systems. Tests of retention of FAAT were made in mice after post-training injection of PREGS into the aforementioned structures. In addition, injections were made into the caudate nucleus, a part of the basal ganglia, as a "control" region, in the sense that it is not considered to play a specific role in retention of learning of conditioned fear responses.

THE REMARKABLE ME EFFECTS OF PREGS

There were significant overall ME effects for intrahippocampal injection of PREGS, DHEAS, and corticosterone (Fig. 1; 8). By far the most potent action was exerted by PREGS, quantities between 10^{-16} g or 2.4×10^{-18} moles/mouse and 10^{-12} g or 2.4×10^{-14} moles/mouse, giving mean trials to criterion which were significantly lower than the vehicle controls ($p < 0.01$). Multiplying moles of PREGS/mouse by Avogadro's number, 6.02×10^{23} molecules/mole, it was calculated that 1.45×10^6 molecules of PREGS were sufficient to cause significant ME on intrahippocampal injection. DHEAS and corticosterone showed significant ME only at much higher concentrations and over smaller concentration ranges than PREGS. Clearly, PREGS was more potent than the other steroids tested and its effects extended over a greater range of concentrations.

When PREGS was tested in the amygdala, mammillary bodies, septum, and caudate nucleus (Fig. 1), there were significant ME effects for amygdala, septum, and mammillary bodies, but not for the caudate. Two-way analysis of variance (ANOVA) showed that the dose-response curves for mammillary bodies and septal injection did not differ significantly from each other, but that both were significantly different from the curves obtained for hippocampus and amygdala.

The retention test scores on intra-amygdalar injection of extremely dilute solutions of PREGS showed that between 15 and 145 molecules of PREGS produced ME. The closely similar results obtained with solutions prepared in two separate laboratories by different

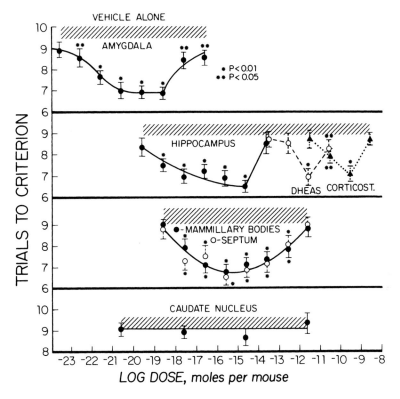

Fig. 1. Effects of post-training intraparenchymal injection of steroids on retention of FAAT in male mice. The mean and SEM for trials to criterion are shown for 15 animals at each dose indicated. Means differing from vehicle alone at $p < 0.01$ (*) or at $p < 0.05$ (**) based on Dunnett's t-tests are indicated. The shaded areas are the mean ± SEM for trials to criterion for vehicle controls. Mice were anesthetized with methoxyflurane, placed in a stereotactic instrument, and a hole was drilled through the skull over each injection site after deflecting the scalp. Mice were trained 48 h after surgery. Four training trials were given using an intertrial interval of 30 s, a warning buzzer of 55 DB, and foot-shock intensity of 0.30 mA. Immediately after training, the test solution containing vehicle or PREGS was injected over a period of 60 s into the target structure. One wk later, T-maze training was resumed until each mouse made five avoidance responses in 6 consecutive training trials. Retention was measured by the number of trials required for each mouse to meet this criterion; the fewer trials required, the greater the retention of learning. The mice in this study were weakly trained so that ME effects on retention of T-maze FAAT could be detected readily. The site of injection then was confirmed histologically using a mouse brain stereotaxic atlas. (*See* ref. *8* for further details.)

dilution procedures and tested under blinded conditions gave confidence in the validity of the results.

CAN THE MEMORIAL PATH OF PREGS IN THE NEUROLABYRINTH BE TRACED?

The finding that so few molecules of PREGS can enhance post-training memory processes when injected into the amygdala in mice established PREGS as the most potent memory enhancer yet reported. In terms of sensitivity, ME caused by PREGS resembles a pheromone-mediated process. For example, the 70 kDa sex-inducing glycoprotein pheromone of the multicellular green flagellate *Volvox carteri*, synthesized and released by sperm cells, exerts its biological response fully at a concentration of $6 \times 10^{-17} M$ (36 molecules/mL) *(11)*. In both of the aforementioned instances, there must occur great amplification of the effects of a very small number of molecules.

In the case of *Volvox carteri*, it was proposed that externally applied pheromone accumulates in the extracellular matrix, whence it enters surface-lying somatic cells. After several hours, a plethora of a protein is released into the extracellular matrix from which is cleaved a greatly amplified quantity of homologue of the original pheromone. The latter then exerts sex-inducing activity in the small number of internally-contained deep-lying asexual reproductive cells. Although the system as a whole requires external contact with only relatively few molecules of pheromone to achieve sex induction, concentrations several orders of magnitude higher are needed for sex induction by direct application of the pheromone to the reproductive cells. Can a mechanism be envisioned by which PREGS similarly might exert an effect in the amygdala, whereby post-training infusion of a small number of molecules of PREGS results in subsequent release from contiguous oligodendrocytes and astrocytes onto neurons of the activated circuits of much greater quantities of PREGS than originally were injected?

Even in minimally active states of mammalian nervous systems, neurons, non-neuronal cells (e.g., glial, ependymal, and endothelial cells), and the extracellular matrix participate in many mutually shaping interactions that range from physical forces they exert on each other *(12)* to exchanges, often through gap junctions, of varieties of trophic and/or inhibitory substances. Much data support the notion that throughout the nervous system there exist gap junctionally coupled astrocytic syncytial networks, enabling rapid passage among the cells of many molecules of up to approximately 1 kDa (e.g., *13*). These interactions are greatly enhanced by nerve activity, during which and for a period after which, members of the system derive from each other and from blood-borne sources various substances required to achieve recovery from preceding activity and to undergo appropriate plastic changes *(14)*. Such interactions among components of a healthy biological system are best described by paraphrase of an old dictum for a healthy social system *(15)*: from each according to its capacities, to each according to its requirements, and together for the benefit of the system as a whole.

Mice used in the ME experiments were weakly trained. Conditions of training are such that, at most, within 2–3 d after training, the vehicle-treated controls show the same numbers of trials to criterion as those observed at initial training of naive animals. Post-training administration of ME substances to such mice results in dose-related decreases by comparison with controls in numbers of trials to criterion at 7 d after initial training. Such substances generally have been found to exert overall physiologically excitatory or depolarizing effects in the systems under study. When during training the strengths of stimuli and numbers of trials are increased sufficiently above those given to the weakly trained animals, maximal retention of learning can be achieved for at least 7 d and sometimes even for many months thereafter. ME is not noted in such strongly trained mice upon post-training administration of substances that are effective in weakly trained animals.

In brief, neural excitation results in increased permeability to cations, thus decreasing the potential across membranes (depolarization). Inward Na^+ current usually is responsible for most of the observed depolarization, but influx of extracellular Ca^{2+} also takes place by entry through voltage-gated Ca^{2+} channels. When there is Ca^{2+} influx into a nerve terminal, neurotransmitter release is facilitated. Increase in cytosolic Ca^{2+} also occurs by release from intracellular Ca^{2+} binding entities. The opening of K^+ channels is activated by the changes in membrane potential. Resultant outward K^+ currents then serve to repolarize the cells and, in some instances, to produce hyperpolarization before the Ca^{2+} balance is restored via the action of Ca^{2+}–Mg^{2+} ATPase, mitochondrial uptake, and by rebinding of Ca^{2+}; and the K^+ channels are closed. The action of Na^+-K^+ ATPase restores the monocation balance.

The time-sequence coordination of the latter events is such that there are pulsatile localized increases in pools of cytosolic free Ca^{2+}, one or more of which reflect accurately the amounts and durations of depolarization to which membranes are subjected. The patterns of such Ca^{2+} transients may have great informational content, their extent and frequency possibly encoding experiential information (16). The free Ca^{2+} either directly or via its interaction with Ca^{2+} binding proteins, of which calmodulin, parvalbumin, troponin C, S-100 and calbindin are examples, releases cascades of many intracellular processes including activation of genes, some of which processes continue after free Ca^{2+} is reduced to the resting level.

Concurrently with the aforementioned, chemical modifications (e.g., phosphorylation or dephosphorylation) of the Ca^{2+} binding proteins and allosteric effects exerted by noncovalent binding of substances to them alter their affinities for Ca^{2+} (17). Relatedly, changes occur in activities of enzymes involved in metabolism of the cyclic nucleotides, cAMP and cGMP, changing their turnovers, relative amounts, and intracellular distributions. There occur changes in activities of protein kinases and phosphatases that act on specific substrate proteins to establish new cell balances. Phosphorylation controls the activity of many enzymes and the conformational states of nonenzymatic proteins. The control of the degrees of protein phosphorylation is the "principal mechanism by which all cell functions in eukaryotic cells are controlled by extracellular signals. Processes as diverse as metabolism, membrane transport and permeability, secretion, contractility, the transcription and translation of genes, cell division and fertilization, neurotransmission, and even memory are all regulated by this versatile posttranslational modification" (18).

Dose-related ME produced by post-training treatment in weakly trained mice causes graded enhancement and/or prolongation of effects of the learning experience that outlast early brief events such as depolarization and the consequential ionic displacements. For example, when mice were trained under conditions giving poor retention in vehicle-injected controls, administration of DHEAS at 2, 30, or 60 min gave significant improvements ($p < 0.01$, $p < 0.01$, and $p < 0.05$, respectively). When injected at 90 and 120 min, DHEAS had no effect (19). Perseverative neuronal activity consisting of reverberation of impulses in neuronal circuits that outlasts the stimulating events is *not* what makes memory-related processes amenable to enhancement long after the first neural events during training have ceased (20).

Calmodulin is the most ubiquitously occurring Ca^{2+}-binding protein and the most extensively studied. Among the changes occurring when free cytosolic Ca^{2+} becomes elevated following stimulation is an increase in Ca^{2+}-calmodulin, which activates many cascade-initiating targets in a coordinated manner so that interlocking cascades throughout the entire activated system result rapidly in effective restorative processes and in adaptive plastic changes. Many substances, including steroids, are known to interact allosterically with calmodulin to regulate activation of calmodulin-dependent targets (17,21,22).

Among the targets activated by Ca^{2+}-calmodulin is the nitric oxide (NO)-producing enzyme, NO synthase. NO, a gaseous free radical formed from the guanidino group of arginine, diffuses freely and rapidly among the matrix, vascular, glial, and neuronal components of the activated neural regions. Notably, NO activates soluble guanylate cyclase and increases rates of turnover and contents of cGMP. NO mediates the stimulation of cGMP formation by glutamate and other NMDA receptor agonists and by a variety of other excitatory influences that act on brain and other tissues. Indeed, the formation of NO from L-arginine is a widespread transduction mechanism for the stimulation of the soluble guanylate cyclase (23–25). Substances with overall excitatory effects, among which are the known memory enhancers, have cGMP as an intracellular messenger for their action (26). In vivo evidence has been adduced supporting the NO-cGMP relationship in rat cerebellum, increases in NO resulting in increases in extracellular content of cGMP (27). By action on presynaptic terminals, cGMP can produce long-term enhancement of transmitter release (28) and, therefore, probably long-term increases in efficacy of information transmittal in activated nerve circuits.

In many instances, it was found that in the effective dose ranges, progressive increases of ME substances first increased responses to a maximum, beyond which decreasing responses were observed until a level was reached at which no significant effects were seen over the controls (29). The decrements observed at higher doses of ME substances possibly may have been attributable to incoordinations induced in management of intracellular free Ca^{2+} and/or calmodulin, leading to chaotogenic effects on release of reaction cascades (30).

The inverted U-shaped dose-response curve previously described usually covers a 2–5-fold dose range. However, in the case of injection of PREGS into limbic system structures, the curves extended over the enormously greater dose ranges of 4 to 6 orders of magnitude (Fig. 1). The latter differentiates the PREGS effects from those of the usual ME substances and suggests that the dose-response curve for PREGS may be a composite of at least two effects. At the upper dose range, PREGS may act like any other excitation-enhancing substance, and at the lower range, in a uniquely special, possibly pheromone-like sensitive fashion. Although to date there has not been identified a specific cellular binding protein with sufficiently high affinity for PREGS to qualify as a saturable high-affinity receptor for PREGS, it has not been ruled out that such an entity exists. The shape of the left-hand portion of the dose-response curve for the amygdala (in Fig. 1) is not inconsistent with such a possibility.

Let us posit that in a manner somewhat analogous to that discussed previously for the flagellate *Volvox carteri*, once binding with an appropriate very high affinity entity occurs, the PREGS administered may participate in activation of a cascade that gives rise to a massive synthesis and/or mobilization of PREGS and its subsequent release. The higher concentrations of PREGS released then could act via much lower affinity, but synergistic, mechanisms to achieve amplification of the effects of the small number of molecules of PREGS initially acting on a presumptive high affinity receptor in a few cells. What might be a mechanism by which such events could occur?

It may be that in weakly trained animals, the post-training "window of opportunity" for ME substances to exert their action is the time during which the effects of initially suboptimally increased levels of Ca^{2+}-calmodulin can be driven to higher levels by increasing cytosolic free Ca^{2+}; or activities of NO synthase and/or guanyl cyclase may be increased directly. In the latter regard, it is particularly interesting that PREGS not only is a negative modulator of the GABA receptor complex and a positive modulator of the NMDA receptor complex, thereby raising excitability of the system as a whole, but that PREGS also greatly amplifies the increase in cytosolic free Ca^{2+} that occurs during stimulation of NMDA receptors (31–35). PREGS also may be a direct activator of soluble guanylate cyclase (36). Thus, PREGS could exert a synergistic amplification of effects of excitatory neural transmission at much lower concentrations than would be expected from action of a given amount of PREGS on any one of the aforementioned systems alone, molar potencies in in vitro measurements made individually on these systems seeming too low to support an important in vivo role for PREGS. Enhancement at multiple sites of the pathway leading from neural excitation to increased metabolism of cGMP might help explain the powerful effects of PREGS on retention of FAAT upon intracerebroventricular or intrahippocampal injection. However, the astonishing results upon intra-amygdalar injection forced a search for an additional amplificatory mechanism by which a minute amount of externally supplied PREGS might result in release of PREGS readily made from preexisting stores of PREG or PREGS, or by synthesis of the latter from cholesterol, cholesterol sulfate, or other precursors.

Biosynthetic pathways for PREG, PREGS, DHEA, and DHEAS in brain may differ from those in extracerebral tissues. The latter substances, found in the brain at higher levels than in blood, largely are localized in astrocytes and oligodendrocytes, and exist therein in the free form and as sulfates and lipoidal esters (37). As yet uncharacterized bound forms of related substances are present in organic solvent extracts of brain, but not of adrenals or testes, that give rise to additional large amounts of PREG and DHEA by processes that are known to produce ketones from hydroperoxides or peroxides (38,39). To date, it has not been technically possible to determine whether or not PREGS and DHEAS also are increased by such treatment (V. V. K. Prasad and S. Lieberman, personal communication). I conjecture that this is likely to take place.

NO, formed in graded amounts on nerve activity, could react with steroidal peroxides or hydroperoxides in a manner similar to that with which NO reacts with superoxide anion to form peroxynitrite (40), to give substances that are not free radicals themselves, but that have great oxidizing power. This could result in enzymatic and/or nonenzymatic cleavage of side chains of cholesterol and cholesterol sulfate to form PREG, PREGS, DHEA, and DHEAS either successively or independently of each other as in the following: cholesterol (or cholesterol sulfate) → PREG (or PREGS) → DHEA (or DHEAS) and/or cholesterol (or cholesterol sulfate) → PREG (or PREGS) and DHEA (or DHEAS). At least a portion of the PREG and PREGS in brain probably comes from cholesterol and cholesterol sulfate via side-chain cleavage catalyzed by cytochrome P450scc; both the enzyme and its mRNA are found in brain. However, it is doubtful that the ketonic DHEA and DHEAS, indigenously formed in brain, arise from PREG or PREGS by side-chain cleavage by the "classical" action of cytochrome P450c17 (17α-hydroxylase/17,20 lyase), because neither the latter enzyme nor its mRNA have been detected in adult brain (7).

HYPOTHESIS: AN AMPLIFICATORY MECHANISM WITH PHEROMONE-LIKE SENSITIVITY PROPOSED FOR THE ME EFFECT OF PREGS

One variant of several potentially experimentally testable scenarios is outlined below. A mechanism is proposed by which a minute quantity of PREGS, externally introduced into the amygdala post-training to mice that have undergone FAAT, attaches with high affinity to receptors on a few glial cells. This induces release of much additional indigenously generated PREGS along the entire extents of nerve circuits that had been activated during the training experience, but which circuits already were electrophysiologically inactive at the time that PREGS was administered. Such a release of PREGS serves as a "now-print" signal, the PREGS acting on all of the neural elements of the participating circuits via relatively low-affinity processes previously described, metaphorically facilitating the "soldering" together of elements of the newly activated circuits by synaptic plastic changes more firmly than would occur otherwise in weakly trained animals. This is reflected in enhanced retention of learning by comparison with controls receiving vehicle alone after training.

Intra-amygdalar administered PREGS associates with astrocytes and oligodendrocytes by binding to a receptor complex that is highly represented on their membranes and in their cytoplasm. This receptor complex consists of an inducible transcription factor (iTF) bound to an inhibitory protein (BP) that keeps the iTF from entering the nucleus (patterned somewhat after NF-kB; *see* ref. *41*). PREGS has a higher affinity for iTF than does the BP, displacing the latter and forming a PREGS–iTF complex that enters from the membrane into the cytoplasm. PREGS has a much higher affinity for iTF than for cytoplasmic PREGS metabolizing enzymes and, therefore, is stabilized in the PREGS–iTF complex, which enters the nucleus readily. In the nucleus, the PREGS–iTF complex or iTF and PREGS separately, after dissociation of the complex, facilitate the transcription of genes coding for enzymes involved in PREGS biosynthesis and in production of iTF and BP, resulting in increases in the relevant mRNAs in the cytoplasm. In this manner, a few molecules of externally administered PREGS, associating with the surfaces of only one or a few cells, lead to enhanced production of PREGS and of its production and control machinery. A portion of the newly formed plethoric supply of PREGS is liberated onto adjacent neuronal elements, and some is transmitted rapidly via gap junctions to neighboring nonneural cells, wherein the process in the cells originally contacted by the exogenously administered PREGS is repeated, except that the PREGS interacts directly with the iTF–BP complex in the cytoplasm. Thus, rapidly and for a brief period, the entire glial blanket surrounding recently activated neural circuitry liberates more PREGS and enhances achievement of maximal connectivities at all levels of the recently activated circuitry.

The aforementioned, at present admittedly a fanciful hypothesis, can be falsified or supported by experiment. At the outset, one could search for an enzyme or enzymes that form PREGS and DHEAS from cholesterol sulfate and DHEAS from PREGS using as cosubstrate peroxynitrite or oxyradicals. Were positive results obtained, tools currently available would permit a rational search to be made for the posited iTF and iTF-binding proteins. Taking another tack, it should be possible to visualize PREGS itself immunocytochemically, at light and electron microscopic levels, in pretraining and posttraining states with and without post-training intracerebral injection of ME-effective amounts of PREGS. The latter would be far below the level of detection by such methods. Elevations in PREGS content produced as suggested might be sufficient to allow PREGS to be noted in brains of PREGS-treated animals in greater amounts than in the vehicle controls, at least for a period of 90 min after training, particularly in the amygdalar region.

CONCLUSIONS

A potentially experimentally testable hypothesis has been outlined here for a mechanism by which a minute quantity of PREGS introduced into the amygdala post-training to mice undergoing FAAT might react with an high-affinity receptor on glial cells, in such a manner as to induce release of much additional PREGS along entire activated nerve circuits. This could serve as a "now-print" signal, the released PREGS acting via relatively low-affinity processes to exert synergistic excitation-enhancing effects, as well as by other pleiotropic effects characteristic of PREGS. Formation in the brain of PROG and derivatives thereof that are positive modulators of the GABA receptor complex by increasing GABAergic inhibition may help prevent occurrence of maladaptive overexcitation at times of PREGS increases (7). It is of considerable interest that among the limbic regions of male rat brain, the highest rate of conversion of PREG to PROG was found in amygdalar tissue (42). The following values were reported for five brain regions (pmoles/10 mg protein/30 min ± SEM): amygdala, 2.5 ± 0.42; septum, 2.2 ± 0.38; hippocampus, 1.2 ± 0.21; hypothalamus, 0.3 ± 0.04; cortex, <0.1.

When injected into the amygdala, PREGS was approximately 10^4 times more potent on a molar basis in producing ME than when injected into the hippocampus, and approximately 10^5 times more potent than when injected into the septum or mammillary bodies. There is much evidence for the belief that processing of sensory data in the amygdala assigns emotional significance to it, and when the stimuli are aversive, elicits behavioral, autonomic, and humoral responses typical of what is commonly known as fear (unconditioned). The amygdala is the central station where unconditioned (e.g., footshock) and conditioned stimuli (e.g., buzzer sound) meet, as in this study. When the two stimuli are experienced simultaneously or the conditioned stimulus is experienced first, fear-conditioned learning takes place, the sounding of the buzzer alone eventually eliciting the fear response, which in our paradigm is the running of the alley of the T-maze to the correct goal box sufficiently rapidly to avoid receiving footshock. The latter type of learning is more complex than a simple conditioned increase of heart rate or eye-blinking, for example, and requires important participation of amygdalar, septo-hippocampal, cerebellar, and cortical structures. It is of interest that PREGS had no effect on the learning and retention of the eye-blink reflex in rabbits when injected into the nucleus interpositus, a key site for the latter type of learning (R. F. Thompson, personal communication).

Sensory information of various modalities enters the amygdala through its basal and lateral nuclei, which communicate bidirectionally with the central nucleus (43,44). From the latter emanate outputs to various neural pathways that trigger unconditioned fear responses, and within it occur the plastic changes that associate the fear responses with nonaversive stimuli that result in conditioned fear responses. However, the site of long-term memory storage may be elsewhere, e.g., the cortex (43). Extensive lesion, pharmacological, and electrophysiological studies establish the central nucleus of the amygdala to be the critical mediator of fear learning. It is in this structure that the mechanism for the remarkable ME effect of PREGS may profitably be sought.

It is presently uncertain as to whether or not the ME observed after injection of PREGS into hippocampus, septum, and mammillary bodies can be attributable to direct effects of PREGS in these structures, or to diffusion from them into the amygdala of small fractions of the amounts administered. The quantities of PREGS required to effect ME in the amygdala are so small that methods employed currently do not possess sufficient sensitivity to give definitive results.

REFERENCES

1. Roberts E. A systems approach to aging, Alzheimer's disease, and spinal cord regeneration. Prog Brain Res 1990;86:339–355.
2. Roberts E, Bologa L, Flood JF, Smith GE. Effects of dehydroepiandrosterone and its sulfate on brain tissue in culture and on memory in mice. Brain Res 1987;406:357–362.
3. Bologa L, Sharma J, Roberts E. Dehydroepiandrosterone and its sulfated derivative reduce neuronal death and enhance astrocytic differentiation in brain cell cultures. J Neurosci Res 1987;17:225–234.
4. Guth L, Zhang Z, Roberts E. Key role for pregnenolone in combination therapy that promotes recovery after spinal cord injury. Proc Natl Acad Sci USA 1994;91:12308–12312.
5. Flood JF, Morley JE, Roberts E. Memory-enhancing effects in male mice of pregnenolone and steroids metabolically derived from it. Proc Natl Acad Sci USA1992;89:1567–1571.
6. Bellino FL, Daynes RA, Hornsby PJ, Lavrin DH, Nestler JE, eds. Dehydroepiandrosterone (DHEA) and Aging. New York Academy of Sciences, New York, NY, 1995.
7. Robel P, Baulieu E-E. Dehydroepiandrosterone (DHEA) is a neuroactive neurosteroid. Ann N Y Acad Sci 1995;774:82–110.
8. Flood JF, Morley JE, Roberts E. Pregnenolone sulfate enhances post-training memory processes when injected in very low doses into limbic system structures: the amygdala is by far the most sensitive. Proc Natl Acad Sci USA 1995;92:10806–10810.
9. Flood JF, Smith GE, Jarvik ME. A comparison of the effects of localized brain administration of catecholamine and protein synthesis inhibitors on memory processing. Brain Res 1980;197:153–165.
10. Flood JF, Baker ML, Hernandez EN, Morley JE. Modulation of memory processing by neuropeptide Y varies with brain injection site. Brain Res 1989;503:73–82.
11. Sumper M, Berg E, Wenzl S, Godl K. How a sex pheromone might act at a concentration below 10^{-16} M. EMBO J 1993;12:831–836.
12. Chen CS, Mrksich M, Huang S, Whitesides GM, Ingber DE. Geometric control of cell life and death. Science 1997;276:1425–1428.
13. Hossain MZ, Peeling J, Sutherland GR, Hertzberg EL, Nagy JI. Ischemia-induced cellular redistribution of the astrocytic gap junctional protein connexin 43 in rat brain. Brain Res 1994;652:311–322.
14. Roberts E, Matthysse S. Neurochemistry: at the crossroads of neurobiology. Annu Rev Biochem 1970;39:777–820.
15. Blanc L. Organisation du Travail. In: Beck EM, ed. Bartlett's Familiar Quotations, 15th ed. Little, Brown, Boston, 1980.
16. Gu X, Spitzer NC. Distinct aspects of neuronal differentiation encoded by frequency of spontaneous Ca^{2+} transients. Nature 1995;375:784–787.
17. Slemmon JR, Martzen MR. Neuromodulin (GAP–43) can regulate a calmodulin-dependent target *in vitro*. Biochemistry 1994;33:5653–5660.
18. Cohen, P. Protein phosphorylation and hormone action. Proc R Soc Lond 1988;234:115–144.
19. Flood JF, Smith GE, Roberts E. Dehydroepiandrosterone and its sulfate enhance memory retention in mice. Brain Res 1988;447:269–278.
20. Baldwin BA, Soltysik SS. The effect of cerebral ischaemia, resulting in loss of EEG, on the acquisition of conditioned reflexes in goats. Brain Res 1966;2:71–84.
21. Gnegy ME. Calmodulin in neurotransmitter and hormone action. Annu Rev Pharmacol Toxicol 1993;33:45–70.
22. Weinstein H, Mehler EL. Ca^{2+}-binding and structural dynamics in the functions of calmodulin. Annu Rev Physiol 1994;56:213–236.
23. Moncada S, Palmer RMJ, Higgs EA. Nitric oxide: physiology, pathophysiology, and pharmacology. Pharmacol Rev 1991;43:109–142.
24. Stuehr DJ, Griffith OW. Mammalian nitric oxide synthases. Adv Enzymol 1992;65:287–346.
25. Schuman EM, Madison DV. Nitric oxide and synaptic function. Annu Rev Neurosci 1994;17:153–183.
26. Drummond GI. Cyclic nucleotides in the nervous system. Adv Cyclic Nucleotide Res 1983;15:373–494.
27. Vallebuona F, Raiteri M. Monitoring of cyclic GMP during cerebellar microdialysis in freely-moving rats as an index of nitric oxide synthase activity. Neuroscience 1993;57: 577–585.

28. Arancio O, Kandel ER, Hawkins RD. Activity-dependent long-term enhancement of transmitter release by presynaptic 3',5'-cyclic GMP in cultured hippocampal neurons. Nature 1995;376:74–80.

29. Cherkin A, Flood JF. Behavioral pharmacology of memory. Opportunities for cellular explanations. In: Woody CD., Alkon DL., McGaugh JL, eds. Cellular Mechanisms of Conditioning and Behavioral Plasticity. Plenum, New York, NY, 1988, pp. 343–354.

30. Mattson MP, Guthrie PB, Kater SB. A role for Na^+-dependent Ca^{2+} extrusion in protection against neuronal excitotoxicity. FASEB J 1989;3:2519–2526.

31. Wu F-S, Gibbs TT, Farb DH. Pregnenolone sulfate: a positive allosteric modulator at the N-methyl-D-aspartate receptor. Mol Pharmacol 1991;40:333–336.

32. Irwin RP, Maragakis NJ, Rogawski MA, Purdy RH, Farb DH, Paul SM. Pregnenolone sulfate augments NMDA receptor mediated increases in intracellular Ca^{2+} in cultured rat hippocampal neurons. Neurosci Lett 1992;141:30–34.

33. Majewska MD. Neurosteroids: endogenous bimodal modulators of the $GABA_A$ receptor, mechanism of action and physiological significance. Prog Neurobiol 1992;38:379–395.

34. Bowlby MR. Pregnenolone sulfate potentiation of N-methyl-D-aspartate receptor channels in hippocampal neurons. Mol Pharmacol 1993;43:813–819.

35. Monnet FP, Mahé V, Robel P, Baulieu E-E. Neurosteroids, via σ receptors, modulate the [^{3}H]norepinephrine release evoked by N-methyl-D-aspartate in the rat hippocampus. Proc Natl Acad Sci USA 1995;92:3774–3778.

36. Vesely DL. Testosterone and its precursors and metabolites enhance guanylate cyclase activity. Proc Natl Acad Sci USA 1979;76:3491–3494.

37. Mathur C, Prasad VVK, Raju VS, Welch M, Lieberman S. Steroids and their conjugates in the mammalian brain. Proc Natl Acad Sci USA 1993;90:85–88.

38. Prasad VVK, Vegesna SR, Welch M, Lieberman S. Precursors of the neurosteroids. Proc Natl Acad Sci USA 1994;91:3220–3223.

39. Lieberman S. An abbreviated account of some aspects of the biochemistry of DHEA, 1934–1995. Ann N Y Acad Sci 1995;774:1–15.

40. Feldman PL, Griffith OW, Stuehr DJ. The surprising life of nitric oxide. Chem Eng News 1993;26–38.

41. Grilli M, Chiu JJ-S, Lenardo MJ. NF-kB and Rel: participants in a multiform transcriptional regulatory system. Int Rev Cytol 1993;143:1–62.

42. Weidenfeld J, Siegel RA, Chowers I. In vitro conversion of pregnenolone to progesterone by discrete brain areas of the male rat. J. Steroid Biochem. 1980;13:961–963.

43. Lavond DG, Kim JJ, Thompson RF. Mammalian brain substrates of aversive classical conditioning. Annu Rev Psychol 1993;44:317–342.

44. Gallagher M, Holland PC. The amygdala complex: multiple roles in associative learning and attention. Proc Natl Acad Sci USA 1994;91:11771–11776.

20

The Neuropsychopharmacological Potential of Neurosteroids

Rainer Rupprecht, MD, Elisabeth Friess, MD, and Florian Holsboer, MD

Contents

Introduction
Nongenomic and Genomic Properties of Neurosteroids
Neuropsychopharmacological Properties of Neurosteroids:
    Behavioral and Clinical Studies
Future Perspectives
References

INTRODUCTION

Steroid hormone action involves binding of the steroids to their respective intracellular receptors, which in turn change their conformation by dissociation from the heat-shock proteins, translocate to the nucleus, and there bind to the respective response elements that are located in the regulatory regions of target promoters *(1)*. Thus, steroid hormone receptors act as transcription factors in the regulation of gene expression. In the last decade, considerable evidence has emerged that certain steroids may alter neuronal excitability via their action at the cell surface through interaction with certain neurotransmitter receptors *(2,3)*. For steroids with these particular properties, the term "neuroactive steroids" has been coined. A variety of neuroactive steroids may be synthesized in the brain itself without the aid of peripheral sources *(4,5)*. Such steroids, which are formed within the brain from cholesterol, are defined as "neurosteroids" *(5)*. Whereas the action of steroids at the genome requires a time period of minutes to hours limited by the rate of protein biosynthesis, the modulatory effects of neuroactive steroids are fast-occurring events of milliseconds to seconds *(6)*. Thus, genomic and nongenomic effects of steroids within the central nervous system (CNS) provide the molecular basis for a broad spectrum of steroid actions on neuronal function and plasticity.

From: *Contemporary Endocrinology: Neurosteroids: A New Regulatory Function in the Nervous System* Edited by: E.-E. Baulieu, P. Robel, and M. Schumacher
© Humana Press Inc., Totowa, NJ

NONGENOMIC AND GENOMIC PROPERTIES
OF NEUROSTEROIDS

In 1986, it was shown for the first time that the neurosteroids allopregnanolone ($3\alpha,5\alpha$-THPROG) and tetrahydrodeoxycorticosterone ($3\alpha,5\alpha$-THDOC) may modulate neuronal excitability via their interaction with the $GABA_A$ receptor complex (2). These steroids are capable of displacing t-butylbicyclophosphorothionate (TBPS) from the choride channel with an affinity superior to that of barbiturates and of enhancing the GABA-evoked chloride current (2). Thus, these neurosteroids may be considered as potent positive allosteric modulators of the $GABA_A$ receptor by increasing the frequency and duration of channel openings of the GABA-gated chloride channel (3,7). Studies concerning the structure-activity relationship of neurosteroids at the $GABA_A$ receptor have revealed that the presence of a 3α-hydroxy group within the A-ring of these molecules is the critical determinant for a positive allosteric activity at the $GABA_A$ receptor (8,9). Steroids lacking these particular properties, e.g., progesterone and the 5α-pregnane steroids 5α-dihydroprogesterone (5α-DHPROG) and 5α-dihydrodeoxycorticosterone (5α-DHDOC), are devoid of any GABA-enhancing potential (8,10) (Fig. 1). Whereas steroids like $3\alpha,5\alpha$-THPROG, $3\alpha,5\alpha$-THDOC, or the synthetic compound alphaxalone are positive allosteric modulators of the $GABA_A$ receptor, dehydroepiandrosterone sulfate (DHEAS) and PREG sulfate (PREGS) display functional antagonistic properties (11,12).

Although the sites of action of neurosteroids at the molecular level have been attributed to unique binding sites on neurotransmitter receptors in the cell membrane (2,3,13), a "neurosteroid binding site" has not yet been determined. Because of the distinct chemical properties of these steroids (14) and their lack of binding to the rat progesterone receptor (PR) (8), up until now these steroids were believed not to possess regulatory properties at the genomic level (3,8). The aim of our studies was to elucidate further molecular mechanisms of neurosteroid action that might be important for the future development of such compounds for potential use in neuropsychopharmacology. Therefore, we addressed the question whether these steroids may be able to regulate gene expression via intracellular steroid receptors (10).

A human neuroblastoma cell line (SK-N-MC) was transiently transfected with a reporter plasmid encoding the mouse mammary tumor virus (MMTV) promoter upstream of the luciferase gene (MMTV-LUC) (15). Expression vectors for the human glucocorticosteroid receptor (hGR) (16), the human mineralocorticosteroid receptor (hMR) (17), and the full-length isoforms of the chicken (cPR_B) (18) and the human (hPR_B) progesterone receptor (19) were cotransfected. Both the cPR_B and hPR_B were strongly activated by $3\alpha,5\alpha$-THPROG and $3\alpha,5\alpha$-THDOC. The cPR_B responded to the neurosteroids in a progestin-like fashion whereas concentrations in the upper nanomolar range were required to activate the hPR_B (Fig. 2) Moreover, the neurosteroids $3\alpha,5\alpha$-THPROG and $3\alpha,5\alpha$-THDOC were able to induce a complete nuclear translocation of the hPR_B, indistinguishable from that achieved by progesterone (PROG) when the hPR_B was expressed in COS-1 cells in immunofluorescence studies. As in previous reports in the rat (8), $3\alpha,5\alpha$-THPROG and $3\alpha,5\alpha$-THDOC did not bind to the PR of either species when the respective steroid receptors were expressed in COS-1 cells. Because the cPR may be activated in a ligand-independent fashion via cyclic AMP or dopamine (20,21), we questioned whether the genomic effects of neurosteroids are mediated via

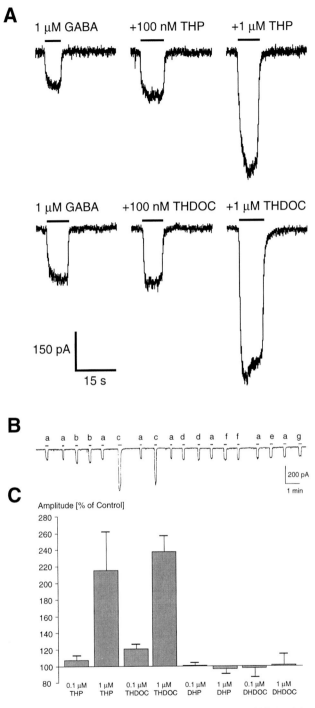

Fig. 1. Modulatory properties of steroids at the GABA$_A$ receptor. (**A**) Positive allosteric modulation of the GABA-evoked chloride current by neurosteroids. The bar indicates the presence of 1 μ*M* GABA. (**B**) Modulatory properties of neurosteroids and of 5α-pregnane steroids at the GABA$_A$ receptor in form of a representative experiment, and (**C**) as the mean ± SD of several independent experiments. (Adapted with permission from ref. *10*.) (THP, 3α,5α-THPROG; THDOC, 3α,5α-THDOC; DHP, 5α-DHPROG; DHDOC, 5α-DHDOC.)

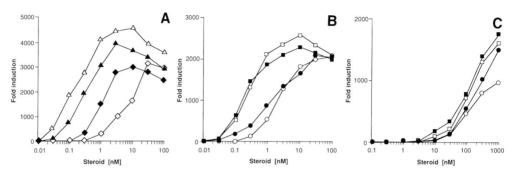

Fig. 2. Progesterone-receptor mediated gene expression by progestins and 5α-reduced neurosteroids. Induction of the MMTV-promoter after cotransfection of cPR$_B$ or hPR$_B$ expression vectors into SK-N-MC cells and incubation with steroids at the indicated concentrations. **(A)** progesterone (closed diamonds) and R 5020 (closed triangles) after transfection of cPR$_B$; progesterone (open diamonds) and R 5020 (open triangles) after transfection of hPR$_B$. **(B and C)** 3α,5α-THPROG (open circles) and 3α,5α-THDOC (closed circles), 5α-DHPROG (open squares) and 5α-DHDOC (closed squares) after transfection of cPR$_B$ (B) and hPR$_B$ (C). The baseline activity of the MMTV-promoter without addition of steroid is set as 1. (Adapted with permission from ref. *10*.)

intracellular kinases. However, this effect was not demonstrable with the hPR. Therefore, a kinase-predominated mechanism seems to be rather unlikely to explain gene expression induced by neurosteroids. Site-directed mutagenesis revealed that the carboxyterminus of the PR is required to confer the genomic effects of neurosteroids. Gel-shift analysis was employed to characterize the DNA-binding properties of the PR induced by neurosteroids. These experiments revealed that, in contrast to PROG, the neurosteroids were able to induce a conformational change of the PR only when added to living cells, but not when added to the band-shift incubation mixture, suggesting that the neurosteroids act indirectly via metabolism in the host cells. In the neuroblastoma cells used for analysis of transactivation, radioactively-labeled 3α,5α-THPROG was converted rapidly into the 5α-pregnane steroid 5α-DHPROG by the 3α-hydroxysteroid oxidoreductase (Fig. 3). The 5α-pregnane steroids 5α-DHPROG and 5α-DHDOC bound to the cPR with considerable affinity, whereas binding to the hPR was less pronounced. Moreover, they were potent inducers of gene expression via cPR and hPR. We could show that the neurosteroids 3α,5α-THPROG and 3α,5α-THDOC not only act through membrane-bound receptors, but may also regulate gene expression via the PR. Intracellular oxidation into 5α-DHPROG and 5α-DHDOC appears to be essential to confer PROG-like induction of DNA binding and regulation of gene transcription. This dual action of brain-derived steroids seems to be of physiological relevance, as the concentrations required for activation of the PR *(10)* and the GABA$_A$ receptor *(3,22)* are in the nanomolar range. Nanomolar concentrations of 3α,5α-THPROG and 3α,5α-THDOC and conversions of these steroids into 5α-DHPROG and 5α-DHDOC were shown to occur in vivo in the rat brain *(14,23)*. Whether genomic or nongenomic effects of these neurosteroids predominate may thus depend on the relative expression of PR *(24,25)*, GABA$_A$ receptors *(26)*, and of metabolizing enzymes *(27,28)* in the target tissues.

In further studies we were able to show that an array of naturally occurring and synthetic neurosteroids may regulate gene expression via the cPR, whereas the hPR displays a more selective transactivation pattern *(29)* (Fig. 4). Of particular interest was the

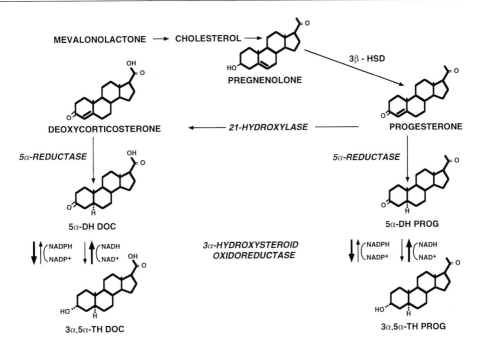

Fig. 3. Biosynthesis and metabolism of neurosteroids.

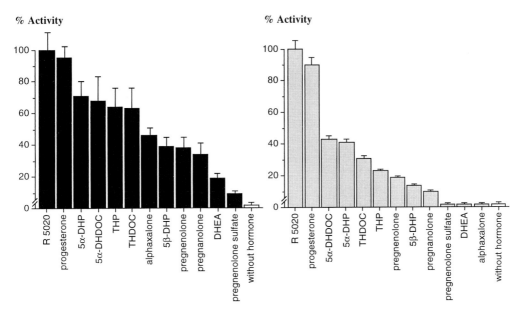

Fig. 4. Maximal biological activity (mean ± SD) of progestins and 5α-reduced neurosteroids at the level of gene expression measured by the induction of the MMTV promoter for the chicken (cPR$_B$) (left panel) and the human progesterone receptor (hPR$_B$) (right panel). (Adapted with permission from ref. 29.) (5α(β)-DHP, 5α(β)-DHPROG; THP, 3α,5α-THPROG; THDOC, 3α,5α-THDOC).

observation that alphaxalone, in contrast to its natural analogue 3α,5α-THPROG, was devoid of any transcriptional activity via the hPR. Thus, modifications within the C-ring of these molecules appear to offer a possibility of creating synthetic neurosteroids that maintain their modulatory activity via the $GABA_A$ receptor, but are devoid of genomic activity via the hPR *(29)*.

NEUROPSYCHOPHARMACOLOGICAL PROPERTIES OF NEUROSTEROIDS: BEHAVIORAL AND CLINICAL STUDIES

The molecular properties of neurosteroids suggest a potential psychopharmacological profile of the different types of neurosteroids. Indeed, preclinical animal studies have suggested potential benefits of various neurosteroids for certain neuropsychiatric disorders. Though clinical studies are thus far rare, first clinical investigations support the results of animal studies.

Systemic Effects of Pregnenolone

Pregnenolone (PREG) may be converted to an array of steroids; nevertheless, behavioral studies have suggested a potential role for PREG, in particular in memory enhancement. Intracerebroventricular administration of PREG and PREGS leads to an amelioration in various memory tasks in rodents *(30)*. These memory-enhancing effects might be attributable to the N-methyl-D-aspartate (NMDA)-agonistic properties of PREGS *(31)*, since NMDA antagonists have been shown to impair cognitive functions in rodents *(32,33)*. However, valid clinical data concerning the memory enhancing properties of PREG in dementia disorders are lacking to date. PREG formation may be increased also indirectly via the diazepam binding inhibitor (DBI) *(34)*, which may offer additional treatment strategies.

Studies of the effects of PREG on sleep in the rat revealed an increase in electroencephalogram (EEG) activity in the delta frequency range that was contrary to the effects of the benzodiazepine hypnotic midazolam *(35)*. In accordance with this animal study, first clinical investigations evaluating the effects of orally administered PREG on sleep-EEG parameters in human volunteers were in line with partial, inverse agonistic properties of PREG at the $GABA_A$ receptor *(36)*. PREG increased the time spent in slow-wave sleep and depressed sigma EEG power during non-REM sleep (36) (Fig. 5). The inverse GABA-agonistic effects of systemically administered PREG as revealed by the sleep-EEG studies may contribute to the understanding of the potential memory enhancing properties of this neurosteroid.

Systemic Effects of Dehydroepiandrosterone (DHEA)

In view of certain similarities in the molecular mechanisms of action between DHEAS and PREGS, memory-enhancing properties should occur also in systemical studies with DHEA. In fact, DHEA has been also shown to enhance memory retention in mice *(37)*. In an animal model of depression, a transgenic mouse model bearing an antisense against the glucocorticosteroid receptor with an impairment of glucocorticoid receptor function, DHEA may reverse cognitive deficits (A. Montkowski et al., unpublished observations). In addition to the effects of DHEA via the cell membrane, potential antiglucocorticosteroid effects of DHEA reported in vivo *(38,39)* may contribute to its behavioral effects. First clinical studies have shown an increase in REM sleep after oral administra-

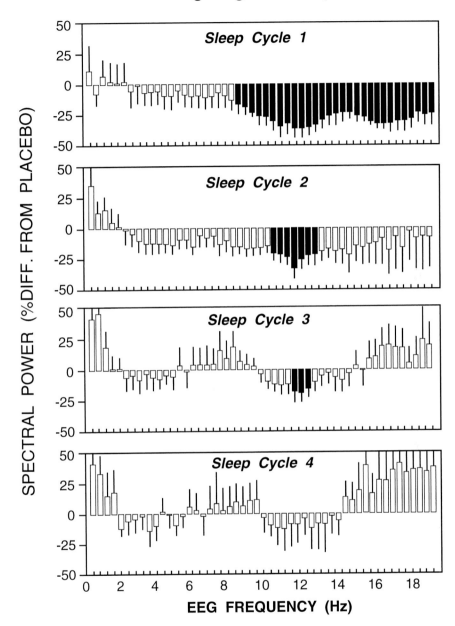

1 mg Pregnenolone p.o.

Fig. 5. Effects of 1 mg PREG on EEG power spectra for the four sleep cycles in healthy adult males. Bars show deviations in percent from the placebo condition as depicted by the zero reference line (mean ± SEM). Solid bars indicate significant differences from the placebo condition ($p < 0.05$). (Adapted with permission from ref. *36*.)

tion of DHEA *(40)*, which is compatible with a potential memory enhancing effect in humans. Moreover, DHEA administration resulted in an increase in EEG activity in the sigma frequency range during REM sleep *(40)* (Fig. 6). Thus, unlike PREG, DHEA

500 mg DHEA p.o.

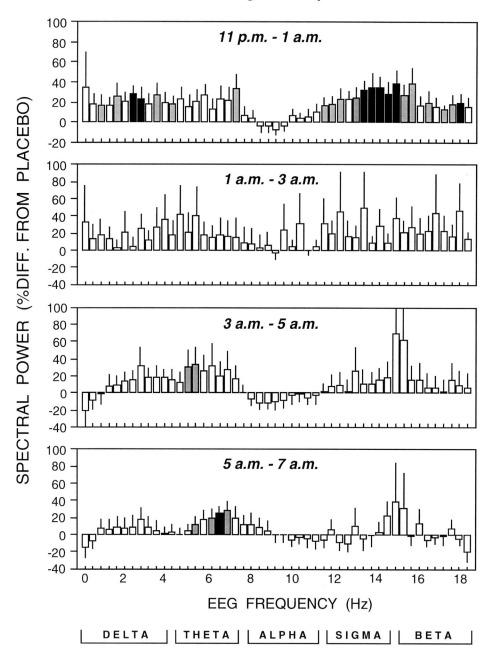

Fig. 6. Effects of 500 mg DHEA on EEG power spectra during REM sleep for 2-h time intervals in healthy adult males. Bars show deviations in percent from the placebo condition as depicted by the zero reference line (mean ± SEM). Solid bars indicate significant differences from the placebo condition ($p < 0.05$). (Adapted with permission from ref. *40*.)

appears to exert mixed GABA-agonistic/antagonistic effects on the sleep-EEG. As DHEA levels decrease with age *(44)*, and decreased concentrations of DHEA were reported in patients suffering from Alzheimer's disease and multi-infarct dementia *(42,43)*, studies are awaited to evaluate the potential benefits of DHEA administration in dementia disorders and in depression in the elderly.

Systemic Effects of 3α-Reduced Neurosteroids

The positive allosteric modulatory properties of 3α-reduced neurosteroids suggest systemic effects of these neurosteroids, which may be beneficial in treating a variety of neuropsychiatric disorders. However, their clinical use has been hampered by their poor water solubility, which can be overcome by the use of certain cylcodextrins in animal studies.

Potential anesthetic properties of these types of neurosteroids were suggested more than 50 years ago *(44)*. These initial observations have been supported by a clinical study employing a pregnanolone emulsion *(45)* and have led to the development of steroid anesthetics such as alphaxalone *(46)*. However, side effects have impaired the development of steroid anesthetics for routine clinical use *(3)*. Nevertheless, intra-cerebroventricular (icv) administration of progesterone and various natural occurring metabolites decreased the pain threshold, probably via a positive allosteric modulation of the GABA$_A$ receptor *(47)*. Moreover, naturally occurring 3α-reduced neurosteroids have been shown to possess anticonvulsant properties *(48,49)*. Such behavioral studies have triggered industrial efforts to develop synthetic compounds which are currently under investigation for the treatment of epilepsy disorders.

Levels of endogenous 3α-reduced neurosteroids are reduced during early ethanol withdrawal *(50)*, which may contribute to the concomitant increase in seizure liability. Reduced plasma levels of 3α-reduced neurosteroids (Romeo et al., submitted) and reduced cerebrospinal fluid (CSF) levels of PREG during depression have also been recently reported *(51)*. Whether the alterations of neurosteroid concentrations are related to the pathophysiology of depression remains to be elucidated. It has been shown that icv administration of 3α,5α-THPROG decreases corticotropin releasing hormone (CRH) concentrations in the hypothalamus *(52)* and an overdrive of CRH and a subsequent hyperactivity of the hypothalamic-pituitary-adrenal (HPA) system plays a crucial role for the pathophysiology of depression *(53)*. Moreover, 3α-reduced neurosteroids may attenuate the response of the HPA system to emotional stress and to adrenaletomy *(54)*. In addition, a preliminary report *(55)* indicates that 3α-reduced neurosteroids are increased during treatment of depression with metyrapone.

The major body of work on the systemic effects of 3α-reduced neurosteroids has focused on the anxiolytic properties of these steroids. Administration of 3α-reduced neurosteroids, e.g., 3α,5α-THPROG *(56–58)*, 3α,5α-THDOC *(59)* or alphaxalone *(60)* clearly reduced anxiety in various tests paradigms in rodents without having sedative effects. The presence of a 3α-hydroxy group was a prerequisite for the anxiolytic effects of these neurosteroids *(56)*, because 3β-reduced steroids were devoid of any anxiolytic properties, as predicted by cellular studies *(61)*. A potential advantage of 3α-reduced neurosteroids as anxiolytics, in comparison to benzodiazepines, might result from their more favorable profile with regard to tolerance and abuse liability in various drug discrimination paradigms (62). Whether the anxiolytic properties of 3α-reduced

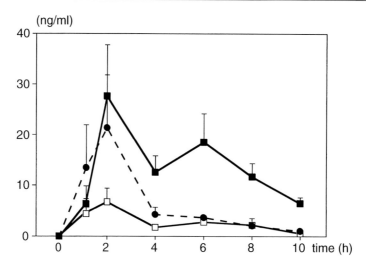

Fig. 7. Plasma concentrations of progesterone (closed circles), 3α,5α-THPROG (allo-pregnanolone) (closed squares) and 3α,5β-THPROG (pregnanolone) (open squares) following the administration of 300 mg micronized progesterone in healthy male volunteers. (Adapted with permission from ref. *76.*)

neurosteroids suggested by animal studies can be confirmed in clinical trials remains to be determined.

Systemic Effects of PROG

Fluctuations in secretion patterns of PROG may be accompanied by mood disturbances, impairment of physical well-being, vigilance state and sleep quality. For example, high levels of PROG precede the clinical symptoms during the premenstrual syndrome (PMS), although there is evidence that PMS does not simply reflect progesterone deficiency *(63,64)*. Dysphoric mood may occur after delivery, which has been attributed to a postpartal "withdrawal" of PROG secretion. Moreover, the frequently reported fatigue during early pregnancy may be related to the enhanced levels of PROG (65).

Administration of exogenous progesterone in various mammalian species has revealed analgesic and anxiolytic effects *(66–68)*. In humans, hypnotic *(69)* and anticonvulsant properties *(70)* have been shown following intravenous administration of progesterone. Studies in women using an oral administration route reported a transient fatigue and a decrease of information processing and verbal memory function *(71–73)*. In view of the poor water solubility and the steroid-receptor-mediated effects of 3α-reduced neurosteroids, the administration of PROG as a precursor molecule appears to be a potential alternative for systemical application of 3α-reduced pregnane steroids. This is supported by animal studies by Smith *(74)* demonstrating a decrease in the spiking of neurons following progesterone injection. Indeed, progesterone is converted very rapidly into 3α,5α-THPROG and also pregnanolone in vivo in rats *(75)* and humans *(76)* (Fig. 7). This in vivo conversion of PROG into 3α-reduced neurosteroids probably accounts for the PROG-induced decrease of epileptic discharges *(70)*, and the GABAergic sleep-EEG patterns with a decrease within the delta frequency range and an increase in the beta frequency range following progesterone adminisitration that has been observed

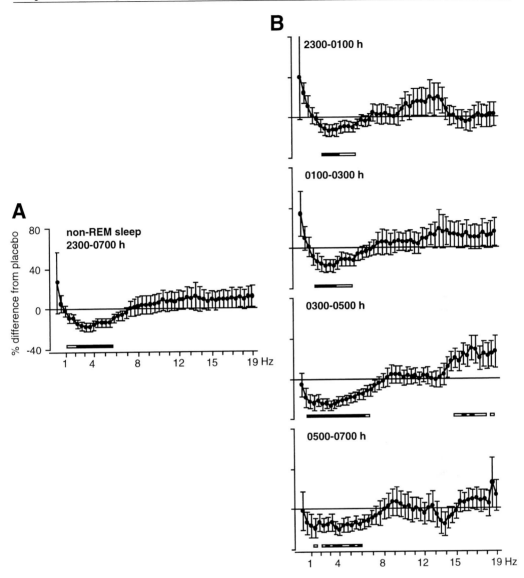

Fig. 8. Effects of 300 mg progesterone administration on EEG power spectra during non-REM sleep of (**A**) the total night and (**B**) four consecutive 2-h periods of night sleep. Data represent the mean (± SE) deviation from placebo condition (= 100%, depicted by the zero reference line). Bars below the abscissa indicate the significance levels of treatment effects compared to the placebo condition (filled bar: $p < 0.05$, open bar: $p < 0.10$, MANOVA for repeated measures, $n = 9$). (Adapted with permission from ref. *76*.)

in rats *(75)* and humans *(76)*. For example, during non-REM sleep (Fig. 8) the slow-wave EEG activity in the delta frequency range declined progressively to a significant decrease between 3 and 5 AM ($p < 0.01$) and was still reduced in the last 2 h of the night following oral administration of micronized progesterone. Similarly, the spectral power in the theta range declined significantly between 3 and 5 AM ($p < 0.02$). In contrast, the EEG activity in the beta frequency range tended to increase during the same time span ($p < 0.07$). Progesterone administration induced changes in sleep architecture and sleep-EEG power spectra *(76)* that are comparable with the well-established effects of agonistic ligands at the GABA$_A$ receptor complex: suppression of REM sleep, an increase in non-REM sleep and especially stage 2 sleep, a prolonged decrease in non-REM sleep-EEG activity in the slow wave frequency range and the largely sleep-stage-independent increase in the spectral power in the higher frequencies of the beta range (>15 Hz) *(35,77–79)*. Within the same study, the effects of PROG administration on sleep could be clearly separated from sedative effects *(80)* following progesterone administration, for which much higher dosages were usually required *(73)*. In addition, spectral analysis of the sleep EEG during the course of pregnancy revealed a progressive reduction of the EEG spectral power, with the largest changes in the spindle frequency range *(81)*; the variations of the spectral power in the upper sigma frequency range have been shown to be related to the menstrual cycle *(82)*.

To date, clinical studies concerning anxiolytic effects of PROG administration are lacking. However, animal studies suggest that potential anxiolytic effects of PROG administration might be gender-specific *(66,83)* and are probably related to an augmentation of GABA$_A$ receptor functioning *(66,67)*. Although PROG administration has been shown to have a clinical benefit in female patients suffering from PMS *(84)*, no relationship could be demonstrated between CSF levels of progesterone or neurosteroids and clinical symptoms in these patients *(63)*. Moreover, in a recently conducted clinical study, there was no significant reduction in symptoms of a benzodiazepine withdrawal following PROG administration *(85)*.

In conclusion, PROG administration may constitute a valuable new therapeutic strategy for various neuropsychiatric disorders. For example, natural PROG may be considered as an alternative to synthetic analogs if an additional agonistic modulation of the GABA-benzodiazepine receptor complex is desired during therapy with progestins. However, the systemic effects of PROG administration are highly complex and may not be simply related to a general increase of GABA$_A$ receptor functioning.

FUTURE PERSPECTIVES

Based on their unique molecular properties, neurosteroids have a promising psychopharmacological profile. Future systemical studies will have to consider both the membrane and the genomic effects of neurosteroids. New synthetic derivatives should allow to separate the transcriptional effects of these steroids from their modulatory effects on neuronal excitability, both with regard to their eventual clinical effects and their potential side effects. For clinical purposes, substances with a sufficient bioavailability after oral administration would be desirable. In addition, pharmacokinetic properties have to be taken into consideration, e.g., linear or U-shaped dose-response curves in animal and clinical studies.

In conclusion, neurosteroids may either modulate neuronal excitability via their interactions with respective neurotransmitter receptors, or may regulate gene expression via PRs (Fig. 9). This intracellular cross-talk between nongenomic and genomic effects of neurosteroids provides the molecular basis for the future development of neurosteroids in neuropsychopharmacology both with regard to clinical effects and to potential side effects.

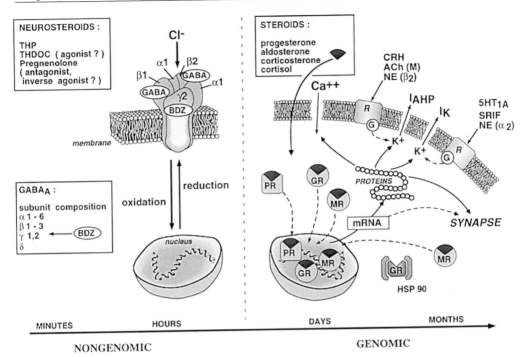

Fig. 9. Nongenomic and genomic properties of neurosteroids. Progesterone receptor (PR), glucocorticoid receptor (GR), mineralocorticoid receptor (MR), heat-shock protein 90 (HSP 90). THP,3α,5α-THPROG; THDOC, 3α,5α-THDOC.

REFERENCES

1. Evans RM. The steroid and thyroid hormone receptor superfamily. Science 1988;240:889–895.
2. Majewska MD, Harrison NL, Schwartz RD, Barker JL, Paul SM. Steroid hormone metabolites are barbiturate-like modulators of the GABA receptor. Science 1986;232:1004–1007.
3. Paul SM, Purdy RH. Neuroactive steroids. FASEB J 1992;6:2311–2322.
4. Akwa Y, Morfin RF, Robel P, Baulieu EE. Neurosteroid metabolism. 7 alpha-hydroxylation of dehydroepiandrosterone and pregnenolone by rat brain microsomes. Biochem J 1992;288:959–964.
5. Baulieu EE. Neurosteroids: A new function in the brain. Biol Cell 1991;71:3–10.
6. McEwen BS. Non-genomic and genomic effects of steroids on neural activity. Trends Pharmacol Sci 1991;12:141–147.
7. Majewska MD. Neurosteroids: endogenous bimodal modulators of the GABA$_A$ receptor. Mechanism of action and physiological significance. Prog Neurobiol 1992;38:379–395.
8. Gee KW, Bolger MB, Brinton RE, Coirini H, McEwen BS. Steroid modulation of the chloride ionophore in rat brain: structure-activity requirements, regional dependance and mechanism of action. J Pharmacol Exp Ther 1988;246:803–812.
9. Harrison NL, Majewska MD, Harrington JW, Barker JL. Structure-activity relationships for steroid interaction with the gamma-aminobutyric acid A receptor complex. J Pharmacol Exp Ther 1987;241:346–353.
10. Rupprecht R, Reul JMHM, Trapp T, van Steensel B, Wetzel C, Damm K, Zieglgänsberger W, Holsboer F. Progesterone receptor-mediated effects of neuroactive steroids. Neuron 1993;11:523–530.
11. Majewska MD, Demigören S, Spivak CE, London ED. The neurosteroid dehydroepiandrosterone sulfate is an allosteric antagonist of the GABA$_A$ receptor. Brain Res 1990;526:143–146.
12. Majewska MD, Mienville JM, Vicini S. Neurosteroid pregnenolone sulfate antagonizes electrophysiological responses to GABA in neurons. Neurosci Lett 1988;90:279–284.
13. Morrow AL, Pace JR, Purdy RH, Paul SM. Characterization of steroid interactions with γ-aminobutyric acid receptor-gated chloride ion channels: evidence for multiple steroid recognition sites. Mol Pharmacol 1990;37:263–270.

14. Purdy RH, Morrow AL, Blinn JR, Paul SM. Synthesis, metabolism, and pharmacological activity of 3α-hydroxy steroids which potentiate GABA-receptor-mediated chloride ion uptake in rat cerebral cortical synaptosomes. J Med Chem 1990;33:1572–1581.

15. Hollenberg SM, Evans RM. Multiple and cooperative trans-activation domains of the human glucocorticoid receptor. Cell 1988;55:899–906.

16. Hollenberg SM, Weinberger C, Ong ES, Cerelli G, Oro A, Lebo R, Thompson EB, Rosenfeld MG, Evans RM. Primary structure and expression of a functional glucocorticoid receptor cDNA. Nature 1985;318:635–641.

17. Arriza JL, Weinberger C, Cerelli G, Glaser TM, Handelin BL, Housman DE, Evans RM. Cloning of human mineralocorticoid receptor complementary DNA: structural and functional kinship with the glucocorticoid receptor. Science 1987;237:268–275.

18. Conneely OM, Kettelberger DM, Tsai MJ, Schrader WT, O'Malley BW. The chicken progesterone receptor A and B isoforms are products of an alternate translation event. J Biol Chem 1989;264:14062–14064.

19. Kastner P, Bocquel M, Turcotte BP, Garnier JM, Horwitz KB, Chambon B, Gronemeyer H. Transient expression of human and chicken progesterone receptors does not support alternative translation initiation from a single mRNA as the mechanism generating two receptor isoforms. J Biol Chem 1990;265:12163–12167.

20. Denner LA, Weigel NL, Maxwell B, Schrader WT, O'Malley BW. Regulation of progesterone receptor-mediated transcription by phosphorylation. Science 1990;250:1740–1743.

21. Power RF, Mani SK, Codina J, Conneely OM, O'Malley BW. Dopaminergic and ligand-independent activation of steroid hormone receptors. Science 1991;254:1636–1639.

22. Puia G, Santi MR, Vicini S, Pritchett DB, Purdy RH, Paul SM, Seeburg PH, Costa E. Neurosteroids act on recombinant human GABA$_A$ receptors. Neuron 1990;4:759–765.

23. Purdy RH, Morrow AL, Moore PH, Paul SM. Stress-induced elevations of γ-aminobutyric acid type A receptor-active steroids in the rat brain. Proc Natl Acad Sci USA 1991;8:4553–4557.

24. Sarrieau A, Dussaillant M, Agid F, Philibert D, Agid Y, Rostene W. Autoradiographic localization of glucocorticosteroid and progesterone binding sites in the human post-mortem brain. J Steroid Biochem 1986;25:717–721.

25. Fox SR, Harlan RE, Shivers BD, Pfaff DW. Chemical characterization of neuroendocrine targets for progesterone in the female rat brain and pituitary. Neuroendocrinology 1990;51:276–283.

26. Olsen RW, Tobin AJ. Molecular biology of GABA$_A$ receptors. FASEB J 1990;4:1469–1480.

27. Krause JE, Karavolas HJ. Pituitary 5α-dihydroprogesterone 3α-hydroxysteroid oxidoreductases. J Biol Chem 1980;255:11807–11814.

28. Melcangi RC, Celotti F, Castano P, Martini L. Differential localization of the 5α-reductase and the 3α-hydroxysteroid dehydrogenase in neuronal and glial cultures. Endocrinology 1993;132:1252–1259.

29. Rupprecht R, Berning B, Hauser CAE, Holsboer F, Reul JMHM. Steroid receptor mediated effects of neuroactive steroids: characterization of structure-activity relationship. Eur J Pharmacol 1996;303: 227–234.

30. Flood JF, Morley JE, Roberts E. Memory-enhancing effects in male mice of pregnenolone and of steroids metabolically derived from it. Proc Natl Acad Sci USA 1992;89:1567–1571.

31. Bowlby MR. Pregnenolone sulfate potentiation of N-methyl-D-aspartate receptor channels in hippocampal neurons. Mol Pharmacol 1993;43:813–819.

32. Flood JF, Baker ML, Davis JL. Modulation of memory processing by glutamic receptor agonists and antagonists. Brain Res 1990;521:197–202.

33. Ungerer A, Mathis C, Mélan C, De Barry J. The NMDA receptor, CPP and γ-L-glutamyl-L-aspartate selectively block post training improvement of performance in a Y-maze avoidance learning task. Brain Res 1991;549:59–65.

34. Korneyev A, Pan BS, Polo A, Romeo E, Guidotti A, Costa E. Stimulation of brain pregnenolone synthesis by mitochondrial diazepam binding inhibitor receptor ligands in vivo. J Neurochem 1993;61:1515–1524.

35. Lancel M, Crönlein TAM, Müller-Preuss P, Holsboer F. Pregnenolone enhances EEG delta activity during non-rapid eye movement sleep in the rat, in contrast to midazolam. Brain Res 1994;646:85–94.

36. Steiger A, Trachsel L, Guldner J, Hemmeter U, Rothe B, Rupprecht R, Vedder H, Holsboer F. Neurosteroid pregnenolone induces sleep-EEG changes in man compatible with inverse agonistic GABA$_A$-receptor modulation. Brain Res 1993;615:267–274.

37. Flood JF, Smith GE, Roberts E. Dehydroepiandrosterone and its sulfate enhance memory retention in mice. Brain Res 1988;447:269–278.
38. Browne ES, Porter JR, Correa G, Abadie J, Svec F. Dehydroepiandrosterone regulation of the hepatic glucocorticoid receptor in the Zucker rat. The obesity research program. J Steroid Biochem Mol Biol 1993;45:517–524.
39. Araneo B, Daynes R. Dehydroepiandrosterone functions as more than an antiglucocorticoid in preserving immunocompetence after thermal injury. Endocrinology 1995;136:393–401.
40. Friess E, Trachsel L, Guldner J, Schier T, Steiger A, Holsboer F. DHEA administration increases rapid eye movement sleep and EEG power in the sigma frequency range. Am J Physiol 1995;268:E107–E113.
41. Thomas G, Frenoy N, Legrain S, Sebag-Lanoe R, Baulieu EE, Debuire B. Serum dehydroepiandrosterone sulfate levels as an individual marker. J Clin Endocrinol Metab 1994;79:1273–1276.
42. Näsman B, Olsson B, Bäckström T, Eriksson S, Grankvist K, Viitanen M, Bucht G. Serum dehydroepiandrosterone sulfate in Alzheimers disease and in multiinfarct dementia. Biol Psychiatry 1991;30:684–690.
43. Sunderland T, Merril CR, Harrington MG, Lawlor BA, Molchan SE, Martinez R, Murphy DL. Reduced plasma dehydroepiandrosterone concentrations in Alzheimers disease. Lancet 1989;8662:570–572.
44. Selye H. The anesthetic effect of steroid hormones. Proc Soc Exp Biol Med 1941;46:116–121.
45. Carl P, Högskilde S, Nielsen JW, Sörensen MB, Lindholm M, Karlen B, Bäckström T. Pregnanolone emulsion: a preliminary pharmacokinetic and pharmacodynamic study of a new intravenous agent. Anaesthesia 1990;45:189–197.
46. Richards CD, Hesketh TR. Implications for theories of anaesthesia of antagonism between anaesthetic and non-anaesthetic steroids. Nature 1975;256:179–182.
47. Frye DA, Duncan JE. Progesterone metatolizes effective at the GABA$_A$ receptor complex modulate pain sensitivity in rats. Brain Res 1994;643:194–203.
48. Belelli D, Lan NC, Gee KW. Anticonvulsant steroids and the GABA/benzodiazepine receptor-chloride ionophore complex. Neurosci Biobehav Rev 1990;14:315–322.
49. Kokate TG, Svensson BE, Rogawski MA. Anticonvulsant activity of neurosteroids: correlation with γ-aminobutyric acid-evoked chloride current potentiation. J Pharmacol Exp Ther 1994;270:1223–1229.
50. Romeo E, Brancati A, De Lorenzo A, Fucci P, Furnari C, Pompili E, Sasso GF, Spalletta G, Troisi A, Pasini A. Marked decrease of plasma neuroactive steroids during alcohol withdrawl. Clin Neuropharmacol 1996;19:366–369.
51. George MS, Guidotti A, Rubinow D, Pan B, Mikalauskas K, Post RM. CSF neuroactive steroids in affective disorders: pregnenolone, progesterone and DBI. Biol Psychiatry 1994;35:775–780.
52. Patchev VK, Shoaib M, Holsboer F, Almeida OFX. The neurosteroid tetrahydroprogesterone counteracts corticotropin-releasing hormone-induced anxiety and alters the release and gene expression of corticotropin-releasing hormone in the rat hypothalamus. Neuroscience 1994;62:265–271.
53. Holsboer F, Spengler D, Heuser IJ. The role of corticotropin-releasing hormone in the pathogenesis of Cushing's disease, anorexia nervosa, alcoholism, affective disorders and dementia. Prog Brain Res 1992;93:385–417.
54. Patchev VK, Hassan AHS, Holsboer F, Almeida OFX. The neurosteroid tetrahydroprogesterone attenuates the endocrine response to stress and exerts glucocorticoid-like effects on vasopressin gene transcription in the rat hypothalamus. Neuropsychopharmacology 1996;15:533–541.
55. Raven PW, O'Dwyer A-M, Taylor NF, Checkley SA. The relationship between the effects of metyrapone treatment on depressed mood and urinary steroid profiles. Psychoneuroendocrinology 1996;21:277–286.
56. Bitran D, Hilvers RJ, Kellogg CK. Anxiolytic effects of 3α-hydroxy–5α [β]-pregnan-20-one: endogenous metabolites of progesterone that are active at the GABA$_A$ receptor. Brain Res 1991;561:157–161.
57. Wieland S, Belluzi JD, Stein L, Lan NC. Comparative behavioral characterization of the neuroactive steroids 3α-OH,5α-pregnan–20-one and 3α-OH,5β-pregnan–20-one in rodents. Psychopharmacology 1995;118:65–71.
58. Wieland S, Lan NC, Mirasedeghi S, Gee KW. Anxiolytic activity of the progesterone metabolite 5α-pregnan-3α-ol-20-one. Brain Res 1991;565:263–268.
59. Crawley JN, Glowa JR, Majewska MD, Paul SM. Anxiolytic activity of an endogenous adrenal steroid. Brain Res 1986;398:382–385.
60. Britton KT, Page M, Baldwin H, Koob GF. Anxiolytic activity of the steroid alphaxolone. J Pharmacol Exp Ther 1991;258:124–129.

61. Prince RJ, Simmonds MA. 5β-pregnan-3β-ol-20-one, a specific antagonist at the neurosteroid site of the GABA$_A$ receptor-complex. Neurosci Lett 1992;135:273–275.

62. Ator NA, Grant KA, Purdy RH, Paul SM, Griffiths RR. Drug discrimination analysis of endogenous neuroactive steroids in rats. Eur J Pharmacol 1993;241:237–243.

63. Schmidt PJ, Purdy RH, Moore PH, Paul SM, Rubinow DR. Circulating levels of anxiolytic steroids in the luteal phase in women with premenstrual syndrome and in control subjects. J Clin Endocrinol Metab 1994;79:1256–1260.

64. Redei E, Freeman EW. Daily plasma estradiol and progesterone levels over the menstrual cycle and their relation to premenstrual symptoms. Psychoneuroendocrinology 1995;20:259–267.

65. Biedermann K, Schoch P. Do neuroactive steroids cause fatigue in pregnancy? Eur J Obstet Gynecol Reprod Biol 1985;58:15–18.

66. Bitran D, Purdy RH, Kellogg CK. Anxiolytic effect of progesterone is associated with increases in cortical allopregnanolone and GABA$_A$ receptor function. Pharmacol Biochem Behav 1993; 45:423–428.

67. Bitran D, Shiekh M, McLeod M. Anxiolytic effect of progesterone is mediated by the neurosteroid allopregnanolone at brain GABA$_A$ receptors. J Neuroendocrinol 1995;7:171–177.

68. Kavaliers M, Wiebe JP. Analgesic effects of the progesterone metabolite 3α-hydroxy-5α-pregnan-20-one and possible modes of action in mice. Brain Res 1987;415:393–398.

69. Merryman W, Boiman R, Barnes L, Rothschild I. Progesterone "anaesthesia" in human subjects. J Clin Endocrinol Metab 1954;14:1567–1569.

70. Bäckström T, Zetterlund B, Blom S, Romano M. Effects of intravenous progesterone infusions on the epileptic discharge frequency in women with partial epilepsy. Acta Neurol Scand 1984;69:240–248.

71. Arafat ES, Hargrove JT, Maxson WS, Desiderio DM, Wentz AC, Andersen RN. Sedative and hypnotic effects of oral administration of micronized progesterone may be mediated through its metabolites. Am J Obstet Gynecol 1988;159:1203–1209.

72. Freeman EW, Weinstock L, Rickels K, Sondhimer SJ, Coutfiaris C. A placebo-controlled study of effects of oral progesterone on performance and mood. Br J Clin Pharmacol 1992;33:293–298.

73. Freeman EW, Purdy RH, Coutifaris C, Rickels K, Paul SM. Anxiolytic metabolites of progesterone: correlation with mood and performance measures following oral progesterone administration to healthy female volunteers. Neuroendocrinology 1993;58:478–484.

74. Smith SS. Progesterone enhances inhibitory responses of cerebellar Purkinje cells mediated by the GABA$_A$ receptor subtype. Brain Res Bull 1989;23:317–322.

75. Lancel M, Faulhaber J, Holsboer F, Rupprecht R. Progesterone administration induces changes in sleep EEG comparable to those of agonistic GABA$_A$ receptor modulators. Am J Physiol 1997;271:E763–E772.

76. Friess E, Tagaya H, Trachsel L, Holsboer F, Rupprecht R. Progesterone-induced changes in sleep in male subjects. Am J Physiol 1997;272:885–891.

77. Borbély AA, Mattmann P, Loepfe M, Lehmann D. Effect of benzodiazepine hypnotics on all-night sleep EEG spectra. Hum Neurobiol 1985;4:189–194.

78. Brunner DP, Dijk DJ, Münch M, Borbély AA. Effect of zolpidem on sleep and sleep EEG spectra in healthy young men. Psychopharmacology 1991;104:1–5.

79. Aeschbach D, Dijk DJ, Trachsel L, Brunner DP, Borbély AA. Dynamics of slow-wave activity and spindle frequency activity in the human sleep EEG: effect of midazolam and zopiclone. Neuro-psychopharmacology 1994;11:237–244.

80. Grön G, Friess E, Herpers M, Rupprecht R. Assessment of cognitive function after progesterone administration in healthy male volunteers. Neuropsychobiology 1997;35:147–151.

81. Brunner DP, Münch M, Biedermann K, Huch R, Huch A, Borbély AA. Changes in sleep and sleep electroencephalogram during pregnancy. Sleep 1994;17:576–582.

82. Driver HS, Dijk DJ, Werth E, Biedermann K, Borbély AA. Sleep and the sleep electroencephalogram across the menstrual cycle in young healthy women. J Clin Endocrinol Metab 1996;81:728–735.

83. Rodriguez-Sierra JF, Hagley MT, Hendricks SE. Anxolytic effects of progesterone are sexually dimorphic. Life Sci 1986;38:1841–1845.

84. Dennerstein L, Spencer-Gardner C, Gotts G, Brown JB, Smith MA, Burrows GD. Progesterone and the premenstrual syndrome: a double blind crossover trial. Br Med J 1980;290:1617–1621.

85. Schweizer E, Case WG, Garcia-Espana F, Greenblatt DJ, Rickels K. Progesterone co-administration in patients discontinuing long-term benzodiazepine therapy: effects on withdrawl severity and taper outcome. Psychopharmacology 1995;117:424–429.

INDEX

A

Acetylcholine (ACh), 210
Acetylcholine receptor, 208
Acetyltransferase, 12–13
Active avoidance
  DHEAS, 326–327
  PREG, 326–327
  PREGS, 327
Acute ethanol intoxication
  neurosteroid levels, 6–7
Adenine nucleotide carrier (ADC), 77, 78
Adhesion molecules
  astroglia signaling
    steroids, 258, 259
Adrenodoxin, 33
Adrenodoxin reductase, 33
Adulthood
P450aro
  sex steroid regulation, 104
Affective disorders
  neuroactive steroids, 149
Afferent system
  midbrain serotonergic system, 237
Aggressive behavior
  DHEA, 323
  neurosteroids, 160, 161
  PREGS, 323
Aging
  neurosteroids, 159, 160
    stress and anxiety, 323, 324
Alcohol dependence
  neuroactive steroids, 147–149
Alcohol withdrawal
  neuroactive steroids, 147–149
Aldosterone synthase, 54t, 57, 58
Allopregnanolone
  aged animals, 324
  burying behavior, 321
  elevated plus maze, 318
  GABA/BZD receptor-chloride ionophore
    complex, 317, 318
  infant animals, 323, 324
  light-dark transition chamber, 319

metabolic pathways, 150f
mirror-chamber test, 320
operant conflict tests, 321
passive avoidance, 326
structures, 145f
swim-stress paradigm, 322, 323
Allopregnolone measurement
  gas chromatographic-mass
    fragmentographic method, 5
  radioimmunoassay, 5
Allosteric model
  predictions, 217f
  schematic diagram, 217f
Allosteric modulation
  ligand-gated channels, 215–217
Alphaxalone
  analysis, 126
Alzheimer's disease, 114
A mER
  estradiol-evoked dopamine release
    female rat striatal tissue, 270–274
Androgen dihydrotestosterone (DHT)
  testosterone, 41
Androgens, 207
Androgens aromatization, 1, 2
Anti-estrogens, 238
Anxiety
  allopregnanolone, 318–321
  DHEAS, 320
  neurosteroid expression, 322, 323
  neurosteroids
    age-related effects, 323, 324
  PREG, 319
  PREGS, 320
  PROG, 318, 320, 321
Anxiety-like measurement paradigms,
    318–322
  burying behavior, 321
  elevated plus maze, 318, 319
  light-dark transition chamber, 319
  mirror-chamber test, 319, 320
  operant conflict tests, 32
Approach-based paradigms, 328–330

nonspatial food/water reinforced tasks, 329, 330
spatial food/water-search tasks, 328, 329
Arachidonic acid, 56
Aromatase, 59
Astrocytes
neurosteroids
trophic effect, 16, 17
Astroglia
hormonal steroids, 256–259
IGF-1 receptors
estradiol, 261
PREG
brain injury, 257
PROG, 256–257
brain injury, 257
synaptic remodeling, 258
sex steroids, 258
steroids
IGF-1, 262–263
Astroglial cells
involvement, 243
Astroglia plasticity
steroid modulation
after brain injury, 257, 258
Astroglia signaling
adhesion molecules
steroids, 258–259
Avoidance, 326–327
Avoidance-based paradigms, 325–328
active avoidance, 326, 327
passive avoidance, 325, 326
water maze, 327

B

Bacteria
PBR mediated cholesterol transport, 82
Benzodiazepine binding
Scatchard analysis, 81
Benzodiazepine receptor, 75–91
Bicuculline-induced seizures, 148
Bile acid synthesizing
P450, 54t
Biological rhythms
neurosteroids, 160
Brain
cell membrane
estradiol-binding sites, 285–288
steroid receptors, 269–289
cholesterol accumulation, 84

developing
ER, 296–298
ERs/signaling proteins, 305–309
estradiol, 294–295
estrogen and neurotrophin signaling
pathways, 304–305
estrogen receptors, 296–298
estrogens, 293–310
neurotrophin-estrogen interactions,
300–303
neurotrophin receptors, 298, 299
neurotrophins, 298
neurotrophin signal transduction
cascades, 299, 300
tyrosine phosphorylation, 303, 304
DHEA and PREG S, 15
DHEA biosynthesis, 11
emotion, 235
HOR, 3alpha, 43
HOR, 11beta, 41
HOR, 17beta, 40
hormone action, 234
hydroxylase, 17alpha, 58
neurosteroids, 3, 3t
quantitation, 3
P450
detection, 52–55
forms, 55–59
reductase, 36
P45019, 59
P450aro, 37, 38, 101–104
P450c11, 36, 37
plasticity
steroid effects, 255–264
P450S
drug, steroid, fatty acid metabolizing,
60–62
P450$_{SCC}$, 84, 85
reductase, 5alpha, 41, 42, 107–109
sex differentiation
neurosteroids, 158
steroid hormones, 1
steroid metabolism, 1, 2
steroids, 51
growth factors, 259–263
steroid synthesis, 84
synaptic plasticity
gonadal hormone regulation, 233–244
Brain-derived neurotrophic factor (BDNF)
developing brain, 298
trkB, 298, 299

Burying behavior
   allopregnanolone, 321
   PROG, 321

C

Calcium channels, 14
   neuronal voltage-gated
      neuroactive steroid modulation, 225–231
Calcium influx, 225
   microspectrofluorimetry studies, 175
Calmodulin, 341–342
CAMP. *See* Cyclic adenosine monophosphate (cAMP)
Catalytic activities
   P450 identification, 55, 56
Catecholestrogens, 115
C6-2B, 84–88
   characterization, 85f
Cellular processes
   circulating hormones, 235, 236
Central nervous system. *See also* Nervous system
   cytochrome P450, 51–62
   development
      neurosteroids, 158
   myelination
      PROG, 19
Channel blockade
   single-channel events, 213
Chlorpromazine
   P450, 61
Cholesterol
   brain, 84
   eukaryotic steroid hormones, 75
Circadian rhythms
   neurosteroid levels, 5, 6
Circulating hormones
   cellular and molecular processes, 235, 236
Clozapine
   P450, 61
Cognition
   neurosteroids, 324–332
CO_2 inhalation, 323
   DHEA, 323
   PREG, 323
   PROG, 323
C17 side chain
   GABA$_A$ receptor, 131

CS-P3
   E-6-^{125}I-BSA, 280–283
CS-P$_3$ membrane
   estradiol
      binding sites, 274–285
C3 substitution
   GABA$_A$ receptor, 130, 131
C20 substitution
   GABA$_A$ receptor, 132

C21 substitution

GABA$_A$ receptor, 132, 133
C-3 sulfate, 178
Cushings' syndrome, 114
Cyclic adenosine monophosphate (cAMP), 79
   neurosteroid biosynthesis regulation, 86, 87
CYP 21, 54t, 58
CYP 7b, 13, 14
Cytochrome P450. *See also* P450
   central nervous system, 51–62
   steroidogenic enzymes, 28
Cytochrome P450$_{SCC}$, 10. *See also* P450$_{SCC}$

D

Dehydroepiandrosterone (DHEA), 2, 28
   aggressive behavior, 15, 323
   biosynthesis, 11
   biosynthetic pathways, 343
   CO_2 inhalation, 323
   ethanol, 7
   GABA/BZD receptor-chloride ionophore complex, 318
   HOR, 17beta, 39, 40
   NMDA receptors, 177
   nongenomic and genomic properties, 350–354
   PREG S
      brain, 15
   REM sleep, 356f
   sigma receptor, 197–199
   systemic effects, 354–357
Dehydroepiandrosterone fatty acids (DHEAL)
   brain, 3t
Dehydroepiandrosterone sulfate (DHEAS). *See also* Dehydroepiandrosterone (DHEA)
   active avoidance, 326, 327

brain, 3, 5, 7, 8
  mirror-chamber test, 320
  passive avoidance, 325
  spatial food/water-search tasks, 329
  water maze, 327
Dendritic spine
  estrogen-induced synaptogenesis, 239
  formation
    molecular events, 242, 243
DES
  DA and NE, 270
Diastereomeric selectivity
  GABAergic steroids, 143–145
Diazepam binding inhibitor (DBI), 88
  amino-acid sequence, 89
  binding to PBRs, 89
  PREG synthesis, 90
  steroid/neurosteroid synthesis, 89–91
Diethylstilbestrol (DES)
  DA, 270
  NE, 270
Dihydrotestosterone (DHT), 55
  5alpha, 2
  testosterone, 41
Dopamine (DA)
  DES, 270
  E, 270–274
  female rat striatal tissue
    A mER, 270–274
Dose-related memory enhancements
  production, 341
Dose-response curve, 342
  allosteric model, 217f
  equation, 217f
  PROG, 216
Drug dependence
  neurosteroids, 160, 161
Drug ligands
  effects, 79–80
Drug metabolizing
  brain
    P450S, 60–62

E

E-6-BSA
  estradiol binding, 284
  proteins, 285, 286
E-17-BSA
  estradiol binding, 284
E-6-^{125}I-BSA

CS-P3, 280–283
  OSCP, 285, 286
Electrophysiological studies
  hippocampal neurons, 175
Elevated plus maze
  allopregnanolone, 318
  PREG, 319
  PREG S, 319
  PROG, 318
Embryogenesis
  P450aro
    sex steroid regulation, 103, 104
Emotion
  hippocampus, 235
Enantiomeric selectivity
  GABAergic steroids, 145–147
Enantioselectivity
  steroid action, 135
Endogenous PBR ligands, 88–91
  PREG formation, 88t
Enzymes
  molecular biology and developmental
    regulation, 27–43
Epoxygenases, 56
ERK
  ER phosphorylation, 308
ERK1
  tyrosine phosphorylation
    estrogen, 304, 305
ERK2
  tyrosine phosphorylation
    estrogen, 304, 305
Escherichia coli, 82
Esterification
  hydroxyl group, 3alpha, 144
Estradiol (E), 2
  astroglia
    IGF-1 receptors, 261
  binding
    E-6-BSA, 284
    E-17-BSA, 284
  binding sites
    brain cell membrane, 285–288
    CS-P$_3$ membrane, 274–285
  brain development, 294, 295
  DA, 270–274
  dopamine
    A mER, 270–274
  GFAP, 256, 258, 259
  glial plasticity
    N-CAM, 259

hypothalamic neurons
  IGF-1, 260
neuroprotective effects, 184
treatment effects, 241
tyrosine phosphorylation
  MAP kinase cascade, 305
Estrogen receptors (ER)
alpha gene, 296
beta gene, 296
brain development, 296–298
developing brain, 296–298
hypothalamic neurons
  IGF-1, 260, 261
serine phosphorylation, 297
signaling proteins
  developing brain, 305–309
tyrosine phosphorylation, 297
  developing brain, 303, 304
Estrogens, 207
brain development, 293–310
dendritic spine formation, 242, 243
effects
  learning and memory, 240, 241
ERK1
  tyrosine phosphorylation, 304, 305
ERK2
  tyrosine phosphorylation, 304, 305
IGF-I, 260
induced synaptogenesis
  dendritic spines, 239
neurotrophins
  developing brain, 300–303
neurotrophin signaling pathways
  developing brain, 304, 305
NGF, 259, 301
nongenomic action, 238
sensitivity
  hippocampus, 236, 237, 238
src
  tyrosine phosphorylation, 306
TRFa, 259
trk, 300, 301
Ethanol
DHEA, 7
P450, 61
Eukaryotic steroid hormones
cholesterol, 75
Exacerbation
PREG S
  NMDA-induced neuronal death, 182, 183

Excitotoxic cell death
modulations
  neuroactive steroids, 182–184
Extracellular regulated kinase (ERK)
ER phosphorylation, 308

F

Fatty acid metabolism
brain
  P450S, 60–62
Flavoprotein, 33
Flunitrazepam, 78, 80, 81

G

GABA$_A$ receptor, 14
alpha subunits, 128, 129
beta subunits, 127, 128
C17 side chain, 131
C3 substitution, 130, 131
C20 substitution, 132
C21 substitution, 132, 133
delta subunits, 129, 130
epsilon subunits, 129, 130
gamma subunits, 129
modulator properties, 351f
multiple steroid-binding sites, 144
neurosteroid antagonists, 155–157
neurosteroids interaction, 125–138
ring system, 130
structure activity relationship, 130–135
water soluble steroids, 133–135
GABA/BZD receptor-chloride ionophore
    complex
DHEA, 318
PREG, 318
GABAergic neurotransmission
steroid
  potentiation, 143–150
GABAergic steroids
diastereomeric selectivity, 143–145
enantiomeric selectivity, 145–147
parturition, 162
structures, 146f
GABA receptor
NMDA receptor, 343
Gamma-aminobutyric acid A (GABA$_A$), 5
NMDA receptors, 177
nongenomic and genomic properties,
    350–354

vs. PBRs, 76
Gamma-aminobutyric acid (GABA)
  antagonistic steroids
    physiological role, 157–162
  serotonergic system, 237
Gamma amino butyric/benzodiazepine
    (GABA/BZD) receptor-chloride iono-
    phore complex
  neurosteroids, 317, 318
Gas chromatographic-mass
    fragmentographic method
  allopregnolone measurement, 5
Genomic actions
  estrogen, 238
Glial cells
  neurosteroids
    trophic effect, 16–19
  steroid hormones
    effects, 17
Glial fibrillary acidic protein (GFAP)
  estradiol, 256, 258, 259
  PREG, 256–257
  testosterone, 256
Glucocoritcosteroids, 207
Glutamate receptors, 14
  endogenous modulators
    neurosteroids, 181, 182
  ionotropic, 136, 137
    neuroactive steroid modulation, 167–
      185
  recombinant
    modulation, 180f
Glycine receptors, 135, 136
Gonadal hormone
  action
    hypothalamus, 234, 235
  IGF-I, 259, 260
  regulation
    brain synaptic plasticity, 233–244
Gonadogenesis, 69
Growth factors
  role, 243
  steroids
    brain, 259–263
Guanine nucleotide proteins
  role, 229, 230

H

Haloperidol
  P450, 61

Herpes Simplex Virus-tyrosine kinase gene,
    83
[^{3}H]-estradiol
  rbOSCP, 287–288
Heterosexual exposure
  neurosteroid levels, 6
Hippocampal formation
  Magnetic resonance imaging (MRI), 114
Hippocampal interneurons, 236, 237
Hippocampal neurons
  electrophysiological studies, 175
Hippocampus
  estrogen sensitivity, 236, 237, 238
  growth factors, 243
  sex hormones, 235
  synaptogenesis, 240
Hormonal steroid
  astroglia, 256–259
  metabolism
    nervous system, 97–115
Hormone action
  brain, 234
Hormone-stimulated steroidogenesis
  PBRs, 80–81
5-HT$_3$ receptors, 137, 138
Hydroperoxide pathway, 11
Hydroxylase
  5alpha, 55
  7alpha, 13, 14
  17alpha, 54t, 57, 58
  3beta, 55
  11beta, 54t, 57, 58
Hydroxyl group, 3alpha
  esterification and oxidation, 144
Hydroxysteroid dehydrogenase (HSD)
  3beta, 13, 38, 39
Hydroxysteroid oxidoreductase (HOR)
  3alpha, 14, 42–43, 110–112
    pathways, 99f, 111f
  20alpha, 14
  11beta, 41, 113, 114
    pathways, 99f, 111f
  17beta, 39, 40, 112, 113
    pathways, 99f, 111f
Hypothalamic astroglia
  steroids
    IGF-1, 262, 263
Hypothalamic neurons
  estradiol
    IGF-1, 260
  IGF-1

estrogen receptors, 260, 261
Hypothalamus
    gonadal hormone action, 234, 235

I

Imipramine
    P450, 61
Immunohistochemical localization
    P4502D4, 61
Immunohistochemistry
    P450$_{SCC}$, 56–57
Infradian rhythms
    neurosteroid levels, 5, 6
Inner mitochondrial megachannel (IMC), 78
Insulin-like growth factor I (IGF-1)
    estradiol
        hypothalamic neurons, 260
    estrogen, 260
    gonadal hormones, 259, 260
    hypothalamic neurons
        estrogen receptors, 260, 261
    steroids
        hypothalamic astroglia, 262, 263
    tanycytes, 262, 263
Insulin-like growth factor I (IGF-1)1 recep-
        tors
    astroglia
        estradiol, 261
Ion channels
    neurotransmitter receptors
        steroid modulators, 168t–174t
    transmitter-gated
        neurosteroids selectivity, 135–138
Ion flux assays
    nAChR, 212
Ionotropic glutamate receptors, 136, 137
    modulation
        neuroactive steroids, 167–185
Isocaproic acid, 29

K

Knockout mouse studies
    steroidogenic factor 1, 70, 71f, 72f

L

Learning
    estrogen effects, 240, 241

neurosteroids, 159, 160, 324–332
Leydig cell, 69, 70
    derived tumors
        pituitary LH secretion, 82
    measurement
        Northern blot analysis and ligand
            binding, 81
Ligand binding
    Leydig cell measurement, 81
Ligand-gated channels, 208–210
    allosteric modulation, 215–217
    characterization, 209
    neuronal nAChR, 210
Light–dark transition chamber, 319
    allopregnanolone, 319
Limbic brain region
    emotion, 235
Lipophilic compounds, 215
Lyase , 54t, 58–59

M

Magnetic resonance imaging (MRI)
    hippocampal formation, 114
Memory
    estrogen effects, 240, 241
    hippocampus, 235
    neurosteroids, 159, 160, 324–332
    performance
        PREG S, 16
Memory enhancement
    PREG S, 337–346
        hypothesis, 343, 344
Menstrual cycle
    neuroactive steroids, 148
Mesolimbic dopamine
    estradiol, 270
Mianserin
    P450, 61
Microspectrofluorimetry
    calcium influx studies, 175
Mineralocorticosteroids, 207
Mirror-chamber test, 319, 320
    allopregnanolone, 320
    DHEAS, 320
    PREGS, 320
    PROG, 320
Mitochondrial PREG formation
    steps, 80
Mitochondrial topography

PBRs, 78–79
Mitogen-activated protein kinase (MAPK)
    cascade
    developing brain, 299
    estradiol
        tyrosine phosphorylation, 305
    Raf kinases, 305–306
Molecular processes
    circulating hormones, 235, 236
Mood
    neurosteroids, 161–162
MP$_2$ fraction
    female rats, 275–279
MP$_3$ fraction
    female rats, 275–279
Mullerian-inhibiting substance (MIS), 69
Myelinating glial cells
    steroid hormones
        effects, 17
Myelin formation
    PROG, 17–19

N

Nerve growth factor (NGF)
    developing brain, 298
    estrogen, 259, 301
    PC2 cells, 299, 300
    trkA, 298–299
    trk signaling cascades, 300
Nervous system. *See also* Central nervous
        system; Peripheral nervous system
    hormonal steroid metabolism, 97–115
    HSD, 3beta, 38, 39
    P450c17
        developmental regulation, 34, 35
    synaptogenesis approaches, 239–241
Neural cell adhesion molecule (N-CAM)
    glial plasticity
        estradiol, 259
Neuroactive steroid
    affective disorders, 149
    alcohol dependence and withdrawal,
        147–149
    concentration-effect curves, 228f
    induced inhibition
        concentration-effect curves, 227f
    inhibition
        whole-cell calcium channel current,
            226f
    modulation

excitotoxic cell death, 182–184
ionotropic glutamate receptors, 167–
    185
neuronal voltage-gated calcium chan-
    nels, 225–231
Neuroendocrine structures, 1
Neurolabyrinth
    PREG S, 339–343
Neuroleptic drugs
    P450, 61
Neuronal nAChR
    PROG, 210, 211f
    steroid inhibition, 210–212, 212
Neuronal regeneration
    PROG and PREG, 17
Neuronal voltage-gated calcium channels
    neuroactive steroid modulation, 225–231
Neurons
    neurosteroids
        trophic effect, 16–19
Neuropeptide gene expression
    regulation, 234
Neuroprotective effects
    estradiol, 184
    PREG hemisuccinate, 183, 184
Neuropsychopharacological potential
    neurosteroids
        future perspectives, 360
Neurosteroids, 2. *See also* Steroids
    3alpha-reduced
        anxiolytic properties, 357
        systemic effects, 357–358
    antagonists
        GABA$_A$ receptors, 155–157
    anxiety
        age-related effects, 323, 324
    astroglia, 256–259
    behavioral studies, 317–333
    beta subunits, 127, 128
    binding sites
        heterogeneity, 127–130
    biosynthesis, 83–88
        PBRs, 87, 88
        rodent brain, 9–14
    biosynthesis and metabolism, 27–43,
        353f
    biosynthesis regulation
        cAMP, 86, 87
    brain and plasma, 3, 3t
    brain quantitation, 3
    CNS development, 158

cognition, 324–332
effects
  myelinating glial cells, 17
endogenous modulators
  glutamate receptors, 181, 182
expression
  anxiety, 322, 323
  stress, 322, 323
GABA/BZD receptor-chloride ionophore
  complex, 317, 318
hormone synthesis
  pathways, 30f
interaction
  GABA$_A$ receptor, 125–138
  molecular mechanism, 126, 127
learning, 324–332
levels
  gender differences, 5
  humans, 8
  monkeys, 7, 8
  rodent brain, 5–7
measurement, 2–9
  humans, 8
  monkeys, 7, 8
  rodent, 2–5
memory, 324–332
neuropsychopharacological potential,
  349–361
  future perspectives, 360
nongenomic and genomic properties,
  350–354
physiological correlates, 14–19
regulatory mechanisms, 9
selectivity
  transmitter-gated ion channel family,
    135–138
sex differentiation
  brain, 158
stress
  age-related effects, 323, 324
trophic effect
  neurons and glial cells, 16–19
Neurotransmitter receptors
  steroid modulators
    ion channels, 168t–174t
Neurotrophins (NT)
  developing brain, 298
  estrogen
    developing brain, 300–303
  receptors
    developing brain, 298, 299

signaling pathways
  estrogen, 304, 305
signal transduction cascades
  developing brain, 299, 300
Nicotinamide-adenine-dinucleotide phosphate (NADPH), 28, 33, 55
Nicotine
  P450, 61
Nicotinic acetylcholine receptor (nAChR)
  characterization, 209
  ion flux assays, 212
  rubidium efflux assays, 212
  steroid modulation, 207–219
Nicotinic receptors, 137
Nigrostriatal dopamine
  estradiol, 270
Nitric oxide producing enzyme
  calmodulin, 342
NMDA-induced neuronal death
  PREG S
    exacerbation, 182, 183
N-menthyl-D-asparate (NMDA)
  induced whole cell currents
    steroid modulations, 183f
  receptor
    electrophysiological investigation,
      176, 177
    GABA receptor, 343
    role, 239, 240
    steroid modulation, 176–179
    structure activity studies, 177–179
  receptor binding sites
    schematic model, 176f
  recombinant receptor
    modulation, 179
Nongenomic action
  estrogen, 238
Non-NMDA receptors
  steroid modulation, 179–181
Non-P450 steroidogenic enzymes, 38–43
Nonspatial food/water reinforced tasks
  PREGS, 330
Nonvoltage-gated calcium influx
  steroid modulation, 230
Norepinephrine (NE)
  DES, 270
Northern blot analysis
  Leydig cell measurement, 81
NT-3
  developing brain, 298
  trkC, 299

NT-4/5
  developing brain, 298
  trkB, 298, 299
NT-6
  developing brain, 298
N-terminal sequencing
  P450S, 60, 61
Nuclear fraction
  female rats, 275–279

O

Oligodendrocyte differentiation process
  P450$_{SCC}$, 84
Ontogenesis
  neurosteroid levels, 5
Operant conflict tests, 321
  allopregnanolone, 321
OSCP
  E-6-^{125}I-BSA, 285–286
  E-mitochondria interactions, 286, 287
Ovarian hormone action, 234
Ovarian hormone modulation, 238
Oxidation
  hydroxyl group, 3alpha, 144

P

P75
  trk, 299
P450
  detection, 52–55
  forms
    brain, 55–59
  identification
    catalytic activities, 55, 56
  nomenclature, 52
P45017, 54t, 58–59
P45019, 59
P45011A, 54t, 56–57
P450aro, 37, 38, 98–104
  brain distribution, 101–104
  mechanism of reaction, 99, 100
  natal development, 102, 103
  pathways, 99f, 111f
  sex steroid regulation, 103, 104
  structural and biochemical properties,
    100, 101
Parturition
  GABAergic steroids, 162
Passive avoidance

allopregnanolone, 326
DHEAS, 325
PREGS, 325, 326
P450 11B1, 54t, 57, 58
P450 11B2, 54t, 57, 58
P4507B, 54t, 56
PBR drug ligand
  P450$_{SCC}$, 90
P450c11, 36, 37
P450c17, 33–35
  developmental regulation
    nervous system, 34, 35
P450c21, 35
PC2 cells
  NGF, 299, 300
P4502D4, 61, 62
  quantitation
    Western blot and immunohistochemi-
      cal localization, 61
Peripheral nerves
  myelination
    PROG, 18
Peripheral nervous system. *See also* Nervous
    system
  P450$_{SCC}$
    developmental regulation, 32, 33
Peripheral-type benzodiazepine receptor
    (PBR), 75–91
Peripheral-type benzodiazepine receptors
    (PBRs)
  binding to DBI, 89
  constitutive steroid producing cell
    model, 82
  drug ligand
    PREG formation, 88t
  vs. GABA$_A$, 76
  hormonal regulation, 81
  hormone-stimulated steroidogenesis, 80,
    81
  ligands, 80
  mediated cholesterol transport
    bacteria, 82
  mitochondrial topography, 78, 79
  molecular modeling, 79
  neurosteroid biosynthesis, 87, 88
  pharmacological and biochemical char-
    acteristics, 76–78
  role
    steroidogenesis, 83
  steroid biosynthesis, 79–83
  steroidogenesis cells

disruption, 82, 83
Personality
  neurosteroids, 160, 161
P_1 fraction
  female rats, 275–279
Phenytoin
  P450, 61
P450 isoforms
  testosterone metabolism, 61t
Pituitary LH secretion
  Leydig cell derived tumors, 82
Plasma
  neurosteroids, 3, 3t
Plasmalemma-microsomal fractions
  female rats, 275–279
Polymerase chain reaction (PCR)
  $P450_{SCC}$, 84–85
Polypeptide diazepam binding inhibitor
    (DBI), 88
Porphyrins, 88
P450 reductase, 35, 36
Pregnenolone (PREG), 2, 28, 79, 227
  active avoidance, 326, 327
  allosteric modulation, 144
  astroglia
    brain injury, 257
  biosynthesis, 10
  CO_2 inhalation, 323
  elevated plus maze, 319
  formation
    endogenous PBR ligands, 88t
    PBRs drug ligand, 88t
  GABA/BZD receptor-chloride ionophore
      complex, 318
  GFAP, 256–257
  hemisuccinate
    neuroprotective effects, 183, 184
  neuronal regeneration, 17
  nongenomic and genomic properties,
      350–354
  sleep cycles, 355
  spatial food/water-search tasks, 329
  synthesis
    DBI, 90
  systemic effects, 354
Pregnenolone sulfate (PREG S), 14, 15, 227
  active avoidance, 327
  aggressive behavior, 15, 323
  DHEA
    brain, 15
  elevated plus maze, 319

exacerbation
  NMDA-induced neuronal death, 182,
      183
memorial path, 339–343
memory enhancement, 337–346
  hypothesis, 343, 344
memory performance, 16
mirror-chamber test, 320
nongenomic and genomic properties,
    350–354
nonspatial food/water reinforced tasks,
    330
passive avoidance, 325, 326
sigma receptor, 197–199
spatial food/water-search tasks, 329
water maze, 327
Presynaptic markers
  synapses, 242
Progesterone 21-hydroxylase, 54t, 58
Progesterone (PROG), 2, 14, 15, 28
  astroglia, 256, 257
    brain injury, 257
  burying behavior, 321
  calcium channel current, 228
  CO_2 inhalation, 323
  dose-response curve, 216
  elevated plus maze, 318
  GFAP, 256
  mirror-chamber test, 320
  myelin formation, 17–19
  neuronal nAChR, 210, 211f
  neuronal regeneration, 17
  neurosteroid vs. endocrine, 2
  nongenomic and genomic properties,
      350–354
  plasma concentrations, 358f
  REM sleep, 359f
  sigma receptor, 197–199
  swim-stress paradigm, 322, 323
  synaptic remodeling
    astroglia, 258
  systemic effects, 358–360
Progestins, 207
Prostate
  P450, 55
Protein sequencing
  P450 detection, 53t
P450S
  brain
    drug, steroid, fatty acid metabolizing,
        60–62

PSA-N-CAM, 259
P450$_{SCC}$, 10, 28–33
  active sites, 79
  C6-2B, 84
  expression, 31
  glia
    transcriptional regulation, 31, 32
  glial cells, 84, 85
  oligodendrocyte differentiation process, 84
  PBR drug ligand, 90
  peripheral nervous system
    developmental regulation, 32, 33

R

Radioimmunoassay
  allopregnolone measurement, 5
Raf kinases
  MAPK cascade, 305, 306
RbOSCP
  [^{3}H]-estradiol, 287, 288
Recombinant glutamate receptors
  modulation, 180f
Reductase
  5alpha, 1, 2, 14, 41, 42, 104–110
    brain distribution, 107–109
    pathways, 99f, 111f
    regulation, 109–110
    structure and biochemical properties, 105–107
REM sleep
  DHEA, 356f
  PROG, 359f
Retina
  DHEA biosynthesis, 11
Ring system
  GABA$_A$ receptor, 130
Rodents
  memory enhancements studies, 339f, 340–343
Rsk
  ER phosphorylation, 308
RT-PCR
  hydroxylase, 17alpha, 58
  P450 detection, 52
  P450S, 60
  P450$_{SCC}$, 10, 56, 57
  steroidogenic factor 1, 70
Rubidium efflux assays
  nAChR, 212

S

Scatchard analysis
  benzodiazepine binding, 81
Seizures
  bicuculline-induced, 148
Serine phosphorylation
  ER, 297
Sertoli cells, 69
Sex steroid
  astroglia, 258
  hormones, 1
    hippocampus, 235
  regulation
    P450aro, 103, 104
Sigma receptor, 14
  assays, 195–197
  binding, 193–195
  function, 198t
    steroidal modulation, 191–199
  molecular studies, 193–195
  NMDA modulation, 196
  steroids, 194t, 197–199
  subtype features, 192t
Signaling proteins
  ERS
    developing brain, 305–309
Single-channel events
  channel blockade, 213
  PROG inhibitions
    schematic diagram, 214f
Sleep cycles
  PREG, 355
Spatial food/water-search tasks
  DHEAS, 329
  PREG, 329
  PREGS, 329
Spinal cord injury, 17
Src
  estrogen
    tyrosine phosphorylation, 306
Steroid hydroxylase expression
  steroidogenic factor 1, 68–70
Steroidogenesis
  PBR role, 83
Steroidogenesis cells
  PBRs
    disruption, 82, 83
Steroidogenic acute regulatory protein (StAR), 83
Steroidogenic cytochromes P450, 28–38
Steroidogenic factor 1

action sites
   target genes, 73t
future directions, 70–73
knockout mouse studies, 70, 71f, 72f
profiles, 68–70
role
   adrenal and gonadal development and
      endocrine function, 67–73
RT-PCR, 70
steroid hydroxylase expression, 68–70
Steroids. *See also* Neurosteroids
action
   enantioselectivity, 135
   sites, 213f
astroglia plasticity
   after brain injury, 257, 258
astroglia signaling
   adhesion molecules, 258, 259
biosynthesis
   PBRs, 79–83
brain, 51
brain plasticity, 255–264
growth factors
   brain, 259–263
hormonal
   astroglia, 256–259
hormones
   brain, 1
   classes, 207
   effects
      myelinating glial cells, 17
   synthesis, 27, 29f
IGF-1
   hypothalamic astroglia, 262, 263
inhibition
   neuronal nAChR, 210–212
   production by, 212–213
   voltage-dependent calcium channels,
      226–229
metabolism
   brain, 1, 2, 60–62
mode of action, 212–215
modulation
   nAChR, 207–219
   nonvoltage-gated calcium influx, 230
   sigma receptor function, 191–199
modulators
   neurotransmitter receptors, 168t–174t
receptors
   brain cell membranes, 269–289
sex

astroglia, 258
sulfonation, 114
synthesizing
   P450, 54t
Steroid sulfatases (SSs), 115
Steroid sulfatase (STS), 12
Stress
   neurosteroid expression, 322, 323
   neurosteroid levels, 6
   neurosteroids, 160
      age-related effects, 323, 324
STs, 114, 115
Suc-associated neurotrophic factor-induced
      tyrosine-phosphorylated target (SNT)
   developing brain, 299
Sulfatase, 12, 115
Sulfotransferases (ST), 11, 12, 114
Sulpiride
   P450, 61
Swim-stress paradigm, 322, 323
   PROG, 322, 323
Synapse density, 243
Synapse formation
   molecular events, 242, 243
Synapses
   presynaptic markers, 242
Synaptic plasticity
   brain
      gonadal hormone regulation, 233–244
Synaptogenesis
   approaches
      nervous system, 239–241
   hippocampus, 240
Systemic effects
   3alpha-reduced neurosteroids, 357, 358
   DHEA, 354–357
   PREG, 354
   PROG, 358–360

T

Tanycytes
   IGF-1, 262, 263
   TGFa, 262, 263
Testosterone
   androgen dihydrotestosterone (DHT), 41
   GFAP, 256
Testosterone metabolism
   P450 isoforms, 61t
TGFa
   tanycytes, 262–263

Thromboxane synthesizing
    P450, 54t
Thyroid hormone treatment, 235
Toluene
    P450, 61
Torpedo nAChR, 209
Transmitter-gated ion channel family
    neurosteroids selectivity, 135–138
Triacontatetraneuropeptide (TTN)
    DBI, 89
Trk
    estrogen, 300, 301
    p75, 299
    signaling cascades
        NGF, 300
TrkA
    NGF, 298, 299
TrkB
    NT-4/5, 298, 299
TrkC
    NT-3, 299
Tuberoinfundibular dopamine
    estradiol, 270
Tyrosine phosphorylation
    ER, 297
Tyrosine 537 phosphorylation
    developing brain, 304

V

Ventromedial nucleus (VMN) neurons, 227,
    228f
Voltage-dependent anion channel (VDAC)
    protein, 77, 78
Voltage-dependent calcium channels
    steroid inhibition, 226–229
Volvox carteri, 340, 342

W

Water maze
    DHEAS, 327
    PREGS, 327
Water-soluble steroids
    GABA$_A$ receptor, 133–135
Western blot
    P4502D4, 61
    P450 detection, 53t, 54
    P450S, 60, 61

X

Xenopus oocytes, 212

ABOUT THE EDITORS

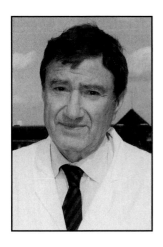

Dr. Etienne-Emile Baulieu is Professor of Biochemistry and Professor of Human Reproduction at the Collège de France in Paris. He is also Research Director of the Unit on Steroid Hormones and Hormonal Communications at the National Institute of Health and Medical Research (INSERM).

He is a cofounder of the World Health Organization (WHO) Program on Human Reproduction and a member of the French Académie des Sciences, National Academy of Sciences of the USA, and the Academia Europea. He is also a Commander of the Legion d'Honneur.

Dr. Baulieu is the recipient of numerous honorary degrees and awards, including the Lasker Research Award (1989). From 1975–1979 he was Chairman of the INSERM Scientific Council.

Dr. Baulieu's research focuses on the role and mode of action, secretion, and metabolism of steroid hormones and neurosteroids, and of the biochemistry and pathophysiology of reproductive processers, nerve myelination, and memory.

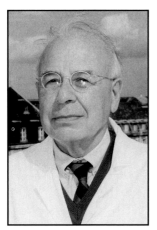

Dr. Paul Robel is Emeritus Research Director at the Centre National de la Recherche Scientifique (CNRS).

He was Vice-Chairman (1975–1978) and Chairman (1982–1986) of the National Institute of Health and Medical Research (INSERM) Committee on Endocrinology, Development, and Reproduction. He is a cofounder of the European Society of Urological Oncology and Endocrinology (ESUOE). He was Chairman of the Association de Recherches sur les Tumeurs Prostatiques, and was a board member of the "Paris-Sud" Medical School (1988–1996).

His awards include the Chevalier de l'Ordre National du Mérite, the Prix Paris (Ligue Nationale contre le Cancer, 1979), and the Prix Breant (French Académie des Sciences, 1986).

Dr. Robel's research focuses on the secretion, metabolism, mode of action, and pathophysiology of androgens and neurosteroids.

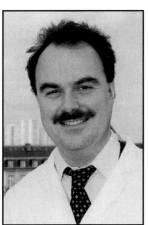

Dr. Michael Schumacher is Research Director of the Unit on Steroids and the Nervous System at the National Institute of Health and Medical Research (INSERM).

He was an Associate Professor at the University of Paris XI. He received his PhD in Biology from the University of Liège in Belgium in 1985 and was a postdoctoral fellow in the laboratory on Endocrinology at the Rockefeller University in New York.

His awards include the Prix Léon Frédéricq (Liége University, 1991) and the Prix Edouard Van Beneden (Royal Society of Sciences, Belgium, 1991).

Dr. Schumacher's research focuses on the actions of gonadal sex steroids in the brain and on the role of steroid hormone metabolism in the developing and adult nervous systems. Since 1991 he has studied the role of neurosteroids in the regeneration of the peripheral nervous system.